Commonsense Approach to Coronary Care

Commonsense Approach to Coronary Care

Sixth Edition

Marielle Vinsant Crawford, RNC, MS
Instructor II, Department of Nursing Education
Baptist Hospital
Miami, Florida

Martha I. Spence, RN, MN, CCRN
Education Coordinator
Mississippi Baptist Medical Center
Jackson, Mississippi

with 385 illustrations

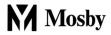 Mosby

St. Louis Baltimore Berlin Boston Carlsbad Chicago London Madrid
Naples New York Philadelphia Sydney Tokyo Toronto

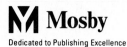
Mosby

Dedicated to Publishing Excellence

Editor: Timothy M. Griswold
Developmental Editor: Jolynn Gower
Project Manager: Linda Clarke
Project Supervisor: Allan S. Kleinberg
Designer: Sheilah Barrett
Manufacturing Supervisor: Karen Lewis

Copyright © 1995 by Mosby–Year Book, Inc.

A Mosby imprint of Mosby–Year Book, Inc.

Sixth Edition

Previous editions copyrighted 1972, 1975, 1981, 1985, 1989

Printed in the United States of America by R.R. Donnelley & Sons
Composition by Clarinda

Mosby–Year Book, Inc.
11830 Westline Industrial Drive
St. Louis, Missouri 63146

Library of Congress Cataloging-in-Publication Data

Vinsant Crawford, Marielle Ortiz.
    Commonsense approach to coronary care / Marielle Vinsant Crawford, Martha I. Spence.—6th ed.
        p.   cm.
    Includes bibliographical references and index.
    ISBN 0-8016-6949-9
    1. Coronary heart disease—Nursing.   I. Spence, Martha I.   II. Title.
    [DLM: 1. Coronary Disease—nurses' instruction.   2. Coronary Disease—programmed instruction.   WG 18 V788c 1994]
    RC685.C6V56   1994
    610.73'691—dc20
    DNLM/DLC
    for Library of Congress   94-14725
                                                                              CIP

95 96 97 98 99 / 9 8 7 6 5 4 3 2 1

Contributors

Darie S. Gilliam, RN, MSN, CCRN
Clinical Nurse Specialist
Critical Care
Baptist Hospital of Miami
Miami, Florida

Laurie Futterman Correa, RN, MSN, CCRN
Coordinator, Cardiac Transplant Program
University of Miami
Miami, Florida

Colleen Counsell, RN, MSN
Nursing Supervisor
Shands Hospital at the University of Florida
Gainesville, Florida

Preface

We first became aware of the need for a new approach to coronary care training while teaching nurses in a course sponsored by the Florida Regional Medical Program and the Florida Heart Association. Initially, we used a traditional, fragmented approach, but this method met with only moderate success. It did not provide the nurse with a basis for realistically and systematically solving patient problems. Subsequently, we developed our own methods for simplification, organization, and practical presentation of the subject matter. When this approach met with success, we wondered if others might also find it meaningful. It has been gratifying to find, through comments made on previous editions, that this approach has been found valid by many of our readers.

For the past twenty years and five editions, we had selected the programmed format for this text in an attempt to simplify the material, encourage participation by the reader, and facilitate self-evaluation. Although many found this format helpful, an equal number have told us over the years that the programmed format was difficult for them to follow due to interruptions in the continuity of the information. These individuals found the information helpful but preferred a different format. Some would not purchase the text specifically because of the programmed format. In response to this feedback, this sixth edition has been converted to the narrative format. As an alternative for those who enjoyed the previous format, self-assessment sections are provided at the end of all units except for Unit 9 (Pharmacologic Intervention). The programmed format is retained in these sections. Practice ECG tracings have also been incorporated when appropriate.

Although comprehensive, in-depth information is provided, this text is designed for beginner or advanced critical care practitioner alike. The text is structured so that the more complex material may be initially omitted without the loss of continuity. This text will be particulary useful for the beginning practitioner who wishes to gradually expand his or her knowledge base without necessarily purchasing multiple additional texts. The information is directed towards practitioners in coronary care units or related settings such as cardiac telemetry/progressive care, critical care, cardiac rehabilitation, cardiovascular laboratories (cardiac catheterization, stress testing, etc.), or the emergency room. Staff nurses, clinicians, clinical specialists, instructors, or case managers in these areas will find information of interest.

Our approach continues to be based on a thorough knowledge of normal anatomy and physiology. Utilizing knowledge of anatomy and physiology, the student is able to deduce the clinical consequences of pathological changes. For example, knowledge of the anatomy of the coronary artery system enables the practitioner to anticipate the type of complications that will be associated with coronary artery occlusion. Knowledge of the role of electrolytes in cardiovascular tissue enables the practitioner to better understand newer diagnostic tests as well as the effects and side effects of recent advancements in drug therapy. The physiology of oxygen radicals in ischemia has been added to Unit 5 in this edition. This particular section may be bypassed by those who do not find it useful without losing the continuity of the chapter.

Although this edition may not appear as simplistic as prior editions, we feel it still retains the intent of the original "common-sense approach" title in its physiologic base and integration of information. The reader is encouraged to think through clinical problems, developing their own critical thinking skills rather than blindly memorizing the solutions of others. We believe memorization is a crutch not an effective learning tool. Therefore, readers are encouraged to use their reasoning powers to a maximum and keep memorization to a minimum. Extensive up to date references are provided allowing the reader to easily obtain more information on the subject matter, independently validate the authors interpretations, and note the extent of recently published information on the subject. References are integrated within the text in this edition.

This text is constructed so that each unit is built on the preceding one. Cross references are provided to maintain the continuity of units. Readers who do not understand a particular section should refer to the previous unit discussing that topic. An index is also provided.

The first four units focus on the physiologic basis of coronary care including normal rhythm and twelve lead ECG patterns. The former two units on fluid and electrolyte balance have been fused into one. Related clinical concepts are intertwined throughout these physiologic units. Unit 3 on Oxygenation has been updated and expanded to incorporate more information on pulse oxime-

try, clinical implications of tissue O2 consumption and newer modes of evaluating effective pulmonary oxygen transport.

Unit 5 on coronary artery disease acts as the turning point of the text focusing more on the pathophysiology, diagnosis, and overall management of angina and acute myocardial infarction. This unit has been heavily updated and expanded to include current pathophysiology concepts, miscellaneous complications, and recent developments in diagnostic testing. Diagnostic tests which have been added include pharmacologic stress testing (nuclear and echocardiographic), SPECT and PET imaging, MRI, and transesophageal echocardiography. Physiological aspects have been expanded and a new section on cardiac rehabilitation has been added to provide a more holistic approach. Nursing process is incorporated throughout this and the remaining units. Specific assessment and intervention for the major electrical and mechanical complications (arrhythmias, heart failure, and shock) are discussed in the remaining chapters. Modifications have been made throughout the text to clarify former illustrations. Legends are now provided.

This sixth edition contains several revisions in the remaining chapters. The new ACLS guidelines have been incorporated into Unit 6 on Electrical Complications and other related chapters. Indications for catheter and surgical ablation are also discussed. Newer arrhythmia terminology is included. The authors' unique approach to ECG interpretations is more thoroughly emphasized and supported with practice ECG traces. A section on signal-averaged electrocardiography has been added. Unit 7 on Interventricular conduction disturbances has been updated and reorganized, ending with a comprehensive discussion of wide QRS tachycardia. The hemodynamic information in Unit 8 has also been reorganized and updated. The section on circulatory assist devices has been expanded to include ventricular assist devices. New illustrations have been added. The new ACLS guidelines have been incorporated into Unit 9 on Pharmacologic Intervention. Recently introduced pharmacologic agents are included. A summary table of agents commonly administered by the IV route has also been added. Information on automatic external defibrillation and temporary DDD pacing has been added to Unit 10 (Electrical Intervention). Recent developments in pacing techniques and troubleshooting are included.

Our primary focus, as with previous editions, is still the patient with acute myocardial infarction in the coronary care unit. However, in this as well as the last edition, we have expanded the scope beyond coronary artery disease to other problems primarily seen with patients in the coronary care units and related areas. These problems include torsades des pointes, pre-excitation syndrome (WPW etc.), cardiomyopathy, and mitral valve prolapse. The former section on malignant ventricular arrhythmias has been replaced by a discussion of sudden cardiac death. Information on electrophysiologic studies has been expanded. A section has also been added on the care of the patient prior to and following cardiac transplantation. Information provided throughout the text on the diagnosis and management of functional disorders such as arrhythmias and congestive heart failure will continue to be valuable in any setting dealing with the patient with heart disease.

We welcome three contributors to this sixth edition: Darie Gilliam, Colleen Counsell, and Laurie Futterman Correa. Their clinical expertise is reflected in Unit 8 (Mechanical Complications), Unit 9 (Pharmacologic Intervention), and Unit 10 (Electrical Intervention). Laurie's expertise in cardiac transplantation has also been incorporated into Unit 11 (Cardiomyopathy).

We continue to strongly recommend that readers of this text supplement their knowl-edge with both a basic and advanced life support course provided by the American Heart Association. The topic of cardiopulmonary resuscitation is critically important in coronary care. Although many components are included in this text, a separate discussion is omitted only because of the excellent training programs already established by the American Heart Association.

We would like to acknowledge and thank: Dr. Louis Lemberg, for his willingness to sponsor us in all our endeavors, for his dedication and committment to coronary care nurse training, and for keeping us clinically oriented; Dr. Azucena Arcebal, for her unique ability to present complex material simply but accurately, for her willingness always to share her knowledge with us, and for treating us as peers; and The Florida Regional Medical Program and Florida Heart Association, for giving us the opportunity to become involved in coronary care nurse training. We would also like to thank Dr. Agustin "Tino" Castellansos, our teacher, philosopher, and friend, for his patience and encouragement in the earlier editions. We have been remiss in previous editions by not acknowledging the invaluable assistance over the years of Dianne Rourke, librarian at Baptist Hospital Medical Sciences Library.

Owing to the multiple revisions in this sixth revisions, we have relied heavily on the support and assistance of the Mosby editorial staff. Their understanding during the added turmoil of Hurricane Andrew's visit was also greatly appreciated. We would like to acknowledge at this time Terry Van Schaik, Jane Petrash, Louann Morrow, and Jolynn Gower.

In addition, we would like to acknowledge others who have taught and encouraged us during the past 20 years: Gloria Steffens, R.N.; Dr. Joan Mayer; Dr. Robert Boucek; Dr. Ramanuja Iyengar; Dr. Ronald Fox; Dr. Charles Roeth; Dr. Andrew Egol; Shirley Mason, R.N.; Judy Mercure, R.N.; Dr. John

Hildreth; Dr. Alvaro Martinez; Barouh Berkowitz; Dr. Hooshang Balooki; Dr. Ruey Sung; Dr. Joseph Civetta; Tina Caruthers, R.N.; Judy Civetta, R.N.; Brenda Sanzobrino, R.N.; Deborah Etter, R.N.; Cheryl Hunneycutt, R.N.; Judith Witmer, R.N.; Virginia Stebbins, R.N.; Marilyn Schactman, R.N.; Jo Ann Pillion, R.N.; Donna Harbin, R.N.; Cheri Contorakes, R.N.; and Georgeanna Quamina, R.N. We thank our contributors Darie Gilliam, Colleen Counsel, and Laurie Futterman Correa for their assistance in this edition. For their encouragement and overall assistance, we acknowledge our parents, Dr. and Mrs. Arturo C. Ortiz and Mrs. Harold Inglis, our husbands Hank and Jerry, and Tracy, Susan, and Sarah Spence.

**Marielle Vinsant Crawford
Martha I. Spence**

Contents

UNIT 1

Anatomy and Physiology

The primary function of the heart is mechanical. The heart serves as a pump to deliver oxygenated blood to the body tissues to meet metabolic or energy demands.

The amount of blood the heart puts out *per minute* is known as the *cardiac output*. Cardiac output is a product of *heart rate × stroke volume*. *Heart rate* is determined primarily by the integrity of the heart's electrical system and the influence of the autonomic (sympathetic and parasympathetic) nervous system. The *stroke volume* is the amount of blood the heart puts out *per beat*. The stroke volume is determined primarily by the efficiency of the heart's mechanical structures and the blood volume returning to the heart.

Normally the body compensates for rises and falls in stroke volume and heart rate so that as one increases the other decreases. For example, when the trained athlete increases muscle mass and thus stroke volume, the heart rate decreases. When the heart muscle has been damaged, as in myocardial infarction resulting in heart failure, the stroke volume decreases. The body compensates to maintain the cardiac output by increasing the heart rate. If the body cannot compensate for a fall in heart rate by increasing the stroke volume or, conversely, for a fall in stroke volume by increasing heart rate, the cardiac output then falls and symptoms develop (see Unit 9).

Normal heart function consists of electrical and mechanical activity. Therefore, abnormal heart function results in disturbances of either electrical or mechanical activity, or both. Abnormal electrical activity may result in arrhythmias. Abnormal mechanical activity may result in heart failure or shock.

ELECTRICAL ACTIVITY: OVERVIEW AND RELATIONSHIP TO MECHANICAL ACTIVITY

The heart has an intrinsic electrical system that allows for initiation and transmission of electrical impulses. Essentially, this electrical activity prepares the heart to contract. The electrical activity of the heart may be recorded on paper. This record is known as the *electrocardiogram (ECG)*.

Electrical activity precedes mechanical activity. Mechanical activity consists of *contraction,* allowing the heart to function as a pump. The mechanical activity of the heart is manifested by a pulse. Mechanical activity is more important than electrical activity because it ensures pump action and cardiac output.

When electrical activity occurs, mechanical activity usually occurs. For every ventricular impulse on the ECG, there is normally a corresponding pulse. However, under selected abnormal conditions, the ECG may show beats without a corresponding pulse. This phenomenon, called *pulseless electrical activity (PEA)* or *electromechanical dissociation (EMD)*, occurs in conditions such as severe congestive heart failure, pneumothorax, severe hypovolemia, and cardiac tamponade. Since pump action is absent, PEA or EMD is considered a form of cardiac arrest.

Primary disturbances in electrical activity occur more frequently than disturbances in mechanical activity and are much easier to correct. For this reason, practitioners place initial emphasis on correcting electrical disorders in the critically ill patient.

MECHANICAL STRUCTURES

The mechanical structures of the heart include its muscle wall, blood vessels, and valves. The heart wall is composed of three major tissue layers. The middle layer, which is the actual heart muscle, is known as the *myocardium*. The thin layer of endothelial cells lining the inside of this muscle wall is known as the *endocardium*. The endocardium is in direct contact with the blood pumped through the heart (Fig. 1-1).

A membranous sac called the *pericardium* surrounds the outside of the muscle wall. The pericardial sac has two linings with a potential space between them—an inner vis-

ceral lining in close contact with the myocardium and an outer parietal lining. The visceral pericardium, which forms the third layer of the heart wall, is referred to as the *epicardium*. A small amount of fluid contained within the pericardial space protects against mechanical friction and excess movement of the heart with changes in posture and thoracic pressure. Excess blood or fluid accumulating between the two linings of this sac is called *pericardial effusion*. If this blood or fluid accumulates rapidly, symptoms of cardiac tamponade can develop.

The heart is divided into right and left sides by a muscular or myocardial structure known as the *septum*. The right and left sides of the heart differ with regard to specific function, musculature, and valvular structure (Table 1-1). The function of the right side is to deliver unoxygenated blood from the body to the lungs. In contrast, the left side delivers oxygenated blood from the lungs to the body (Fig. 1-2). Blood enters the right side of the heart via the superior vena cava and the inferior vena cava. Blood leaves the right side via the pulmonary artery. Blood enters the left side of the heart via four pulmonary veins (two from each lung) and leaves via the aorta. (Note that veins carry blood toward the heart; arteries carry blood away from the heart.) The right side of the heart has thinner musculature because it projects its volume against minimal resistance in the pulmonary circulation. The left side of the heart has thicker musculature

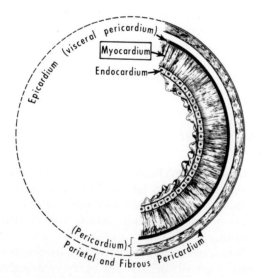

Fig. 1-1 Layers and linings of the heart wall. The myocardium is differentiated from the endocardium and the double-layered pericardial lining.

because it projects its volume against greater resistance in the peripheral circulation.

Each side of the heart has two sets of valves. Valves serve as separators and further divide each side of the heart into a receiving chamber, the *atrium,* and an ejecting chamber, the *ventricle.* Atrioventricular (AV) valves separate the atria from the ventricles. Semilunar valves separate the ventricles from the blood vessels leaving them (Fig. 1-2).

The AV valve in the right side of the heart is called the *tricuspid valve,* after its three major sections or "cusps." It separates the right atrium from the right ventricle. The AV valve in the left side of the heart is the *mitral valve.* It is a bicuspid valve that separates the left atrium from the left ventricle. The AV valves on both sides of the heart are supported by ropelike structures known as *chordae tendonae,* which attach to papillary muscles.[5,11] The papillary muscles are extensions of the ventricular myocardial wall and contract with the ventricular wall, allowing for valve closure. The chordae prevent excessive movement of the valve cusps up into the atria during ventricular contraction (Fig. 1-3). Since the papillary muscles are composed of myocardial cells, these muscles may become damaged in myocardial infarction,

Table 1-1. Comparison of right and left sides of the heart

Right ventricle	Left ventricle
A. Function	
1. Delivers unoxygenated blood from body to lungs	1. Delivers oxygenated blood from lungs to body
2. Projects its volume against minimal resistance—the lungs	2. Projects its volume against maximal resistance—the body
B. Musculature	
1. Thin walls	1. Thick walls
C. Valves	
1. AV valve; tricuspid	1. AV valve: mitral
2. Semilunar valve; pulmonary	2. Semilunar valve: aortic

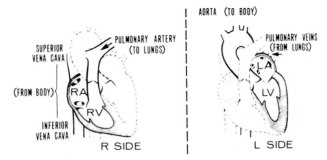

Fig. 1-2 Major structures carrying blood into and out of the right side versus the left side of the heart. The similar roles of the atrioventricular (AV) and semilunar (SL) valves in each side are also illustrated.

weakening the structure of the valves and altering their function.

The semilunar valve in the right side of the heart is the *pulmonary* or *pulmonic valve*. It separates the right ventricle from the vessel leaving it, the pulmonary artery. The semilunar valve in the left side of the heart is the *aortic valve*. It separates the left ventricle from its outflow vessel, the aorta. The semilunar valves appear cuplike, have three cusps each, and have no supporting structures.[5,12] These valves open with ventricular contraction and close passively after ventricular ejection as the backflow of blood fills the cusps (Fig. 1-3). The aortic valve is significant because it contains the origin of the coronary arteries.

In the adult, cardiac disorders affecting the left side of the heart are more frequent and are the focus of this text. Myocardial infarction predominantly involves the left ventricle. Mitral and aortic valve disease also is more common than tricuspid and pulmonary valve disease.

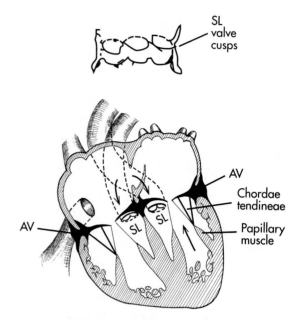

Fig. 1-3 Differences in atrioventricular (AV) valve and semilunar (SL) valve structure. Note that the papillary muscles are extensions of the myocardial wall. Closure of the mitral and aortic valves is compared, although it does not occur simultaneously. The coronary artery openings in the aortic valve are omitted here for simplicity.

NORMAL MECHANICAL ACTIVITY

The heart's mechanical activity consists of a period of contraction with ejection, known as *systole,* and a period of relaxation with filling, known as *diastole.* Atrial contraction can also be called atrial systole. Ventricular contraction can also be called ventricular systole. (Note that *ventricular* systole is manifested as the apical pulse and represents the ejection of blood to the body.)

The right and left atria fill and contract together. For practical purposes, then, they can be considered a single functional unit. The right and left ventricles fill and contract together, so they similarly can be considered a single functional unit. The heart sounds serve as clinical parameters for outlining the

heart's mechanical events. Heart sounds essentially are produced by closure of the valves, although the exact mechanics involved in producing these sounds are more complex.

During ventricular systole, the valves between the atria and ventricles (AV valves) close, so that blood is ejected into the blood vessels and not back into the atria. Since ventricular systole is considered the first mechanical event, the sound produced during closure of these valves is known as the first heart sound, or S_1 (Fig. 1-4). S_1 is the "lub" heard with a stethoscope and marks the onset of ventricular systole. Closure of the AV valves occurs as a result of not only ventricu-

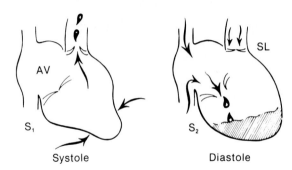

Fig. 1-4 Relationship of normal heart sounds to systole and diastole. Closure of the atrioventricular (AV) valves (S_1) marks the onset of systole. Closure of the semilunar (SL) valves (S_2) marks the onset of diastole.

lar contraction but also pressure changes in the ventricular chamber. Pressure increases in the ventricular chambers as they fill. As a result of this pressure, the valves begin to close passively. When the ventricles contract, this mechanical event actively completes closure of the valves. During a brief period after the AV valves close and before the semilunar valves open, pressure is generated but no actual ejection of blood volume occurs. This phase of systole where no blood is actually ejected is known as *isovolumetric (isovolumic) contraction*.

At the onset of ventricular diastole, the semilunar (SL) valves close so that blood enters the ventricle only from the atria. The sound produced during closure of these valves is known as the second heart sound, or S_2 (Fig. 1-4). S_2 is the "dubb" heard with a stethoscope and marks the onset of ventricular diastole. Two clinically significant periods occur during ventricular diastole. During early diastole, the ventricles fill passively from the atria, which have been acting as a reservoir until the AV valves open. At the end of diastole, atrial contraction occurs, contributing a last boost of blood into the ventricles before systole (Fig. 1-5). This atrial contraction is also called "atrial kick". Atrial contraction is not necessary for ventricular filling to occur and contributes only 15% to 25% of normal stroke volume and cardiac output.[13] If atrial contraction does not occur, cardiac output is merely reduced by that amount.

The effectiveness of the heart as a pump is reflected by the blood ejected *per minute*. The cardiac output is determined by both the electrical structures, which maintain the rate and rhythm, and the mechanical structures, which maintain the stroke volume or the volume of blood ejected by the ventricles *per beat*. Stroke volume is specifically determined by three major factors: *preload*, *afterload*, and *contractility* (Fig. 1-6).[6,12] Preload is more closely related to diastole. Contractility and afterload are more closely related to systole. Preload refers to the stretching of the heart fibers prior to contraction during ventricular filling, or *diastole*. The stretching (lengthening) of these fibers depends on two major factors: (1) the volume returning to the heart (i.e., circulating volume or *venous return*) and (2) the distensibility of the cardiac muscle fibers, also referred to as *compliance* (see Unit 8).

As mentioned, stroke volume is also determined by cardiac contractility and by afterload, which are associated with ventricular *systole*. Contractility refers to the shortening of the myocardial fibers; it is also called the *inotropic* property of these cells. Contractility depends on the integrity of the myocardial cellular structures. Afterload refers to the load placed on the myocardium after the cells have begun to contract or the resistance to ventricular ejection associated with aortic valve opening.[6,12] Resistance to aortic valve opening is generated by the *systemic vascular resistance* (SVR) or *aortic diastolic pressure* and is also reflected in the *mean aortic pressure*. Afterload initially is affected to a lesser extent

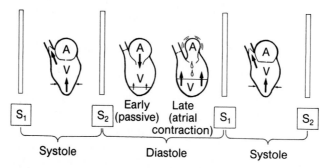

Fig. 1-5 Summary of major events occurring in systole and diastole in relation to normal heart sounds. Events in early versus late diastole are illustrated, including atrial contraction ("atrial kick").

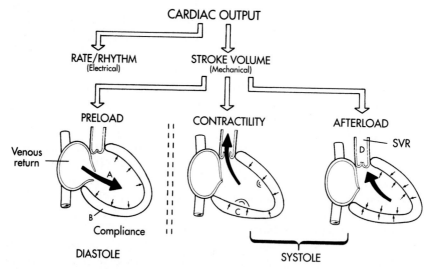

Fig. 1-6 Determinants of cardiac output, including specific determinants of stroke volume. Major factors affecting preload include venous return *(A)* and myocardial fiber distensibility or compliance *(B)*. The major factor affecting contractility is the ability of the muscle fiber to shorten *(C)*. Factors affecting afterload include preload *(C)* and especially the systemic vascular resistance or arterial pressure *(D)*.

by the preload, since the myocardial cells have to overcome the ventricular filling pressure before attempting aortic valve opening (Fig. 1-6).

RELATED CELLULAR STRUCTURES

Cardiac muscle cells contain inner cores of contractile proteins known as *myofibrils*. Each myofibril is wrapped in a meshlike tubular network that runs the length of the cell. These tubules are known as *longitudinal*, or *L, tubules.* The L tubules completely surround the muscle fiber, and they, in turn, are surrounded by a layer of mitochondria, which store the adenosine triphosphate (ATP) used as an energy source for contraction. Single tubules called *transverse*, or *T, tubules* run perpendicular to the muscle cell. These tubules link the outside of the cell with the inside of the cell (Fig. 1- 7). The points at which the L tubules contact the T tubules serve as calcium storage sites. The tubules also carry the electrical signal into the myocardial cell.

The contractile proteins are separated by the T tubules into contractile units known as *sarcomeres*. The L tubules that surround these contractile units are also called the *sarcoplasmic reticulum*.[1,4,6,10] The contractile proteins, actin and myosin, are arranged together in parallel bands, giving the muscle a striped, or striated, appearance (Fig. 1-8).

Small projections, known as *cross-bridges*, extend from the myosin within the muscle cell and serve as potential contact points between the contractile proteins.

The electrical signal mobilizes calcium from outside and inside the cell and causes it to bind with actin. This binding activates the myosin cross-bridges, which pull the actin toward the myosin, causing them to overlap. This sliding and overlapping of the contractile proteins cause the muscle fiber to shorten, or *contract*.[10,12]

The chemical energy required for sliding and shortening of the muscle proteins is obtained from the splitting of phosphate from ATP, which is produced in the muscle cell. When contraction is over, calcium is pumped out of the active areas, and relaxation occurs. The pumping out of calcium also requires energy from ATP. ATP is most effec-

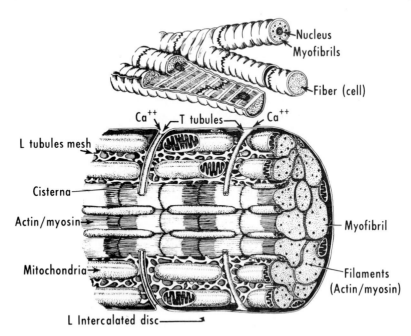

Fig. 1-7 Cardiac muscle cell. The contractile unit or sarcomere is located between every two T tubules. The L tubule or sarcoplasmic reticulum surrounds each sarcomere.

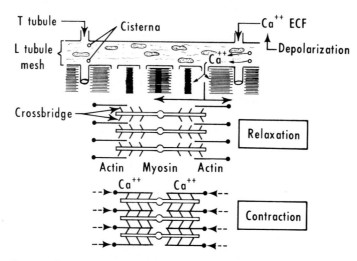

Fig. 1-8 Contractile unit or sarcomere. The position and interaction of the contractile proteins during relaxation and contraction are illustrated.

tively produced by the breakdown of fats or glucose in the presence of oxygen. In reduced oxygen states, less ATP is produced.

Thus both myocardial contraction and relaxation are impaired (see Unit 5).

ELECTRICAL STRUCTURES

In the normal heart, the electrical impulse begins in the *sinoatrial (SA) node*. Because the SA node initiates the electrical stimulus, it is called the *pacemaker of the heart*. The SA node is located superficially, high in the right atrium, and next to the superior vena cava[13] (Fig. 1-9).

After leaving the SA node, the impulse is thought to travel through the specialized conduction tissue in the atria to the atrial muscle cells, causing them to contract. The specialized atrial conduction fibers that lie between the SA node and the AV node are called the *internodal* tracts. One specialized conduction tract, known as *Bachmann's bundle* or the *interatrial tract*, branches off from the anterior internodal tract and carries the impulse between the right and left atria. The

existence of these specialized tracts is currently under dispute. Atrial impulses may spread along less well-defined pathways.[13]

The normal sequence of activation in the heart is the (1) SA node, (2) atria, (3) AV node, (4) bundle of His, (5) right and left bundle branches, (6) Purkinje fibers, and (7) ventricular musculature (Fig. 1-9). The *supraventricular* structures (located above the ventricle) include the SA node, atria, AV node, and bundle of His. The conduction structures in the *ventricles* consist of the structures below the bundle of His, including the right and left bundle branches and the Purkinje fibers.

The *AV node* is located in the back of the right atrium close to the septal leaflet of the tricuspid valve. The AV node and the sur-

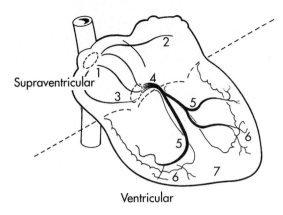

Supraventricular

Ventricular

Fig. 1-9 Normal conduction structures and conduction sequence. Supraventricular structures are differentiated from ventricular structures.

rounding conduction tissue, including the *bundle of His*, are commonly referred to as the *AV junction*. Although moving anteriorly, penetrating the septum, the bundle of His is still located for the most part within the atria

NORMAL ELECTRICAL ACTIVITY

The cardiac conduction structures have three main electrical properties that allow for the generation and transmission of electrical activity:

1. *Automaticity*—the ability to *initiate* an impulse or stimulus.
2. *Excitability*—the ability to *respond* to an impulse or stimulus.
3. *Conductivity*—the ability to *transmit* impulses to other areas.

The SA node is a specialized piece of tissue that can periodically initiate its own impulse. The SA node is therefore said to have the property of *automaticity*. Normally, the SA node initiates its own impulses at a rate of 60 to 100 beats per minute. The AV junctional tissue (i.e., the AV node and the bundle of His) and the ventricular conduction structures also have the property of automaticity. The AV junction fires at an inherent

above the ventricles and is therefore regarded as supraventricular.[4] The heart's electrical impulse slows briefly at the AV junctional tissue. This delay allows for atrial contraction to precede ventricular contraction, ensuring the atrial contribution to cardiac output.

As mentioned, the ventricular conduction structures consist of the bundle branches as well as the Purkinje fibers. Two major bundle branches emerge from below the His bundle: the *right bundle branch,* which carries the electrical impulse to the right ventricle, and the *left bundle branch,* which carries the electrical impulse to the left ventricle. The main left bundle branch separates almost immediately into two divisions: an anterosuperior division and a posteroinferior division. The Purkinje fibers emerge from the three ends of the bundle branches and carry the impulse through each ventricle to the ventricular muscle cells.

rate of 40 to 60.[4,13] The ventricular conduction structures fire at an inherent rate of 20 to 40.

Under normal conditions, the impulse from the SA node is released before either the AV junctional tissue or the ventricular conduction structures can spontaneously fire. The SA node, therefore, usually dominates the AV junctional tissue and sets the pace for the heart. However, if the SA node is injured or depressed, the AV junctional tissue can assume control. When the AV junctional tissue assumes the role of pacemaker, the heart rate usually is slower than when the heart is under the SA node's control. If both the SA node and the AV junctional tissue are unable to maintain control of the rhythm, the ventricular conduction structures assume control as the dominant pacemaker of the heart. The heart rate then is significantly slower. Ventricular pacemaker cells are less reliable than those of the AV junctional tissue and may not fire at all.

Automaticity may be either enhanced or suppressed in the natural pacemaker areas by the autonomic nervous system, which innervates the heart. The autonomic nervous system is composed of the sympathetic and parasympathetic nerves. The *sympathetic* nerves innervate the entire myocardium and generally enhance automaticity. The *parasympathetic* nerves selectively innervate the structures within the atrium and generally suppress automaticity. (Note that although parasympathetic fibers have been identified within the ventricles, they are not clinically significant.)[9,13]

Under sympathetic stimulation the heart rate may increase to 150 beats per minute and yet remain under the control of the SA node. Beyond this point, abnormal pacemakers often assume control of the rhythm. SA node activity may be suppressed by the parasympathetic nervous system, resulting in heart rates of less than 60 beats per minute. Both AV junctional and ventricular activity also may be enhanced by the sympathetic nervous system. The parasympathetic nervous system suppresses AV junctional activity but usually does not affect ventricular activity.

Both the normal cardiac muscle cells in the atria and ventricles and the normal conduction structures possess the properties of *excitability* and *conductivity*, allowing them to respond to and transmit electrical signals. Cardiac cells respond to and transmit electri-

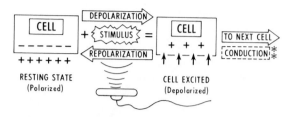

Fig. 1-10   Normal process of excitability and conduction.

cal impulses by the process of *depolarization* (Fig. 1-10).

At rest, cardiac cells are negatively charged on the inside with respect to the outside. In this state they are said to be *polarized*. This charge is maintained by the distribution of the electrolytes (see Unit 4). In response to advancing electrical impulses, positive charges move into the cells. The insides of these cells become electropositive, and the cells are depolarized. This change in cell charge signals adjacent cells, causing their depolarization. In this way the impulse is transmitted and spreads throughout the conduction tissue and myocardium. If adjacent cells are normal, the excitation process (depolarization) automatically results in conduction. Thus the term *depolarization* is often used synonymously with *conduction*. Once depolarized, the cell prepares for another electrical impulse by recharging, or *repolarizing* (Fig. 1-10). Sensing electrodes placed on the skin surface can detect these changes in charge, producing deflections on recording paper. The deflections form the ECG complex (see Unit 2).

POSITION OF THE HEART WITHIN THE CHEST

The heart is rotated and positioned on its side within the chest cavity. The right ventricle lies *anteriorly,* and the left ventricle lies *posteriorly* (Fig. 1-11). The left ventricle can be further isolated within the chest cavity for identification of the major left ventricular

surfaces: *anterior, lateral,* and *inferior* (Fig. 1-12). Because the inferior surface of the left ventricle lies just above and parallel to the diaphragm, it is also called the *diaphragmatic* surface.

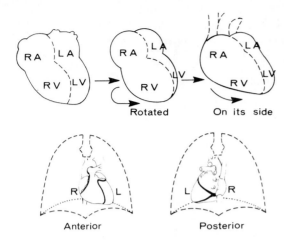

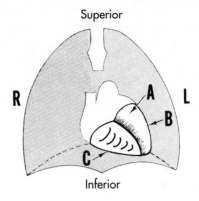

Fig. 1-11 Position of heart within chest cavity.

Fig. 1-12 Position of left ventricle (LV) within chest cavity. The major LV surfaces are illustrated: anterior *(A)*, lateral *(B)*, and inferior or diaphragmatic *(C)*.

CORONARY ARTERIES

Like other organs in the body, the heart has its own rich blood supply. The heart receives blood for its own maintenance from two *coronary arteries*, the right and the left. The coronary arteries are the first branches off the aorta, originating from the spaces within the cusps of the aortic valve called the *sinuses of Valsalva*. The coronary arteries exit from within the aortic cusps and travel along the outer surface of the heart. They provide blood for both the electrical and mechanical structures of the heart.

Right coronary artery

The right coronary artery branches off from the right sinus of Valsalva and proceeds to the heart's anterior surface, winding around to the right in the groove between the *right atrium* and the *right ventricle* (Fig. 1-13). Before reaching the surface of the heart, it emits a branch that partially supplies the SA node. The right coronary artery then winds around the back of the heart, dividing the right atrium and the right ventricle posteriorly. At this point an important branch descends posteriorly in the groove separating the right and left ventricles; this branch is therefore named the *posterior descending branch.*[11,13] The right coronary artery gives a branch to the AV node at about the same level as the origin of the posterior descending branch. The right

coronary artery, then, supplies both the SA and AV nodes. The posterior descending branches that perforate the septum supply portions of the bundle of His and of the posteroinferior division of the left bundle branch.

The right coronary artery also supplies the muscle cells of the right atrium and right ventricle and a portion of the left ventricle. When rotated and positioned within the chest cavity, most of the posterior portion of the left ventricle becomes the inferior or diaphragmatic surface (Fig. 1-14).[4,7,11] The posterior descending branch of the right coronary artery supplies the posteroinferior surface of the left ventricle and sends out perforating branches that supply the posterior one third of the septum.

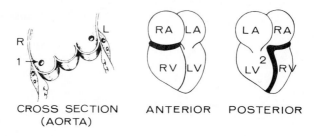

CROSS SECTION
(AORTA) ANTERIOR POSTERIOR

Fig. 1-13 Right coronary artery: origin *(1)*, pathway, and major posterior descending branch *(2)*.

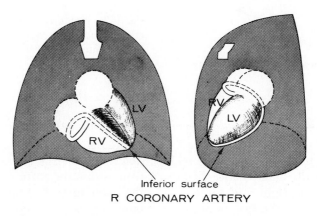

Inferior surface
R CORONARY ARTERY

Fig. 1-14 Left ventricular (LV) surface supplied by the right coronary artery.

In summary: The right coronary artery supplies the following:

1. SA node (55%*)[7,13]
2. AV node (90%*)[7,13]
3. Bundle of His (a portion)
4. Posteroinferior division of the left bundle branch (a portion)
5. Posterior third of septum
6. Right atrial/ventricular muscle
7. Posteroinferior wall of the left ventricle

Left coronary artery

The left coronary artery supplies a larger portion of the left ventricle than does the right coronary artery. The left coronary artery emerges from the left sinus of Valsalva. The initial portion of this artery is known as the *left main coronary artery*. The left coronary artery divides into two main branches as it reaches the surface of the heart. One of these branches descends anteriorly, separating the right ventricle from the left ventricle. This branch is thus called the *left anterior descending* (LAD) branch (Fig. 1-15). The LAD supplies most of the right bundle branch and the anterosuperior division of the left bundle branch.[4,7]

The second branch winds or twists around

---

*Percentage of hearts in which these conduction structures are supplied by the right coronary artery.

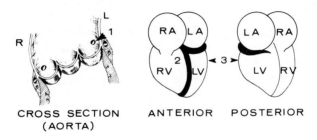

CROSS SECTION
(AORTA)　　ANTERIOR　POSTERIOR

Fig. 1-15 Left coronary artery: origin *(1)*, pathway, and major branches—anterior descending *(2)*, and circumflex *(3)*.

the left side and the back of the heart, dividing the left atrium and the left ventricle anteriorly and posteriorly. This branch is thus called the *circumflex* branch (see Fig. 1-15). The circumflex may or may not descend posteriorly. If the circumflex branch descends significantly in a given individual, that person is said to have a dominant left coronary system. The circumflex supplies the SA node in 45% of the general population and also supplies a portion of the posteroinferior division of the left bundle branch. (Note that the posteroinferior division has a dual blood supply—from both the right and left coronary arteries.)

The left coronary artery also supplies the muscle cells of the left atrium and a portion of the left ventricle. The diagonal branches from the LAD supply the anterior portion of the left ventricle. The LAD also gives off penetrating branches called septal perforators, which supply the anterior two thirds of the septum. The circumflex branch of the left coronary artery travels toward the left, supplying the muscle cells of the left atrium and the lateral portion of the left ventricle. The left coronary artery is most significant because it provides the blood supply to the anterior and lateral walls of the left ventricle (Fig. 1-16).[4,7]

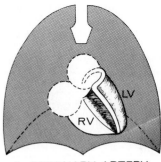

L CORONARY ARTERY

Fig. 1-16 Left ventricular (LV) surfaces supplied by the left coronary artery.

In Summary: The left coronary artery supplies the following:

Anterior descending	Circumflex
1. Anterior two thirds of septum	1. SA node (45%*)
2. Right bundle branch (RBB) (major portion)	2. Posteroinferior division of left bundle (a portion)
3. Anterosuperior division of the left bundle	3. Lateral wall of the left ventricle (LV)
4. Anterior wall of the left ventricle (LV)	

*Percentage of hearts in which this conduction structure is supplied by the left coronary.

CORONARY VEINS

The heart receives its oxygenated blood via the coronary arterial system. Deoxygenated blood returns to the right atrium via the coronary venous system. The opening through which the coronary veins drain into the right atrium is known as the *coronary sinus*. This opening is located in the lower posterior portion of the right atrium.

SELF-ASSESSMENT

1 The heart has both _____ and _____ activity. Electrical activity of the heart is detected by the _____. Mechanical activity of the heart is best detected by the _____.

electrical
mechanical
ECG
pulse

Mechanical activity is significant because it ensures _____ action. For every beat on the ECG, there should be a corresponding _____.

pump

pulse

2 Electrical activity of the heart begins in the _____. The supraventricular electrical structures include the _____, _____, and _____.

SA node
SA node,
atria; AV junction

The ventricular electrical structures include the _____ _____ and _____ fibers.

bundle
branches; purkinje

The electrical properties of the heart consist of (1) the ability to *initiate* an impulse (_____), (2) the ability to *respond* to an impulse (_____), (3) the ability to *transmit* an impulse (_____). When the inside of the cell is electrically positive with respect to the outside, the cell is said to be (depolarized/repolarized).

automaticity
excitability
conductivity
depolarized

3 Mechanical activity of the heart begins with a period of contraction, or _____, followed by a period of relaxation, or _____.

systole; diastole

S$_1$ marks the onset of (systole/diastole) and is produced by closure of the (AV/semilunar) valves. S$_2$ marks the onset of (systole/diastole) and is produced by closure of the (AV/semilunar) valves.

systole
AV; diastole
semilunar

The AV valve on the left side of the heart is the _____ valve. The semilunar valve on the left side of the heart is the _____ valve. Chordae tendonae and papillary muscles support the (AV/semilunar) valves.

mitral
aortic
AV

4 Cardiac output is the amount of blood put out by the heart per _____. Cardiac output is a product of heart _____ and _____ volume, which in turn depends on the heart's _____, _____, and _____.

minute; rate
stroke
preload; contractility
afterload

Preload is dependent on (venous return/SVR) and is primarily associated with ventricular (systole/ diastole).

venous return
diastole

Afterload is dependent on (venous return/SVR) and is primarily associated with ventricular (systole/diastole).

SVR
systole

5 The contractile unit of the myocardial cell is known as the _____ and contains the contractile proteins referred to as _____ and _____. Calcium acts as a trigger to cause overlapping of these proteins, resulting in (shortening/lengthening) of the muscle fibers, or _____.

sarcomere
actin; myosin
shortening
contraction

Both contraction and relaxation require energy in the form of _____.

ATP

6 Within the chest wall the heart is _____ and positioned on its _____. The left ventricle therefore becomes the (anterior/posterior) ventricle.

rotated
side; posterior

Myocardial infarction occurs almost exclusively in the (right/left) ventricle. In the setting of coronary care, the primary concern is therefore the (right/left) ventricle.

left

left

7 Review the blood supply of the left ventricle (LV) (Fig. 1-17):

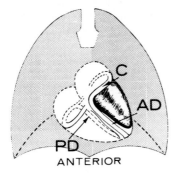

Fig. 1-17 Branches of right and left coronary arteries and relationship to the left ventricle. The anterior descending (AD) and circumflex (C) branches of the left coronary artery are contrasted with the posterior descending (PD) branch of the right coronary artery.

The anterior descending branch (AD) of the (right/left) coronary artery supplies the _____ wall of the LV. The circumflex branch (C) of the (right/left) coronary artery supplies the _____ wall of the LV. The left coronary artery as a whole supplies both the _____ + _____ walls of the LV and is thus associated with (AWMI/IWMI). Since the left coronary artery supplies a portion of each bundle branch, anterior wall myocardial infarction (AWMI) is associated with _____ _____ block.

left
anterior
left; lateral

anterior; lateral
AWMI

bundle branch

The posterior descending (PD) branch of the (right/left) coronary ar-

right

tery supplies the _____ wall of the LV and is thus asso-   inferoposterior,
ciated with (AWMI/IWMI). Since the right coronary artery supplies a por-   IWMI
tion of both the _____ and _____ nodes, inferior wall   SA; AV
myocardial infarction (IWMI) is associated with _____ bradycar-   sinus
dia and blocks at both the _____ and _____ nodes.   SA; AV

REFERENCES/SUGGESTED READINGS

1. Alspach JG: AACN core curriculum for critical care nursing, ed 4, Philadelphia, 1991, WB Saunders.
2. Anthony CP, Thibodeau GH: Textbook of anatomy and physiology, ed 11, St. Louis, 1983, CV Mosby.
3. Berne RM, Levy MN: Physiology, ed 6, St. Louis, 1992, Mosby–Year Book.
4. Conover MB: Understanding electrocardiography, ed 6, St. Louis, 1992, Mosby–Year Book.
5. Darovic GO: Hemodynamic monitoring: invasive and noninvasive clinical application, Philadelphia, 1987, WB Saunders.
6. Guyton AC: Textbook of medical physiology, ed 8, Philadelphia, 1991, WB Saunders.
7. Hanisch PJ: Identification and treatment of acute myocardial infarction by electrocardiographic site classification, Focus on Critical Care 18:480, Dec. 1991.
8. Huszar RJ: Basic dysrhythmias: interpretation and management, St. Louis, 1988, Mosby–Year Book.
9. Levick JR: An introduction to cardiovascular physiology, London, 1991, Butterworths.
10. Lindemann JP: Contractile protein alterations in heart failure, Hosp Pract 26:47, 1991.
11. Schlant RC, Silverman ME, Roberts WC: Anatomy of the heart. In Hurst JW, Schlant RC, editors: The heart, arteries, and veins, ed 7, New York, 1990, McGraw-Hill.
12. Schlant RC, Sonnenblick EH: Normal physiology of the cardiovascular system. In Hurst JW, Schlant RC, editors: The heart, arteries, and veins, ed 7, New York, 1990, McGraw-Hill.
13. Underhill SL et al: Cardiac nursing, ed 2, Philadelphia, 1989, JB Lippincott.

UNIT 2

The Normal
Electrocardiogram

The electrocardiogram (ECG) is a record of the wave of depolarization and repolarization spreading through the heart. The changes in cell charges occurring during depolarization and repolarization produce deflections either on an oscilloscope (cardiac monitor) or on recording paper, forming the ECG complex.

ECG COMPLEX

The largest deflection in the ECG record is the *QRS complex*. This complex may be either upright or inverted and still be normal (Fig. 2-1). The electrical impulses spreading through the ventricles produce the QRS complex, which represents ventricular depolarization. This ECG deflection is the easiest to identify initially and is the most clinically significant, since it triggers ventricular contraction which produces the pulse.

After depolarization, the heart must recover before it can receive another impulse. This process is known as *repolarization*. Ventricular repolarization is represented on the ECG by the *T wave*, which follows the QRS complex (Fig. 2-1). The T wave may also be upright or inverted in the presence of a normal rhythm, and it may not always be clearly visible. However, if consecutive QRS complexes are visible, T waves may be assumed to be present because depolarization cannot occur without repolarization from previous impulses.

The electrical impulses spreading through the atria produce the *P wave*, which precedes the QRS complex (see Fig. 2-1). The P wave represents atrial depolarization, which precedes ventricular depolarization. Atrial repolarization usually does not appear on the ECG because it is of such low voltage. Identification of both the T wave and P wave is facilitated by first identifying the larger and more distinct QRS complex.

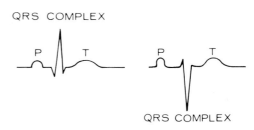

Fig. 2-1 Major deflections of the normal ECG complex.

Let us consider the QRS complex in more detail, beginning with the positive and negative deflections. A positive deflection is defined as one that points above the baseline, and a negative deflection is one that points below the baseline (Fig. 2-2). The baseline is the horizontal line immediately preceding the vertical QRS complex deflection. This line is also called the *isoelectric line*.

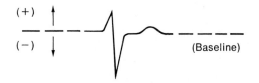

Fig. 2-2   The baseline as determined from the beginning of the QRS complex. It acts as a reference point for determining positive (+) and negative (−) deflections. This baseline is less likely to be affected by patient movement and increases in heart rate than the horizontal point preceding the P wave.

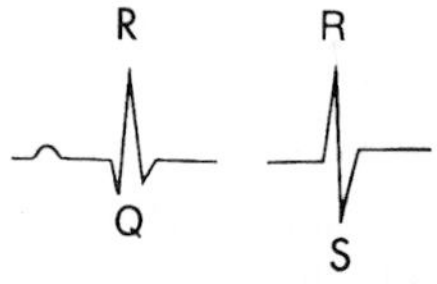

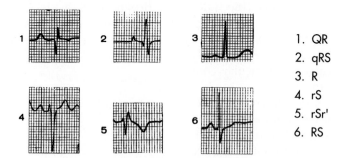

Fig. 2-3   Specific deflections of the QRS complex.

The *R wave* is defined as the first positive deflection in the QRS complex. A *Q wave* is defined as a negative deflection preceding the R wave. An *S wave* is defined as a negative deflection following the R wave (Fig. 2-3). A completely negative QRS complex is commonly referred to as a *QS complex*. (Q waves and S waves are always negative; R waves are always positive.) Although not every QRS complex has Q, R, and S waves, the wave representing ventricular depolarization is collectively known as the QRS complex, regardless of its configuration.

Each wave in the QRS complex can be further described according to its size. A large wave is denoted by a capital *Q, R,* or *S.* A small wave is denoted by a small *q, r,* or *s* (Fig. 2-4).[4,8,11,16] Specific labeling of the QRS complex is not critical when identifying normal rhythms, but it becomes more clinically significant when assessing normal or abnormal 12-lead ECG patterns.

1. QR
2. qRS
3. R
4. rS
5. rSr'
6. RS

Fig. 2-4   Practice labeling QRS complexes. The fifth example shows a second positive deflection. When this occurs the wave is labeled *R prime* or *R'.*

Intervals and segments

Certain intervals on the ECG are significant. The *P–R interval,* measured from the beginning of the P wave to the beginning of the QRS complex (Fig. 2-5), begins with atrial depolarization and ends with the beginning of ventricular depolarization. The P–R interval represents the delay between

atrial and ventricular depolarization, or the time it takes an impulse to travel from the sinoatrial (SA) node to the ventricles. This normal delay between atrial and ventricular conduction occurs within the artrioventricular (AV) conduction tissue (AV node, bundle of His, and bundle branches).[4,11,16] This de-

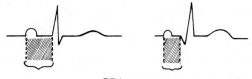

PR interval

Fig. 2-5 The P–R interval. This interval always begins with a P wave and ends with the initial portion of the QRS complex whether or not it is literally an "R" wave. The second interval is actually a "P–Q" interval.

lay allows time for atrial contribution to cardiac output. The P–R interval correlates the electrical impulse of the atria with that of the ventricles and allows for detection of AV conduction blocks. The normal P–R interval is from *0.12 to 0.20 seconds.*

Another less frequently measured interval is the *Q–T interval* (Fig. 2-6). The Q–T in-

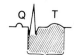

Fig. 2-6 Q–T interval.

terval includes ventricular depolarization (the QRS complex) plus ventricular repolarization (the T wave). The Q–T interval thus may be altered by any change in ventricular activity such as those occurring with electrolyte imbalances and the use of selected drugs.

A more significant portion of the Q–T interval is the QRS duration. The duration of the QRS complex is measured from the be-

ginning of the QRS complex to the end of the QRS complex (Fig. 2–7). The normal

Fig. 2-7 QRS complex duration or width.

QRS complex duration is less than 0.10 second.[4,8,13,16] However, significant abnormalities are usually not confirmed unless the QRS duration exceeds 0.12 second.[15] If no Q wave is present, the "QRS" is measured from the beginning of the first deflection in the complex.

Another important portion of the Q–T interval is the S–T segment. The *J,* or junction point, marks the end of the QRS complex and the beginning of the S–T segment[4,8,16] (Fig. 2-8). The S–T segment rep-

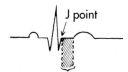

Fig. 2-8 S–T segment.

resents the heart's resting period between ventricular depolarization and repolarization. When the T wave is not clearly visible, the beginning of the S–T segment or J point is easier to determine than the end. This segment is normally level with the baseline or isoelectric but may be displaced above or below the baseline in angina or acute myocardial infarction.

Refractory periods and vulnerable period

During repolarization, the individual cardiac cells go through periods of varying excitability until their normal excitability is restored. These periods are called the *refractory periods.* Excitability is the ability of the heart to respond to an electrical impulse. The refractory periods of the heart are times during which the heart is unable to respond *nor-*

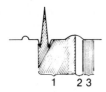

Fig. 2-9 Refractory periods: absolute (1), relative (2), supernormal (3).

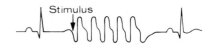

Fig. 2-10 Vulnerable period. Stimulus produces chain reaction response.

mally to a second electrical impulse.

The refractory periods of the ventricles are represented by certain areas within the Q–T interval (Fig. 2-9). The *absolute* refractory period is that time during the cardiac cycle when the cardiac cells are unable to respond to a second stimulus, regardless of the strength of the stimulus. In the normal heart the absolute refractory period includes the QRS and the initial part of the S–T segment. An electrical stimulus that reaches the ventricles during the absolute refractory period will not cause a myocardial response. The *relative* refractory period is that time during repolarization when only a strong stimulus can cause a response. The *supernormal* period is that time during repolarization when even a weak stimulus can cause a response.

The refractory periods refer to single responses to electrical stimuli. However, at a critical point during repolarization, the heart may respond to a stimulus with more than one response. This period of *altered excitability* is known as the *vulnerable period*. The vulnerable period is that portion of the cardiac cycle when a stimulus may produce *repetitive firing*, also referred to as a *chain reaction response* (Fig. 2-10). With acute myocardial ischemia the vulnerable period of the heart occurs on the apex of the T wave.[4]

ECG GRAPH
Calculating intervals

On an ECG recording paper at a standard paper speed of 25 mm per second, each large box (between two dark lines) equals 0.20 second. Each small box (between two light-colored lines) equals 0.04 second (Fig. 2-11). To determine the duration or width of the QRS complex, multiply the number of small boxes occurring during this period by 0.04 second. Focusing on the complex with an asterisk shown in Fig. 2-11, there are two small boxes from the beginning to the end of the QRS complex. Thus, the duration or width of the QRS complex in this trace is 0.08 second (2 × 0.04 second) and is within normal limits. Determine the duration of the P–R interval in the same way. Using the same complex, the number of small boxes from the beginning of the P wave to the beginning of the QRS complex is three. Thus, the duration of the P–R interval in this complex is 0.20 second (5 × 0.04 second), also equal to one large box, and is within normal limits.

Calculating heart rates

Measurement of the ventricular rate is made from one QRS complex to the next QRS complex (commonly called the *R–R interval*). When measuring ventricular rate, you may use any component of the QRS complex as a reference point. However, make the measurement between two consistent points, that is, R to R, Q to Q, or S to S.

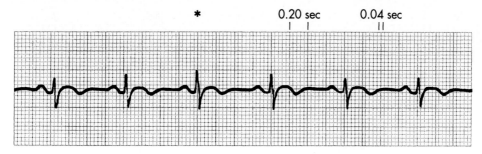

Fig. 2-11   Using the ECG graph to calculate the duration of the QRS complex and the P–R interval.

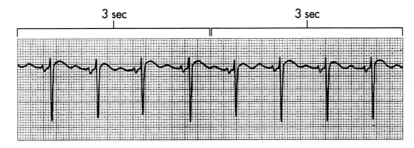

Fig. 2-12   Six-second trace. The ventricular rate in this trace is estimated at 80 beats per minute (8 complexes in 6 seconds × 10 = 60 seconds).

Measure atrial rate from one P wave to the next P wave; this interval is referred to as the *P–P interval.*

ECG paper is often divided by markings into intervals that represent spans of 1 second or, more commonly, 3 seconds (Fig. 2-12). If using unmarked ECG paper, determine 3-second intervals by counting and marking every 15 large boxes. A 6-second tracing, which is commonly used for rhythm analysis, would contain 30 large boxes or two 3-second segments. Determine 1-second intervals by counting and marking every five large boxes. (Note: 3 seconds = 15 × 0.20; 1 second = 5 × 0.20.)

You can rapidly estimate the ventricular rate for 1 minute by counting the number of QRS complexes occurring in a 6-second trace and multiplying this number by 10 (see Fig. 2-12).[4,15] This figure gives the number of QRS complexes occurring in 60 seconds, or 1 minute. You can also obtain the ventricular rate for 1 minute by multiplying the number of QRS complexes occurring in one 3-second span by 20. You can use this method with both regular and irregular rhythms.[13,16]

A more accurate method for calculating rates is also available. This method is preferred when normal and abnormal beats or rhythms are interspersed or when the ventricular rate of a sustained abnormal rhythm remains regular. When the ventricular rate of an abnormal rhythm is irregular, the earlier method is preferred.

To calculate rates by this more accurate method, first look for a portion of the QRS complex that falls on a dark line or at the beginning of a large box. Estimate the rate from this reference point (Fig. 2-13). If a

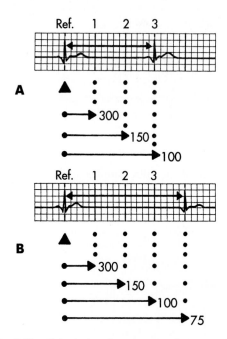

Fig. 2-13 Calculating heart rates. In example **A,** the heart rate is 100 beats per minute. In example **B,** the heart rate is 75 beats per minute.

QRS complex occurs at the first dark line after the reference point (i.e., every dark line), it means a ventricular impulse is occurring every 0.20 second or 300 times per minute (60 seconds per minute divided by 0.20 second between complexes). If, instead, a QRS complex occurs at the second dark line after the reference point, the rate is slower—exactly half as fast—or 150 beats per minute (see Fig. 2-13). If the next QRS complex occurs at every third dark line, the rate is one third of 300, or 100, and so on.[8,11,13,15]

Line	Rate value	Line	Rate value
1	300	6	50
2	150	7	43
3	100	8	37
4	75	9	33
5	60		

Each large box is composed of five smaller boxes. Consider these smaller components

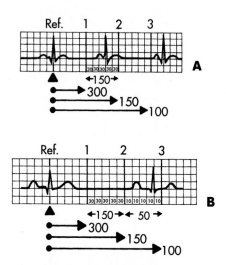

Fig. 2-14 Calculating heart rates. In example **A,** the heart rate is 210 beats per minute (150 + 30 + 30). In example **B,** the heart rate is 110 beats per minute (100 + 10).

when calculating rates that fall between the previously designated values (Fig. 2-14). In Fig. 2-14, the first complex that occurs after the reference point is located *between* the first and second dark lines after the reference complex. Therefore, the ventricular rate in this example falls between 300 and 150 beats per minute. The rate is less than 300 and greater than 150. There are five smaller boxes, represented by light-colored lines, within each large box or between two dark lines. To obtain the value of each small box between 300 and 150, subtract 150 from 300 and divide the difference (150) by 5 for a value of 30 per small box. Since the QRS complex after the reference complex falls between two light-colored lines (or small boxes) before 150, add the value of these two boxes to 150 (or subtract the value of three boxes from 300). To obtain the value of each small box between 150 and 100, subtract 100 from 150 and divide the difference (50) by 5 for a value of 10 per box.

A third method for rate calculation is to divide 1500 by the number of small squares between two QRS complexes. This system is based on a QRS complex occurring every 0.04 second or 1500 times per minute (60 sec per minute divided by 0.04 second between beats).[3,4,15,16] This method provides for more accurate calculation of rapid heart rates and may be preferable in children.

SINUS RHYTHMS

A sinus rhythm originates in the SA node. The ECG pattern produced confirms this origin. When interpreting ECG patterns, the authors suggest using the following systematic approach:

1. Analyze the QRS complex.
2. Analyze the P wave.
3. Analyze the P–R interval.

Although this approach by beginning with the QRS complex purposefully does not follow the normal conduction sequence, it has many practical advantages and may be used consistently when interpreting both normal and abnormal rhythms. The QRS complex is the most clinically significant component of the ECG pattern since it initiates ventricular contraction and is the major determinant of cardiac output. Analysis of the rate and configuration of the QRS complex alone are often sufficient to determine the immediate clinical significance of and initial therapy for cardiac rhythms (see Unit 6). The QRS complex is also the easiest deflection to identify and can facilitate the identification of the smaller P wave, which should immediately precede it.

The QRS complex is analyzed first to determine if the origin of the rhythm is ventricular or supraventricular. The ventricular rate may be simultaneously assessed to detect a critically slow or fast rhythm. The label *supraventricular* refers to a rhythm originating above the ventricles (see Unit 1). Since the SA node is considered supraventricular, the configuration of the QRS complex in a sinus rhythm should be consistent with that of a supraventricular rhythm. Supraventricular impulses are usually transmitted through the

	ATRIAL RATE
NORMAL SINUS RHYTHM	60–100
SINUS BRADYCARDIA	LESS THAN 60
SINUS TACHYCARDIA	101 – 150

Fig. 2-15 Classification of sinus rhythms by rate.

normal AV conduction pathways to the ventricles. When an impulse reaches the ventricles through these normal AV pathways, the ventricular musculature is depolarized rapidly. The resulting QRS complex is narrow, that is, less than 0.12 second.[15] In a single patient, *all* impulses arising *above* the ventricles should be conducted similarly through the AV conduction system to reach the ventricles. Therefore, all supraventricular impulses in a particular patient should produce QRS complexes having the same configuration. Supraventricular impulses may therefore be described as producing QRS complexes that are narrow and unchanging. The QRS complex in a sinus rhythm is typically narrow and unchanging. The QRS complex may be either positive or negative depending on the lead.

Analysis of the P wave and calculation of the atrial rate aid in the differential diagnosis of supraventricular rhythms. Supraventricular rhythms may originate not only in the SA node but also in other areas of the atria or in the AV junction. If the P wave pattern is normal, it can be assumed that the impulse originated within the normal place in the atria—the SA node. Thus, it is the *P wave* characteristics that confirm the diagnosis of sinus rhythm.

In sinus rhythm a P wave should be visible, preceding each QRS complex, with no sudden irregularities in the P–P interval, and a P wave rate of 150 or less. If the P wave rate is greater than 150 in an adult, the rhythm may not be sinus. (Remember that under sympathetic stimulation, the heart rate may increase *up to* 150 beats per minute and yet remain under the control of the SA node. Beyond this point, abnormal pacemakers often assume control of the rhythm.) Confirm that the P wave is upright (positive) in lead II, signifying its origin in the upper portion of the atria where the SA node is located rather than in the lower portion of the atria where the AV junction is located.

Identifying a normal P–R interval confirms that the sinus impulse is related to the ventricular impulse and has been conducted without any AV delay or block. Consider the P–R interval normal if a QRS complex follows every P wave at constant intervals of normal duration.

In summary, diagnose sinus rhythm according to the following criteria:

1. *QRS complex*—narrow and unchanging (origin supraventricular)
2. *P wave*—visible preceding each QRS complex, no sudden irregularities in P–P interval, P wave rate 150 or less, upright in lead II (origin sinus).
3. *P–R interval*—QRS complex following each P wave at constant intervals of normal duration (no AV delay or block).

The most flexible of these criteria is the width of the QRS complex. Sinus rhythm can occur in the presence of an abnormal, or wide, QRS complex. Width merely implies a delay. A wide QRS complex occurring in a constant relationship with a normal P wave (as evidenced by a constant P–R interval) means that the normal sinus impulse has been delayed in the ventricles, usually as a result of bundle branch block (see Unit 7). In the presence of a bundle branch block, the QRS complex configuration, although wide, typically remains the same.

After identifying the origin of a rhythm as sinus, further classify it according to atrial rate as either normal sinus rhythm, sinus tachycardia, or sinus bradycardia. In each of these sinus rhythms, the atrial rate and the ventricular rate are usually the same, so the P wave rate will correspond to the more easily measured QRS rate.

Normal sinus rhythm

Normal sinus rhythm (NSR), also referred to as regular sinus rhythm (RSR), has all the ECG characteristics of a sinus rhythm. In addition, the P wave rate (and QRS rate) is between 60 and 100 (Fig. 2-16).

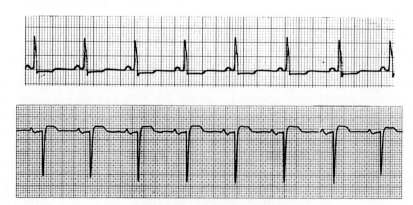

Fig. 2-16 Normal sinus rhythm (NSR) or regular sinus rhythm (RSR).

Sinus tachycardia

When automaticity in the SA node is enhanced, impulse discharge increases. Increased automaticity in the SA node may result in an arrhythmia known as sinus tachycardia (ST). Sinus tachycardia fulfills all the ECG criteria for sinus rhythm; however, the heart rate generally falls in the range of 101 to 150 beats per minute (Fig. 2-17).

Researchers have identified some factors that enhance automaticity in the SA node. With acute myocardial infarction, the most significant factors are (1) sympathetic stimulation (fever, pain, anxiety, activity); (2) heart failure; (3) dehydration (hypovolemia); (4) hypoxia; and (5) drugs (atropine, epinephrine, aminophylline). Initial therapy in the management of sinus tachycardia is to correct the underlying cause rather than to depress automaticity. For example, if the sinus tachycardia is associated with heart failure, initial therapy should attempt to improve cardiac function and decrease cardiac work load.

NURSING ORDERS: The patient with sinus tachycardia

RELATED NURSING DIAGNOSES: Alteration in cardiac output, anxiety, activity intolerance, alteration in comfort

1. Is patient symptomatic from the fast rate?
   —Check sensorium, skin color and temperature, blood pressure.
   —Assess for angina.
2. Is oxygenation adequate?
   —Observe character and rate of respirations.
   —Assess O_2 saturation (pulse oximetry) or arterial blood gas values.
3. Is the tachycardia associated with heart failure or dehydration (hypovolemia)?
   —Auscultate lungs for crackles.
   —Check fluid balance, pulmonary capillary wedge pressure.
   —Assess for dyspnea.
4. Is the tachycardia associated with drug therapy?
   —Check whether the patient is receiving isoproterenol (Isuprel), atropine, aminophylline, epinephrine, or dopamine.
   —If so, consider discontinuing or turning down the intravenous drip.
5. Are there any stressors that may elicit a sympathetic response and thus increase the heart rate?
   —Consider antipyretics if fever present and determine cause.
   —Initiate measures to decrease anxiety.
   —Medicate for pain.

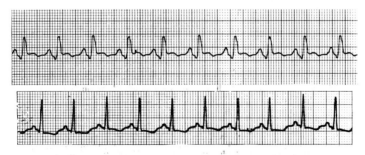

Fig. 2-17   Sinus tachycardia (ST).

Sinus bradycardia

When automaticity is depressed in the SA node, the rate of impulse discharge from this area decreases. Slowing of the sinus rate to less than 60 beats per minute results in an

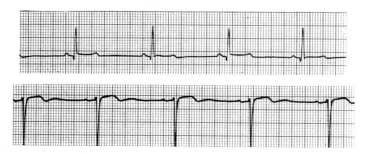

Fig. 2-18   Sinus bradycardia (SB).

arrhythmia known as *sinus bradycardia* (SB) (Fig. 2-18). Sinus bradycardia is normal in athletes. It fulfills all the ECG criteria for sinus rhythms except that the heart rate is slower.

Several factors depress automaticity and conduction in the SA node. With acute myocardial infarction, the most significant factors are (1) ischemia (to the SA node); (2) parasympathetic or vagal stimulation (ischemia to the vagal fibers, carotid sinus pressure, Valsalva maneuver); and (3) drugs (digitalis, beta blockers, verapamil). Sinus bradycardia is clinically significant when it causes a symptomatic fall in cardiac output. (Remember that cardiac output = *heart rate* × stroke volume.) Sinus bradycardias may also be significant because slow rates may precipitate the development of dangerous tachyarrhythmias. Initial therapy in the management of sinus bradycardia involves accelerating the ventricular rate.

NURSING ORDERS: The patient with sinus bradycardia

RELATED NURSING DIAGNOSES: Alteration in cardiac output

Sinus arrhythmia

Both the SA node and the lung are innervated by the parasympathetic nervous system via the vagus nerve. The SA node may therefore be affected by respirations. The rate of the SA node may *gradually* increase with inspiration and *gradually* decrease with

1. Is the patient symptomatic from the slow rates?
   —Watch for the development of hypotension, changes in level of consciousness, and syncope.
   —Assess for changes in skin color and temperature and for diaphoresis.
   —Assess for angina or dyspnea.
   —Assess for ventricular arrhythmias associated with the slow rate.
2. Is the bradycardia associated with infarction of the inferior wall?
   (Note that slow rates classically accompany this type of infarction.)
3. Is the sinus bradycardia associated with any drug therapy?
   —Check whether the patient is receiving digitalis, Calcium channel blockers, or a beta blocker.
4. Is the patient hypoxic?
5. Have atropine at the bedside.
6. Is bradycardia associated with Valsalva maneuvers or other vagal stimulation?
7. Refer to Unit 6 for the incorporation of advanced cardiac life support protocols.

expiration.[14,16] If these effects are marked, the overall rhythm appears irregular. This irregularity is considered a normal physiologic process and is especially marked in young people (Fig. 2-19).

This physiologic variation in heart rate has

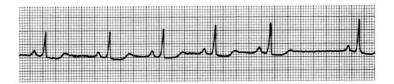

Fig. 2-19 Sinus arrhythmia.

been attributed to the *Bainbridge reflex*, which is activated by volume receptors located in both atria. Distention of these receptors by a sudden increase in atrial volume increases impulse transmission to the vasomotor center via *vagal* (parasympathetic) *sensory pathways.* The motor response is via sympathetic pathways and results in an increase in the heart rate. This sympathetic response appears to be selective in that other sympathetic effects, such as increased contractility and vasoconstriction, do not occur simultaneously. This increased heart rate occurring in response to increased atrial volume promotes emptying of the atria and prevents congestion of blood.

12-LEAD ECG

A lead is an electrical system used to record electrical activity. Leads are used in cardiac monitoring systems as well as in standard 12-lead ECG recording systems. A lead is composed of a negative and a positive electrode. These electrodes sense the magnitude and direction of electrical forces and record surface information from the cardiac borders.

The positive electrode is the most sensitive electrode. Electrical forces traveling toward a positive electrode produce a predominantly positive deflection on the ECG monitor or record. Electrical forces traveling away from a positive electrode (or toward a negative electrode) produce a predominantly negative deflection on the ECG monitor or record. Forces traveling perpendicular to the positive electrode inscribe small or biphasic (half positive and half negative) deflections on the ECG record or monitor (Fig. 2-20).[3,16]

In the normal heart, the left ventricle has the most muscle mass and the most electrical forces. For this reason, the sum of all the electrical forces traveling through the ventricles is usually represented by a force shifted

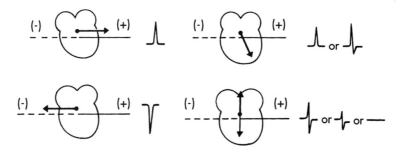

Fig. 2-20 Lead electrodes, cardiac electrical forces, and corresponding ECG deflections.

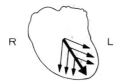

Fig. 2-21 The normal summation force (vector) or *axis* of the heart.

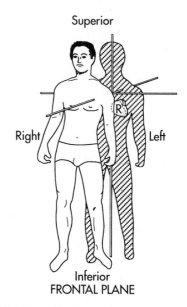

Fig. 2-22 Frontal plane dimensions and corresponding cardiac borders.

slightly to the left (Fig. 2-21). Arrows called vectors represent both the magnitude and direction of electrical forces. The summation force (large arrow) is known as the *summation vector,* or *axis.* The ventricular, or QRS, axis in the normal heart is shifted toward the left. The ventricular axis, or ventricular summation vector, is reflected on the ECG as the QRS complex.[4,11,14] The more exact range of normal axis is discussed in Unit 7.

Planes of the heart

A plane is an imaginary, flat, two-dimensional surface with four borders that can act as reference points for recording cardiac electrical and mechanical activity. Monitoring electrodes are placed at the borders of planes to form the leads that record electrical activity.

Standard limb leads

A standardized method of electrode placement was devised by Einthoven. In devising this method, he first used the frontal plane. Einthoven selected positions on the arms and legs as potential electrode sites (Fig. 2-24). With the use of two electrodes at a time, he derived three standard *bipolar leads.* When both the positive and the negative electrodes are located on the body surface, this lead is called a *bipolar lead.* An ECG recorder with a recording cable attached utilizes lead principles to record information from the body surfaces. The cable endings are attached to monitoring electrodes placed in the designated positions: right arm (RA),

Planes slice through the body, providing cross-sectional views at different angles. Three planes are used to record cardiac electrical activity—the *frontal, sagittal,* and *horizontal* planes (Figs. 2-22 and 2-23). The frontal and horizontal planes are referred to most frequently in electrocardiography.

left arm (LA), left leg (LL). The electrode placed at the right leg (RL) position functions as a ground, or neutralizing, electrode. The electrode placed at the LL position is also called the foot (F) electrode.

To obtain lead I, the two arm positions are used. The left arm (LA) is designated positive and the right arm (RA) is designated negative by programming the cable endings that are marked LA and RA (Fig. 2-25). Lead II is obtained by using the RA and the LL or F electrodes. The RA is designated negative and the LL or F positive (Fig. 2-25). Lead III is obtained by using the LA and the LL or F electrodes. The LA is designated

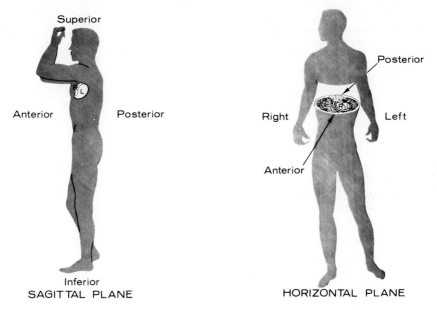

Fig. 2-23 Sagittal and horizontal plane dimensions and corresponding cardiac borders.

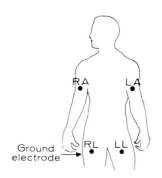

Fig. 2-24 Limb electrode positions.

negative and the LL or F positive (Fig. 2-25). The three bipolar leads can be joined to form a triangle with the heart as a central source of electricity within this triangle (Fig. 2-26).[8,14]

Three more leads may be derived from the frontal plane positions. Each position is designated separately as a positive electrode. The two other limb positions share the role of negative electrode to augment the voltage

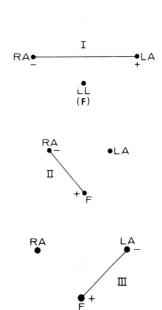

Fig. 2-25 The bipolar limb leads (leads I, II, and III): positive and negative electrode positions.

29

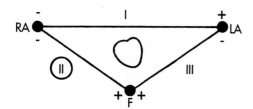

Fig. 2-26 Summary of all three bipolar limb leads.

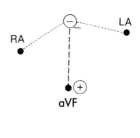

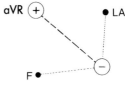

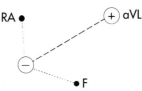

Fig. 2-27 The unipolar limb leads (leads aVF, aVR, and aVL): positive and negative electrode positions.

of the recorded forces. Thus the negative electrode extends directly as an imaginary line between the two other electrode positions through a central zero reference point.[3,4,13,14,16] Since only the positive electrode is actually on the body surface, these leads are called *unipolar leads*.

Lead aVF is created by making the LL or F electrode positive. The negative electrode extends in an imaginary direction between the two other electrode positions. The electrical forces recorded in a unipolar system are small and must use augmented voltage or extra electrical energy. For this reason, this lead is known as the *augmented voltage (aV) foot (F) lead,* or *lead aVF*. Lead aVF has one visible electrode on the body. It is therefore called a *unipolar lead*. Using the same principles, the RA and LA electrodes are used to obtain leads aVR and aVL (Fig. 2-27).

The three bipolar limb leads may be moved to a central point so that they intersect (Fig. 2-28). The three unipolar limb leads may then be added. The final diagram shown in Fig. 2-29 is a representation of all six limb leads or frontal plane leads and is called the *hexaxial reference system*.[3,4,11,14,16]

By superimposing the ventricular forces of a particular patient's heart over a lead such as lead I, you can deduce the morphology of the QRS complex in this lead (Fig. 2-30). The ventricular forces of this person's normal heart travel toward the positive electrode in lead I. Therefore, you can expect

that a normal QRS complex in lead I will have a predominantly positive deflection. Conversely, when a patient has a predominantly positive QRS complex in lead I, you can expect that the ventricular forces of this person travel toward the positive electrode in lead I and thus could be normal. Confirmation of these forces as normal requires the assessment of at least one additional lead such as lead aVF (see Unit 7).

Using these principles of electrophysiology, you can deduce the QRS morphology in each of the limb leads. In Fig. 2-31, the patient's ventricular forces are traveling toward the positive electrodes of all the standard limb leads except for lead aVR. Thus, the QRS complex for this patient is positive in all leads except lead aVR. Since the ventricular forces are traveling most directly toward the positive electrode of lead II, the largest positive deflection should be on lead II.

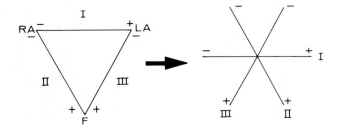

Fig. 2-28   Intersection of the bipolar limb leads at a central reference point.

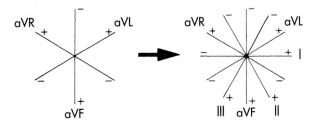

Fig. 2-29   Intersection of both bipolar and unipolar limb leads at a central reference point.

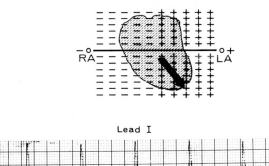

Lead I

Fig. 2-30   Normal ventricular forces as recorded on lead I.

Since the ventricular forces are traveling away from the positive electrode of lead aVR, the QRS complex in lead aVR is negative. When forces are traveling perpendicular to a lead, the QRS complex is smaller and is half positive and half negative as in lead aVL. This pattern is referred to as *biphasic*.

On the ECG, the P wave represents the atrial electrical forces or the P wave axis.

When the SA node activates the atria, the forces of the atria travel directly towards the foot and positive electrode of lead II. Therefore, in a sinus rhythm, the P wave is positive in lead II and is often most clearly visible in this lead. In a sinus rhythm, the P wave in lead aVR is also negative because the atrial forces move directly away from the positive electrode (Fig. 2-32).[4,8]

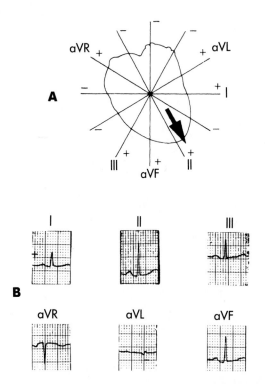

Fig. 2-31 Normal ventricular forces: relationship to all limb leads **(A)** and corresponding QRS complex configurations **(B).**

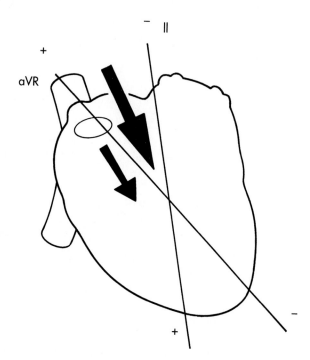

Fig. 2-32 Leads II and aVR: role in validating normal (sinus) P wave configuration.

Standard chest leads

The limb leads provide six views of the heart in the frontal plane. The chest leads provide six other standard views of the heart's electrical activity within the horizontal plane. The horizontal plane slices the body transversely, anterior to posterior (Fig. 2-33).

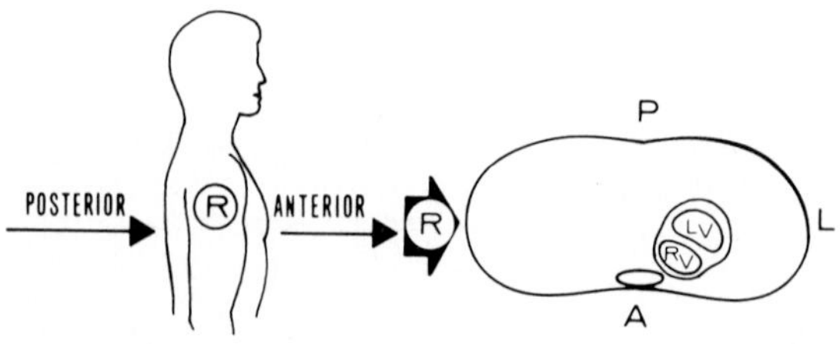

The chest leads are derived using the principle of the unipolar leads. These leads also represent augmented voltage of vector forces and are known as *V leads* or *precordial leads.* In the V leads, the positive electrode is placed on the front or side of the chest wall; the negative electrode extends in an imaginary line posteriorly toward a central reference point created by the limb electrodes. The positive electrode of lead V_1 is located

Fig. 2-33 The horizontal plane: cross-sectional view.

just to the right of the sternum in the fourth intercostal space. The positive electrode is then moved along the chest wall toward the left to form leads V_2 to V_6 (Fig. 2-34).[3,6,14,16]

The left ventricle lies rotated posteriorly in the chest. Therefore, the QRS forces in

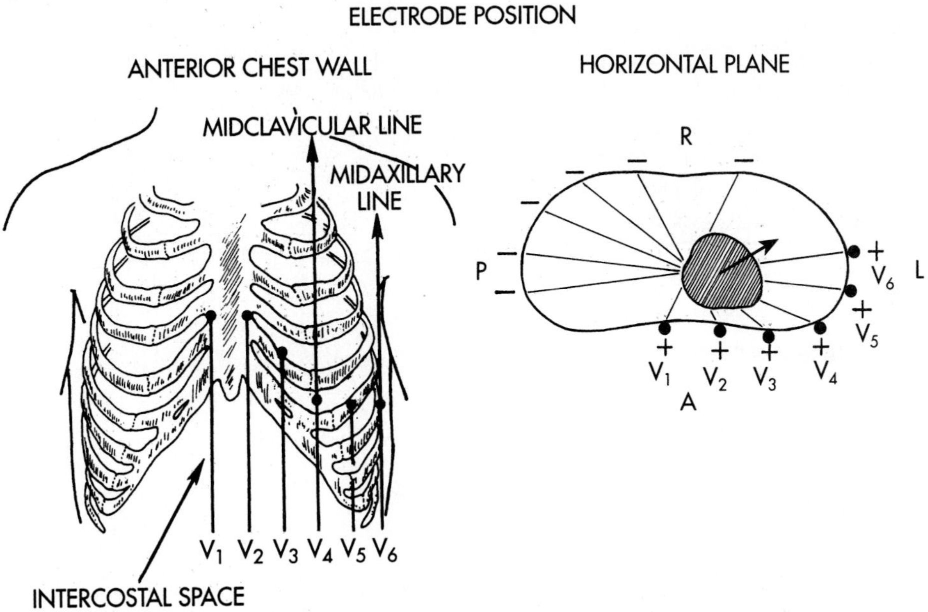

ELECTRODE POSITION

ANTERIOR CHEST WALL

MIDCLAVICULAR LINE

MIDAXILLARY LINE

V_1 V_2 V_3 V_4 V_5 V_6

INTERCOSTAL SPACE

HORIZONTAL PLANE

R

P

L

V_6

V_5

V_1 V_2 V_3 V_4

A

Fig. 2-34   The chest leads: location of the positive electrodes for leads V_1 to V_6. The summation ventricular force is also illustrated. The positive electrode of lead V_1 is placed at the fourth intercostal space to the right of the sternum with lead V_2 immediately opposite to the left of the sternum. Lead V_4 is placed at the fifth intercostal space, midclavicular line with lead V_3 in between V_2 and V_4. Lead V_6 is placed at the fifth intercostal space, midaxillary line, with lead V_5 in between V_4 and V_6.

the horizontal plane travel posteriorly as well as to the left. (Remember that the summation ventricular forces travel toward the left ventricle.) In lead V_1, the ventricular forces travel away from the positive electrode. Therefore, the normal QRS in lead V_1 should be predominantly negative. The ECG patterns on leads V_2 to V_5 are a transition from the V_1 pattern to the V_6 pattern. The R wave becomes larger and the S wave becomes smaller as the progression occurs (see Fig. 2-35). The tallest R waves generally appear in lead V_5.[14]

The force of septal depolarization is best confirmed on the chest leads. This force, although small, contributes to the QRS complex. The septum is the first portion of the

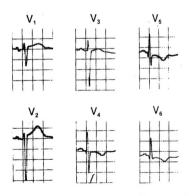

Fig. 2-35   Chest leads: normal QRS complex configurations.

33

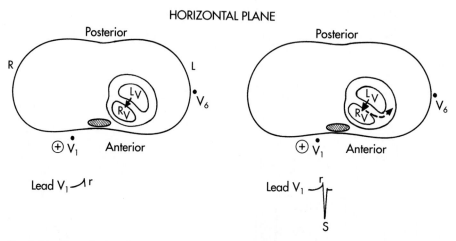

Fig. 2-36 Ventricular depolarization, including septal depolarization, as recorded in lead V_1.

ventricle to be depolarized. Septal depolarization occurs from left to right and posteriorly to anteriorly. (The major portions of the ventricles are depolarized from right to left and anterior to posterior. Thus septal depolarization occurs in the opposite direction.)

In lead V_1 the initial, or septal, force is represented by a small r wave.[4,11] It is caused by the wave of septal depolarization traveling toward the right and thus toward the positive electrode of this lead. The major

ventricular forces travel in the opposite direction, toward the left or away from the positive electrode. This force is represented by a large S wave (Fig. 2-36).

In lead V_6 the initial, or septal, force is represented by a small q wave, indicating the wave of septal depolarization traveling away from the positive electrode of this lead.[4,11] The major ventricular forces travel in the opposite direction, producing a large R wave (Fig. 2-37).

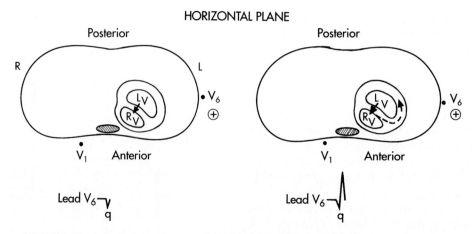

Fig. 2-37 Ventricular depolarization, including septal depolarization, as recorded in lead V_6.

Recording surface information

Let us consider the outer or epicardial surfaces of the left ventricle and correlate the leads with the surface they reflect. (Remember that the most sensitive electrode is the positive electrode.) The foot electrode of the frontal plane looks directly up toward the inferior surface of the left ventricle. The leads that use the foot electrode as a positive, or sensing electrode are leads II, III, and aVF. These leads then reflect the electrical activity of the inferior surface of the left ventricle (Fig. 2-38).[11,14,16] These leads can best detect inferior wall myocardial infarction (IWMI).

Let us now discuss the anterior surface and the leads that reflect its electrical activity. The LA electrode of the frontal plane looks directly at the lateral portion of the anterior surface of the left ventricle. The leads that use the left arm as the positive electrode are leads I and aVL (Fig. 2-39). Leads I and aVL, then, reflect the lateral surface of the left ventricle.[11,14,16] The positive electrodes of the chest leads border the septal and lateral portions of the anterior surface of the left ventricle within the horizontal plane. Leads I, aVL, and V_1 to V_6 reflect the electrical activity of the entire anterior wall (Fig. 2-39). Therefore, extensive anterior wall myocardial infarctions (AWMIs) appear most clearly in leads I and aVL and in the

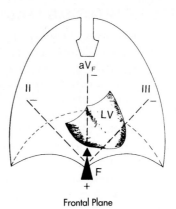

Fig. 2-38 Leads reflecting the inferior wall of the left ventricle.

chest leads. If an infarction is confined to the septal area of the anterior wall, it is most visible in leads V_1 through V_4.[8,11,14] If an infarction is confined to the lateral portion of the anterior wall, it is most visible in leads I, aVL, and V_4 to V_6.[11,14]

Lead aVR uses the RA as its positive electrode. Unlike the other limb electrodes, the RA electrode does not look directly at any outer surface of the left ventricle. This electrode, however, does look at the inside of the heart. Lead aVR reflects the inside of the left ventricle and is also called an *intracavitary lead* (Fig. 2-40). Subendocardial changes are most visible in lead aVR.

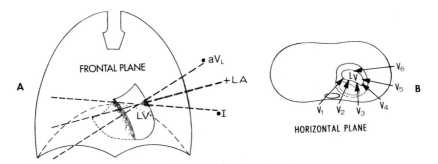

Fig. 2-39 Leads reflecting the anterior wall (septal and lateral) of the left ventricle.

CARDIAC MONITORING LEADS/SYSTEMS

Cardiac monitoring systems usually require three major components: (1) *electrodes,* (2) a *monitoring cable,* and (3) an *oscilloscope display.* A bedside or central *recorder* is a critical option in a coronary care unit. Another valuable option is an electronic or tape memory bank with the ability to play back a record of the onset of rhythm disturbances, ECG changes, or both.

Monitoring systems are available in the form of large bedside units or small portable units. The small units may be connected to radio transmitters (telemetry) or to recorders that are later connected to oscilloscope displays for playback (Holter monitoring). In coronary care units the larger "hardwire" or fixed bedside units are most common. The portable units are popular in convalescent (progressive care) cardiac units.

All cardiac monitoring systems use lead concepts to obtain the ECG record or display. Knowledge of lead concept allows the nurse to select optimal electrode positions and facilitates problem solving.

A minimum of three electrodes is usually required to obtain an ECG record from a hardwire bedside unit. An external ground electrode may not be necessary with telemetry units, leaving two major electrodes. Three-electrode monitoring systems are popular in many coronary care units. The two-electrode systems used with telemetry units incorporate the same principles. These systems cost less and are less cumbersome than four-electrode or five-electrode systems. However, to obtain their maximal efficiency, two-electrode and three-electrode systems require more ingenuity and adjustment from the nurses using them. In determining proper electrode position, first consider positions that most closely mimic the standard lead positions such as the limb leads (Fig. 2-41).[15] Then move the limb electrodes in toward the chest to allow for patient movement with minimal muscle artifact. You can also place the leads on flat, bony surfaces instead of muscle surfaces to minimize artifact (see p. 39).

Designations on the cable usually identify the negative and positive electrodes. These designations are far more useful in monitoring systems than the cable ending markings RA, LA, or LL, which are often best disregarded. After you identify the cable ending that programs the positive electrode, you can connect it to electrodes placed in any limb position to obtain a variety of leads. A lead selector is not necessary. Systems recommending RA, LA, and RL limb positions require moving the *positive electrode* (LA) to obtain leads other than lead I. The RL cable ending always functions as ground. Systems with the three major limb positions indicated on the cable (RA, LA, and LL) usually employ a lead selector that automatically adjusts the positive and negative electrodes as necessary to obtain standard limb lead equivalents.

You also can obtain chest lead equivalents from either three-electrode or two-electrode monitoring systems. (Keep in mind that the chest leads are unipolar leads.) Three-electrode monitoring systems function as bipolar systems. Therefore, these chest lead equivalents are *modified bipolar* chest leads

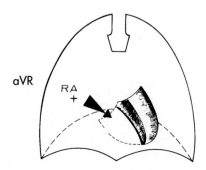

Fig. 2-40 Lead reflecting the endocardial surface of the left ventricle.

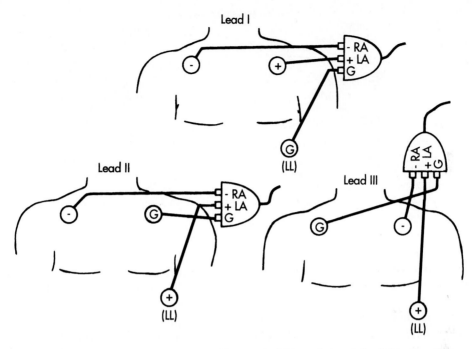

Fig. 2-41 Monitoring electrode positions mimicking the standard bipolar limb leads.

and are called *MCL leads*. The "CL" designation actually refers to "chest–left arm,"[4,11] which are the bipolar electrode positions used. Place the negative electrode on the left arm. Place the positive electrode in the appropriate "V," or chest lead position; it acts as the exploring or sensing electrode.[5,14,15] The most common chest lead positions are V_1 and V_6 (Fig. 2-42). To obtain modified chest leads with an RA, LA, RL system, identify the positive and negative electrodes by leaving the lead selector in the lead I position. The LA cable ending is thus designated as positive and the RA cable ending as negative. In RA, LA, LL systems, you can leave the lead selector in the lead I position as was just discussed or in the lead II position. However, when in the lead II position, the LL cable ending (instead of the LA ending) would become positive with the RA cable ending negative. In monitoring systems

without lead selection capabilities, the LA cable ending usually designates the positive electrode, and the RA cable ending usually designates the negative electrode. Do not rely on color coding of the cable endings, since colors are not standard and cable endings may be moved.[6]

By obtaining equivalents of the standard ECG leads on the monitoring leads, you can initially detect many of the same changes on these leads and later verify them on a standard 12-lead ECG. This concept is particularly important because significant ECG changes are often transient and can be missed if not documented immediately. Whenever possible, obtain a multilead record from the monitor. Multiple ECG views facilitate the interpretation of changes in the direction of electrical forces associated with such factors as bundle branch blocks, hemiblocks, and arrhythmias. Multiple views

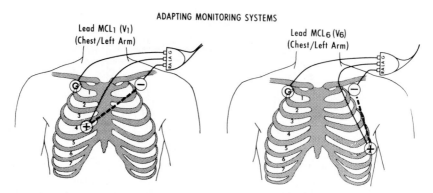

Fig. 2-42   Monitoring electrode positions mimicking the chest leads.

may also document significant surface information indicative of ischemia or infarction (see Unit 5). The unipolar leads provide the most direct surface information. However, the bipolar equivalents are usually adequate in an emergency. Therefore, in a patient who has an acute MI or in a situation in which you need to rule out a possible MI, keep electrodes in the LA (lead I—lateral position), LL (lead II—inferior position), and V_1 and V_2 or MCL_1 and MCL_2 (anterior position) configuration. If these patients complain of chest pain, obtain a record from each of these leads by adapting the cable endings to the appropriate electrode positions, as mentioned earlier.

There is no single ideal monitoring lead for every patient. For this reason, a multilead system is recommended. Although lead II usually records clear, upright P waves, lead V_1 (MCL_1) may also record clear (although not necessarily upright) P waves in a given patient. Lead I often records less artifact in a mechanically ventilated patient than either V_1 or lead II because there is less movement of the positive electrode. Leads V_1 (MCL_1) and V_6 (MCL_6) are often helpful in detecting bundle branch blocks associated with acute AWMI (see Unit 7) or in detecting improper positioning of pacing catheters (see Unit 11). Lead V_1/MCL_1, particularly when

combined with lead V_6/MCL_6, can be helpful in differentiating ventricular rhythms from supraventricular rhythms with aberrant conduction (see Unit 7).[5,6] Verify acute myocardial injury detected on a monitoring lead with a standard 12-lead ECG. Use your judgment in selecting the best monitoring lead for a given patient situation. This choice should be part of the nursing plan of care.

The oscilloscope display in a monitoring system provides a menu of multiple options to facilitate arrhythmia diagnosis.[5] Figure 2-43 illustrates some of the most commonly available adjustments. The *size,* or *sensitivity,* dial/selection adjusts the *amplitude* of the ECG pattern. The *position* dial/selection may be provided in older models centering the trace. The *rate meter* records an approximation of the heart rate and allows setting high and low *alarms.* This terminology may vary slightly from brand to brand. For example, the rate meter may be referred to as "digital heart rate." The systole light allows evaluation of monitor sensing. Additional modules can display and/or record venous or arterial pressure, temperature, cardiac output, arterial and/or venous saturation, respirations, and end tidal CO_2. Computerized systems allow for gross rhythm analysis, trending of information, and correlation with intervention.

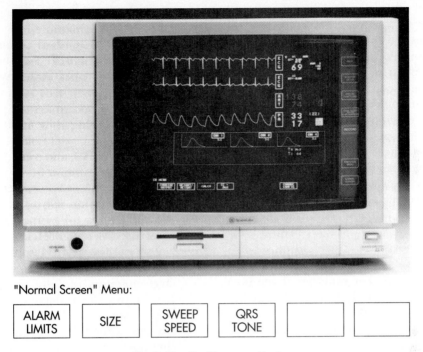

"Normal Screen" Menu:

| ALARM LIMITS | SIZE | SWEEP SPEED | QRS TONE | | |

Fig. 2-43   Oscilloscope display.

ECG ARTIFACTS

Electrical interference or poor electrical conduction can often distort the ECG trace. This distortion is called *artifact*.[2,4,5] Figures 2-44 through 2-48 provide a few examples of artifact with corresponding corrective nursing action.

NURSING ORDERS: 60-Cycle Interference (Fig. 2-44)

1. Check for crossing of cable wires with other electrical wires, such as call light, bed control, or transducer cables.
2. Check contact of cable with conductive

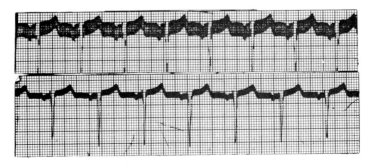

Fig. 2-44   Sixty-cycle interference artifact.

parts of other electrical equipment, such as side rails of electrical beds or metal portions of ventilators.

3. Try momentarily pulling the plug of any other electrical equipment in contact with the patient.
4. Try turning the sensitivity (size/gain) control down to minimize the effect.
5. Check for loose connections at cable or electrode sites.
6. Try pressing on each electrode to temporatily improve contact. If baseline is corrected, change that electrode only. Check the positive electrode of each lead first.
7. If a wide baseline is present only on selected leads, solve the problem using lead concepts. For example, if the trace on leads II and III has a wide baseline but lead I does not, the faulty electrode or cable wire is designated by the LA cable ending.
8. Reapply new electrodes using a drying agent, such as alcohol, deodorant, or benzoin, if not previously used.
9. Rub the skin with a gauze pad or the abrasive tip on the disposable electrode, if not previously done, to lower skin resistance.
10. Check for frayed or broken wires, and change the cable.
11. Verify grounding of all electrical equipment.
12. If a five-lead cable is being used for three-lead monitoring, plug the cable's unused receptacles.
13. Remember when first connecting a patient to a monitor that has not been previously turned on, there may be a period of 60-cycle interference as the machine is "warming up."

NURSING ORDERS: Movement/Muscle Activity (Fig. 2-45)
1. Check to see if the patient is moving or having tremors.
2. Prevent excessive cable movement by clipping the cable to the patient's clothing.
3. Ask the patient to hold still momentarily.
4. If artifact is still present, check to see whether the electrodes are positioned over skin folds, large muscle masses, large amounts of fatty tissue, or joints. If so, move electrode(s) to another site.
5. Select another lead if necessary.
6. Do not attempt to diagnose atrial arrhythmias in the presence of this type of artifact.
7. For clues in differentiating ventricular arrhythmias, see Fig. 2-46.

NURSING ORDERS: Mimicking Ventricular Arrhythmias (Fig. 2-46)
1. Never defibrillate from a tracing record before checking the patient for absence of pulse. Patient or cable movement artifact can mimic this pattern as well as tremors.
2. Premature ventricular contractions may be distinguished from artifactual QRS complexes if:

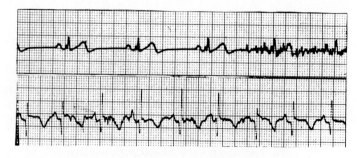

Fig. 2-45   Movement and muscle activity artifact.

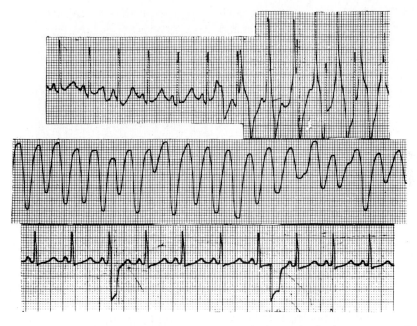

Fig. 2-46   Artifact mimicking ventricular arrhythmias.

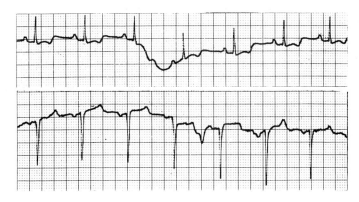

Fig. 2-47   Wandering baseline artifacts.

—They reset the natural QRS interval. Artifact does not.

—Sharp deflections coinciding with the QRS interval can be measured throughout the pattern change (suggests artifact).

NURSING ORDERS: Wandering Baseline (Fig. 2-47)

1. Take measures to prevent excessive cable movement.

2. Note if the patient is moving.

3. Select another lead.

4. Select the monitoring rather than diagnostic mode on the monitor.

5. If baseline is moving in a cyclic fashion, consider possible effects of respiratory chest wall movement. Move the positive electrode away from the diaphragm (that is, higher) or change the lead.

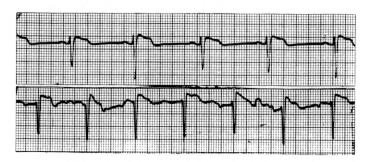

Fig. 2-48 Respiratory artifact.

6. Check to see if the electrodes are firmly attached to the skin. If not, reapply them with proper skin preparation.
   NURSING ORDERS: Respiratory Effects (Fig. 2-48)
1. Differentiate these gradual QRS changes occurring with respiration from sudden, noncyclic QRS changes, which may indicate arrhythmias.
2. No action is indicated since this artifact results from normal movement of the heart with respiration and does not significantly distort the trace. However, switching to another lead usually can abolish it.

Lead I

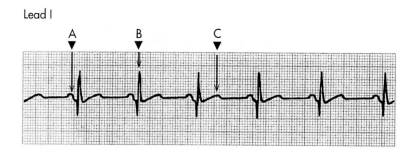

Fig. 2-49 Self-assessment trace 1.

SELF-ASSESSMENT

1 The QRS complex in the above trace is designated by the letter _____ and indicates _____ depolarization. This QRS complex (does/does not) have a Q wave. Its exact configuration on this lead may be described as _____. The width of the QRS complex is _____ small boxes or _____ second.

The QRS complex (is/is not) normal because it is _____ and _____. This indicates that the origin of this impulse is (ventricular/supraventricular).

B; ventricular

does

QR

2; 0.08

is; narrow

unchanging

supraventricular

2 The P wave in the above trace is designated by the letter _____ and indicates _____ depolarization. The P wave (is/is not) normal because it is _____, (regular/irregular), and (upright/inverted), with a rate less than _____. This indicates that the origin of this impulse is _____.

A; atrial
is; visible; regular
upright; 150
sinus

3 A QRS complex (does/does not) follow each P wave at a constant interval. This interval is called the _____ interval. The duration of this interval is _____ small boxes or _____ second. Thus this interval (is/is not) normal and indicates the absence of abnormal _____ delay or block.

does
P–R

4 The rate of both the P and QRS complexes in this trace is _____. Thus the rhythm may be completely interpreted as (NSR/SB/ST).

60–63
NSR

5 The QRS complex is slightly more positive than negative in the lead depicted in the above trace. Thus you can assume that the patient's ventricular forces are traveling slightly (toward/away from) the positive electrode of this lead. Since the positive electrode in lead I is on the _____, this means the ventricular forces are traveling slightly toward the _____ and thus (are/are not) considered to be traveling in the normal direction.

toward

LA
left; are

Lead V_1 (HCL$_1$)

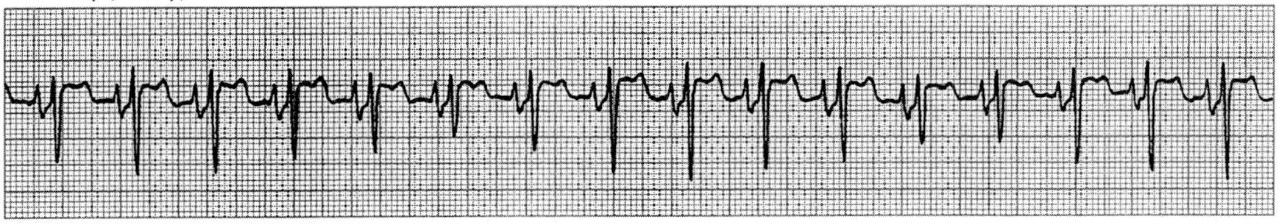

Fig. 2-50   Self-assessment trace 2.

6 QRS Complex
   a. appearance:_____   narrow, no significant change
   b. rate (vent):_____   110
   P Wave
   a. appearance:_____   visible, regular, biphasic
   b. rate (atrial):_____   110
   P–R Interval:_____   constant, normal duration
   Interpretation:_____   ST

Comments: The cyclic QRS changes are compatible with respiratory artifact (see Fig. 2-48) and thus do not represent an abnormal ventricular focus. The QRS complex is normally negative in lead V_1. Although the P wave is not upright, this rhythm may still be considered sinus since the trace is not on lead II. In the presence of a normal P–R interval, the rhythm is unlikely to be junctional. In the presence of a regular P wave at a rate of less than 150, the rhythm is unlikely to arise at another site in the atria. The only possible remaining supraventricular origin is the SA node. Biphasic and inverted P waves are common in lead V_1 because of the relationship of the positive electrode to the pathway of the SA node. A P wave rate of 115 is considered a tachycardia for the SA node.

Lead V_1 (MCL$_1$)

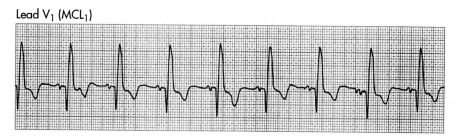

Fig. 2-51   Self-assessment trace 3.

7 QRS Complex

   a. appearance:_____ wide, unchanging

   b. rate (vent):_____ 66

   P Wave

   a. appearance:_____ visible, biphasic, regular

   b. rate (atrial):_____ 66

   P–R Interval:_____ constant, normal duration

   Interpretation:_____ NSR

Comments: From the QRS complex alone, determining whether this rhythm is ventricular or supraventricular is difficult, since the complex is abnormally wide but does not change. Remember, sinus rhythm can occur in the presence of a wide QRS complex when bundle branch block is present. Sinus rhythm is confirmed when the QRS complex is related to a normal P wave at a constant P–R interval as in this trace. Although biphasic, the P wave is considered normal since the P–R interval is normal and biphasic P waves are common on lead V_1.

8 Leads I, II, III, aVR, aVL, and aVF are (limb leads/chest leads) and are obtained from electrodes in the (frontal/horizontal) plane. Leads aVR, aVL, and aVF are (unipolar/bipolar). In self-assessment trace 4 (Fig. 2-52) the QRS complex is predominantly (positive/negative) in both leads I and aVF. Since the positive electrode in lead I is on the _____ and the positive electrode in lead aVF is on the _____, this means the ventricular forces are traveling (up/down) and toward the (right/left). These forces (are/are not) considered normal.

   Leads V_1 and V_6 are referred to as (limb leads/chest leads) and are obtained from electrodes in the (frontal/ horizontal) plane. The QRS pattern

limb leads

frontal

unipolar

positive

LA

LL (F)

down; left

are

chest leads

horizontal

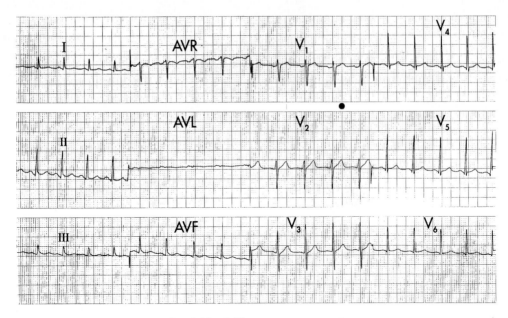

Fig. 2-52 Self-assessment trace 4.

in V_1 above (is/is not) normal because it has a _____ configuration.
     The P wave is normal because it is upright in lead _____ and
inverted in lead _____.
     The inferior wall of the LV is reflected on leads _____. The
anterior wall of the LV is reflected by leads _____ (lateral), and
leads _____ (septal).

is; rS

II,
aVR

II, III, aVF
I, aVL, V_4–V_6
V_1–V_4

REFERENCES/SUGGESTED READINGS

 1. Andrews LK: Tracking electrical impulses, Am J Nurs 89(3):370, 1989.
 2. Atchinson JJ: Arrhythmia or artifact? Am J Nurs 89(2):210, 1989.
 3. Caine R: Essentials of monitoring the electrocardiogram, Nurs Clin North Am 22(1):77, 1987.
 4. Conover MB: Understanding electrocardiography, ed 6, St. Louis, 1992, Mosby–Year Book.
 5. Decker S: Continous EKG monitoring systems, Nurs Clin North Am 22(1):1, 1987.
 6. Drew BJ: Using cardiac leads the right way, Nursing 22(5):50, 1992.
 7. Fenstermacher RN: Arrhythmia recognition and management, Philadelphia, 1989, WB Saunders.
 8. Grauer K: A practical guide to ECG interpretation, St. Louis, 1992, Mosby–Year Book.
 9. Hill NE, Goodman JS: Importance of accurate placement of precordial leads in the 12-lead electrocardiogram, Heart Lung 16(5):561, 1987.
10. Johantgen MA: Quick reference to dysrhythmias: identification and intervention, Gaithersburg, MD, 1991, Aspen Publications.
11. Marriott HJ: Practical electrocardiography, ed 8, Baltimore, 1988, William & Wilkins.

12. Rowlands DJ: Clinical electrocardiography, Philadelphia, 1991, JB Lippincott.
13. Scheidt S: Basic electrocardiography: ECG, 1986, West Caldwell, Ciba-Geigy.
14. Sweetwood HM: Clinical electrocardiography for nurses, ed 2, Gaithersburg, MD, 1989, Aspen Publications.
15. Textbook of advanced cardiac life support, ed 2, Dallas, 1990, American Heart Association.
16. Underhill SL et al: Cardiac nursing, ed 2, Philadelphia, 1989, JB Lippincott.

Oxygenation and Acid-Base Balance

OXYGENATION: AN INTRODUCTION

Tissue oxygenation depends on *oxygen delivery,* or the arterial O_2 supply, and *oxygen demands.* Oxygen delivery, in turn, is dependent on (1) the *blood supply* to the tissues per minute and (2) the *oxygen supply* within that blood. The blood supply (cardiac output) is determined by the integrity of the cardiovascular system. The available oxygen supply within the blood is determined by the integrity of the pulmonary system and the hemoglobin (red blood cell) content of the blood (Fig. 3-1).

Oxygen demands are determined by the metabolic needs of the cells. Metabolic needs and O_2 demands can increase dramatically by simple nursing procedures such as position changes (31%), weighing (36%), bathing (23%), electrocardiogram (ECG) (16%), and endotracheal tube (ET) suctioning (22%). O_2 demands increase further by complications such as fever (10% for each degree C), sepsis (50% to 100%), and visitors (22%).[13,52] A normal response to these increased O_2 demands is to increase the cardiac output and thus increase the O_2 supply. However, a weakened heart muscle cannot increase cardiac output to provide for these demands. As a result, the tissues become hypoxic more easily. Inadequate tissue oxygenation in the patient with coronary artery disease can occur as a result of either decreased cardiac output, pulmonary congestion, or increased metabolic demands.

Hypoxemia versus hypoxia

Inadequate oxygenation is detected from signs and symptoms of either hypoxemia or hypoxia. The state in which there is a low Pao_2 (less than 80 mm Hg or, more critically, less than 60 mm Hg) and a potentially lowered O_2 content in the blood is known as *hypoxemia.*[24,38] The state in which there is insufficient oxygen at the *tissue* level is known as *hypoxia* (see Fig. 3-1).

Hypoxemia is initially determined from alterations in the arterial Po_2 reported on an arterial blood gas sample. Correlate the arterial Po_2 with the O_2 saturation levels and the serum hemoglobin levels to determine the O_2 content. A critically low arterial O_2 saturation (Sao_2) is less than 90%.[13]

Hypoxia is determined from the signs and symptoms of inadequate tissue oxygenation. Inadequate tissue oxygenation is manifested by cellular metabolic changes and cerebral symptoms. Significant tissue hypoxia results in cellular metabolic changes leading to acidosis. Acidosis may be detected from the pH and bicarbonate values tested on either an

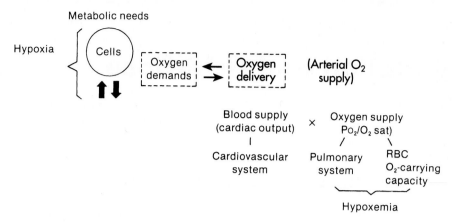

Fig. 3-1 Tissue oxygenation: major determinants and roles of the cardiovascular and pulmonary systems. The significance of hypoxemia is also illustrated.

arterial or a venous blood gas sample. The venous O_2 saturation (Svo_2) is also helpful in detecting changes in tissue oxygen demands or cardiac output that could result in hypoxia.

Hypoxia also results in cerebral symptoms because the brain is sensitive to lack of oxygen.[26] These symptoms include restlessness, agitation, irritability, syncope, and other alterations of consciousness. Dizziness, tremors, or convulsions may also occur. Collectively, these cerebral symptoms may be referred to as *sensorium changes*. The alterations in consciousness fall into two categories: (1) alterations in mental function, such as confusion and disorientation; and (2) alterations in arousal, such as lethargy, stupor, and coma.

Symptoms associated with reflex cardiovascular and respiratory responses may accompany either hypoxemia or hypoxia and are the result of chemical stimulation of nerve receptor areas known as *chemoreceptors*. The central chemoreceptors, located in the medullary area of the brainstem, respond to the changes in pH associated with hypoxia. The peripheral chemoreceptors, located in the aorta and carotid arteries, respond to the changes in arterial Po_2 associated with hypoxemia.[16,46] The peripheral chemorecep-

tors may also respond to hypoxia resulting from severe drops in cardiac output (see Unit 4).

As the result of chemoreceptor stimulation, the sympathetic nervous system and the cardiovascular and respiratory centers are activated. The cardiovascular response includes an elevated blood pressure, tachycardia, arrhythmias, cool and moist skin, and decreased urine output.[20] The respiratory response includes increased respiratory rate and respiratory effort. The individual uses accessory muscles during inspiration and diaphragmatic muscles during the normally passive expiration.

When cardiovascular disorders result in the hypoxic state, the symptoms may differ slightly from those typically associated with hypoxia. The blood pressure, which indicates gross cardiovascular function, is typically lower. Heart rate may be slow or fast since it may be the cause of the decreased cardiac output. The clinical state of hypoxia resulting from inadequate cardiac output is also known as *shock* (see Unit 9).

Hypoxia typically occurs as a consequence of hypoxemia. Hypoxemia occurs in the presence of pulmonary congestion associated with congestive heart failure (CHF), resulting in impaired oxygen transport. Evaluate the effectiveness of oxygen transport in the lungs by assessing arterial Po_2. Hypoxemia related to pulmonary congestion may lead to hypoxia in patients with a compromised myocardium. These patients are unable to compensate for decreased oxygen in the blood by increasing cardiac output. The ar-terial Po_2 and O_2 saturation can be normal in the hypoxic patient if the lungs are normal, but the cardiac output is low.[24,39] Thus, hypoxia can occur in the absence of hypoxemia. Hypoxemia can also occur in the absence of hypoxia in a patient with an adequate cardiac output and abnormal lungs.

EVALUATING OXYGEN TRANSPORT IN THE LUNGS: ROLE OF Pao_2

Arterial Po_2 (Pao_2) may be used as an indicator of O_2 content based on an assumed correlation with O_2 saturation. However, its major value is in evaluating O_2 transport in the lungs as a potential cause of hypoxemia. Pao_2 reflects the pressure of the oxygen dissolved in solution. The pressure of the dissolved oxygen in arterial blood depends on the pressure of O_2 gas delivered to the alveolus, the presence or absence of airway obstruction, and the integrity of the alveolar capillary membrane.

Room air is 21% oxygen. The *fraction* of *inspired* air that is composed of oxygen gas is 0.21. A clinical term frequently used to express inspired O_2 concentration is FIo_2, or *fraction of inspired oxygen.* The remainder of gas in room air is predominantly nitrogen. At sea level, a gas that completely fills the atmosphere exerts a barometric pressure of 760 mm Hg. At room air the inspired O_2 pressure is about 150 mm Hg or 760 mm Hg minus the humidity or water vapor pressure of the larger airways (47 mm Hg) × the FIo_2 (0.21).[3,20,31,51]

The oxygen pressure (Po_2) drops to 100 mm Hg when oxygen reaches the alveolus. This is due to imbalances in alveolar O_2 delivery and uptake by the blood and the presence of CO_2.[31,51] Normal arterial Po_2 at room air (FIo_2 21% or 0.21) ranges from 80 to 100 mm Hg. Pao_2 is 10 to 20 mm Hg less than alveolar Po_2 (PAo_2) as a result of normal disparities in the alveolar capillary mem-brane. Pao_2 levels below 80 mm Hg are abnormal and may be considered hypoxemic.[20,37] Pao_2 levels below 60 mm Hg indicate significant hypoxemia (see section on Evaluating Blood Oxygen Content: Role of O_2 Saturation (Sao_2)).

When you give 100% O_2 to a patient, O_2 particles completely fill the atmosphere. Therefore, at sea level, they should exert a pressure of 760 mm Hg. However, carbon dioxide and water vapor occupy the air passages, limiting the available space for oxygen. CO_2 and water vapor particles combined exert a pressure of 87 mm Hg, which allows 673 mm Hg to be occupied by oxygen. Allowing for normal limitation in gas exchange and the presence of minimal disease, PAo_2 and Pao_2 at an FIo_2 of 1.00 (100%) are at least 500 mm Hg, or five times the FIo_2. The normal Pao_2 of 100 mm Hg at room air is also five times the FIo_2 (0.21). Therefore, at any FIo_2 *the expected Pao_2 should be approximately five times the FIo_2* (Fig. 3-2).[3,38] This correlation is less accurate as FIo_2 increases and is only a gross initial assessment tool.

The difference between the PAo_2 and the actual Pao_2 is known as the *alveolar-arterial O_2 difference* (A-aDo_2), or the *A-a gradient* (see Fig. 3-2). You may assume an abnormal A-aDo_2 in the presence of any Pao_2 significantly lower than expected for its corresponding FIo_2. Significant gradients can lead to hypoxemia. For example, at an FIo_2 of

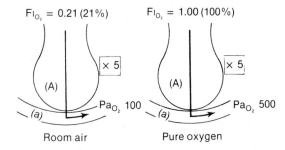

$FI_{O_2} = 0.21\ (21\%)$ $FI_{O_2} = 1.00\ (100\%)$

× 5   × 5

(A)   (A)

Pa_{O_2} 100 Pa_{O_2} 500

(a)   (a)

Room air   Pure oxygen

Fig. 3-2 Role of the Pa_{O_2} in evaluating oxygen transport. The normal Pa_{O_2} is five times the FI_{O_2}. The difference between the alveolar P_{O_2} (PA_{O_2}) and arterial P_{O_2} (Pa_{O_2})—known as the A-aD_{O_2} or A-a gradient—is normally only 10 to 20 mm Hg, although it increases to some extent at higher FI_{O_2}'s. Greater differences imply impaired pulmonary oxygen transport.

0.40 (40%), the PA_{O_2} and expected Pa_{O_2} are each 200 mm Hg, allowing for a slight difference of 10 to 20 mm Hg. If the patient's

Oxygen therapy

Minimal amounts of supplementary oxygen are usually adequate in maintaining blood O_2 levels in the patient who has an acute myocardial infarction. This is true even in the presence of moderate CHF. Low-flow O_2 systems, such as nasal prongs (cannula), are relatively comfortable and provide an average FI_{O_2} range between 24% and 44%, depending on the flow rate and the patient's respiratory pattern.[6,26,45] Irregular patterns may cause this amount to fluctuate from breath to breath. The goal of O_2 therapy is to maintain the Pa_{O_2} greater than 60 mm Hg and O_2 saturation greater than 90%.[34]

When selecting appropriate modes of O_2 therapy, consider the following: (1) degree of hypoxemia, pulmonary dysfunction, or both; (2) the desired FI_{O_2}; (3) the need for a constant FI_{O_2}; (4) patient comfort; (5) the patient's respiratory pattern; (6) the need for concurrent moisture and/or ventilatory sup-

actual Pa_{O_2} is 100 mm Hg, pathologic interference with gas transport is present, resulting in an abnormal alveolar-arterial O_2 difference of 100 mm Hg (200 − 100 mm Hg). At a lower FI_{O_2}, hypoxemia (Pa_{O_2} less than 60 to 80 mm Hg) would be present.

Alveolar-capillary changes contributing to a widened A-a gradient and hypoxemia include the following changes in pulmonary function: (1) alveolar collapse or compression; (2) alveolar congestion with mucus, fluid, or both; (3) interstitial fluid accumulation; (4) bronchospasm; (5) emboli; and (6) alterations in pulmonary blood flow associated with changes in cardiac output. In the presence of CHF with pulmonary edema, Pa_{O_2} is usually low, and the A-a gradient increases. You may be required to supplement oxygen on a temporary basis to maintain the Pa_{O_2} at the minimal critical level of 60 mm Hg.

port; (7) the possibility of a hypoxic respiratory drive; and (8) arterial blood gas (ABG) response to previously used O_2 measures. Table 3-1 compares and contrasts the different modes of O_2 therapy that might be used in a coronary care unit (CCU).

Oxygen has the potential for being both therapeutic and toxic. Toxic actions of oxygen affect the lungs and the central nervous system (CNS), cardiovascular system, eyes, and red blood cells.[20,21] Toxic pulmonary changes include atelectasis and increased capillary permeability with pulmonary edema. Early symptoms of toxicity include chest pain, cough, sore throat, and paresthesias.[21,26] The amount of oxygen toxic to lung tissue remains controversial. *Significant* damage probably does not occur until inspired O_2 concentrations of more than 50% with their corresponding high alveolar oxygen pressures have been delivered for longer than 24 hours.[20,21,26,34] However, after suffi-

Table 3-1. Modes of oxygen administration in the patient without intubation or tracheotomy[6,45]

O₂ system	Liter flow	FIo₂	Advantages	Potential disadvantages
1. Nasal cannula/prongs or nasal catheter	6 L	24%–44%	Most comfortable, simplest	FIo₂ varies with respiratory pattern (↓ with ↑ rate and depth).
2. Face masks	5–8 L	40%–60%	Higher FIo₂	Less comfortable and falls off easier than cannula
3. Face tents	15 L	82%–88%	Higher FIo₂; more comfortable than face mask; better tolerated; less variation with respiratory pattern	Can fall off
4. Mask with reservoir (nonrebreathing mask)	10–12 L	60%–100%	High FIo₂	Less comfortable
5. Ventimask	4 L	24%, 35%, 28%, 40%	Less variation with respiratory pattern because of flow that fills lungs more completely; greater range of selection for FIo₂, especially in low ranges	FIo₂ may still vary slightly (e.g., 21% to 23%); highly uncomfortable.
6. Face mask with nebulizer at 100% setting	10 L	26%–39% or 41%–53% or 42%–62%	Greater range of selection for FIo₂ especially in high ranges; provides particulate moisture as well as O₂	FIo₂ still varies with respiration (diluted with rate and depth).
7. Face mask with nebulizer at 100% setting plus nasal prongs	15 L each	66%–86%	Higher FIo₂	FIo₂ still varies with respiration.
Manual resuscitators				
8. Bag-valve mask resuscitator (Ambu/Hope/Air-Shields) with O₂ reservoir cap over inlet	O₂ source at 15 L	90%–100%	No spontaneous respiration required; more aseptic for rescuer than mouth-to-mouth; extra O₂ can be provided to O₂ source.	Difficult to obtain seal; tidal volume may be less than by mouth-to-mouth.
9. O₂-powered mechanical resuscitator (Elder valve/Robert Shaw)	40 L/min	100%	Less effort required for rescuer	Rescuer unable to feel changes in resistance because of obstruction; can cause gastric distention; not recommended for less than age 12 because of inspiratory pressures (40 mm Hg)

51

cient oxygen is delivered to maximally saturate the hemoglobin and raise Pao_2 to 80 to 100 mm Hg, the benefit of extended exposure to larger inspired O_2 concentrations is questionable. Exposure to 100% O_2 concentration can cause temporary atelectasis, which may further compromise oxygenation.[20,21,26] However, oxygen should never be withheld during a cardiac arrest for fear of either O_2 toxicity or respiratory depression.[20,45]

Role of pulmonary function

The major function of the lungs is to exchange oxygen and carbon dioxide between the blood and the external environment. This process may be referred to as *external respiration*. The process of exchanging oxygen and carbon dioxide between the blood and the tissue cells is referred to as *internal respiration*.[39] Internal respiration occurs as a consequence of external respiration (Fig. 3-3) and is dependent upon cardiac function. External respiration depends on the processes of (1) *ventilation* (movement of air); (2) *perfusion* (movement of blood); and (3) *diffusion* (movement of gas particles between air and blood).

The pulmonary structures are composed of airways that transport the air (structures of ventilation) and airways that actually come into contact with the blood and participate in gas exchange (structures of respiration). Structures of ventilation are also known as *conducting airways* because their major function is to transport air. These structures heat, humidify, filter, and transport O_2-containing air. The structures of ventilation include the upper airways (nasopharynx), larynx, trachea, bronchi, and larger bronchioles. These airways subdivide into smaller airways, assuming a treelike appearance. The last level of bronchioles before gas exchange takes place is known as the *terminal bronchiole* level.

The gas-exchange, or *respiratory*, airways include the respiratory bronchioles, alveolar ducts, and alveolar sacs (Fig. 3-4). The alveoli contain three types of cells. Type I and II pneumocytes alternate to form the alveolar lining. Macrophages act as scavengers, floating between alveoli to remove foreign substances that have not been filtered by the conducting airways. The type II pneumocytes secrete *surfactant*, a substance that forms a film which lines the inner surface of the alveoli. Surfactant lowers the surface tension of the alveoli, limiting their tendency to collapse on expiration.

The alveoli and the respiratory bronchioles are wrapped by meshes of capillaries that contact the lung cells at key sites (see Fig. 3-4). Within this capillary network, large interstitial spaces exist, which may accumu-

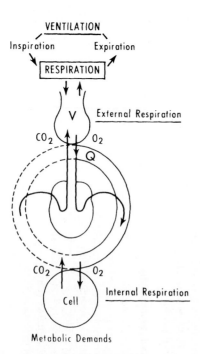

Fig. 3-3 External versus internal respiration: role of the lungs.

late fluid. The interstitial fluid spaces in the lung exist, more specifically, between the capillaries and their contact points with the alveolar surface and also between the capillaries themselves. The *lymphatic system* constantly drains this interstitial fluid space, exerting a vacuum effect.

The movement of gas particles across the alveolar-capillary membrane is limited by fluid accumulation in this interstitial space, particularly in the small spaces between the alveolar and capillary contact surfaces. Diffusion of oxygen and carbon dioxide is also limited by the permeability of the alveolar-capillary membrane. This membrane permits carbon dioxide to diffuse more easily than oxygen. Therefore, pulmonary congestion interferes with O_2 transport first. Hypoxemia occurs before CO_2 retention and is usually severe when there is CO_2 retention. CO_2 retention in the patient with acute myocardial infarction is usually an indicator of severe congestive heart failure, extensive pulmonary congestion, and significant hypoxemia.

The primary function of the lungs is mechanical. The lungs serve as a pump to deliver oxygen to the blood and to remove carbon dioxide from it to meet metabolic demands. The amount of air pumped or exchanged by the lungs in one minute is called *minute ventilation*. Minute ventilation is to the lungs what cardiac output is to the heart.

Minute ventilation is a product of respiratory rate and tidal volume. The tidal volume is the volume of air exchanged with each normal breath. The normal tidal volume is 10 to 15 ml/kg of body weight in the mechanically ventilated patient.[46] The tidal volume is limited by changes in airway resistance or compliance, including the integrity of the pleural linings and thoracic cage. Airway resistance may be defined as interference to air flow in the bronchial tubes. An increase in airway resistance occurs with constriction or obstruction of the bronchial tubes. In the patient who has had an acute myocardial infarction, bronchial obstruction may occur secondary to the fluid accumulation and bronchospasm associated with pulmonary edema.

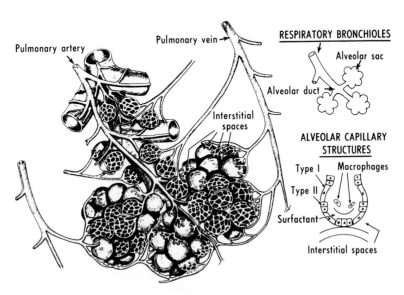

Fig. 3-4 Respiratory airways.

Compliance is a natural property of the chest wall, alveoli, bronchi, and bronchioles. Healthy lung tissue can stretch to accommodate the entering lung volume without a significant rise in pressure. Compliance is more accurately expressed as changes in pressure for a given change in volume ($\Delta V/\Delta P$). Accumulation of interstitial fluid caused by CHF makes the lung tissue less compliant. For the same changes in volume, the airway pressure required to ventilate the lung increases, limiting maximum filling of the airways. In the presence of an increase in airway resistance or a decrease in compliance, the tidal volume decreases and/or the inspiratory airway pressure increases, indicating potentially impaired gas exchange.

The normal stimulus for respiration is the level of CO_2 in the blood and the cerebrospinal fluid. CO_2 forms carbonic acid, which in turn increases the H^+ ion concentration and lowers the pH. The pH (H^+) level is sensed by specialized chemically sensitive nerve cells located in the brainstem on each side of the medulla.[3,16,44,46] These cells, known as *chemoreceptors*, are bathed by the cerebrospinal fluid. An increased CO_2 level stimulates these cells to transmit nerve signals to the inspiratory center in the medulla. Chemically sensitive nerve fibers that play a role in regulating respiration are also located peripherally in the carotid arteries and aorta. These areas are called *peripheral chemoreceptors*. In contrast, those in the brain are called *central chemoreceptors* (Fig. 3-5). The peripheral chemoreceptors are primarily sensitive to lack of oxygen.[16,46] They respond by stimulating the cardiovascular system and play a secondary role in regulating respiration. Signals from the medulla descend within the spinal cord, exiting first at the cervical level. The cervical spinal nerves join to form the phrenic nerve and innervate the diaphragm. The impulse then descends to the thoracic region. The intercostal nerves exit from the thoracic region and innervate the intercostal muscles. The diaphragm and intercostal muscles contract in response to nervous stimulation. As the chest wall expands, providing a greater potential space for air, the intrathoracic pressure becomes negative. This negative pressure acts as a vacuum, drawing air into the airways. The normal process of inspiration is active. During expiration the chest wall relaxes, allowing air to leave the lung passively. The use of abdominal muscles during expiration indicates forced expiration and is an early sign of respiratory distress in the patient who has congestive heart failure (CHF).

Normal and abnormal imbalances in ventilation (V) and perfusion (Q) prevent all the inspiratory volume from participating in gas exchange. The air in the conducting airways does not come into contact with the blood. Therefore, this air does not participate in gas exchange and may be considered "wasted air" or *dead space*.[37,46] The amount of normal (anatomic) dead space is approximately equal to a person's body weight in pounds. For example, 110 pounds equals 110 ml of dead space. If the patient's tidal volume is 500 ml, only 390 ml of each inspiration is available to the respiratory airways for gas exchange. Additional dead space may exist in pathologic states. The two most common examples are pulmonary embolism and decreased cardiac output.[38,46] In pulmonary embolism, the blood flow to the respiratory airways is occluded. Air flow to these areas cannot participate in gas exchange. Ventilation in these areas exceeds perfusion (Fig. 3-6). Decreases in cardiac output can also result in areas where ventilation exceeds perfusion.[31]

When no air (ventilation) is available for gas exchange, the *blood flow* (perfusion) is *wasted* and a *shunt* exists. The total or *physiologic shunt* consists of the anatomic shunt, capillary shunt, and venous admixture.[20,32,37] Certain blood vessels within the lungs completely bypass the respiratory airways, creating a

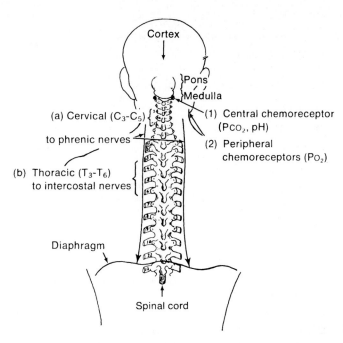

Fig. 3-5 Neurologic control of respiration: role of central versus peripheral chemoreceptors. The level of P_{CO_2} and/or pH (H^+) in the arterial blood and cerebrospinal fluid is sensed by the central chemoreceptors in the medulla, which generate an electrical signal. This signal is transmitted down the spinal cord, exiting at the cervical level to eventually form the phrenic nerves and at the thoracic level via the intercostal nerves. The peripheral chemoreceptors, located in the aorta and carotid arteries, can also activate these signals in response to a low Pa_{O_2}.

normal amount of *anatomic* shunting.[20,32,37] Additional pathologic shunting may occur with disorders resulting in alveolar collapse (atelectasis), compression (pneumothorax), or occlusion (consolidation). The characteristic blood gas pattern is a significant decrease in Pa_{O_2} in spite of increases in FI_{O_2} up to 60% to 100%.[20,31,32,34] Increased oxygen concentrations do not penetrate completely obstructed or collapsed alveoli and do not reach the arterial blood. Only measures that reopen the alveoli restore the Pa_{O_2}. This form of shunt is referred to as a *capillary shunt*. The sum of the anatomic and capillary shunt is known as the *absolute shunt*.[32]

When airways are partially obstructed with bronchospasm, pulmonary edema, or mucus, some air (ventilation) reaches the alveoli (see Fig. 3-6). However, since the blood flow is not affected, the amount of ventilation to the airways is less than the perfusion. This phenomenon is described as *V/Q mismatch*, a *low V/Q unit* (V < Q), *venous admixture,* "relative shunt," "incomplete shunt," or "shunt effect."[20,32,39] The major difference between this and a capillary or absolute shunt is that the airways are partially rather than completely obstructed. The hypoxemia of V/Q mismatch or venous admixture is responsive to increases in the FI_{O_2} since some of the oxygen reaches the alveolus and capillary blood.[20,34] These changes can occur in the patient with acute myocardial infarction

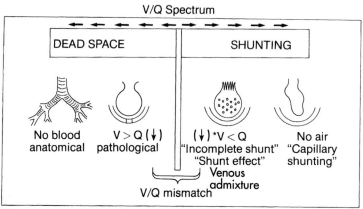

V/Q Spectrum

DEAD SPACE

SHUNTING

No blood
anatomical

V > Q (↓)
pathological

(↓)*V < Q
"Incomplete shunt"
"Shunt effect"

No air
"Capillary
shunting"

Venous admixture

V/Q mismatch

*Most common cause of hypoxemia

Fig. 3-6 V/Q imbalances: dead space versus shunting. In dead space the air is "wasted" because it comes into contact with either no blood or reduced amounts. The most extreme form, although normal, is anatomic dead space. In shunting, the blood is "wasted" because it comes into contact with either no air or reduced amounts. The most extreme form is the true capillary shunt, which is usually abnormal.

complicated by CHF. Increased cardiac output can potentiate venous admixture since there is more blood (perfusion) than air (ventilation).[31,32]

Blood bypassing the lungs because of cardiac defects (for example, ventricular septal defect) is a pathologic form of anatomic shunting. Both cardiac and pulmonary shunting complicate acute myocardial infarction. The most common form of pulmonary shunting complicating acute myocardial infarction is venous admixture or incomplete shunt secondary to pulmonary edema. Pulmonary shunting is referred to as *right to left shunting* to distinguish it from the *left to right shunting* typical of cardiac mechanisms.

Mismatching of V and Q creates areas of dead space (wasted air) and shunting (wasted blood) and interferes with effective gas exchange. Oxygen transport is impaired and hypoxemia occurs. The causes of hypoxemia include hypoventilation, diffusion defects, V/Q mismatch, and shunt (capillary). Of these, the most common is V/Q mismatch.[3,20,51] Hypoxemia is more severe with capillary shunt than with V/Q mismatch (venous admixture).

A wide A-a gradient (A-aDo$_2$) is a reflection of shunting (both capillary and venous admixture).[20] However, the A-aDo$_2$ is affected by increases in the FIo$_2$, changes in cardiac output, and pulmonary changes.[20,38] Other more accurate measures of pulmonary shunting have been suggested. These include the Pao$_2$/PAo$_2$ (a/A) ratio, Pao$_2$/FIo$_2$ ratio, and the respiratory index (A-aDo$_2$/Pao$_2$).[9,20,32,38] The physiologic shunt equation or shunt fraction (Qs/Qt), although less practical, is the most accurate. It takes both cardiac output and O$_2$ content into account. However, more complex formulas are required as well as a mixed venous sample, which must be obtained from a pulmonary artery (PA) catheter.[9,20] A 10% shunt is considered normal, and a 20% to 29% shunt is consistent with significant pulmonary disease since it indicates that 20% to 29% of the

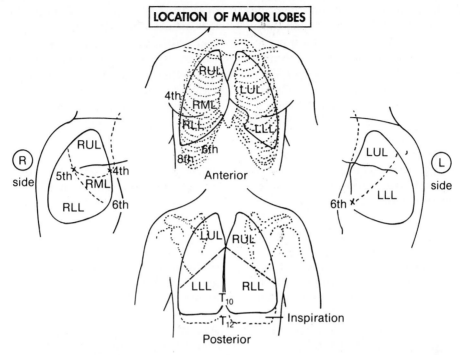

Fig. 3-7 Location of major lobes for auscultation: anterior, posterior, and lateral views.

blood flow or cardiac output is not ventilated.[32,38] Of the other measurements, the a/A ratio is the most accurate. The PaO_2/PAO_2 ratio varies less with increases in FIO_2.[9] The normal ratio is less than 0.75 to 0.80 and decreases with increasing shunt.[20,32] The PaO_2/FIO_2 ratio does not consider CO_2 changes. Data regarding its accuracy are contradictory.[9,38]

Auscultation of the lungs

Auscultation is the most widely used repiratory assessment parameter in the coronary care unit. However, the information gained by the *inspection* process is also valuable. Information gained from inspection includes respiratory rate, effort, and symmetry, evidence of shallow or forced respiration, abnormal respiratory patterns such as Cheyne-Stokes, and sputum characteristics.

Respiratory failure exists when the lung fails to exchange either oxygen or CO_2 effectively. Therefore, either a PaO_2 less than 50 to 60 mm Hg or a PCO_2 greater than 50 mm Hg may indicate respiratory failure. Respiratory failure usually occurs secondary to heart failure in acute myocardial infarction.

To perform inspection and auscultation, you should know certain anatomic landmarks that outline the lungs and their major lobes within the thoracic cavity (Fig. 3-7). Auscultation of the anterior chest wall provides information about all three lobes of the right lung and the upper lobe of the left lung. The sixth rib marks the lower rim of the right and left lung anteriorly. The fourth rib marks the dividing point between the upper and middle lobes on the right. Posteriorly, the lower border of the lung coincides with the twelfth thoracic vertebra on inspiration. Auscultation of the posterior chest wall provides information about the lower lobes of the lungs. Auscultation of each chest wall laterally provides information about the upper and lower lobes.

Characteristic breath sounds are produced within the alveoli and larger bronchial tubes. The normal *bronchial* sounds are tubular or hollow with a prolonged expiration. They are best mimicked over the trachea. The normal alveolar sounds are soft and whispery with a prolonged inspiration and short expiration. They are known as *vesicular* and are best heard over the major lung fields.[27]

By auscultating the lungs of patients who have heart failure, you may detect areas of *decreased breath sounds* and the presence of *adventitious* ("extra") sounds. Bilateral, symmetrically decreased breath sounds may occur in the presence of the decreased tidal volumes associated with shallow breathing or emphysema. Localized areas of decreased breath sounds may occur with pleural effusion associated with the interstitial fluid accumulation of CHF.

Abnormal extra sounds heard in patients with CHF include *crackles* (formerly called rales) and *wheezes*. Crackles are produced by the movement of air through fluid in the terminal air passages, or alveoli.[20,27] Crackles may also be produced by pressure variations occurring during the opening of small or medium airways that are atelectactic.[20,27] Fluid in the alveoli and interstitial spaces is typically associated with CHF in the patient with an acute myocardial infarction. When crackles occur in the patient with an acute myocardial infarction, they are best heard at the end of inspiration and do not disappear with coughing.[20] The movement of air through narrowed bronchial tubes produces *wheezing*. The wheezes of CHF occur because of congestion and narrowing of the respiratory bronchiole and are heard first on expiration. With severe obstruction, you may hear wheezes throughout inspiration and expiration. Wheezes caused by CHF are usually associated with moderately dense crackles.[20]

You may distinguish the abnormal lung sound of CHF, at times, from those of primary pulmonary disease or infection by differences in their onset, intensity, and timing in the respiratory cycle. The movement of air through the mucus in larger bronchial tubes produces a third adventitious sound known as a *rhonchus*.[20] Rhonchi are related to wheezes but sound distinctly different from them. Although some authorities recommend grouping rhonchi and wheezes together as wheezes,[5,46] the 1987 International Symposium on Lung Sounds supports the separation of these adventitious sounds into separate categories in the United States nomenclature.[23] Many clinicians continue to differentiate between three adventitious sounds.[20,27,28,49] However, the use of rhonchi is the least precise or consistent.[53] The rhonchus sounds like a coarse rumbling or snoring mingled with crackling and may at times sound like a coarse crackle. However, you will first hear these sounds on expiration, then on early inspiration. The end of inspiration usually remains clear. The respiratory timing is more critical than the quality of the sound in determining the type of sound.

In primary asthma, you will usually hear wheezes before the onset of any other abnormal sound. Later, they are typically accompanied by rhonchi because of an increased mucus production in the same airways. In CHF, wheezes usually accompany crackles. Abnormal lung sounds caused by primary pulmonary disease usually begin during expiration and eventually affect inspiration. Alveolar congestion caused by pulmonary disorders cannot be distinguished from the alveolar congestion of CHF by auscultation.

Both small and large airway congestion and obstruction may exist in the patient who has either cardiac or primary pulmonary disease. In these patients you may not be able to distinguish crackles from rhonchi.

Changes in the *intensity* of the normal breath sounds may provide further distinguishing characteristics. Localized areas of decreased breath sounds may be associated with either the pleural effusion of CHF or a large area of atelectasis, or pneumothorax.[5,20] However, areas of localized increased breath sounds are more typically associated with primary lung disease. Increased breath sounds indicate a complete alveolar obstruction (consolidation) or collapse (microatelectasis).[5,20] The louder, more hollow bronchial sounds are no longer muffled by alveolar sounds. Additional characteristics of bronchial sounds include egophony (*e* to *a* changes) and whispered pectoriloquy (magnified transmission of whispered sounds).

EVALUATING BLOOD OXYGEN CONTENT: ROLE OF O_2 SATURATION (Sao_2)

Oxygen is carried within the blood in two forms: (1) dissolved in solution and (2) bound to hemoglobin in the red blood cell for storage. The Po_2 reflects the pressure, or tension, exerted by the small amount of oxygen in solution. The O_2 saturation reflects the amount of oxygen bound to hemoglobin.

Oxygen first enters the blood plasma as dissolved gas particles by the process of diffusion (Fig. 3-8). Diffusion is defined as the movement of particles from a region of greater concentration to a region of lesser concentration. O_2 particles move from a region of greater concentration in the alveolar

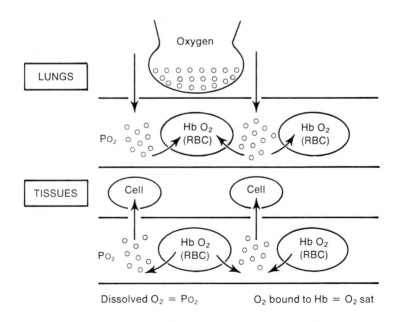

Dissolved O_2 = Po_2 O_2 bound to Hb = O_2 sat

Total normal arterial capacity: 20 ml

Fig. 3-8 Oxygen content of blood; relationship between Po_2 and O_2 saturation.

air to a region of lesser concentration in the venous blood. Because gas particles exert pressure both in the atmosphere and in solution, a pressure gradient exists across the alveolar capillary membrane, which facilitates the movement of oxygen into the blood. As the pressure of oxygen dissolved in the blood increases, some of the oxygen is pushed into the red blood cell for storage. Eventually most of the oxygen in the blood is carried in the storage form. Therefore, the greatest amount of information about the O_2 content in the blood is obtained from the O_2 saturation. Oxygen leaves the blood at the tissue level from the content dissolved in the plasma first. As the dissolved oxygen is removed, it is replaced from the amount stored in the red blood cells.

The *total O_2 content* of the blood equals the amount bound to hemoglobin plus the amount of oxygen in solution. The normal *arterial O_2 content* of the blood is about 20 ml of oxygen per each 100 ml of blood, assuming a hemoglobin content of 15 g.[25] Each gram of hemoglobin, fully saturated, has the ability to store 1.34 to 1.39 ml of oxygen. A patient with 15 g of hemoglobin has the *capacity* to carry 20.10 ml of oxygen bound to hemoglobin in each 100 ml of blood (that is, 15 g Hb × 1.34 ml O_2/g Hb)[42] when fully saturated. Determine the actual content bound to hemoglobin by multiplying this figure by the patient's percent saturation.[25] A patient's O_2 content will be less than his or her O_2 capacity whenever the O_2 saturation is less than 99%. Each mm Hg of pressure exerted by the oxygen in solution represents only 0.003 ml of oxygen or only 3% of the total oxygen content.[13,40] If this same patient had an arterial Po_2 of 100 mm Hg, the amount of oxygen represented by this pressure would be only 0.3 ml of oxygen in each 100 ml of blood (that is, Po_2 of 100 mm Hg × 0.003 ml of O_2 per mm Hg). Thus the amount of oxygen in solution represents only a small amount of oxygen exerting a large amount of pressure. Since about 98% of the blood O_2 content is represented by the O_2 saturation,[13,17,40,42] clinicians often consider assessment of the O_2 saturation alone sufficient to evaluate blood O_2 content.

Determine the percentage of O_2 saturation by comparing the actual O_2 content of a patient's hemoglobin with the potential O_2 capacity of that hemoglobin. Calculate O_2 saturation based on an assumed relationship to a measured Po_2 or, more accurately, measure it directly with an oximeter.

The percentage of O_2 saturation and oxygen content, when measured directly, is highly dependent on the patient's serum hemoglobin level. In the presence of anemia, fewer hemoglobin sites are available. These sites become quickly filled with even small amounts of oxygen. Thus the O_2 saturation may be normal or high, although the O_2 content is low.[24,42] In the presence of polycythemia, excess hemoglobin sites are available. These excess sites become difficult to fill, even in the presence of adequate amounts of oxygen. Thus the O_2 saturation is low, whereas the blood O_2 content is normal.

When at least 5 g of capillary hemoglobin becomes unsaturated, *cyanosis* appears. The equivalent level of desaturated arterial hemoglobin is about 3.45 g.[9a] In the presence of a normal serum hemoglobin of 15 g, the onset of cyanosis corresponds to an arterial saturation of about 80% (1/5 or 20% desaturated hemoglobin) and a paO_2 of 45 mm Hg.[9a] In the presence of a low serum hemoglobin level, cyanosis may not appear, although the blood O_2 content is low, until the hypoxemia is even more severe. Elevated hemoglobin levels may be associated with asymptomatic cyanosis at only slightly higher O_2 saturations but normal O_2 content. Thus the presence of cyanosis accurately reflects a low O_2 saturation but is not an accurate, early sign of either hypoxia or hypoxemia. Peripheral cyanosis alone is also often related to vasoconstriction in response to cold.

The amount of oxygen bound to hemoglobin is dependent to a great extent on the pressure exerted by the particles in solution (Po_2). The pressure of these particles pushes oxygen into the red blood cell, where it can combine with hemoglobin for storage. The lower Po_2 levels occurring at the tissue level allow the oxygen to dissociate from the hemoglobin, replacing some of the dissolved oxygen that has already been used. This relationship may be displayed graphically (Fig. 3-9). At a Po_2 of 60 mm Hg, the expected O_2 saturation is 90%. Below this level small changes in Po_2 are associated with large decreases in O_2 saturation and content.[20,25,42,48] For this reason these levels of Po_2 and O_2 saturation are considered critical. The graphic representation of the relationship between the Po_2 and O_2 saturation levels is known as the Hb-O_2 (oxyhemoglobin) dissociation curve.[18,40,48]

Normally, hemoglobin and oxygen bind together ("associate") tightly. However, certain factors, when in excess, may alter this relationship and cause oxygen and hemoglobin to dissociate from each other. These factors alter the expected O_2 saturation percentage associated with a given Po_2. Changes in pH (H^+ ion concentration), carbon dioxide pressure (PCO_2), temperature, or red blood cell phosphates can alter the hemoglobin-oxygen relationship. Hydrogen ions and carbon dioxide push oxygen off hemoglobin and loosen the hemoglobin-oxygen relationship (Fig. 3-10). Therefore, in the presence of decreased pH (increased H^+ ion) and increased carbon dioxide, the O_2 saturation should be lower than expected, for example, a Po_2 of 60 with O_2 saturation of 85% (less than 90%). Although the lower O_2 saturation facilitates O_2 removal from the red blood cell and its delivery to the tissues, it impairs the uptake and storage of oxygen at the alveolar-capillary level.

The red blood cell phosphate 2,3-diphosphoglycerate (2,3-DPG) also pushes oxygen off hemoglobin. This phosphate, unlike other more commonly known cellular phosphates, such as adenosine triphosphate (ATP), accumulates during the preaerobic phase of glucose breakdown. Therefore, during hypoxia, 2,3-DPG continues to be produced and maintains a loose relationship between hemoglobin and oxygen to promote O_2 delivery to the tissues (see Fig. 3-10). In the presence of hypoxia, the level of cellular 2,3-DPG increases, O_2 saturation decreases, and O_2 delivery to the tissue is enhanced. An increase in cellular temperature produces a similar effect on O_2-Hb binding to make more oxygen available for the increased metabolic demands. The increased temperature may reflect an increased CO_2 production

RELATIONSHIP OF O_2 SAT TO Po_2 (ASSOCIATION/DISSOCIATION)

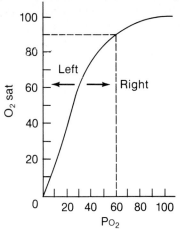

NOTE: At Po_2 of 60 (mm Hg), expected O_2 sat is 90%

Fig. 3-9 Graphic representation of the relationship of the Po_2 to hemoglobin-O_2 binding or the O_2 saturation. This graph is also referred to as the hemoglobin-O_2 dissociation curve and may be said to represent association of oxygen as well when tracking the upstroke of the curve. A key relationship illustrated is the O_2 saturation of 90%, which corresponds with a Po_2 of 60 mm Hg when pH, PCO_2, temperature, and 2,3-DPG are normal.

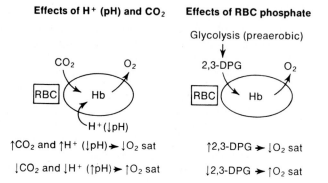

Effects of H⁺ (pH) and CO₂   Effects of RBC phosphate

$\uparrow CO_2$ and $\uparrow H^+$ ($\downarrow pH$) ➤ $\downarrow O_2$ sat $\uparrow 2,3$-DPG ➤ $\downarrow O_2$ sat

$\downarrow CO_2$ and $\downarrow H^+$ ($\uparrow pH$) ➤ $\uparrow O_2$ sat $\downarrow 2,3$-DPG ➤ $\uparrow O_2$ sat

Fig. 3-10 Clinical factors altering hemoglobin-O_2 binding.

secondary to the accelerated metabolic rate.[38] If the lower saturation is plotted graphically on the Hb-O_2 dissociation curve, the lower saturation level would occur at a point to the right of the standard curve. For this reason, a decrease in O_2 saturation occurring with decreased pH, increased P_{CO_2}, increased temperature, and hypoxia is known as a "shift to the right" in the Hb-O_2 dissociation curve.[18,36,40,46,48]

In the presence of increased pH, decreased P_{CO_2}, decreased temperature, or decreased 2,3-DPG levels, the converse is true. The O_2 saturation will be higher than expected. If the higher saturation level is plotted graphically on the Hb-O_2 dissociation curve, the higher saturation level would occur at a point to the left of the standard curve. For this reason, the higher O_2 saturation for a given P_{O_2} in these settings is known as a shift to the left.[18,36,40,47,48] Red blood cell phosphates, including 2,3-DPG, deteriorate in blood stored longer than 7 to 10 days because of the effects of storage and the preservatives added.[34] Therefore, relatively fresh blood may be more desirable in settings such as coronary bypass surgery. A high O_2 saturation facilitates O_2 uptake at the alveolar level but inhibits O_2 delivery at the cellular level. Any extreme high or low impairs O_2 transport at some level and should be corrected as quickly as possible to promote efficiency of O_2 utilization.

EVALUATING TISSUE OXYGENATION: ROLE OF AVDO_2, SvO_2, VO_2

Tissue oxygenation depends on both oxygen supply and oxygen demands. The oxygen supply to the tissues is dependent upon not only the arterial O_2 content, which is determined to a great extent by the pulmonary function, but also upon the blood supply or cardiac output, which is determined by cardiovascular function.[34] The normal O_2 supply or O_2 *delivery* at rest is 1000 ml/minute. The O_2 delivery is calculated by multiplying the arterial O_2 content (20 ml/100 ml times a constant of 10 to convert milliliters to liters) by the cardiac output in liters (5).[18,25,52]

The amount of oxygen actually used by the tissues is the O_2 *consumption*. O_2 consumption is based on the amount of O_2 which is actually extracted or used by the tissues. The O_2 extracted by the tissues is determined by comparing the arterial and venous O_2 contents. The O_2 content of venous blood represents the amount of oxygen remaining in the blood after the tissues have

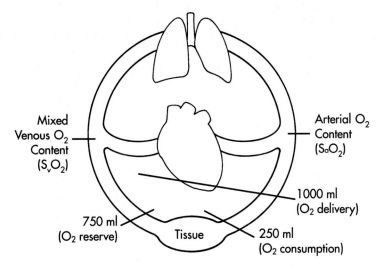

Fig. 3-11   Role of AVD_{O_2} and Sv_{O_2} in evaluating tissue oxygenation. Tissue O_2 extraction is determined by subtracting the venous O_2 content from the arterial O_2 content to obtain the A-V O_2 difference (AVD_{O_2}). This difference is a reflection of cardiac function (cardiac output) as well as tissue O_2 demands. Tissue O_2 demands and cardiac output may also be determined by assessing the Sv_{O_2}, especially when Sa_{O_2} values are also available.

extracted the amount they need. The difference between the arterial and venous O_2 contents is called the *A-V O_2 difference* (AVD_{O_2}) and is a measure of tissue extraction. Until the last decade, the AVD_{O_2} was regarded as the best reflection of tissue oxygenation. However, the venous O_2 content alone, as reflected by the venous O_2 saturation, or Sv_{O_2}, also accurately reflects tissue O_2 extraction or oxygenation and can be continuously monitored (Fig. 3-11).

To obtain an accurate reflection of the average tissue extraction from all parts of the body, a mixed venous sample is required. A mixed venous sample is best obtained from a catheter in the pulmonary artery where blood returning from all parts of the body has been optimally mixed before being oxygenated (see Unit 8). Tissue oxygenation may be assessed by intermittently or continuously measuring the O_2 saturation of this mixed venous sample (Sv_{O_2}). The normal venous O_2 saturation (Sv_{O_2}) is 60%

to 80%.[18,25,35,52] Determine the exact tissue O_2 extraction (AVD_{O_2}) by calculating the venous O_2 content and subtracting it from the arterial O_2 content (p. 60). The normal Av_{O_2} difference at a hemoglobin of 15 g is 5 ml.[25]

If a cardiac output measurement is available, the exact tissue O_2 consumption (V_{O_2}) can be calculated. The amount of oxygen consumed by the tissues per minute (V_{O_2}) depends on the amount of O_2 extracted from each 100 ml of arterial blood (AVD_{O_2}) and also the amount of blood supplied to the tissues per minute—the cardiac output (Fig. 3-12). Determine tissue O_2 consumption by multiplying the AVD_{O_2} (5 ml/100ml × a constant of 10 to convert to milliliters to liters) by the cardiac output in liters (5). The normal tissue O_2 consumption is 50 × 5 or 250 ml/minute.[18,25]

When tissue O_2 consumption increases or the cardiac output decreases, the tissue must extract a greater amount of oxygen from

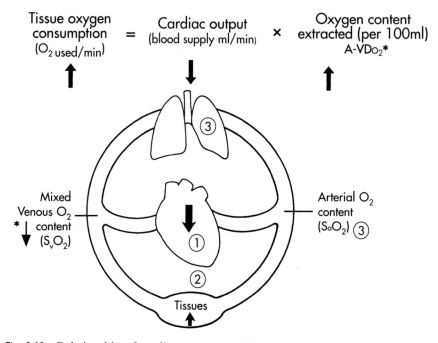

$$\underset{(O_2\ used/min)}{\text{Tissue oxygen consumption}} = \underset{\text{(blood supply ml/min)}}{\text{Cardiac output}} \times \underset{\substack{\text{extracted (per 100ml)} \\ \text{A-VDo}_2*}}{\text{Oxygen content}}$$

Mixed Venous O_2 content (S_vO_2)

Arterial O_2 content (S_aO_2) (3)

Tissues

Fig. 3-12 Relationship of cardiac output to $AVDo_2$ and Svo_2. A fall in Svo_2 indicates the cardiac output is decreased *(1)*, tissue O_2 demands have increased *(2)*, or the arterial O_2 content is low *(3)*, usually secondary to pulmonary dysfunction. If Sao_2 is available, the effects of the lungs may be eliminated and the $AVDo_2$ may be obtained. A high $AVDo_2$ reflects a fall in cardiac output when tissue O_2 demands remain constant. Measurements of both the cardiac output and $AVDo_2$ allow for tissue O_2 consumption to be determined.

the blood O_2 reserve to meet O_2 needs (see Figs. 3-11 and 3-12). This principle is referred to as the *Fick principle*. The venous O_2 saturation and content decrease, resulting in an increased $AVDo_2$ difference. Thus when the $AVDo_2$ increases, or when the Svo_2 decreases, either tissue O_2 demands have increased or else cardiac output has decreased.

A normal Svo_2 implies that O_2 delivery has effectively met any increased O_2 demands without depleting the venous O_2 reserve. Use of the venous O_2 reserve is less efficient and is thus associated with tissue symptoms.[25,52] Normal persons can increase their cardiac output significantly to meet increasing oxygen demands or compensate

for decreases in arterial O_2 content.[18,25] The critically ill cardiac patient may be unable to compensate by this mechanism as a result of a limited cardiac function or heart failure. Determination of the $AVDo_2$ or Svo_2 provides a means to estimate changes in cardiac output. In the patient who has a severely damaged myocardium resulting from an acute myocardial infarction, the cardiac output is usually low. To compensate for the low cardiac output, more oxygen is extracted from the arterial blood. Thus the $AVDo_2$ is high and the Svo_2 is low.[25] Tissue O_2 demands are incorrectly assumed to remain stable. If concurrent measurements of cardiac output are available, changes in tissue O_2 demands and

O_2 consumption may be detected and correlated with nursing measures, physiologic or psychological changes, and medical intervention.

OXIMETRIC MONITORING

The evolution of bedside oximetric monitoring over the past few years has revolutionized the assessment of oxygenation in the critically ill patient. *Oximeters* are photoelectric devices that measure the oxygen saturation of the blood. These devices allow for continuous measurement and display of either arterial or venous saturation. The use of arterial or pulse oximetry (Sao_2/SpO_2) is currently more popular, since the techniques used to measure it are noninvasive while those used to measure venous saturation (Svo_2) are invasive.

Oximetric analysis of both arterial and venous oxygen saturation is based on the principle that oxygenated hemoglobin absorbs or reflects a different wavelength of light than does unoxygenated hemoglobin.[8,35,40] This method of analysis is known as *spectrophotometry*. Two wavelengths of light, red and infrared, are emitted from a light source that is directed through and illuminates the blood. The light absorbed by or reflected from the oxygenated and unoxygenated blood is transmitted via a photodetector to a processor for analysis. To obtain *arterial* saturation readings, the light source and photodetector are contained within a sensor that is attached to a pulsatile extremity or the bridge of the nose, which contains pulsatile blood flow. To obtain *venous* saturation readings, the light source and photodetector are contained within an optical module and are transmitted via a catheter inserted directly into the blood.

You may compare both arterial and venous readings with arterial blood gas laboratory readings for accuracy. However, expect some discrepancy since these laboratories measure saturation using *co-oximetry*. Co-oximetry is a more accurate process using four or more wavelengths of light instead of two or three.[8,35] Abnormal hemoglobins such as carboxyhemoglobin and methemoglobin, detected by co-oximetry, are not detected by simple oximetry and produce inaccurate readings.[13,29,35,40,42,48] Methemoglobin levels can increase with injury, ingestion of toxins, or administration of nitrates.[13] The presence of other intravascular substances that absorb light such as bilirubin (greater than 20 mg%) and dyes can also result in inaccurate readings.[8,13,29,35,36]

In these settings false low values may occur. Compare oximeter readings more frequently with co-oximetry values. In the presence of dyes such as indocyanine green (Cardio-Green) or methylene blue, do not use oximeters.[42]

Continuous Sao₂ Monitoring (Pulse Oximetry)

In pulse oximetry the light source is contained within a probe usually clipped to or folded over a finger or earlobe and secured with adhesive. The probe or sensor may also be placed over the bridge of the nose. A dual wavelength of light is emitted from the top of the sensor and is projected through the pulsating blood (Fig. 3-13). A photodetector located on the opposite side registers the difference in light absorption by oxygenated and deoxygenated hemoglobin.[8,35,40] This information is displayed numerically on an oscilloscope or monitor. You may obtain a retrievable hard-copy record when a printer is attached.

Arterial O_2 saturation correlates roughly with the Pao_2 and reflects the effectiveness of pulmonary gas transport. Indications for

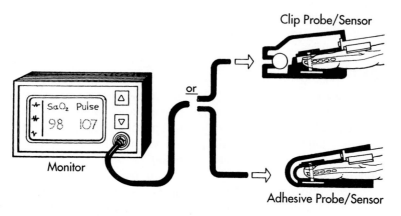

Fig. 3-13 Components of Sao_2 monitoring systems (pulse oximetry).

pulse oximetry include patients with hypoxemia related to respiratory depression, pulmonary congestion, or pulmonary disease, patients receiving or being weaned from O_2 or ventilator therapy, patients undergoing sedation or anesthesia, and transport of patients with unstable pulmonary status. In patients with borderline pulmonary reserve, significant changes have been reported with nursing measures such as suctioning, bathing, turning, other activity, and chest physical therapy.[13,35,48] These changes can suggest the need for rest periods, increased supplemental oxygen, or longer preoxygenation times. Changes in Sao_2 are correlated with pain, fever, agitation, positional changes, and arrhythmias, indicating the need for O_2, analgesics, sedation, antipyretics, or repositioning.[13,36]

Limitations include the inability to reflect tissue O_2 and changes in acid-base, cardiac output, or CO_2.[11,29,35] Arterial blood gas measurements are still indicated for these reasons as well as to confirm the accuracy of Sao_2 readings. Simultaneous Svo_2 monitoring allows correlation with tissue O_2 changes, thus compensating for this limitation. Arterial O_2 content is reflected only when adjusted for hemoglobin levels. In the presence of anemia, Sao_2 may be normal in spite of a low O_2 content, since there is less hemoglobin to saturate.[40,42] Oximeters may lose their reliability at hemoglobins lower than 5 g.[42]

Arterial blood is differentiated from venous blood as a result of fluctuations in blood flow, oxyhemoglobin, and light absorption occurring with systole and diastole.[8,35] A pulse rate and O_2 saturation are computed from these fluctuations. A wave form display is available in some models.[48] The pulse rate and wave form are indicators of the effectiveness of the pulsatile flow. The accuracy of the Sao_2 measurement is limited by a weak pulse signal. Weak pulse signals can occur secondary to hypothermia, administration of vasoconstricting drugs, edema, and peripheral vascular disease.[8,35,36,40,42] Massage the finger or earlobe to increase local blood flow. Some oximeter models have heating elements within the probe with sensors to monitor skin temperature.[36] Blood pressure cuffs, restraints, and arterial lines may also result in weak pulse signals.[13,42] Compare the heart rate periodically with the patient's actual heart rate on an ECG trace or by auscultation. Some oximeter models integrate the ECG pattern to improve accuracy.[13,35,40] External light,

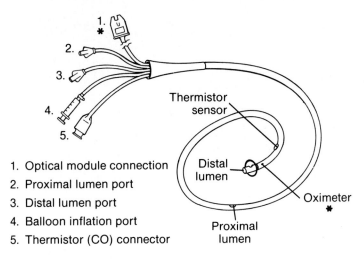

1. Optical module connection
2. Proximal lumen port
3. Distal lumen port
4. Balloon inflation port
5. Thermistor (CO) connector

Fig. 3-14   Fiberoptic PA catheter.

improper positioning of the probe, and patient movement may also interfere with the accuracy of the pulse oximeter (see Nursing Orders).[8,13,36,40,48]

Most oximeter modes have alarms for both saturation and heart rate. Pulse oxime-

try values may be up to 2% to 3% higher than the more accurate co-oximeter measurements. For this reason, lower limits of 92% rather than 90% have been suggested.[29,35,48]

Continuous SvO_2 monitoring

Venous oximetric monitoring uses fibers that transmit light waves and are known as *fiberoptics*. These fibers can be contained within vascular catheters. Light waves of two or three different wavelengths are projected by an optical module, which is connected to the fiberoptic port of a specialized PA catheter (see Fig. 3-14).[35] Calibrate the fiberoptic catheter against a controlled color reference before insertion or calibrate after insertion by comparing the readout with an actual PA blood sample sent to a blood gas laboratory.[35] A fiberoptic channel transmits light waves to the catheter tip and illuminates the blood passing by the distal or pulmonary artery lumen (see Fig. 3-14). The light reflected by the hemoglobin is transmitted back to the photodetector in the optical module using the principle of *reflection spectrophotometry*.[18,35] The microprocessor calcu-

lates the ratio of oxyhemoglobin (HbO_2) to total hemoglobin. It also computes the SvO_2 data, displays the data numerically and/or graphically on an oscilloscope or monitor, and provides a hard copy when a printer is attached. Cardiac output is usually simultaneously obtained and displayed.

A *light intensity bar record* is also graphically displayed on the monitor trace and chart record (Figs. 3-14 and 3-15). This bar record allows the operator to evaluate the quality of the light signals being reflected and to proceed with troubleshooting should the intensity be poor. A low-intensity light signal reading may mean the catheter is kinked, the distal lumen is occluded, or the connection with the optical module is poor.[35] A high-intensity signal reading may mean the catheter tip is against a vessel wall and needs repositioning. A damped intensity may mean

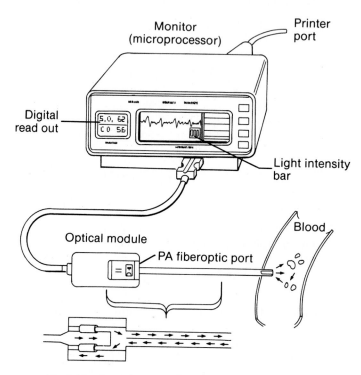

Fig. 3-15 Components of Svo$_2$ monitoring systems.

the catheter has become wedged or there is clotting over the tip of the catheter.

Changes in the Svo$_2$ usually precede critical changes in the patient's condition and thus alert the nurse to the risk of decompensation before it occurs. The normal Svo$_2$ is 60% to 80%.[18,25,52] Consider any rise or fall in the Svo$_2$ of 10% or greater for 10 minutes or longer significant, and investigate the situation.[11,18] Condense or expand time frames on the monitor trace or chart record as desired (Fig. 3-16). Indications for Svo$_2$ monitoring include acute myocardial infarction, trauma, cardiac surgery, sepsis, and titration of positive end-expiratory pressure (PEEP).[11]

A fall in the Svo$_2$ may occur in the presence of factors that decrease cardiac output, decrease arterial oxygen content, or increase oxygen demands and thus compromise tissue oxygenation.[2,25,35] Svo$_2$ reflects the in-

teraction of these parameters as well as the effects of single components.[2] Factors that decrease the Svo$_2$ secondary to a decrease in cardiac output include heart failure, hypovolemia, a decrease in inotropic, vasoactive, or intraaortic balloon support, arrhythmias, mechanical ventilation with PEEP, acute ventricular septal defect, papillary muscle rupture, cardiac tamponade, and cardiac arrest.[11,18,25,35]

Factors that decrease the Svo$_2$ secondary to a decrease in arterial oxygen content include anemia and impaired pulmonary gas transport. Although anemia does not alter the Sao$_2$, the Svo$_2$ is affected secondary to the decreased oxygen content and compromised tissue oxygenation. Factors that may interfere with pulmonary gas transport in the patient with coronary artery disease include respiratory depression, hypoventilation, and pulmonary edema sec-

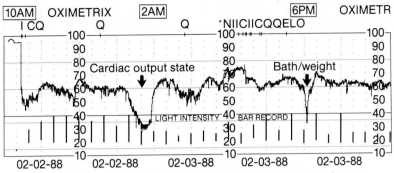

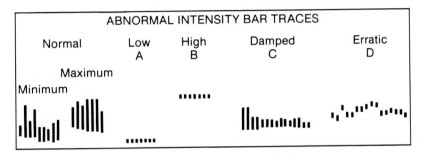

Fig. 3-16 Graphic changes in Svo_2 and abnormal light intensity bar changes.

ondary to CHF. Impaired pulmonary gas transport may be confirmed by concomitant monitoring of the Sao_2 with pulse oximetry.

Factors increasing oxygen demands may also compromise tissue oxygenation, causing a fall in the Svo_2. These factors include fever, pain, shivering, seizures, agitation, anxiety, increased respiratory effort, family visits, and nursing measures such as bathing, turning, weighing, and dressing changes.[11,18,25,52]

Although less commonly seen, an increase in Svo_2 may occur in the presence of increased cardiac output or decreased oxygen demands. The major clinical condition causing this change is sepsis. Tissue oxygen extraction is impaired secondary to vasodilation and peripheral shunting, cellular impairment in O_2 uptake, and the high cardiac output that may limit time for hemoglobin unloading.[18,25,35] A PA catheter in the wedge position may also result in an increased Svo_2.[11,25] Cyanide poisoning secondary to nitroprusside (Nipride) toxicity is also associated with a high Svo_2.[11,25] High Svo_2 secondary to decreased O_2 demands occurs with hypothermia or the use of paralytic agents.[11,18,25]

NURSING ORDERS: Oximetric monitoring (Sao_2/Svo_2)

RELATED NURSING DIAGNOSES: Impaired gas exchange, ineffective airway clearance, alteration in cardiac output, impaired tissue perfusion

1. In the presence of Sao_2 values less than 92% via pulse oximetry:
   a. Provide suppplemental O_2.
   b. Report values to physician.
   c. Note any correlation with pain, agitation, fever, or arrhythmias, and administer sedation or antipyretics as ordered. Provide verbal reassurance also.
   d. Note correlation with nursing mea-

sures such as suctioning, bathing, activity, or chest physical therapy. Provide rest periods or longer preoxygenation times if needed. Repositioning may also be indicated.

e. If change occurs following sedation, verify that airway is open and support respirations as needed.

2. To ensure the accuracy of Sao_2 readings via pulse oximetry:

a. Assess the circulation of the earlobe or finger. If cool and pale with capillary refill greater than 3 seconds, massage the site before attaching the probe, or select an alternate site. Remove fingernail polish and artificial nails.[36,40,42] Do not place probe over edematous areas.

b. Position probe so that the light source and photodetector are directly opposite each other.[42] Use designated markings to determine.[40] Ensure probe is securely in place. Change position of adhesive probes every 24 hours and clip probes every 4 hours.[42] Use the index, middle, or ring fingers. Watch for skin breakdown or allergic reactions to the adhesive.[40]

c. Instruct the patient to limit movement of finger and not keep finger dependent. Change location if movement interferes with readings.[42] Observe for constricting movements such as bending the elbow or holding the siderails tightly.[13]

d. Periodically compare the patient's actual heart rate by ECG or auscultation with the heart rate displayed on the oximeter. Light bars and waveform displays are provided in some models to evaluate the strength of the pulsation.[40,48]

e. Protect probe from bright lights, including sunlight, fluorescent lights, and infrared heating lamps. Cup hand over probe to test if readings are affected.

Cover probe, if necessary, with opaque material such as a washcloth or move away from light source.[13,36,42]

f. When using blood pressure cuffs, restraints, and arterial line, select opposite extremity or earlobe.[42]

g. Periodically recheck values with standard co-oximetry samples and/or test on yourself.[13]

h. Verify alarms are active.

i. Note the presence of abnormal hemoglobins such as carboxyhemoglobin or methemoglobin and serum bilirubin greater than 20%.

3. In patients with anemia or compromised cardiac output or those receiving vasoconstricting medications, consider simultaneous monitoring of Svo_2.

4. In the presence of a 10% decrease in Svo_2 sustained for 10 minutes or longer, assess the patient for:

a. Fall in cardiac output
   • Check the urine output.
   • Auscultate the lungs for increased crackles.
   • Auscultate the heart for the presence of a new S3 gallop or systolic murmur indicative of papillary muscle rupture or ventricular septal defect.
   • Check wedge pressure and validate with thermodilution cardiac output measurements.
   • Check for a decrease in inotropic support or change in intraaortic balloon pump assist ratio.

b. Decreased arterial oxygen content
   • Check hemoglobin content and potential bleeding.
   • Assess patient for a decrease in pulmonary oxygen transport, pulmonary edema, pneumonia, decrease in FIo_2, bronchospasm, sedation. Open airway, suction, or support respirations as needed.

5. Note correlation of a fall in Svo_2 with pain, fever, agitation, or nursing mea-

sures such as bathing, turning, or weighing, and adjust nursing care accordingly as with SpO_2 findings. Note the effects of respirations, vasoactive or inotropic drugs, circulatory assist devices, and ventilatory modes that may increase arterial content while compromising cardiac output. Correlate with pulse oximeter readings if available.

6. In the presence of a 10% increase in SvO_2 sustained for 10 minutes or longer, assess the patient for:
   a. increased cardiac output
      • Assess patient for signs of sepsis, including a decreased systemic vascular resistance.
      • Check for excessive inotropic support.

   b. decreased tissue oxygen demands— Check for hypothermia or paralyzing drugs.

7. To ensure the integrity of the PA catheter and accuracy of SvO_2 readings:
   a. Periodically check the quality of the light intensity bars.
   b. Assess the PA waveform for normal amplitude and contour. With a dampened tracing, check for wedging, and flush catheter.
   c. Infuse fluids through ports of fiberoptic pulmonary artery lines at rates no greater than 100 ml/hour. Do not infuse blood owing to the small size of the lumina.
   d. Coil catheter loosely when applying dressings.

ACID-BASE BALANCE
Introduction

An *acid* is a H^+ donor.* Consider the following equation as an example: (A)H_2CO_3 = (B)H^+ + (C)HCO_3. In this equation, a hydrogen ion (proton) is given up by substance A. Therefore, this substance is an *acid* and is more specifically the formula for carbonic acid. A *base* is a H^+ acceptor.* In the same equation, a hydrogen ion can be accepted by substance C. Therefore, this substance is a *base* and is more specifically the formula for bicarbonate. The base bicarbonate and carbonic acid are closely related, since one converts into the other simply by the addition or removal of H^+. Many acids and bases in the body are similarly related to each other, forming acid-base "partnerships."

Changes in the hydrogen ion concentration are measured by the *serum pH*. The pH is a mathematical representation of the H^+ concentration. It is not a direct measurement of the H^+ ion in the blood. The pH reflects the H^+ ion concentration in an inverse, or reciprocal, manner. Therefore, a decreased pH equals an increased H^+ concentration. An increased pH equals a decreased H^+ ion concentration. Regulation of the H^+ concentration is important because many cellular chemical reactions are pH dependent.

An *increased* H^+ concentration indicates *acidosis*. Acidosis is an acid-base imbalance resulting from *increased acid* or *decreased base*. A *decreased* H^+ concentration, or *increased* pH, indicates *alkalosis*. Alkalosis is a state of *increased* base or *decreased* acid. The normal pH of arterial blood is 7.35 to 7.45. A pH of 7.2 indicates acidosis. A pH of 7.6 indicates alkalosis (Fig. 3-17).

Acids are normally generated in the body as a result of cellular metabolism.[24] Carbonic acid (H_2CO_3) is a major by-product of cellular metabolism.[50] Carbonic acid may be converted into carbon dioxide (CO_2), which is excreted by the lungs as a volatile gas.[20,33,37,45] Since the volatile gas CO_2 is

---

*References 3, 20, 24, 33, 45, 55.

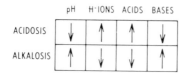

	pH	H-IONS	ACIDS	BASES
ACIDOSIS	↓	↑	↑	↓
ALKALOSIS	↑	↓	↓	↑

Fig. 3-17 Comparison of acidosis and alkalosis.

formed from and may be converted back into H_2CO_3, it is considered a *volatile acid*.[24]

Noncarbonic acids are also produced as by-products of normal cellular metabolism. The noncarbonic metabolic acids are *nonvolatile* and are excreted by the *kidneys*. These non-volatile by-products are also known as *fixed acids*.[24] Some examples of normal fixed acids are sulfuric acid, phosphoric acid, ketoacids, and lactic acids.[20,37]

Although the source of all normal acids in the body is metabolic, these metabolic acids may be regulated by either respiratory or nonrespiratory body mechanisms. Carbonic acid is the only acid excreted by both mechanisms (Fig. 3-18). In clinical usage, the term *metabolic* is reserved for *nonrespiratory* mechanisms or imbalances.[3,16]

Bases are formed from substances contained in most foods that are absorbed via the gastrointestinal tract, and are normally generated within the red blood cells, lower gastrointestinal tract, and kidneys. The primary base generated by the body is *bicarbonate*. Bicarbonate is generated from the breakdown of carbonic acid in the red blood cells and kidney tubules (see Fig. 3-18).[33] Free hydrogen ions are also produced. This H^+ is excreted in the urine or may attach to, and thus be absorbed by, the hemoglobin molecule in the red blood cells. Other body bases include phosphate, lactate, hemoglobin, and ammonia, which may be obtained from protein breakdown.

Buffering is the body's first line of defense against changes in pH caused by acid-base imbalance. Buffers minimize or absorb the changes in pH associated with excess acids or bases, acting as "chemical sponges."[3,16,20,55] Buffers may be single acids or bases, a combination of an acid and its related base, or a substance that can convert into either an acid or a base as needed. Some of the body's buffers include hemoglobin, the carbonic acid–bicarbonate system, the phosphoric acid–phosphate system, and proteins, which can convert to an acid or base as needed.[3,16,20,45]

The carbonic acid–bicarbonate buffer system is the major buffer in the body.[20] For the pH to be maintained within normal limits, the ratio of bicarbonate (HCO_3^-) and carbonic acid (H_2CO_3) must be in a balance of 20:1 (Fig. 3-19).[33,45,50]

Respiratory imbalances

Respiratory disorders produce disturbances in acid-base balance either by interfering with or by accelerating the excretion of CO_2 in the lungs. When hypoventilation occurs, CO_2 is retained and H_2CO_3 accumulates. Acidosis resulting from respiratory disorders that cause carbonic acid accumulation is known as *respiratory acidosis*. When hyperventilation occurs, there is an excessive loss of CO_2 by the lungs, and H_2CO_3 levels fall. This loss of acid results in alkalosis. Alkalosis resulting from respiratory disorders that cause hyperventilation with H_2CO_3 excretion is known as *respiratory alkalosis*.

ABG values most useful in the assessment of respiratory imbalances (Fig. 3-20) are the pH and the PCO_2. The pH confirms the presence of an imbalance and differentiates between an acidosis and an alkalosis. The PCO_2 reflects the pressure of the dissolved CO_2 gas in solution within the plasma. Actual H_2CO_3 levels in the plasma are usually very small and thus are not separately measured clinically.

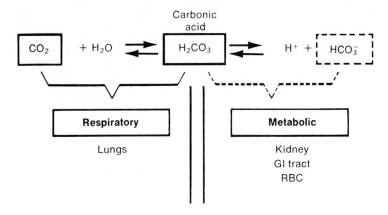

Fig. 3-18   Respiratory and nonrespiratory regulation of acid-base balance.

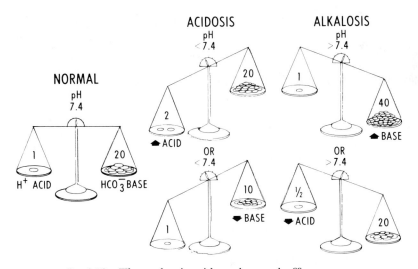

Fig. 3-19   The carbonic acid—carbonate buffer system.

Metabolic imbalances

The term *metabolic* is used clinically to refer to *nonrespiratory* regulating mechanisms or imbalances. *Metabolic acidosis* occurs from the accumulation of metabolic acids not readily excreted by the lungs. These acids are nonvolatile or fixed. Excess fixed acids accumulate as a result of abnormal metabolism, exogenous ingestion, or impaired excretion. Metabolic acidosis may also occur because of excessive loss of bicarbonate via the lower gastrointestinal tract.

Excessive elimination of both carbonic acids and fixed acids occurs in the presence of either upper gastrointestinal or renal excretion. Loss of acid results in a relative excess of bicarbonate and other bases, producing a

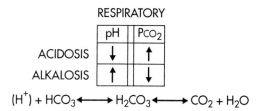

RESPIRATORY

	pH	PCO_2
ACIDOSIS	↓	↑
ALKALOSIS	↑	↓

$$(H^+) + HCO_3 \longleftrightarrow H_2CO_3 \longleftrightarrow CO_2 + H_2O$$

Fig. 3-20 Key blood gas changes in respiratory imbalances.

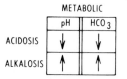

METABOLIC

	pH	HCO_3
ACIDOSIS	↓	↓
ALKALOSIS	↑	↑

Fig. 3-21 Key blood gas changes in metabolic imbalances.

metabolic alkalosis. Direct intravenous administration or oral ingestion of bicarbonate or other alkaline substances may also produce a metabolic alkalosis.

The ABG values most useful in the assessment of metabolic imbalances are the *pH, bicarbonate levels,* and base excess (or deficit). The pH confirms the presence of an imbal-

Compensation and electrolyte changes

The respiratory system may assist the kidneys in the regulation of metabolic acid-base imbalances. This assistance is known as the *compensatory* effort of the lungs. The respiratory system begins to compensate within minutes for a metabolic acidosis by excreting H_2CO_3 in the form of CO_2.[3,16,24,33] In acute situations the compensatory effort by the lungs represents a *secondary defense system* and is rarely completely effective in normalizing the pH. Compensatory efforts for metabolic alkalosis are limited by the effect of an increase in CO_2 on the respiratory centers. The kidneys also assist the lung in the regulation of respiratory acid-base imbalances. However, renal or metabolic compensation for respiratory disorders is slow (12 to 48 hours) and is usually not seen in acute disorders.[3,16,20,24,33]

The three electrolytes directly affected by acid-base imbalances are K^+, Ca^{++}, and Cl^-. The serum levels of these electrolytes appear *high* in a state of *acidosis.* In contrast, serum

ance and differentiates between an acidosis and an alkalosis. Fixed acid levels are not routinely measured. Their presence is implied by their effect on the bicarbonate and base excess (deficit) levels.[16,20,38] Zero base excess corresponds with the base present in the blood at a normal pH (7.4) and normal PCO_2 (40 mm Hg) and reflects the effects of all the body's buffers, including bicarbonate. See Fig. 3-21.[20]

levels of K^+, Ca^{++}, and Cl^- are usually *low* in a state of alkalosis. The total body levels of K^+ and Ca^{++} may be normal, but their *location* may be altered. In an acidosis, K^+ moves from the intracellular to the extracellular fluid (serum) in exchange for H^+. In alkalosis, Ca^{++} may change from a state of *free* to *bound* (see Unit 4). The serum Cl^- level increases in selected forms of metabolic acidosis associated with increases in the level of hydrochloric acid. The serum Cl^- level decreases in metabolic alkalosis with the excretion of hydrochloric acid.

Changes in pH may directly or indirectly enhance cardiac automaticity via its related electrolytic changes, causing arrhythmias. Arrhythmias may be associated with either a high or low pH. Acidosis also decreases the effect of sympathetic drugs and may increase the sensitivity to toxic effects.[22,38,45] When acidosis exists, defibrillation is less effective because of the inevitable cardiac depression.

Respiratory acidosis

Respiratory acidosis occurs when there is impaired excretion of CO_2 by the lungs, and it is confirmed clinically by the presence of a low pH and a high P_{CO_2}. Bicarbonate and base excess changes are present primarily in chronic states. Carbon dioxide and carbonic acid may be retained when the *rate, depth,* or *effectiveness* of ventilation is *decreased.* Impaired ventilation occurs in the presence of any the following: (1) suppression of the respiratory centers; (2) obstruction or collapse of the airways; and (3) compression of the airways.[20]

Suppression of the respiratory centers may be associated with the effects of narcotic administration, postcardiac arrest, brain damage, or the chronic CO_2 retention associated with chronic obstructive pulmonary disease (COPD). Patients with chronic bronchitis have severe V/Q mismatching, causing impaired CO_2 excretion and chronic CO_2 retention. Eventually, the central chemoreceptors lose their sensitivity to CO_2. The peripheral chemoreceptors, which respond to lack of oxygen, assume control of respiration. Administration of oxygen at high concentration in these patients abolishes their respiratory drive and may cause excessive CO_2 retention and respiratory arrest. It is important to consider that not all patients with COPD retain CO_2. However, until the absence of CO_2 retention is confirmed, O_2 administration in a patient with COPD should be confined to low flow rates (1 to 2 L/minute) or low concentrations. The exception is when these patients are being either manually or mechanically ventilated on a continuous basis.

CO_2 retention may also occur as the result of *severe* obstruction or collapse of the conducting, or respiratory, airways. Obstruction of the airways may be caused by mucus, bronchospasm, or the fluid of pulmonary edema. In the early stages of pulmonary edema caused by CHF, the patient hyper-ventilates in response to hypoxemia. Carbon dioxide continues to be excreted in the presence of minimally to moderately dense fluid because it diffuses across the alveolar-capillary membrane more easily than oxygen. Therefore, hyperexcretion of carbon dioxide occurs. Excess CO_2 excretion results initially in respiratory alkalosis. As the pulmonary congestion becomes more severe in the later stages of CHF, interference with diffusion of both oxygen and carbon dioxide occurs. Respiratory acidosis occurs. Respiratory acidosis also occurs when severe pulmonary edema complicates adult respiratory distress syndrome (ARDS) or with extensive atelectasis. Atelectasis, or collapse of the airways, may be caused by shallow breathing, the effects of anesthesia and cardiopulmonary bypass, or damage to the alveolar cells with loss of surfactant.

Compression of the airways, limiting CO_2 excretion, may result from a *severe* pneumothorax or pleural effusion. The effect of this compression on the airways is also referred to as compression atelectasis. Pneumothorax may occur as a complication of aggressive cardiopulmonary resuscitation or subclavian catheter placement. Pleural effusion may occur in the setting of CHF when the excess interstitial fluid exceeds the ability of the lymphatic system to drain the interstitial space. The excess interstitial fluid moves into the pleural linings.

The *clinical signs* of respiratory acidosis are decreased rate and depth of respirations and sensorium changes. The patient's respirations represent the primary cause of the imbalance rather than compensatory efforts. The patient experiences headache and sensorium changes or alterations in level of consciousness because of the toxic effect of acidosis and CO_2 on the CNS.[20,44,55] Generally, as the respiratory acidosis becomes more severe, the level of consciousness decreases. The kidneys attempt to compensate for the imbalance by retaining base in the form of bicarbonate. However, renal compensation for respiratory disorders is slow and is usually not seen in acute disorders. In acidosis, whether respiratory or metabolic, K^+ moves into the serum, resulting in ECG changes and cardiac effects of hyperkalemia.[44]

Intervention attempts to improve ventilation and stabilize the pH.[20] Avoid bicarbonate unless the pH is <7.2. Perform the fol-

Respiratory alkalosis

Respiratory alkalosis occurs when there is an increased excretion of carbon dioxide by the lungs, and it is confirmed clinically by the presence of a high pH and low CO_2. Since most causes are acute, bicarbonate and base excess levels are usually within normal limits. Carbon dioxide is lost when the respiratory *rate* or *depth* is increased, as when the following occur: (1) pain; (2) anxiety; (3) flail chest; (4) respiratory therapy; and (5) *early phases* of pulmonary edema and other acute respiratory conditions as mentioned earlier.[20,38,43]

In the early phases of acute respiratory disorders, respiratory rate and depth are stimulated in response to hypoxemia.[20] CO_2 excretion may continue in the absence of effective O_2 transport because carbon dioxide diffuses more easily than oxygen. Hyperventilation may also result from stimulation of juxtopulmonary capillary receptors in the alveolar wall by increased interstitial fluid or the end products of platelet and thrombin degradation, even in the absence of hypoxemia. Acute respiratory disorders that may result initially in hypoxemia and increased CO_2 excretion include pulmonary edema due to CHF, asthma, pneumonia, pulmonary emboli, pneumothorax, ARDS, and flail chest secondary to chest trauma.

The CNS exerts a stimulating effect on the respiratory center in the presence of stress associated with pain or anxiety. Respiratory alkalosis has been reported in patients in

lowing therapies: (1) treat the CHF, with specific measures to decrease pulmonary congestion (e.g., high Fowler's position with legs dangling, diuretics, vasodilators, and morphine sulfate); (2) use chest physical therapy (e.g., moisture, saline instillation, percussion or vibration, bronchodilators, incentive inspirometers, coughing techniques); (3) use mechanical ventilation with PEEP to reverse atelectasis; and (4) drain air or fluid.

CCUs in the absence of hypoxemia or hypoxia. The presence of chest pain, anxiety, or both is thought to be the mechanism.[10] Anxiety associated with the effects of mechanical ventilation exerts a similar influence. Use of large tidal volumes during mechanical ventilation can also contribute to hyperventilation and respiratory alkalosis.[47]

The low CO_2 and high pH associated with mild respiratory alkalosis are beneficial in patients with increased intracranial pressure (ICP) since they produce cerebral vasoconstriction. These patients are purposefully hyperventilated manually or during mechanical ventilation.[5] However, care must be taken not to exceed PCO_2 and pH limits to avoid clinical signs and symptoms of respiratory alkalosis.

The *clinical signs* of respiratory alkalosis are deep and/or rapid respirations and tremors, tetany, seizures, and paresthesias, caused by Ca^{++} binding and decreased ionized Ca^{++}.[10,20]

Coronary spasm may also be triggered by respiratory alkalosis.[10] The deep, rapid respirations represent the *cause* of the imbalance. Alkalosis causes an increase in bound Ca^{++} and thus a decrease in free or ionized Ca^{++} (see Unit 4). This results in symptoms of hypocalcemia. However, the total serum Ca^{++} level is not affected. Techniques for measuring ionized calcium levels, if available, may be helpful.

Perform the following *therapies* or *inter-*

ventions: (1) relieve pain; (2) relieve hypoxemia by positioning the patient for optimal chest expansion and ventilation; (3) administer supplementary oxygen; (4) select more comfortable modes of oxygen therapy; (5) treat CHF (see Unit 8); (6) use chest physical therapy techniques; (7) use bronchodilators; and (8) drain air or fluid. Airway-splinting measures such as PEEP are critical in ARDS. With suspected pulmonary emboli, anticoagulation prevents further clot accumulation and degradation and may curb hyperventilation. Support the patient psychologically to relieve anxiety.

Metabolic acidosis

Metabolic acidosis may result from increased levels of fixed acids or decreased levels of base, and it is confirmed clinically by the presence of a low pH, low bicarbonate, and decreased base excess (deficit).[22] The P_{CO_2} is commonly low, reflecting compensatory efforts of the lung. The accumulation of fixed (nonvolatile) acids may occur as a result of abnormal metabolism, decreased excretion, or exogenous ingestion. Loss of bicarbonate (base) from selected gastrointestinal disturbances or bicarbonate deficits associated with drug therapy may also result in a metabolic acidosis.

Metabolic acidosis caused by abnormal metabolism may occur with diabetes, hypoxia, and shock. In diabetes, fats may be preferentially metabolized for energy because insufficient insulin is available to metabolize glucose. The increased breakdown of fats releases an excess of ketoacids. Acidosis associated with excess ketoacids is called *ketoacidosis* and is a form of metabolic acidosis.

In shock, which is a form of hypoxia, metabolism takes place in the absence of sufficient oxygen. This anaerobic metabolism produces lactic acid and creates a state of lactic acidosis. Lactic acidosis also occurs in liver failure, certain forms of tumors, and excess alcohol intake.[22] Elevated blood lactate levels help confirm the diagnosis.[22]

Metabolic acidosis also results from decreased excretion of fixed acids and loss of base. Since the primary route of excretion of fixed acids is the kidney, renal failure results in accumulation of these acids and the production of metabolic acidosis. Decreased levels of the base bicarbonate can occur with either direct loss or decreased formation. Clinical examples of these factors include diarrhea and administration of acetazolamide (Diamox). Diarrhea results in loss of lower gastrointestinal secretions rich in bicarbonate.[16] Administration of the diuretic Diamox results in the inhibition of carbonic acid breakdown into bicarbonate and free H^+. Bicarbonate is not reabsorbed and H^+ is not eliminated. Na^+ is excreted in exchange for H^+ to maintain electrical equilibrium, thus allowing for Diamox's diuretic effect.

The *clinical signs* of metabolic acidosis are sensorium changes and deep, rapid respirations. The sensorium changes are a manifestation of the toxic effect of acidic substances on the CNS. These sensorium changes include alterations in consciousness, restlessness, agitation, dizziness, and confusion. The deep, rapid respirations seen in metabolic acidosis are the respiratory system's attempt to assist the kidneys in excreting acid.[22] These respirations are called *Kussmaul's respirations*. The respiratory system compensates, at least partially, for a metabolic acidosis by excreting acid in the form of carbon dioxide. The serum K+ increases in exchange for H^+, producing ECG signs of hyperkalemia and cardiac depression (see Unit 4).

The *therapy* for metabolic acidosis partly depends on the degree of pH alteration. If you administer sodium bicarbonate aggressively, you may overcorrect the problem. A pH shift may occur too rapidly for the brain to adjust, while creating a metabolic alkalosis that is far more difficult to correct. Arrhythmia may also be generated, and Hg-O_2 binding may occur, decreasing O_2 availability to the tissues.[22,30] Thus, administer sodium bicarbonate in small amounts when the drop in pH is severe (pH less than 7.2) or the base deficit is less than 10 mEq/L.[30,38] With cardiac arrest, the American Heart Association recommends that Na^+ bicarbonate be used only after defibrillation, CPR, and antiarrhythmic therapy (@ 10 minutes). Administer further dosages 10 minutes apart as indicated by blood gas changes.[45] When the pH is greater than 7.2, correct the underlying cause.[22] Supplement oxygen along with modes of respiratory and cardiovascular support for the CCU patient with a lactic acidosis caused by hypoxia. Perform antibiotic therapy with the patient in septic shock. A new drug, sodium dichroacetate (DCA), stimulates the cellular breakdown of lactic acidosis and is still under investigation.[22]

Role of anion gap

The anion gap may be helpful in the differential diagnosis and prompt management of metabolic acidosis. Not all charged particles in the blood are measured on a set of routine serum electrolyte tests. The two cations, or positively charged particles, measured on routine serum electrolytes, are Na^+ and K^+. The two anions, or negatively charged particles, measured on routine serum electrolytes, are Cl^- and HCO_3^-. The bicarbonate is often measured and reported as the CO_2 content (see Unit 4).

According to the law of electroneutrality, the total number of positively and negatively charged particles in the serum must remain equal. However, the sum of the Cl^- and HCO_3^- levels does not equal the serum Na^+ level (serum K^+ levels are so small that they are usually not considered).[17,30,55] There are usually fewer negative charges. This is the *anion gap*. The normal anion gap is 8 to 16 mEq/L but can differ with at least two of the newer laboratory analyzers.[17,20,55] It is composed of small amounts of albumin and other protein, $HPO_4^=$, and fixed acids.[22]

Consider the following example: Na^+ 147 mEq/L, K^+ 4.6 mEq/L, Cl^- 105 mEq/L, CO_2^- 18 mEq/L. The normal CO_2 content is 24 to 30 mEq/L. The CO_2 content in this example is low, indicating the presence of metabolic acidosis. Calculating anion gap in the absence of an acidosis can produce spurious findings of no significance. The sum of the anions (Cl^- and CO_2^-) equals 123 mEq/L. The sum of the anions does not equal the serum Na^+ level. There is a gap of 24 mEq/L (147 − 123 mEq/L). This difference indicates an abnormal, large anion gap.

The causes of metabolic acidosis can be grouped into two categories: (1) those associated with the accumulation of acid in the form of HCl and (2) those associated with accumulation of organic or fixed acids such as lactic acid, ketoacid, or other uremic acids. The presence of exogenous acids, such as acetylsalicylic acid (ASA) or alcohol may also contribute.[30] In the patient with an acute myocardial infarction, the most common cause of an abnormal anion gap is lactic acidosis secondary to hypoxia especially in the presence of a normal blood glucose, which rules out diabetic ketoacidosis.[20,22]

When HCl accumulates, causing metabolic acidosis, the serum Cl^- level is high. This change usually compensates for the drop in CO_2 content, and the gap remains normal.[30] Causes of metabolic acidosis with a normal anion gap include diarrhea or excessive intestinal drainage, renal tubular acidosis, adrenal insufficiency, administration of certain drugs such as acetazolamide (Diamox) and mafenide (Sulfamylon), and administration of certain types of hyperalimentation fluid.[20,30] These causes of are not commonly seen in the CCU and thus, when found, eliminate more commonly associated complications. An abnormally small anion gap may indicate either low serum levels of anions such as albumin or high serum levels of Na^+ or other cations such as Ca^{++}.[17,30,55] In these cases, acidemia is usually not present.

Evaluate the anion gap to obtain a differential assessment of acidosis in a set of routine serum electrolytes. Electrolyte changes noted before ABG changes may enhance the importance of an ABG sample. Determine the anion gap on routine electrolytes in between ABG samples to assess acid-base improvement or deterioration.

Metabolic alkalosis

Metabolic alkalosis results from increased levels of base (bicarbonate), excess loss of fixed acids, or both. It is confirmed clinically by the presence of a high pH, high bicarbonate, and increased base excess. The Pco_2 is usually normal since compensatory efforts of the lung are limited by the effects of a rising Pco_2 on the central respiratory center.

Bicarbonate accumulation may occur as a result of exogenous ingestion in the form of antacids, overzealous correction of an acidosis with intravenous sodium bicarbonate, or loss of acid (H^+) and chloride via the gastrointestinal tract or kidneys. Both acid and chloride may be lost secondary to diuresis, vomiting, or upper gastrointestinal suction. When chloride (an anion) is lost from the body, bicarbonate is retained by the kidneys to maintain the body's electroneutrality. Accumulation of this bicarbonate may result in a metabolic alkalosis.

The *clinical signs* of metabolic alkalosis are slow, shallow respirations and symptoms of decreased calcium effect. The slow, shallow respirations represent the respiratory system's attempt to assist the kidneys in conserving acid. However, these efforts are limited by the normal respiratory centers and are only minimally effective.[20] Alkalosis also causes increased binding of free calcium, producing symptoms of hypocalcemia. These symptoms include tremors, tingling or other paresthesias, muscle spasms, and seizures.

Perform the following *therapies* or interventions: (1) stop administration of diuretics; (2) replace KCl; (3) administer acetazolamide (Diamox); and (4) implement seizure precautions. Administer direct intravenous dilute hydrochloric acid solutions to correct severe metabolic alkalosis.[37,38] Acidifying agents such as ammonium chloride may correct the serum pH but can increase K^+ excretion and further potentiate arrhythmias.[38] However, these agents are not usually necessary in coronary care. Metabolic alkalosis is the most difficult imbalance to correct and is most effectively managed by prevention.

ARTERIAL BLOOD GASES: CORRELATION OF OXYGENATION AND ACID-BASE BALANCE

Because alterations in acid-base balance are not necessarily associated with states of inadequate oxygenation, you may want to consider acid-base and oxygenation values separately when analyzing a set of ABG values.

The following are the normal values assigned to acid-base parameters: pH 7.35 to 7.45, Pco_2 35 to 45 mm Hg, HCO_3^- 22 to 26 mEq/L, and base excess ±2 to 3 mEq/L. When analyzing the acid-base component of ABG values, follow these steps:

Step 1: Check the pH. Is the value above or below normal? The pH indicates whether the primary problem is acidosis or alkalosis.

Step 2: Check the values that reflect the respiratory component. Is the Pco_2 normal, in-

	RESPIRATORY		METABOLIC	
	pH	P_{CO_2}	pH	HCO_3
ACIDOSIS	↓	↑	↓	↓
ALKALOSIS	↑	↓	↑	↑

Fig. 3-22 Comparison of key blood gas changes in respiratory and metabolic imbalances.

creased, or decreased? Does this potentially represent acidosis or alkalosis?

Step 3: Check the value that reflects the metabolic, or nonrespiratory, component. Are the HCO_3^- and base excess normal, increased, or decreased?

Step 4: Determine the primary disorder by comparing the pH change with the corresponding respiratory or metabolic change (Fig. 3-22).

Step 5: Note whether any compensatory efforts are present. These are indicated by respiratory or metabolic changes that do not correspond with the pH.

Step 6: Evaluate why this patient's blood gas values are abnormal and determine nursing action to be taken.

Consider the following ABG example:

pH	7.31	Pao_2	55 mm Hg
Pco_2	72 mm Hg	FIo_2	55% (0.55)
HCO_3^-	16 mEq/L	Sao_2	85%
Base excess	−6 mEq/L	Hg	24 g/dl

In the preceding example, the pH is decreased, indicating a primary acidosis. The Pco_2 is increased, indicating high acid (carbonic) and potential respiratory acidosis. The HCO_3^- and base excess levels are high, indicating high base and potential metabolic alkalosis. The pH indicates that the primary disorder is most likely the respiratory imbalance, or respiratory acidosis. The other metabolic changes most likely reflect the body's attempts at compensation. The presence of metabolic compensation indicates a chronic respiratory disorder. Related nursing diag-

noses for acid-base imbalances include alteration in cardiac output, alteration in tissue perfusion, impaired gas exchange, ineffective airway clearance, ineffective breathing pattern, alteration in elimination, anxiety, knowledge deficit, and electrolyte imbalance. Acid-base findings in arterial and venous blood gases are usually the same except in the setting of CPR when ventilation is established. In this setting, acidosis may be present on venous gases with respiratory alkalosis present on ABGs.[37,45]

When analyzing the oxygenation component of blood gas values, follow these steps:

Step 1: Analyze the Pao_2 to determine the effectiveness of O_2 transport in the lungs. Is the Pao_2 critically low (less than 60 mm Hg)? Is the Pao_2 at 5 times the FIo_2? Estimate the A-a gradient.

Step 2: Analyze the O_2 saturation to determine the arterial O_2 content. Is the O_2 saturation critically low (less than 90%)? Correlate with the patient's hemoglobin. Relate to the Pao_2.

Step 3: Analyze the pH and mixed venous saturation (Svo_2), if available, to determine the presence of hypoxia. Correlate with any hypoxemic changes, cardiac output measurements, and signs and symptoms.

Step 4: Determine potential mechanism and modes of intervention.

In the example provided, the critically low Pao_2 indicates hypoxemia. At an FIo_2 of 55% (0.55), the expected Pao_2 should be aproximately 275 mm Hg (5 × 55 = 275). The actual Pao_2 of 55 mm Hg indicates a wide A-a gradient (at 220 mm Hg) and significant impairment of pulmonary O_2 transport. The low saturation (Sao_2) reflects an apparent deficit in O_2 content. However, this patient's serum hemoglobin level is high. The actual O_2 content is 18.34 ml O_2/dl (1.39 ml O_2/g Hb × 24 g Hb/dl × 55% saturation). Thus the O_2 content is only slightly low. The low O_2 saturation reflects the difficulty in filling the excess hemoglobin sites.

The arterial O_2 supply is actually adequate. Symptoms of hypoxia may not be apparent because of the compensation provided by this high hemoglobin content. Refer to the nursing orders on oximetric monitoring for nursing diagnoses related to oxygen imbalances. Venous blood gases might be helpful in determining if the cardiovascular system is compromised. However, hypoxia is unlikely in the presence of a normal bicarbonate and base excess.

The complete interpretation of this blood gas example is chronic respiratory acidosis with impaired O_2 transport. A major disorder that may result in this clinical picture is chronic bronchitis (COPD). Nursing action attempts to improve ventilation. Supplemental bicarbonate is not indicated. The compensatory efforts of the cardiovascular system may be impaired in the patient with an acute myocardial infarction and chronic respiratory disease.

SELF-ASSESSMENT

The third day after his admission to the coronary care unit for acute anterior wall myocardial infarction, Mr. J became short of breath and developed sinus tachycardia with increased crackles on auscultation. His blood pressure dropped to 98/50 and he became cold and clammy. Intravenous dopamine was initiated. A pulmonary artery catheter was inserted and the following arterial and venous blood gases were obtained:

pH	7.27	Pao_2	58 mm Hg	Pvo_2	30 mm Hg
Pco_2	26 mm Hg	FIo_2	40%	Hb	12 g/dl
Hco_3^-	12 mEq/L	Sao_2	84%	Svo_2	40%
Base excess	−13	Temperature	101° F		

1 The pH is (high/low/normal), indicating a(n) _____. The Pco_2 is (high/low/normal), indicating respiratory(acidosis/alkalosis). Both the bicarbonate (Hco_3^-) and base excess are (high/low/normal), indicating metabolic (acidosis/alkalosis).

low; acidosis
low; alkalosis
low
acidosis

The pH indicates that the primary disorder is most likely the _____. The other changes most likely reflect the body's attempts at _____. Symptoms in this disorder include central _____ system depression, (hypoventilation/hyperventilation), and (increased/decreased) serum K^+.

metabolic acidosis
compensation
nervous; hyperventilation
increased

2 The Pao_2 is critically (high/low) since it is less than _____ mm Hg, indicating significant _____. At an FIo_2 of 40% (0.40), the expected PAo_2 is _____ mm Hg with a Pao_2 within _____ mm Hg of this value. The difference between the expected and actual Pao_2 is _____ mm Hg, indicating a (normal/wide) A-a gradient (A-aDo_2) and decreased or impaired pulmonary O_2 _____.

low; 60
hypoxemia
200
10 to 20
142; wide

transport

In a patient with CHF and pulmonary congestion, a wide A-a gradient most likely reflects (capillary shunting/venous admixture), which is also referred to as _____ mismatch. Since (some/no) air reaches the blood, an increase in FIo_2 (should/should not) result in an increased Pao_2. The low cardiac output contributes to (dead space/shunting), which may also interfere with gas exchange.

venous admixture
V/Q; some
should
dead space

3 The Sa_{O_2} is (high/low/normal), indicating potential abnormal arterial O_2 (content/transport). This patient's arterial O_2 content is _____ ml O_2/100 ml (1.39 ml O_2/g Hg × _____ g Hg × _____ % saturation). The Sa_{O_2} is (higher/lower) than expected for the Pa_{O_2} of 58 mm Hg, indicating a "shift to the _____." In this patient the most likely cause is the presence of _____, and it may be further affected by the patient's _____.

low

content; 14

12; 84

lower

right

acidosis

temperature

4 The Sv_{O_2} is (high/low/normal), reflecting (high/low) cardiac output or high _____ O_2 demands as well as the low arterial O_2 content. These changes are compatible with (hypoxemia/hypoxia). The A-V O_2 difference (AVD_{O_2}) is about _____ ml O_2/100 ml, which is (high/low/normal).

low; low

tissue

hypoxia

7

high

5 The complete interpretation of the set of blood gases is metabolic acidosis with hypoxemia and hypoxia. In this patient the most likely cause is (hypovolemic/cardiogenic) shock secondary to congestive _____ failure. Crackles in this setting are usually end (inspiratory/expiratory) and represent (fluid/mucus) in the airways.

cardiogenic; heart

inspiratory

fluid

6 Potential intervention could include (increasing/decreasing) the FI_{O_2}, (fluid/diuretics), and cardiovascular support. Na^+ bicarbonate (should/should not) be administered since the pH is greater than _____.

increasing

diuretics; should not

7.2

Mrs. H was admitted to the coronary care unit complaining of severe retrosternal chest pain. Vital sign were blood pressure 160/80, pulse 96, respirations 26. The lungs were clear and the cardiac rhythm was sinus rhythm with occasional PVCs. Intravenous D5W was started and morphine sulfate, 2.5 mg, was administered. The following arterial blood gases were obtained:

pH	7.6	Pa_{O_2}	82 mm Hg
P_{CO_2}	22 mm Hg	FI_{O_2}	21%
$H_{CO_3}^-$	22 mEq/L	Hb	14
Base excess	O	Temperature	98.8° F

7 The pH is (high/low/normal), indicating a(n) _____. The CO_2 is (high/low/normal), indicating respiratory (acidosis/alkalosis). Both the bicarbonate ($H_{CO_3}^-$) and the base excess are (high/low/normal).

The pH indicates that the disorder is _____. Compensation (is/is not) present, indicating the respiratory change is (acute/chronic). The Pa_{O_2} is (high/low/normal). Therefore, in this patient the cause of the imbalance is most likely _____. Later, Mrs. H became more short of breath. End-inspiratory crackles were present on auscultation. O_2 was started via nasal cannula at 5 L, and pulse oximetry was initiated. The Sa_{O_2} (Sp_{O_2}) was 94%.

high; alkalosis

low; alkalosis

normal

respiratory alkalosis

is not; acute

normal

pain

8 This pulse oximetry reading is (high/low/normal). A limitation of pulse normal oximetry is that it (does/does not) reflect hypoxia, especially in the presence of a (high/low) cardiac output.

normal
does not
low

REFERENCES AND SUGGESTED READINGS

1. Ahrens T: Blood gas assessment of intrapulmonary shunting and deadspace, Crit Care Nurs Clin North Am 1(4):641, 1989.
2. Ahrens T: SvO$_2$ monitoring: is it being used appropriately? Crit Care Nurse 10(7):70, 1990.
3. Alspach JG, editor: Core curriculum for critical care nursing, Philadelphia, 1991, WB Saunders.
4. Anderson S: ABG's. Six easy steps to interpreting blood gases, Am J Nurs 90(8):42, 1990.
5. Bates B: Guide to physical examination, ed 4, Philadelphia, 1987, JB Lippincott.
6. Bolgiano CS, Buntin K, Shoenberger MM: Administering oxygen therapy: what you need to know, Nursing 20(6):47, 1990.
7. Brown LH: Pulmonary oxygen toxicity, Focus Crit Care 17(1):68, 1990.
8. Brown M, Vender JS: Noninvasive oxygen monitoring, Crit Care Clin 4:493, 1988.
9. Cane RD et al: Unreliability of oxygen tension based indices in reflecting intrapulmonary shunting in critically ill adults, Crit Care Med 16(12):1243, 1988.
9a. Carpenter KD: A comprehensive review of cyanosis, Crit Care Nurse 13(4):66, 1993.
10. Chelmowski MK: Hyperventilation and myocardial infarction, Chest 93(5):1095, 1988.
11. Copel LC et al: Continous SvO$_2$ monitoring. A research review, Dimens Crit Care Nurs 10(4):202, 1991.
12. Enger EL et al: Perspectives on the interpretation of continuous mixed venous oxygen saturation, Heart Lung 19(5 Pt2):578, 1990.
13. Ehrhardt BS et al: An easy way to check oxygen saturation, Nursing 20(3):50, 1990.
14. Fallat RJ: Welcome the new era of oximetry, Intens Care Med 14:357, 1988.
15. Gawlinski A et al: Evaluating oxygen delivery and oxygen utilization with mixed venous oxygen saturation monitoring: a case study approach, Heart Lung 19(5 Pt2):566, 1990.
16. Guyton AC: Textbook of medical physiology, ed 8, Philadelphia, 1991, WB Saunders.
17. Handerhan B: Computing the anion gap, RN 54(7):30, 1991.
18. Hardy G: Svo$_2$ continuous monitoring techniques, Dimens Crit Care Nurs 7(1):8, 1988.
19. Janusek LW: Metabolic alkalosis, Nursing 20(6):52, 1990.
20. Kersten LD: Comprehensive respiratory nursing, Philadelphia, 1989, WB Saunders.
21. Lodato RF: Oxygen toxicity, Crit Care Clin 6(3):749, 1990.
22. Lorenz A: Lactic acidosis: a nursing challenge, Crit Care Nurse 9(4):64, 1989.
23. Mikani R et al: International symposium on lung sounds, Chest 92(2):342, 1987.
24. Mims BC: Interpreting ABG's, RN 54(3):42, 1989.
25. Mims BC: Physiologic rationale of SvO$_2$ monitoring, Crit Care Nurs Clin North Am 1(3):619, 1989.
26. Mims BC: The risks of oxygen therapy, RN 50(7):20, 1987.
27. Murray JF: History and physical examination. In Murray JF, Nadel JA, editors: Textbook of respiratory medicine, Philadelphia, 1988, WB Saunders.
28. Pasterkamp H et al: Nomenclature used by health care professionals to describe breath sounds in asthma, Chest 92(2):346, 1987.
29. Peters K et al: Increasing clinical use of pulse oximetry, Dimens Crit Care Nurs 9(2):107, 1990.
30. Pfister SM et al: Arterial blood gas evaluation: metabolic acidemia, Crit Care Nurse 9(1):70, 1989.
31. Reischman RR: Review of ventilation and perfusion physiology, Crit Care Nurse 8(7):24, 1988.
32. Reischman RR: Impaired gas exchange related to intrapulmonary shunting, Crit Care Nurse 8(8):35, 1988.
33. Russell JM: Successful methods for arterial

blood gas interpretation, Crit Care Nurse 11(4):14, 1991.

34. Rutherford KA: Advances in the treatment of oxygenation disturbances, Crit Care Nurs Clin North Am 1(4):659, 1989.

35. Rutherford KA: Principles and application of oximetry, Crit Care Nurs Clin North Am 1(4):649, 1989.

36. Schroeder CH: Pulse oximetry: a nursing care plan, Crit Care Nurse 8(8):50, 1988.

37. Shapiro BA et al: Clinical application of blood gases, ed 4, Chicago, 1989, Year Book Medicl Publishers.

38. Shapiro BA: Arterial blood gas monitoring, Crit Care Clin 4(3):479, 1988.

39. Shapiro BA et al: Clinical application of respiratory care, ed 3, Chicago, 1985, Year Book Medical Publishers.

40. Sonnesso G: Are you ready to use pulse oximetry? Nursing 21(8):60, 1991.

41. Spotlight on acid-base balance, Nursing 20(3):32HH, 1990.

42. Spyr J et al: Pulse oximetry: understanding the concept, knowing the limits, RN 53(5):38, 1990.

43. Taylor DL: Respiratory alkalosis, Nursing 19(3):60, 1990.

44. Taylor DL: Respiratory acidosis, Nursing 20(3):52, 1990.

45. Textbook of advanced cardiac life support, ed 2, Dallas, 1990, American Heart Association.

46. Thelan LA, Davie JK, Urden LD: Textbook of critical care nursing: diagnosis and management, St. Louis, 1990, Mosby–Year Book.

47. Vaughn S, Puri VK: Cardiac output changes and continuous mixed venous oxygen saturation measurement in the critically ill, Crit Care Med 16(5):495, 1988.

48. Von Rueden KT: Noninvasive assessment of gas exchange in the critically ill patient, AACH Clin Issues Crit Care Nurs 1(2):239, 1990.

49. Ward JJ: Lung sounds: easy to hear, hard to describe, Respir Care 34(1):17, 1989.

50. Weldy NJ: Body fluids and electrolytes: a programmed presentation, ed 6, St. Louis, 1992, Mosby–Year Book.

51. West WB: Ventilation, blood flow, and gas exchange. In Murray JF, Nadel JA, editors: Textbook of respiratory medicine, Philadelphia, 1988, WB Saunders.

52. White KM: The physiologic basis for continuous mixed venous oxygen saturation monitoring, Heart Lung 19(5 Pt2):548, 1990.

53. Wilkins RL et al: Lung sounds terminology used by respiratory care practitioners, Respir Care 34(1):36, 1989.

54. Wilkins RL et al: Lung sounds: a practical guide, St. Louis, 1988, Mosby–Year Book.

55. Winter SD et al: The fall of the serum anion gap, Arch Intern Med 150(2):311, 1990.

Fluid and Electrolyte Balance

The body's fluid is located within two major compartments: inside the cells (*intracellular fluid,* or ICF) and outside the cells (*extracellular fluid,* or ECF). The extracellular fluid compartment contains both intravascular fluid and interstitial fluid. Intravascular fluid is located within the blood vessels and is synonymous with the blood plasma or "serum." (*Serum* is literally defined as plasma without the clotting factors.) Intravascular fluid surrounds the blood cells. Interstitial fluid surrounds the tissue cells (Fig. 4-1). Excess fluid accumulating in the interstitial space is referred to as *edema.*

The many types of particles found within the body fluid compartments contribute to fluid concentration. These particles may be either electrically charged or noncharged. Examples of noncharged particles include glucose, fats, urea, O_2, CO_2, and hormones. The most significant of these in determining fluid concentration are glucose and urea.[8,13] Urea is measured by the blood urea nitrogen, or serum BUN.

Charged particles are known as *ions* or *electrolytes. Cations* are positively charged particles, and *anions* are negatively charged particles. The major role of cations is to determine the electrical events of living cells, especially cardiac cells. Anions play a major role in acid-base balance either by accepting or donating hydrogen (H^+) ions (see Unit 3).

The exact distribution of electrolytes varies between the body fluid compartments. The two major cations located primarily but not exclusively within the intracellular fluid compartment are potassium (K^+) and magnesium (Mg^{++}) (Fig. 4-2). The two major anions within the intracellular fluid compartment are protein (PRO^-) and phosphate ($HPO_4^=$). The two major cations located primarily but not exclusively within the extracellular fluid compartment are sodium (Na^+) and calcium (Ca^{++}) (see Fig. 4-2). The two major anions within the extracellular fluid compartment are chloride (Cl^-) and bicarbonate ($HCO_3^=$). The most important electrolyte in determining serum (extracellular) fluid concentration is Na^+.

The distribution of electrolytes between the two extracellular fluid compartments (plasma and interstitial fluid) is identical, except for the presence of a greater amount of protein in the plasma (see Fig. 4-2). This protein difference is a major factor responsible for fluids staying within the plasma rather than in the interstitial space, thus preventing the development of edema (see Fluid Shifts: Mechanisms of Edema Formation and Inflammation).

ROUTINE SERUM ELECTROLYTES

Serum electrolyte levels reflect the ion concentrations within the intravascular fluid or plasma, which is part of the extracellular fluid compartment. The two cations mea-

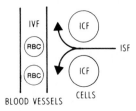

Fig. 4-1 Major fluid compartments. The extracellular fluid (ECF) = interstitial fluid (ISF) + intravascular fluid (IVF) or plasma. The intracellular fluid (ICF) = tissue cells + RBCs.

sured on routine serum electrolyte tests are Na+ and K^+. Since a greater distribution of Na^+ exists within the extracellular fluid, the normal serum Na^+ concentration (135 to 145 mEq/L) is greater than that of K^+ (3.5 to 5 mEq/L).

The two anions measured on routine serum electrolyte tests are Cl^- and HCO_3, the two major extracellular anions. The HCO_3^- level is often reported as the CO_2 content and thus may not be as clearly apparent as the Cl^- level. Carbon dioxide is carried within the blood in three forms: (1) freely dissolved as a gas, (2) combined with water to form carbonic acid (H_2CO_3), and (3) converted to bicarbonate to facilitate acid excretion and buffering. About 95% of the carbon dioxide in the blood actually is in the form of bicarbonate, instead of free carbon dioxide as the name suggests. Thus the measurement of CO_2 content essentially reflects bicarbonate levels. The normal serum levels of 24 to 30 mEq/L corresponds roughly with the normal bicarbonate levels obtained on an arterial blood gas.

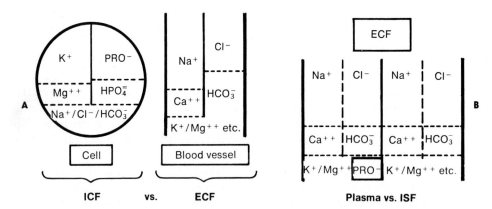

Fig. 4-2 Distribution of electrolytes within the fluid compartments. The ICF versus ECF compartments are first compared (A), then the two ECF compartments (B).

CELLULAR HOMEOSTATIC MECHANISMS

Many interacting forces in the body combine to maintain physiologic equilibrium, or *homeostasis*. Equilibrium of gas and fluid concentrations is maintained by processes that allow the movement of either particles or fluid across the cell membranes.

Diffusion is the movement of particles from a region of greater concentration to a region of lesser concentration (Fig. 4-3). An example is the gaseous exchange in the lungs. Oxygen particles move from a region of greater concentration (in the air) to a region of lesser concentration (in the venous blood). Since gas particles exert pressure both in the atmosphere and in solution, a pressure difference or gradient also exists that facilitates the movement of oxygen into the blood (see Unit 3). The process of diffusion is therefore influenced not only by concentration gradients but by pressure gradients.

Energy is required to actively move particles in the absence gradient or against a concentration gradient. This process is called *active transport*.[28] The major example of active transport in the body is the Na^+-K^+ pump, which establishes a concentration gradient so that electrical events may occur.[8]

Osmosis is the movement of water from a region of lesser concentration (of dissolved particles) and more water to a region of greater concentration (of dissolved particles) and less water (see Fig. 4-3). Within the body cells, semipermeable membranes limit the free movement of some particles.[19] In this setting, the movement of water by osmosis aids in stabilizing the fluid concentration.[28]

The concentration of particles per unit of water is measured by either osmolality or osmolarity. The concentration of intravenous (IV) solutions is measured by their *osmolarity* (mOsm/L), or particles per *liter* of water. The concentration of the plasma or serum is measured by the serum *osmolality* (mOsM/kg), i.e., particles per *kilogram* of water.[13,28] Since one liter of water weighs 1 kilogram, the measurements are interchangeable. When referring to body fluids, *osmolality* is preferred since it correlates more directly with osmotic pressure.[13]

The normal serum osmolality is 280 to 295 mOsm/kg. The major factors determining serum osmolality are the serum Na^+ (a charged particle) and the glucose and blood urea (two noncharged particles).[9,23] The serum Na+ is the most significant factor.[8,13] For the more specific role of protein, refer to pages 93 and 94.

Fluids or solutions having the same concentration in relation to each other are called *isoosmolar* or *isotonic*. Administering an isotonic solution into the plasma does not alter the osmotic concentration. A *hyperosmolar* or *hypertonic* solution has a greater concentration of dissolved particles when compared with that of another solution. A *hypo-osmolar* or *hypotonic* solution has a lesser concentration of dissolved particles when compared with that of another solution. In the human body, changes in plasma concentration often occur before either interstitial or intracellular changes. Plasma is also more easily accessible for fluid replacement therapy. Fluid movements and intracellular changes result from any changes in plasma concentration.

An example of a clinical state that may result in hypertonicity or hyperosmolality of the plasma is diabetes mellitus. In the presence of a hypertonic plasma, water moves out of the cells into the plasma (Fig. 4-4). Fluid also moves out of the interstitial space, probably before moving out of the cells. The circulating blood volume and urine output initially are increased. However, in time the circulating volume decreases and cells may become dehydrated. Hypertonic solutions may be useful in the acute cardiac patient to mobilize excess fluid from the interstitial and intracellular fluid compartments or in hypo-

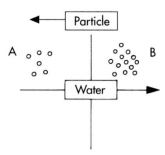

Fig. 4-3 The processes of diffusion and osmosis. In diffusion, *particles* move from an area of greater concentration to an area of lesser concentration. In osmosis, *water* moves from an area of lesser concentration to an area of greater concentration (or more water to less water).

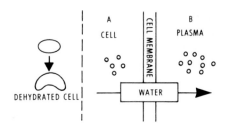

Fig. 4-4 Fluid shifts in the presence of hypertonic serum or plasma.

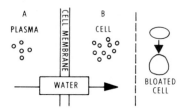

Fig. 4-5 Fluid shifts in the presence of hypotonic serum or plasma.

volemic shock states to increase circulating blood volume. However, fluid overload can occur if renal function is impaired. The practitioner should monitor urine output, pulmonary status, and hemodynamic parameters, if available.[11]

Clinical states resulting in hypotonic plasma concentrations are very common, especially in a coronary care unit. They include congestive heart failure (CHF), hepatic failure, certain stages of renal failure, and the effects of popular diuretic agents. Hypotonic states may be associated with either volume overload or volume depletion (see Fluid Imbalances). In the presence of a hypotonic plasma, water moves from the plasma or serum into the cell and interstitial spaces (Fig.

4-5). In hypovolemic states, this further depletes the circulating blood volume. Hypotonic hypovolemic states are associated with more rapid onset of shock and more significant symptoms for the same amount of fluid loss. Hypotonic solutions are not very effective in maintaining circulating blood volume, since the fluid administered quickly moves out of the plasma.[11,25] However, they may be used to rehydrate the cells, when the circulating volume is no longer critically low.[12] In hypervolemic states such as CHF, extra fluid moves into the interstitial space, potentiating the edema. In this setting fluid movements occur in response to other vascular changes as well as the changes in plasma tonicity.

SYSTEMIC HOMEOSTATIC MECHANISMS: ROLE OF RECEPTORS

Fluid and electrolyte balance is also regulated systemically by special areas in the body known as *receptors*. Receptors are specialized cells or sensory nerve endings that send messages to the hormonal and cardiovascular centers in the brain. They also help regulate heart rate, blood pressure, and respiratory rate.

Increases or decreases in intravascular fluid and/or Na^+ result in changes in plasma concentration (tonicity or osmolality). Special cells in the body known as *osmoreceptors* are sensitive to these changes in serum osmolality. The osmoreceptors are located in the hy-

pothalamus and are bathed by the body's fluid. They send signals to the posterior pituitary gland to control the release of *antidiuretic hormone* (ADH). ADH inhibits excretion of water by the kidneys, thereby causing water conservation.[13]

In the presence of plasma hypotonicity, or decreased osmolality, the osmoreceptors bloat and in this way sense the increased body fluid.[19,28] ADH is inhibited, leading to diuresis. In the presence of plasma hypertonicity, or increased osmolality, the osmoreceptors shrink and in this way sense decreased body fluid. ADH is released, leading to water resorption. Alcohol blocks the effect of ADH in the kidney, resulting in loss of free water and a hypertonic serum.

The hypothalamus is also sensitive to decreases in cardiac output. Lowered cardiac output stimulates the osmoreceptors, resulting in secretion of ADH and water resorption. A concurrent change in osmolality is not necessary.[13] This effect may also be mediated by the pressoreceptors.[13,16]

The *pressoreceptors*, also called *baroreceptors*, are sensitive to pressure exerted on the vascular walls as they are stretched by the volume of blood leaving the heart—i.e., the *cardiac output.* They are located in the walls of the aortic arch, the internal walls of the carotid arteries,[3,16] and the juxtaglomerular apparatus in the kidneys. Stretch receptors have also been identified in the atria and in the superior and inferior vena cava.[13,16,17] Stimulation of the pressoreceptors ultimately results in both hormonal and nervous responses. The hormone released is *aldosterone,* which is secreted by the adrenal cortex. Aldosterone causes the kidney to retain Na^+ and water and excrete K^+. The *parasympathetic* nervous system is affected via the vagus nerve.[3,13,16] The sympathetic nervous system may also be affected.[3,16] Vagal stimulation causes slowing of the heart and decreases the cardiac output. An *increased cardiac output* inhibits the release of aldosterone and stimulates the vagus nerve to slow down the heart. Inhibition of the sympathetic nervous system may also occur, resulting in vasodilation and decreased contractility.[3,16] A *decreased cardiac output* stimulates the release of aldosterone and inhibits the vagus nerve, allowing the heart rate to increase.

Aldosterone release is controlled by mechanisms involving both the brain and the kidneys. Changes in cardiac output are sensed by the pressoreceptors in the aorta and carotid arteries, which send signals to the brain (hypothalamus). The hypothalamus, in turn, regulates the release of adrenocorticotropic hor-

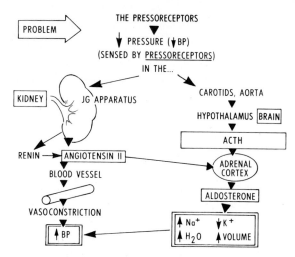

Fig. 4-6 Effects of pressoreceptor stimulation in the kidneys, carotids, and aorta.

mone (ACTH). This hormone stimulates the adrenal cortex to produce aldosterone. The juxtaglomerular apparatus in the kidneys also acts as a pressoreceptor area, although it is not strictly classified as one (Fig. 4-6). Decreased pressure and ischemia are sensed, causing stimulation of the renin-angiotensin mechanism.[19,20] Renin is released into the blood and acts as a catalyst in the synthesis of angiotensin I. Angiotensin I is carried by the circulating blood to the lungs, where an enzyme present in lung tissue converts it to angiotensin II, in the presence of a converting enzyme. Angiotensin II causes vasoconstriction and aldosterone secretion.[13,16] Increased renal perfusion and pressure inhibit the renin-angiotensin mechanism. Atrial stretch receptors cause the release of atrial natriuretic peptide (ANP), which also inhibits this mechanism and causes Na^+ excretion and vasodilation.[2,13,19,50]

The *chemoreceptors* are sensitive to lack of oxygen in the blood as reflected by the pressure of the dissolved oxygen or pO_2, increased CO_2, and increased H^+.[3,7,13] Lack of oxygen may be associated with either a de-

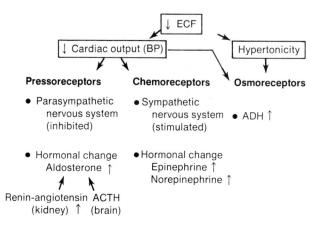

Fig. 4-7 Pressoreceptor, chemoreceptor, and osmoreceptor responses.

crease in the actual amount of oxygen in the blood or a decrease in the cardiac output, which can result from severe fluid depletion.[16] The chemoreceptors are located in the walls of the aortic arch and carotid arteries. When the arterial pressure drops to approximately 40 to 80 mm Hg, the influence of the chemoreceptors becomes more powerful than that of the pressoreceptors.[16] Stimulation of the chemoreceptors results in both hormonal and nervous responses that sup-

port each other (Fig. 4-7). The sympathetic nervous system is stimulated.[16,34] The adrenal medulla releases the hormones epinephrine and norepinephrine, which act as mediators for sympathetic activity (see Unit 9). These hormones cause stimulation of heart rate and contractility and constriction of the peripheral blood vessels. These changes are responsible for the signs and symptoms of shock, which result from severe volume depletion as well as other causes.

FLUID IMBALANCES
Hypervolemia

Hypervolemia is a condition in which excess fluid volume accumulates in the extracellular fluid compartment. It is also called *circulatory overload* or *fluid overload*. The major related nursing diagnosis is alteration in fluid volume:excess. The excess volume typically accumulates first in the vascular compartment or plasma, then in the interstitial space. The plasma concentration may be either hypotonic, isotonic, or hypertonic depending on whether both Na^+ and water are retained in equal amounts. Thus serum osmolality is not a good single indicator of volume overload. Weight gain can be more indic-

ative. A sudden weight gain of 2 pounds within 24 hours may indicate that a patient has retained as much as 1000 ml of fluid since 1 liter of water weighs 1 kg, or 2.2 pounds.

The most common cause of hypervolemia in the coronary care unit (CCU) is *congestive heart failure*. In CHF, the initial change is a fall in cardiac output due to a weakened heart. Initially no volume imbalance exists. However, the fall in cardiac output is quickly sensed by both the pressoreceptors and the osmoreceptors. The pressoreceptors trigger a sequence of events that causes the release of aldosterone. Aldosterone causes both Na^+

and water retention and K^+ excretion. The osmoreceptors and pressoreceptors cause the release of ADH, which causes additional water retention without Na^+. Although both Na^+ and water are retained, more water than Na^+ is retained. Thus the serum (plasma) becomes hypotonic.[2,7] The serum osmolality, hematocrit, and serum Na^+ usually are low. The atrial stretch receptors are stimulated with the release of ANP but are unable to fully compensate.[2] This type of pseudohyponatremia is called *dilutional hyponatremia* and should not be treated as a true low serum Na^+. The effects of mechanical ventilation produce similar changes.

The clinical symptoms associated with CHF are related to the excess fluid and hypotonicity, decreased cardiac output, and pressure changes within the heart and blood vessels. Hemodynamic monitoring provides the most accurate information regarding these changes (see Unit 8). The excess fluid in the vascular compartment places an added work load on the heart. Some of this excess fluid moves first to the interstitial space and eventually into the cell, potentiating the pulmonary and systemic edema produced primarily by cardiovascular pressure changes. The hypotonicity promotes further fluid movement into these areas. Signs of in-

creased intracellular fluid include headache, nausea and vomiting, confusion, and seizures. These are also signs and symptoms of hyponatremia and may be referred to as signs and symptoms of water intoxication (see Sodium Imbalances).

The symptoms associated with the decreased cardiac output mimic those of hypovolemic states and include a decreased urine output, low blood pressure, and, when severe, signs of shock. Many signs and symptoms of shock result from a chemoreceptor response.

Because of the effects of aldosterone and ADH on the kidney, urine specific gravity, urine osmolality and urine K^+ levels are high, whereas the urine Na^+ level is low.[4,9] If renal damage (secondary renal failure) occurs, the serum and urine osmolality as well as the urine Na^+ and K^+ levels become equal.[4,9] The serum BUN and creatinine levels are also useful indicators.

The primary therapy for hypervolemia is fluid restriction with strict intake and output and diuretics. Treatment may also involve dialysis or hemofiltration to remove fluid excess.[22,27] Additional therapy is directed toward the primary cause. For a complete discussion of CHF therapy, refer to Unit 8.

Hypovolemia

Hypovolemia is a condition in which a fluid deficit exists in the extracellular fluid compartment. It is also called *fluid depletion* or *dehydration*. The major related nursing diagnosis is fluid volume deficit. The plasma concentration may be hypotonic, isotonic, or hypertonic, depending on whether both Na^+ and water are lost in equal amounts.[4,9] Thus serum osmolality is not a good indicator of hypovolemia. Hemodynamic changes provide the most accurate information (see Unit 8).

The most common cause of hypovolemia in the coronary care unit is excessive diure-

sis. With excessive diuresis, blood volume decreases and therefore cardiac output falls. The fall in cardiac output is sensed by the pressoreceptors and osmoreceptors so that both aldosterone and ADH are released. Na^+ and water are retained. Although this response is helpful, it is insufficient to correct the problem. When volume losses exceed the ability of the receptors to compensate for them, symptoms appear and supportive intervention is indicated.

The clinical symptoms associated with excessive diuresis are related primarily to the cellular dehydration and the decrease in cardiac output. Acute symptoms associated with dehydrated cells include thirst[13,19] and elevated temperature. Chronic symptoms of dehydration include dry mucous membranes and decreased skin turgor.[19,20] However, the practitioner should not use skin turgor to assess dehydration in the elderly, since it normally decreases with aging.[28]

Symptoms associated with decreased cardiac output mimic those of hypervolemia and include decreased venous filling, decreased urinary output, hypotension (orthostatic, early), and, when severe, signs of shock.[19,20] Many signs and symptoms of shock are due to a chemoreceptor receptor response. Diuretics may result in a greater loss of Na^+ than water and a hypotonic serum. With decreased cardiac output, the serum Na^+ and osmolality are low. The vascular volume becomes more compromised as fluid moves inside the cell. The signs and symptoms of shock may appear earlier than in other forms of fluid loss. The hematocrit is high in all forms of hypovolemia.[28] Because of the effects of aldosterone, urine osmolality, specific gravity, and urine K^+ levels are high, whereas the urine Na^+ level is low.[1,15] The BUN and creatinine levels and ratios are helpful in detecting secondary renal failure.[20] An elevated BUN alone is compatible with hypovolemia.

Elderly patients are more susceptible to hypovolemia because of the effects of medications, chronic illness, an impaired thirst mechanism, and a smaller percentage of total body water. Fluid losses are also intensified in the patient who has taken nothing by mouth or is comatose, who has an altered level of consciousness with limited water access, or who is receiving tube feedings without supplemental water. Diaphoresis and hyperventilation may also contribute to fluid losses.

The primary mode of therapy in the critically ill hypovolemic patient is intravenous fluid replacement. In the patient with cardiac disease, accomplish this most safely in conjunction with invasive hemodynamic monitoring. You may administer fluid "boluses" of up to 200 ml over 10 minutes. Isotonic fluids are most common. You may also use hypertonic fluids since they can mobilize extra fluids out of the cells and interstitial space into the plasma. You may also administer crystalloids or colloids. Common glucose and/or electrolyte fluids are referred to as crystalloids because of their tendency to crystallize.[25] Examples of colloids include albumin (5%/25%) and synthetic plasma expanders such as dextran and hetastarch (Hespan). Colloids are larger molecules (proteins or large starches) that remain in the plasma longer than glucose or saline.[7,25] These agents act primarily by mobilizing fluids out of the interstitial space (edema) into the vascular compartment.[9] This effect can expand the vascular compartments with lower volumes than required of crystalloids,[10,21] and colloids may be especially indicated when hypovolemia is accompanied by fluid shifts or edema. The multiple side effects associated with dextran limit its current use. Side effects include bleeding due to inhibition of platelets and clotting factors, renal failure due to tubular obstruction, anaphylaxis, and interference with type and crossmatching.[9,25] Hespan has fewer side effects,[9,21] is usually less expensive, and is more easily available than albumin (5%/25%).[7,9] Side effects include primarily transient, asymptomatic alterations in clotting parameters and serum amylase.[21] Albumin can bind calcium, lowering the ionized level, and thereby decrease cardiac contractility.[7]

FLUID SHIFTS: MECHANISMS OF EDEMA FORMATION AND INFLAMMATION

Edema is strictly defined as excess fluid in the interstitial fluid compartment[16] (extracellular). It occurs commonly as the result of volume and circulatory changes. However, the term is also used clinically to describe the accumulation of fluid inside the cell occurring as the result of cellular damage.[13] The most familiar clinical example of this phenomenon is cerebral edema, the intracellular accumulation of fluid in brain cells. Cerebral edema as a result of cerebral hypoxia may occur in the patient with coronary artery disease secondary to cardiac arrest, severe CHF, and shock.

The practitioner should attempt to distinguish fluid accumulation occurring as the result of volume overload and circulatory changes from the intracellular and interstitial fluid accumulation associated with direct cellular damage. This second process, more commonly called *inflammation*, is discussed in the second portion of this section. Both processes occur in the patient who has either angina or an acute myocardial infarction (MI).

Edema formation

Factors predisposing to edema formation include the following changes in addition to extracellular fluid excesses: (1) increases in capillary pressure; (2) inadequate lymphatic drainage or overload; (3) decreased serum albumin levels; and (4) increased capillary permeability (Fig. 4-8).[13,19] Capillary pressure is generated as the result of the heart's pumping action and is also affected by the heart's filling pressures. The capillary pressure tends to push fluid from the vascular compartment into the interstitial space. Two factors are responsible for holding fluid within the vascular compartment, thus offsetting the effects of the capillary pressure: the serum proteins and the intact capillary membranes that keep them within the vascular compartment. More proteins exist inside the vascular compartment than in the interstitial space, creating an osmotic pressure gradient. Because proteins are considered colloids, this force or pressure is called the *serum colloid osmotic pressure* or *oncotic* pressure. The protein primarily responsible for the plasma oncotic (colloid osmotic) pressure is *albumin*. The osmotic role of protein differs from that of Na^+ since it controls fluid movements between the vascular and interstitial compartments (i.e., within the ECF) rather than between the vascular compartment and the cells.[19]

In acute MI complicated by heart failure, left ventricular filling pressure—and consequently pulmonary capillary pressure—

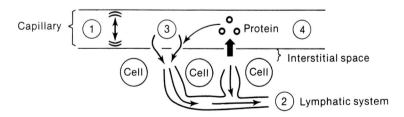

Fig. 4-8 Capillary dynamics favoring edema: (1) increasing capillary pressure, (2) overloaded lymphatic drainage, (3) increasing capillary permeability, and (4) decreasing serum protein levels.

93

rises. When the capillary pressure exceeds the plasma oncotic pressure, fluid moves out of the blood vessels and into the interstitial spaces. Lymphatic drainage increases in the body's efforts to minimize edema formation. However, overload soon occurs.

Lowered serum albumin levels may exist in the patient with coronary artery disease due to inadequate nutrition, liver failure, or stress. In response to corticosteroid release during stress, protein reserves are converted to glucose for energy, resulting in a protein deficit. Lowered serum albumin levels facilitate edema formation. Pulmonary and systemic edema may occur at capillary pressures that individuals usually tolerate well. Administering supplementary albumin may be helpful.

Increased capillary permeability is not usually a factor in the pulmonary or systemic edema of the patient with coronary artery disease. However, it is implicated in the myocardial inflammatory response associated with angina or acute MI.

Inflammation

Local damage to tissue results in a combination of intracellular and interstitial fluid accumulation known as *inflammation* (Fig. 4-9). Inflammation is a patterned, nonspe-

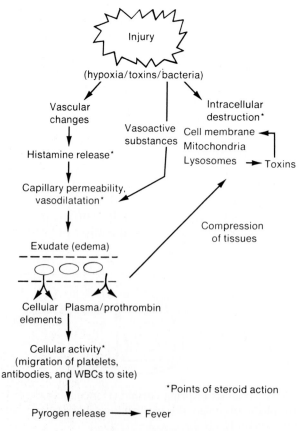

Fig. 4-9 Inflammatory response to injury.

cific response to any type of cellular injury, and it is considered part of the stress response (see Unit 5). An immediate inflammatory response occurs secondary to the localized myocardial hypoxia associated with angina and acute MI.

The intracellular fluid accumulation occurs as the result of damage to the cell membranes,[13] mitochondria, lysosomes, or all of these. In hypoxic cellular damage, intracellular fluid accumulation and swelling also occur as a result of inactivation of the Na^+–K^+ pump. The interstitial fluid—true edema—occurs as a result of an increase in capillary permeability. Increased capillary permeability is associated with histamine release from storage sites located in specialized cells embedded among most common tissue cells. Other vasoactive substances, such as bradykinin and serotonin, may also cause myocardial injury.

CATIONS: ROLES IN ELECTRICAL ACTIVITY

In the *polarized,* or resting, state, the inside of the cell is electrically negative with respect to the outside. All of the body's charged particles, or *ions,* contribute to the cell's charge. However, the cations play a more significant role in determining this charge.

In the polarized or resting state the cell has a net negative charge. The major factors responsible for this electronegativity are (1) the presence of *nondiffusible* intracellular proteins, which act as *anions,* and (2) enhanced membrane permeability to K^+, allowing for diffusion of K^+ out of the cell (Fig. 4-10).[3,5,16,18,26]

In the resting state, the cell membrane is 50 to 100 times more permeable to K^+ than to Na^+. The K^+ particles move by diffusion from the area of greater concentration inside the cell to the area of lesser concentration outside the cell. As the positively charged K^+ particles leave the cell, the inside of the cell becomes more electronegative with respect to the outside. Thus the cation K^+ is the most important electrolyte in determining the polarized state.[5,16]

Excitation and conduction of electrical impulses in the heart depend on the process of *depolarization.* In response to advancing electrical impulses, positively charged particles move into the cells. The inside of these cells becomes *electropositive* and the cells are said to be depolarized.

Both Na^+ and Ca^+ play major roles in the process of *depolarization.* When an electrical impulse reaches a ventricular resting cell membrane, the permeability to K^+ decreases and the permeability to Na^+ suddenly increases. The Na^+ "gates" open. Sodium ions rush into the cell by the process of diffusion, upsetting the previous electronegativity. The inside of the cell becomes electropositive with respect to the outside and is thus *excited.* This local electrical response then acts as an electrical signal and stimulates adjacent cells, spreading the original electrical stimulus throughout the heart. The spread or transmission of electrical signals throughout the heart is known as *conduction.* Both excitation and conduction, then, depend on the process of depolarization.

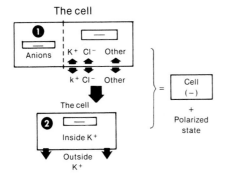

The cell

Anions

K^+ Cl^- Other

k^+ Cl^- Other

The cell

Inside K^+

Outside K^+

= Cell (−)
+
Polarized state

Fig. 4-10   Factors creating the polarized state.

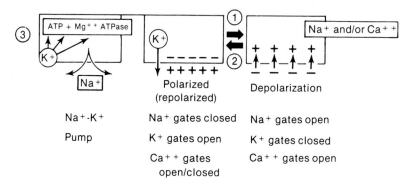

Fig. 4-11 Depolarization (1) and repolarization (2): role of electrolytes. The $Na^+ - K^+$ pump (3) returns Na^+ and K^+ to their original sites.

The cells of normal atrial and ventricular musculature and Purkinje fibers depolarize and conduct impulses rapidly. Therefore they are called *fast cells*. Depolarization in fast cells is caused by the rapid influx of Na^+ and is referred to as *fast-channel electrical activity*.[3,5,6,18,29]

This rapid influx of Na^+ is followed by a secondary slower inward movement of Ca^{++}, which aids further in depolarization (Fig. 4-11). Like Na^+, Ca^{++} is a positively charged particle located primarily outside the cell. The cell membrane permeability to Ca^{++} also changes when an electrical impulse reaches it, opening the Ca^{++} gates, usually after the Na^+ gates. The slow, inward Ca^{++} movement during depolarization is logically called *slow-channel electrical activity*. Slow-channel activity dominates in the SA and AV nodes, which are referred to as *slow cells*.[3,5,6,18,29]

Before the cells can respond to another impulse, they must return to their previous resting or polarized state. This process is known as *repolarization* (see Fig. 4-11). During repolarization the Na^+ gates close and the K^+ gates reopen. As the K^+ gates open, diffusion occurs, causing some of the intracellular K^+ to move out of the cell. Because of this positive ion loss, the inside of the cell again becomes electronegative with respect to the outside. Thus the electrolyte K^+ is responsible for both the initial polarization and the subsequent repolarization of cardiac cells. The Ca^{++} gates remain open during early repolarization and then close, extending the total period of repolarization, allowing for the refractory periods.

The Na^+ that enters the cell during depolarization is returned to its extracellular site by the $Na^+ - K^+$ pump, which also returns K^+ to its intracellular site. The contribution of the $Na^+ - K^+$ pump to cell charge is minimal in the normal cell since most of the Na^+ pumped out is replaced by the equivalently charged K^+ pumped into the cell. The pumping of Na^+ and K^+ against their concentration gradients is an active transport process requiring energy in the form of adenosine triphosphate (ATP). The cation Mg^{++} is important in the breakdown of ATP for energy. Therefore, Mg^{++} is necessary for normal functioning of the $Na^+ - K^+$ pump (Fig. 4-12). A separate but closely related Ca^{++} pump returns Ca^{++} to its extracellular site. This Ca^{++} pump also requires energy, or ATP.

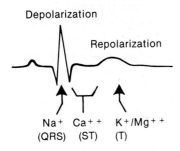

ECG CORRELATION

Depolarization

Repolarization

Na⁺   Ca⁺⁺   K⁺/Mg⁺⁺
(QRS) (ST)   (T)

Fig. 4-12   Effects of electrolytes on the ECG.

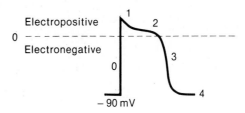

Fig. 4-13   The action potential or single-cell ECG.

ECG correlation

On the electrocardiogram (ECG) the QRS complex represents ventricular depolarization. Na^+ has its major effect during depolarization, thus potentially affecting the *QRS complex*. The T wave represents ventricular repolarization. K^+ has its major effect during polarization and repolarization, thus initially affecting the *T wave*. Mg^{++} affects the level of intracellular K^+ by controlling the Na^+–K^+ pump. Therefore, Mg^{++} also affects the T wave (see Fig. 4-12).

The effects of Ca^{++} begin during depolarization and extend into repolarization. However, during depolarization the effects of Na^+ are more pronounced. During active repolarization the effects of K+ are more pronounced. In between depolarization and active repolarization, the effects of Ca^{++} are unopposed by more significant movements of either Na^+ or K^+. Therefore, Ca^{++} effects are best detected in between the QRS complex and T wave or during the *ST segment* (see Fig. 4-12).

Action potential

In the resting or polarized state, the cardiac cell has the potential for electrical activation—a resting potential. Normal resting potential varies, depending on the type of cell. The level of the resting membrane potential depends on both the integrity of the cell membrane and its resting permeability to K^+. Atrial and ventricular muscle cells normally have a resting membrane potential of approximately −90 millivolts (mV). When a single cell is activated by a stimulus, local electrical changes occur that produce an action current, or *action potential*. This action potential from a single cell may be recorded on graph paper, producing a pattern (Fig. 4-13).

Let us first consider the electrical characteristics of stable atrial and ventricular muscle cells. The phase of electrical action denoted by O represents a change in cellular polarity from electronegative to electropositive. Therefore, *phase O* represents the process of *depolarization*. The phase of electrical action denoted by *phases 1, 2, and 3* represents the return to electronegativity, or *repolarization*. The resting electronegative state is called *phase 4*.[1,5,6,26] The action potential represents the electrical activity of single cells. It correlates roughly with the surface ECG, which represents the electrical activity of many cardiac cells or many action potentials (Fig. 4-14).

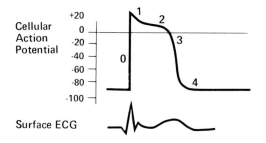

Fig. 4-14 Correlation of action potential events with the surface ECG.

Let us now correlate the phases of the muscle action potential with the corresponding electrolyte movements. *Phase 0* of the action potential represents depolarization and occurs because of the rapid influx of Na^+ followed by the slower influx of Ca^{++} (Fig. 4-15). The effects of Na^+ subside immediately after phase 0, when the Na+ gates close. In contrast, the effects of Ca^{++} extend into repolarization as the Ca^{++} gates remain open and then slowly close. At the end of phase 0 the inside of the cell is electropositive with respect to the outside.

Phase 1 represents an early brief phase of repolarization. It is thought to be caused by inward movement of the negatively charged particle Cl^- into the cell[6] or a transient outward movement of K^+.[5,18] During this phase the action potential experiences a small negative deflection. *Phase 2* in the repolarization process is a plateau period. This plateau occurs because of a persistent, slow, inward movement of Ca^{++} balanced by an early, outward movement of K^+. The plateau corresponds roughly to the absolute refractory period.[1,18,26]

Phase 3 represents the rapid phase of repolarization, in which K^+ rapidly leaves the cell and the Ca^{++} currents are eventually inactivated. The cell thus becomes progressively more electronegative. *Phase 4* represents the return to maximum electronegativity or the resting membrane potential. During this phase the Na^+–K^+ pump is most active, although Na^+–K^+ pump activity may occur throughout the repolarization process.[6,18]

All the phases of electrical action (1, 2, and 3) may be referred to collectively as *electrical systole*. The resting phase (4) between electrical activity is known as *electrical diastole* and corresponds to the resting membrane potential, or the polarized state.

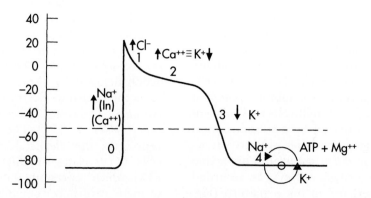

Fig. 4-15 Correlation of electrolyte movements with action potential events.

Automaticity

Automaticity is a normal property of conduction structures such as the sinoatrial (SA) node, atrioventricular (AV) junction,[16] and ventricular Purkinje fibers. Automatic cells are characteristically *unstable* and not able to sustain this electronegative state until a stimulus arrives. Instead, they spontaneously start to lose their electronegativity and begin to depolarize (Fig. 4-16). These cells do not require a stimulus to alter their resting state and initiate depolarization. Automatic cells depolarize spontaneously during electrical diastole, represented by phase 4 of the action potential graph. Therefore, the property of automaticity is also called *phase 4 depolarization*, or *spontaneous diastolic depolarization*. This spontaneous depolarization is associated with the influx of Na^+ and/or Ca^{++} depending on the exact resting cell charge (Fig. 4-16).[18]

The resting cell charge of automatic cells is typically lower or less negative than that of nonautomatic cells. Therefore, automatic cells are referred to as *hypopolarized*. The resting membrane potential is lowest in the

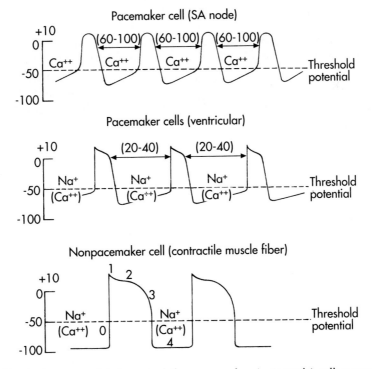

Fig. 4-16 Action potential characteristics: pacemaker (automatic) cells versus nonpacemaker (stable muscle) cells.

SA node and AV node, characteristically in the −60 to −50 mV range.[3,13,18] Since hypopolarization favors the opening of Ca^{++} gates or channels,[3,5,6,29] depolarization in the SA node or AV junction is predominantly Ca^{++} dependent rather than Na^+ dependent (see Fig. 4-16). Hypopolarized cells also depolarize slowly in response to electrical stimulation. Thus the slope of phase O is more gradual.[3,5,6] Ca^{++}-dependent depolarization is called *slow-channel depolarization*.

The slope or incline of phase 4 determines

the rate of diastolic depolarization or the rate of the pacemaker. The more gradual the slope, or incline, the slower the rate of automatic discharge. The steeper the slope, or incline, the faster the rate of automatic discharge (see Fig. 4-16). The level of membrane potential at which an action potential is generated is called its *threshold*.[18] The higher the threshold, the harder it is for the automatic cell to generate an action potential or actual impulse. Lowering the threshold makes it easier for the cell to generate an impulse.

SODIUM IMBALANCES

Sodium (Na^+) is the primary extracellular cation. Sodium plays a major role in both fluid balance and the electrical events of the heart, smooth muscle (gastrointestinal [GI] tract), skeletal muscle, and nervous system. Sodium's major electrical role is during depolarization (see the preceding section). Local Na^+ changes caused by the effects of some antiarrhythmic agents can result in QRS widening. However, serum Na^+ changes are not associated with significant ECG effects, perhaps because of the large amount of extracellular Na^+.

The normal serum Na^+ is 135 to 145 mEq/L. Serum Na^+ levels are regulated by the hormone aldosterone, which is released in response to cardiac output changes and serum Na^+ and K^+ changes. Na^+ is excreted by the kidneys, skin, and GI tract. Foods rich in Na^+ include canned and frozen vegetables (especially tomatoes), cheese, catsup, olives, pickles, luncheon meats, and chocolate.

Hyponatremia

Hyponatremia, or low serum Na^+, may be associated with hypervolemia, hypovolemia, or normal ECF volumes.[4,9,15,23] In most cases, serum osmolality is low or hypotonic.[9,23] The major exception is the presence of high serum glucose, proteins, or fats.[7,9,23]. Hyponatremia occurs in hypervolemia in response to a low cardiac output or inappropriate ADH secretion (SIADH). Pseudohyponatremia due to a low cardiac output occurs in CHF and liver failure and is also called *dilutional hyponatremia*. Although both Na^+ and water are retained, more water is retained. The total body Na^+ is actually high. Dilutional hyponatremia can also occur in renal failure.[7,9,14,23]

Hyponatremia occurs in hypovolemia when Na^+ loss is greater than fluid loss. This condition can result from diuresis, vomiting, diarrhea, GI drains, and some forms of renal failure.[15,23]

The signs and symptoms of hyponatremia are generally related to the hypervolemia or hypovolemia present[9] or to the low serum Na^+ itself. Signs and symptoms directly related to the low Na^+ include skeletal muscle changes, GI changes, and central nervous system (CNS) changes. The skeletal muscle changes include muscle weakness, fatigue, and depressed deep tendon reflexes. The GI changes include anorexia, nausea, vomiting, abdominal cramps, and diarrhea. The CNS changes, including headache and altered level of consciousness, are more likely to develop with sudden acute drops in the serum Na^+.[23] Focal signs such as hemiparesis, tremor, and rigidity are less common. The most serious symptoms are seizures due to increased electrical instability in the brain. These are associated with a mortality exceeding 50%.[23]

Therapy in hyponatremia is directed towards the underlying disorder and the associated fluid imbalance. Supplemental Na^+, especially in the form of strongly hypertonic solutions (i.e., 3% to 5% NS), is administered with caution only in true low Na^+ states. Rapid correction may be associated with further neurologic complications.[23]

Hypernatremia

Hypernatremia, or high serum Na^+, is less common than hyponatremia, especially in the CCU. Hypernatremia is associated primarily with hypovolemia and a high serum osmolality or hypertonic serum.[9] The most common causes in the critically ill patient are diabetes insipidus, administration of osmotic diuretics, alcohol intoxication, and renal failure. These conditions are typically associated with a greater fluid loss than Na^+.[1,9,14,15]

The signs and symptoms of hypernatremia mimic those of hypovolemia. They are associated with the high osmolality and both cellular and extracellular dehydration. Specific symptoms include thirst,[13] elevated temperature, CNS changes,[15,23] flushed skin, dry mucous membranes, and decreased urine output. The CNS changes include lethargy, irritability, hallucinations, and coma. Seizures may occur, especially during rehydration.[23]

Therapy in hypernatremia consists of fluid replacement, restriction of Na^+ intake, and correction of the primary disorder (e.g., vasopressin (Pitressin) therapy for diabetes insipidus).

POTASSIUM IMBALANCES

Potassium (K^+) is the primary intracellular cation. Potassium's major roles in electrical events are producing repolarization and maintaining the polarized state. Potassium also plays a significant role in acid-base balance and cellular metabolism. The normal serum K^+ is 3.5 to 5.0 mEq/L.

Let us consider the role of K^+ in acid-base balance in more detail. The positively charged particles H^+ and K^+ are closely related. K^+ and H^+ have the ability to exchange with one another if there are excesses or deficits of either ion in the plasma. For example, if excess H^+ ions exist in the plasma as in an acidosis, K^+ will trade for H^+ and move into the plasma, allowing H^+ to leave and move into the cell (Fig. 4-17). Thus the serum K^+ will be high in an acidosis with all the corresponding ECG effects. However, the total body K^+ will not be high. This effect commonly results in at least mild increases in serum K^+ in hypoxic lactic acidosis and diabetic ketoacidosis and, less commonly, in respiratory acidosis.[7,57]. In acidotic states such as diabetic ketoacidosis, other factors such as serum hyperosmolality and/or prerenal failure may contribute to the development of high serum K^+ levels and typical ECG changes.[57] Likewise, if a deficit of H^+ occurs with high HCO_3^- levels in the plasma as in alkalosis, some of the K^+ will leave the plasma and move into the cell in exchange for H^+. Thus the serum K^+ will be low in an alkalosis. Hypokalemia may be either the cause or the result of an alkalosis. Sympathetic (beta-2 adrenergic) stimulation has also been implicated in causing hypokalemia by stimulating the $Na^+ - K^+$ pump.[7,31,33,57]

Potassium is also necessary for anabolic

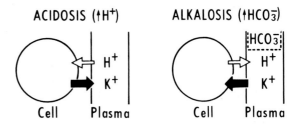

Fig. 4-17 Serum potassium shifts in the presence of acid-base imbalance. The serum K^+ is high in the presence of an acidosis and low in the presence of an alkalosis.

processes within the cells that use *amino acids* and *glucose*. K^+ is transported into the cells together with glucose and insulin for this purpose.

The serum potassium level is regulated by the hormone aldosterone, which is released by the adrenal cortex in response to stress, cardiac output changes, and serum Na^+ and K^+ changes. A high serum potassium stimulates the release of aldosterone, which in turn causes the retention of Na^+ and water and the excretion of K^+. Potassium is excreted by the kidneys and GI tract.

Hypokalemia

Hypokalemia, or low serum K^+, may occur as a result of increased K^+ loss, decreased K^+ intake, alkalosis, sympathetic stimulation, hormonal influences, metabolic factors, or hypomagnesemia (p. 113). Hypokalemia commonly occurs because of increased K^+ loss with diuretic therapy, especially in elderly women and hypertensive patients.[55] During chest pain, this effect is often combined with the effects of sympathetic stimulation.[55,57] Loss of K^+ may also occur with GI suction or vomiting, diarrhea, laxatives, intestinal drains, and excessive diaphoresis. Administration of potassium-free solutions or diets deficient in potassium may also result in hypokalemia.

Medications promoting renal K^+ excretion or K^+ shifts may potentiate hypokalemia. In addition to diuretics, medications promoting K^+ excretion include penicillin, carbenicillin, gentamicin, and amphotericin.[7,31] The IV administration of sympathetic-stimulating agents such as dopamine or epinephrine may potentiate hypokalemia by promoting the movement of K^+ into the cell.[53,55]

The signs and symptoms of hypokalemia generally are divided into those relating to skeletal muscle, smooth muscle, and the heart. The skeletal muscle signs and symptoms of hypokalemia are similar to those in hyperkalemia. They include generalized skeletal muscle weakness, aching, and tenderness, which may be perceived as muscle cramping. The weakness may progress to paralysis if the hypokalemia is severe. Hyporeflexia and respiratory arrest may also occur.[31,41,43,44] These symptoms are compatible with peripheral rather than CNS involvement.[47]

The effects of hypokalemia on the smooth muscle of the GI tract are slightly more specific. Hypokalemia decreases smooth muscle tone in the GI tract and may result in atony of the bowel (paralytic ileus), abdominal distention, and constipation.[44,53] CNS changes may also occur but are not as typical.[41,43,53]

The adverse effects of hypokalemia on electrical activity in the heart are potentially life-threatening. Cardiac cells with unstable cell membranes and automatic properties are particularly sensitive to hypokalemia's effects. Life-threatening ventricular arrhythmias may occur as a result of enhanced automaticity in the His-Purkinje or ventricular conduction fibers. Hypokalemia increases the sensitivity of the heart to the automaticity and triggered arrhythmias of digitalis toxicity and may also enhance ectopic impulse formation by its effects on repolarization. In the presence of hypokalemia, repolarization is prolonged. Prolonged repolarization makes recovery and subsequent conduction in adjacent myocardial cells nonuniform, and it may allow ectopic impulses to develop because of altered conduction or reentry as well as automaticity (see Unit 6). Ventricular arrhythmias with torsades des pointes patterns have also been associated with hypokalemia (see Unit 11).

The ECG effects of hypokalemia may be attributed to the delayed repolarization. In the presence of hypokalemia, the T wave flattens and a prominent U wave appears. The T and U waves fuse into one wave, giv-

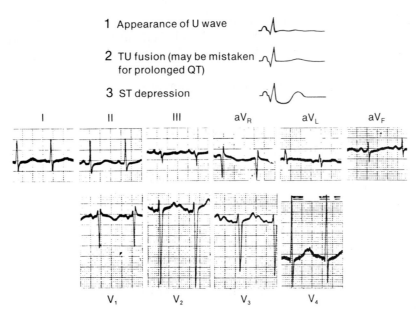

1 Appearance of U wave

2 TU fusion (may be mistaken for prolonged QT)

3 ST depression

I II III aV$_R$ aV$_L$ aV$_F$

V$_1$ V$_2$ V$_3$ V$_4$

Fig. 4-18   ECG changes in hypokalemia. Note the differences between V$_1$ and V$_2$.

ing the appearance of a prolonged Q–T interval (Fig. 4-18). TU wave fusion may be distinguished from normal U waves, which remain separated from their related T waves and occur for unknown reasons. Some investigators have proposed repolarization of the Purkinje fibers as a possible mechanism for normal U waves. However, this theory does not explain why they do not occur in most individuals. In severe hypokalemia the ST segment is also depressed.

The authors have personally observed that early ECG changes caused by K$^+$ can be most clearly detected on leads V$_2$ to V$_4$ (see Fig. 4-18). These changes may be totally invisible on routine monitoring leads or on their standard lead equivalents, including V$_1$ (MCL1). We have no explanation other than possibly the proximity of the heart to the chest wall in these leads.

Potassium replacement therapy consists of administering potassium salts by oral and parenteral routes and increasing nutritional sources. In acute hypokalemia, the dose of intravenous K$^+$ is usually 10 to 40 mEq per hour diluted in at least 50 ml of fluid using an infusion pump.[33,37,44,53,57] Administer IV potassium with caution if the patient requires more than 40 mEq per hour. Obtain the approval of the pharmacist whenever greater concentrations are ordered. Also consider monitoring on a lead V$_2$ equivalent (see Unit 2). Because parenteral potassium may irritate the blood vessels, administer it in large central veins when using high concentrations. Report complaints of "burning" with parenteral administration so that flow rate, concentration, or dosages can be adjusted. If the low K$^+$ is due to low Mg^{++}, K$^+$ replacement may not be effective until the Mg^{++} is corrected.

Commonly administered oral potassium salts include Kaon-Cl, Kaochlor Preps, K-Lyte/Cl, Slow-K, and Kay Ciel. Enhance palatability of the dissolvable oral preparations with fruit juice. Monitor for ulcerations of the stomach and small bowel, which have been reported with the use of some oral preparations. Decrease GI irritation by administering K^+ during or after meals.[53]

Many foods are rich in K^+ in addition to the classically cited orange juice and bananas. Examples include prunes, raisins, other dried fruits, fresh tomatoes, potatoes, and dark green vegetables such as broccoli and peas.[43,44,53] Encourage the use of salt substitutes rich in K^+.[53] Substitute potassium-sparing diuretics for those promoting K^+ loss.[7]

Hyperkalemia

Hyperkalemia may occur as a result of decreased K^+ excretion, acidosis, hyperosmolality,[57] overzealous replacement therapy, hypoaldosteronism, tissue trauma, or administration of multiple units of stored blood. The most common causes of hyperkalemia in the CCU are failure to discontinue potassium supplements when no longer necessary and parenteral replacement therapy without careful monitoring of serum K^+ levels and renal function. Careful monitoring of urine output as well as serum creatinine and BUN levels is important during replacement therapy. End-stage renal failure and diabetic or lactic acidosis are also common causes of hyperkalemia.

Salt substitutes[52] and various medications commonly potentiate hyperkalemia, especially in high-risk individuals. These medications include antibiotics containing K^+, ACE inhibitors, nonsteroidal antiinflammatory agents, cyclosporine, heparin, nonselective beta blockade, succinylcholine (Anectine), and mannitol. The ACE inhibitors, nonsteroidal antiinflammatory agents, cyclosporine, and heparin result in hypoaldosteronism via a variety of mechanisms. Beta blockade and Anectine mobilize K^+ out of the cells into the serum. The increased serum osmolality resulting from mannitol administration may produce increased serum K^+ levels.[33,57]

The effects of hyperkalemia on skeletal muscle are similar to those of hypokalemia. Hyperkalemia also causes skeletal muscle weakness. Hyperreflexia and paresthesias may occur.[41,43,52] The effects on the GI tract are more specific. Hyperkalemia increases smooth muscle tone and irritability in the GI tract. Increased irritability may result in intestinal cramping and diarrhea. CNS changes may also occur but are not as typical.[1,31] Distinguishing K^+ imbalances on the basis of clinical symptoms alone is difficult. Hyperkalemia is often asymptomatic.[57] Serum values and ECG evidence provide more information.

Unlike hypokalemia, hyperkalemia is an electrical *depressant*. Hyperkalemia alters electrical activity so that the cardiac cells repolarize more rapidly *but* less effectively. The normal level of electronegativity (resting potential) is never reached. Mild hyperkalemia may enhance automaticity and ectopic impulse formation. However, as the imbalance progresses, automaticity becomes rapidly *depressed*, a more common effect. End-stage hyperkalemia is associated with ectopy related to decreased conduction and asystole.

The earliest ECG sign of hyperkalemia is peaked T waves, which characteristically are symmetrical and are best visualized in leads V_2 to V_4. When repolarization is disturbed, depolarization is eventually affected. The next ECG sign of hyperkalemia is an effect on ventricular depolarization, widening of the QRS complex, followed by an effect on atrial depolarization, and disappearance of the P wave (Fig. 4-19). End-stage hyperkalemia is associated with rounding off of the T wave and marked QRS slurring. This effect also appears with a dying heart, as the cell membrane is no longer able to contain the intracellular K^+. Hyponatremia, hypocalcemia, and/or hypermagnesemia can

ECG evidence of hyperkalemia

1 Peaked T waves
  (note symmetry)

2 QRS widening

3 P wave disappearance

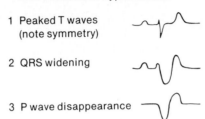

Early hyperkalemia

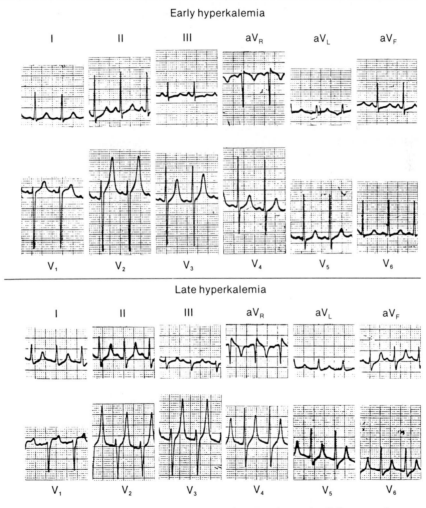

Late hyperkalemia

Fig. 4-19 ECG changes in hyperkalemia. Note the dramatic differences between V$_1$ and V$_2$.

Continued.

End-stage hyperkalemia

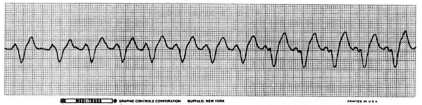

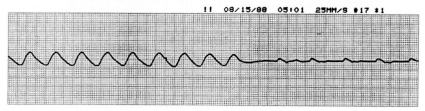

Fig. 4-19, cont'd.   For legend see p. 105.

Table 4-1. Potassium imbalances

	↓ K⁺ Hypokalema	↑ K⁺ Hyperkalemia
Neuromuscular	• Weakness • Hyporeflexia • Paralysis • Respiratory arrest • Paralytic ileus	• Weakness • Hyperreflexia • Paresthesias • Abdominal cramps • Diarrhea
Heart	• ↑ Electrical instability (automaticity) • PVCs/VT/VF • Torsades de pointes • ↑ Digitalis toxicity	• Cardiac depression • Ideoventricular rhythm/AIVR • Asystole
ECG*	• ↓ T wave (flat) • Appearance of U wave • TU fusion • ST depression	• ↑ T wave (peaked) • QRS widening • Disappearance of P wave
Therapy	• IV/oral KCl • Mg^{++} • Salt substitute • K⁺-sparing diuretics • ↑ Dietary K⁺	• Glucose • Insulin • Na^+ Bicarbonate • Inhaled B_2 agents • Ca^{++} Cl/gluconate • Ion exchange resins • Diuretics • Dialysis
Dietary Sources	• Orange juice/bananas/potatoes/tomatoes • Dried fruits (e.g., prunes/raisins) • Dark green vegetables (e.g., broccoli/peas)	

*Leads V_2–V_4 (MCL_2-MCL_4) best.

potentiate any of these ECG effects.[57]

Therapy for acute hyperkalemia involves counteracting the depressant effects on the heart and mobilizing the K^+ from the plasma. Mobilize K^+ from the plasma into the cardiac cells, as well as into cells throughout the body, by administering *glucose (10% to 50%), insulin,* and *Na^+ bicarbonate.* (Remember, K^+ is transported into cells in the presence of glucose and insulin for use in anabolic processes.) Insulin also stimulates the Na^+-K^+ pump, which causes more K^+ to be pumped back into the cell.[31,57] Administering bicarbonate produces an alkalotic effect, which also moves K^+ into the cells in exchange for H^+. This mode of therapy is particularly indicated when the mechanism of the hyperkalemic ECG changes is an acidosis. Administering inhaled beta-2 sympathetic stimulating agents such as albuterol (Ventolin) may move K^+ into the cell.[33,57]

Also consider giving sodium (bicarbonate) and calcium (chloride or gluconate) in hyperkalemia as cardiac stimulants. Calcium acts to lower the threshold potential, thus enhancing excitability, and may counteract some of the calcium binding produced by the bicarbonate administration.[57] Therapy for chronic hyperkalemia is directed towards removing K^+ from the body. This goal is accomplished with dialysis or cation exchange resins such as sodium polystyrene sulfonate (Kayexalate). Kayexalate exchanges Na^+ for K^+ in the GI tract. Administer it rectally or orally, together with sorbitol, which exerts an osmotic effect, further promoting K^+ excretion and preventing constipation. Diuretics can also be administered in the presence of an adequate urine output.[7,41,52,57] Table 4-1 summarizes potassium imbalances.

CALCIUM IMBALANCES

The calcium ion is important in electrical impulse conduction and in cardiac, vascular, and smooth muscle contractility. Calcium acts as the link between electrical and mechanical activity (Fig. 4-20). Ca^{++} is also important in blood clotting and in bone matrix formation. The first two effects are the major considerations in coronary care. The normal serum Ca^{++} is 8.5 to 10.5 mg/dl.

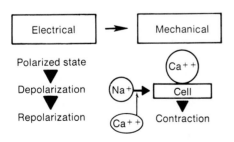

Fig. 4-20   Role of calcium in linking electrical and mechanical activity.

Calcium is carried within the blood in three forms: (1) *free or ionized,* (2) *bound to serum proteins* (primarily albumin), and (3) *bound to other anions* such as citrate, phosphate, and bicarbonate.[7,40,54,59] The ionized fraction is the most important because it causes virtually all of the physiologic effects of calcium. About one half of the total serum calcium is normally ionized. Commonly reported serum Ca^{++} levels usually reflect *total* serum Ca^{++} and do not differentiate between ionized and bound calcium. Methods for measuring ionized calcium levels are available at some institutions and allow for more complete analysis of Ca^{++} imbalances. The normal *ionized* serum Ca^{++} is 4.0 to 5.0 mg/dl (1.17 to 1.29 mm/L).[7,31,38,54]

GI absorption of calcium requires vitamin D. Calcium is excreted by the kidneys as well as regulated by the hormones parathormone, which is secreted by the parathyroid gland, and calcitonin, secreted by the thyroid gland. *Parathormone* secretion requires magnesium. Parathormone raises the serum calcium in three ways: (1) by promoting Ca^{++} absorption from the GI tract, (2) by promoting Ca^{++} release from bone stores, and (3) by promoting Ca^{++} resorption in the renal tubules in exchange for phosphate ($HPO_4^=$) excretion. Generally, if Ca^{++} levels increase, $HPO_4^=$ levels decrease. If $HPO_4^=$ levels increase, Ca^{++} levels decrease. *Thyrocalcitonin* (calcitonin) blocks mobilization of Ca^{++} from bone stores, therefore lowering the serum Ca^{++}.

Hypocalcemia

Hypocalcemia may occur as a result of protein loss, alkalosis, renal failure, transfusions of stored blood, hemodilution secondary to cardiopulmonary bypass, acute pancreatitis, or surgical resection of the parathyroid or thyroid gland. Calcium may also be lost as a result of diarrhea or the effects of diuretics such as furosemide (Lasix). The most common cause of hypocalcemia in coronary care is probably an underlying alkalosis. Alkalosis promotes the binding of calcium to serum proteins. The level of free or ionized calcium then falls, resulting in symptoms of hypocalcemia. The total blood calcium level usually remains unchanged, so the serum Ca^{++} level may appear normal without a separate measurement of the ionized portion.

Patients with chronic renal failure often have arteriosclerotic vascular disease involving the heart and may undergo treatment in the CCU. In chronic renal failure, hypocalcemia results from decreased excretion of $HPO_4^=$ and decreased activation of vitamin D. In hyperphosphatemia, calcium levels decrease as a result of binding with the phosphate, precipitation, and subsequent excretion.[1,7,41]

The signs and symptoms of hypocalcemia are generally divided into those related to skeletal and smooth muscle, those affecting the cardiac muscle or electrical activity, and those affecting the ECG. The effect of hypocalcemia on skeletal and smooth muscle is related to the ion's effect during depolarization. When the serum Ca^{++} levels fall, less Ca^{++} is available to repel Na^+ entry. As a result, repetitive depolarization of nerve cells occurs, resulting in increased motor neuron firing. This increase in neuromuscular irritability may result in the repetitive skeletal muscle contractions known as *tetany*. Skeletal muscle contraction remains normal with decreased serum Ca^{++} levels because of rich intracellular calcium stores. In addition to tetany, the symptoms of increased motor and/or sensory nerve discharge include tremors, skeletal muscle spasms, numbness or paresthesias of the fingers, toes, and face,[41] and intestinal cramps. Skeletal and smooth muscle spasms may be manifested by the typical carpopedal spasm or by bronchospasm, laryngospasm, dyspnea, or difficulty in talking. Positive Chvostek's and Trousseau's signs are also associated with the skeletal muscle irritability of hypocalcemia. A *positive Chvostek's sign* is twitching of the facial muscles in response to tapping of the facial nerve in front of the ear. A *positive Trousseau's sign* is spasm of the thumb muscle precipitated by occlusion of blood flow to the hand with a blood pressure cuff, temporarily decreasing the available Ca^{++} further.[32] Decreased vascular smooth muscle contraction can result in vasodilation and hypotension. Bruising and bleeding may also occur with hypocalcemia because of impaired coagulation. Investigators have also reported CNS changes.[59] Thus, both the peripheral and central nervous systems may be involved.[47]

In cardiac muscle, contraction is *directly* and primarily dependent on extracellular

Ca^{++} movement since intracellular Ca^{++} stores are minimal. Thus the effects of hypocalcemia on cardiac muscle are primarily related to the role of the ion in contractility—that is, mechanical activity. When ionized calcium decreases, myocardial contractility decreases, potentiating heart failure. Neuromuscular symptoms need not be present for this effect to occur.[59] All inotropic agents also depend on Ca^{++} to work. They may, therefore, be ineffective in the presence of hypocalcemia.[31] Electrical effects may also appear. Electrical instability occurs, resulting in cardiac arrhythmias.

Calcium effects on the ECG are most noticeable between depolarization and active repolarization or within the *ST segment*. In the presence of hypocalcemia, the ST segment is prolonged (Fig. 4-21). This change is equally visible on all standard leads. Since the ST segment is contained within the QT interval, changes in the ST segment also affect the QT interval. There is no effect on either the T wave or the QRS complex. In renal failure, hypocalcemia often occurs in combination with hyperkalemia. A clear ST segment in combination with T wave peaking is diagnostic.

Therapy for hypocalcemia consists of correcting the underlying problem and administering calcium, magnesium, vitamin D, and/or protein supplements. In renal failure, control calcium levels by lowering the serum phosphate with phosphate binders such as Amphojel and Basojel. Always evaluate hypocalcemia in light of acid-base findings. Reserve calcium administration for symptomatic patients.[59] The calcium salts most commonly used for acute replacement therapy are calcium chloride and calcium gluconate. In the adult, calcium chloride is usually preferred because of its higher calcium content and its more consistent effect on ionized Ca^{++}.[31] Administer calcium by the intravenous route *slowly* (except in a cardiac arrest situation to avoid vagal effects on the SA node and/or blocking of Na^{+}-dependent fibers). The usual suggested dose of IV calcium is 100 to 200 mg of "elemental" calcium, or 4 to 7 ml of 10% calcium chloride,[31,40,59] diluted in 50 to 100 ml and administered over 10 to 20 minutes.[1,7] Some

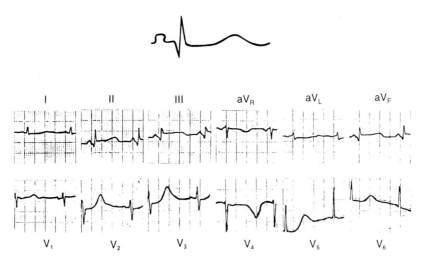

Fig. 4-21 ECG changes in hypocalcemia.

authors recommend faster administration rates of up to 2 to 5 minutes.[31,54] Because of calcium's short half-life, follow these IV bolus doses by a drip of 50 to 200 mg of elemental Ca^{++} (1 to 2 mg/kg) per hour.[7,31,59] For treatment of hyperkalemia, typically administer slightly higher concentrations (ie, 10 to 20 ml of 10% CaCl) over 5 to 10 minutes.[31] Do *not* administer calcium intravenously in conjunction with sodium bicarbonate, because precipitation will occur. A variety of oral calcium supplements are also available. These include Ca^{++} carbonate, Ca^{++} lactate, Ca^{++} gluconate, Os-Cal, Tums, and Titralac. Dietary supplements include milk and dairy products.

Hypercalcemia

Hypercalcemia occurs most commonly in the presence of malignancies and in conditions that promote release of Ca^{++} from bone stores. Parathormone-like chemicals are secreted by a variety of tumors, resulting in an increased serum Ca^{++}. Disorders associated with bone demineralization and Ca^{++} release include hyperparathyroidism secondary to renal failure, immobility, and multiple fractures.[32] Practitioners should encourage patients to ambulate as soon as possible to decrease the effects of immobility. Both hypercalcemia and hypocalcemia may occur in renal failure, although the latter is more common.[41] Hypercalcemia is *uncommon* in the CCU. However, hypercalemia may occur in certain collagen diseases affecting the heart (e.g., sarcoidosis) and in myocardial tumors. Both of these disorders are associated with increased serum protein, increased total serum calcium, and increased bound calcium.

The signs and symptoms of hypercalcemia are generally opposite to those of hypocalcemia. In hypercalcemia, more Ca^{++} is available to line pores of the cell and repel the Na^+ ion. Therefore, depolarization and neuromuscular activity are depressed. Signs of skeletal muscle depression include lethargy and muscle weakness. Signs of smooth muscle depression include the GI symptoms of constipation, nausea, and vomiting. Symptoms of neurologic depression reflect involvement of the CNS and the peripheral nervous system.[47] These include headache, apathy, and altered levels of consciousness.

The effects of Ca^{++} on the heart muscle reflect the role of Ca^{++} during mechanical activity. When ionized Ca^{++} increases, myocardial contractility decreases. Although mild increases in contractility may be beneficial, excess serum levels of Ca^{++} may result in extreme spastic contraction of the myocardium and interfere with relaxation. The ECG effect of Ca^{++} is on the ST segment. Hypercalcemia causes the ST segment to shorten and/or disappear (Fig. 4-22). Little if any space is visible between the QRS complex and the T wave. However, hypercalcemia does not affect either the QRS complex or the T wave.

With hypercalcemia, Ca^{++} deposits may be evident in body tissues, especially within the *renal medulla*. An early sign of hypercalcemia is polyuria caused by impaired renal concentrating ability. Renal calculi may also form. Osteoporosis with pathologic fractures and bone pain may result from depletion of bone Ca^{++} stores in response to increased demands for Ca^{++} release into the serum.

Therapy for hypercalcemia consists of the following: (1) correcting the underlying cause; (2) promoting Ca^{++} excretion by the kidneys; (3) directly suppressing serum Ca^{++} levels; and (4) binding excess ionized calcium. To facilitate elimination of Ca^{++} by the kidneys, administer saline and diuretics. Accomplish direct suppression of serum Ca^{++} levels by adminstering *calcitonin* or *steroids* or both. Steroids promote the movement of Ca^{++} into the cells and compete with vitamin D to minimize GI resorption

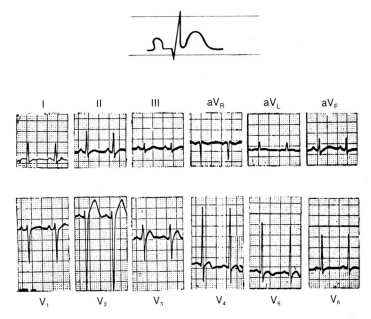

I   II   III   aV_R   aV_L   aV_F

V_1   V_2   V_3   V_4   V_5   V_6

Fig. 4-22   ECG changes in hypercalcemia.

and inhibit osteoclast activity[7] to prevent mobilization of Ca^{++} from bone stores. One method of binding excess ionized calcium is by administering sodium bicarbonate. The chemotherapy agent plicamycin (mithramycin) is effective in controlling the hypercalcemia associated with a variety of neoplasms via a toxic effect on the osteoclasts.[7,36,40] Side effects include bone marrow depression and toxic effects on the liver and/or kidney.[36] The biphosphonate etidronate

(Didronel) also inhibits the function of the osteoclasts.[7,36,40] Reduce the dose of this agent and mithramycin by one half in the patient with renal failure[36]. Also consider dialysis to treat hypercalcemia. Administering IV or oral phosphates such as Neutra-Phos or Fleet's Phospho-Soda to bind calcium and facilitate its excretion[32,41] is not a preferred mode of therapy because of the risk of toxic hyperphosphatemia.[36,40] Table 4-2 summarizes calcium imbalances.

MAGNESIUM IMBALANCES

Magnesium is closely related to other cations involved in the electrical and mechanical activity of the heart and is equally important. It is a necessary activator of the enzyme ATPase, which causes splitting of the ATP molecule with energy release. Thus, Mg^{++} is important in the normal function of the Na^+-K^+ pump, which requires ATP to function. Through this function, Mg^{++} controls serum K^+ levels. Splitting of ATP is required for *mechanical* activity as well as *electrical* activity. Energy from ATP breakdown is required to move the contractile proteins actin and myosin. Energy is also required for the transfer of Ca^{++} out of the myofibrils to allow for muscle relaxation.[55]

Mg^+ is also necessary for parathormone secretion and thus influences serum Ca^{++}

Table 4-2. Calcium imbalances

	↓ Ca^{++} Hypocalcemia	↑ Ca^{++} Hypercalcemia
Neuromuscular	• Tetany/tremors • Carpopedal spasm • Numbness • Paresthesias • + Chvostek's • + Trousseau's • Abdominal cramps • Bronchospasm • CNS changes	• Weakness • Constipation • Nausea/vomiting • CNS changes (headache/apathy/ LOC)
Heart	• ↓ Contractility • Arrhythmias	• ↑ Contractility

ECG	Prolonged
	  ST segment
		Shortened
		  ST segment

Other	• Bruising • Bleeding	• Renal calculi • Osteoporosis
Therapy	• IV/Oral Ca^{++} • Mg^{++} • Vitamin D • PKO supplements • Phosphate binders • Correct alkalosis • ↑ Dietary Ca^{++}	• Saline • Diuretics • Calcitonin • Steroids • Na$^+$ bicarbonate • Mithramycin • Didronel • Dialysis • IV/oral phosphates
Dietary Sources	Milk/dairy products	

levels, altering both the electrical and mechanical effects of Ca^{++}. Thus, Mg^{++} controls both serum K$^+$ and serum Ca^{++} levels. The practitioner should suspect hypomagnesemia in the presence of a combined hypokalemia and hypocalcemia.

In addition to influencing serum calcium levels, magnesium directly influences calcium transport in skeletal muscle, smooth muscle, and cardiac electrical and mechanical structures. Magnesium inhibits both the cardioactive and vasoactive effects of calcium. Its actions mimic those of calcium channel blockers except Mg^{++} is less selective[42,48,55,56] (see Unit 9). In the patient with an acute MI, magnesium may have an antiarrhythmic and anti-hypertensive effect, reverse coronary spasm, inhibit the release of catecholamines (sympathetic chemicals) and thrombus formation, and prevent the accumulation of intracellular calcium associated with reperfusion injury (see Unit 5).[34,46,48,49,51] Magnesium infusion may be beneficial in myocardial preservation and reperfusion injury. Two current studies—LIMIT-2 (Leicester Intravenous Magnesium Trial) and ISIS-4 (Fourth International Study of Infarction Survival)—are testing this hypothesis.[45] Mg^{++} may also offer protection against the formation of atherosclerotic lesions. This effect is at least partially due to Mg^{++} binding with fats in the intestinal tract with decreased fat absorption and circulating lipoproteins.[51] Investigators have also reported bronchodilating effects.[49]

Mg^{++} is primarily an intracellular cation. In addition to its role in the Na^+–K^+ pump, it is used in protein synthesis and acts as a co-factor in @ 300 enzymatic reactions.[41,49] Therefore, *serum* Mg levels are normally low.

Hypomagnesemia

Mg^{++} deficits may occur as a result of deficient intake, increased loss, or decreased absorption. The critically ill patient may have an incidence as high as 60% to 65%.[35] In the coronary care setting the most common cause of decreased Mg^{++} levels is *diuretic therapy*. Mg^{++} is excreted by the kidneys and GI tract. With diuretic therapy, Mg^{++} loss generally parallels K^+ loss. Investigators have postulated that effective therapy for diuretic-induced hypokalemia may also require supplementary magnesium administration. Low serum Mg^{++} levels unrelated to renal losses typically occur in the first 48 hours after MI,[45,46,49] and have been associated with significant ectopy.[31] These low levels may be due to an intracellular Mg^{++} shift with formation of Mg^{++} soaps in response to the release of catecholamines (sympathetic chemicals).[7,35,46] Low Mg^{++} levels can potentiate coronary vasospasm and hypertension and have been associated with sudden cardiac death.[49,56]

Hypomagnesemia[49] may also be associated with GI losses from diarrhea, vomiting, intestinal drains, or the excessive use of laxatives common in the elderly. Hypomagnesemia commonly occurs in chronic alcoholism, probably resulting from a combination of predisposing factors, such as inadequate dietary sources, impaired absorption or GI loss caused by associated GI disturbances, pancreatitis, and renal losses associated with alcohol's diuretic effects. The elderly alcoholic patient receiving laxatives, diuretics, or both may easily have an acute MI. At that time, this patient is at risk for devel-

The normal serum Mg^{++} level is 1.8 to 2.4 mg/dl. Magnesium's effect on the ECG is less characteristic than that of potassium and calcium, although it often affects the T wave, which may be due to its close relationship to K^+. Calcium effects may also contribute to the ECG effects.[6,51]

oping the side effect of hypomagnesemia, aggravating the complications of acute MI. Hypomagnesemia is also common in patients with chronic obstructive pulmonary disease (COPD) and respiratory failure.[39,42] Medications associated with renal Mg^{++} losses in addition to the diuretics include aminoglycosides, cardiac glycosides (digitalis), cyclosporine, amphotericin, and terbutaline.[35,39,49,55]

The signs and symptoms of hypomagnesemia are linked with neuromuscular irritability and instability. Increased smooth muscle, skeletal muscle (peripheral nervous system), and central nervous system irritability occur in response to related Ca^{++} deficits. Increased cardiac instability (automaticity) and chronic myopathies occur in response to related K^+ deficits. Skeletal muscle symptoms of hypomagnesemia include leg cramps, muscle spasms, twitching, tremors, hyperreflexia, paresthesias, and tetany. Low-magnesium tetany has been reported even with normal serum Ca^{++} levels. CNS symptoms include confusion, disorientation, coma, and seizures. Delirium tremens has been attributed to low Mg^{++} in some cases. Patients have also reported nausea, vomiting, and diarrhea.[32]

The most commonly cited cardiac symptoms are ventricular arrhythmias, leading to or potentiating ventricular fibrillation (VF) especially with the *torsades de pointes* pattern (see Unit 11). Magnesium therapy has been effective in selected cases of "refractory" VF and should at least be considered in such cases. Hypomagnesia enhances the potential for developing digitalis toxicity, since digitalis also has an effect on the Na^+-K^+ pump (see Unit 9). Hypomagnesemia enhances the myocardial uptake of digitalis. Patients also have experienced supraventricular arrhythmias.[42,46,48,49] Prophylactic magnesium infusions and/or bolus injections administered in the first 24 to 48 hours of acute MI can decrease the incidence of both significant ventricular and supraventricular arrhythmias.[34,35,45,46] These infusions may become part of the routine management of acute MI in the near future.[46] The ECG effects of hypomagnesemia may be similar to those in either hypokalemia or hypocalcemia[51] but are more variable. Flattening of the T wave, appearance of a U wave, and TU fusion[1,30,32,55] can result, especially with severe Mg^{++} deficiency.[51] ECG effects may also include inverted T waves,[1,3,31,49] wide QRS complexes,[31,40] prolonged P–R intervals,[31,32,40] and ST depression,[1,49] although the mechanism is unclear. Early K^+ losses from the cell can result in peaked T waves secondary to a transient elevation in serum K^+.[51]

Therapy for Mg^{++} deficits consists of magnesium sulfate administered by parenteral routes and dietary supplementation. (Dietary sources include meat, seafood, nuts, green vegetables, whole grains, dairy products, and chocolate.[1,51,58]) Note that magnesium is administered significantly differently when used for arrhythmia control as opposed to correction of low serum values. For management of ventricular arrhythmias such as torsades de pointes, administer Mg^{++} in higher dosages of 1 to 2 g of magnesium sulfate salt over 1 to 2 minutes, IV,[31,40,40a,42] followed by a second bolus of 2-4 g after 10-15 min, if necessary (see Unit 11).[7] Consider prophylactic infusions of 8 g in 500 ml of D5W at 8 ml per hour in acute MI.[34] For low serum Mg levels, generally administer IV magnesium sulfate at a dose of 32 to 48 mEq Mg^{++} or 4 to 6 g of magnesium sulfate, diluted at least 1:10 to avoid venous sclerosis, over 1 to 3 hours.[31,32,34,54,55] Monitor serum Mg^{++} levels after each 16 mEq.[32] Intramuscular magnesium replacement or oral replacement as in the form of magnesium-containing antacids may also be beneficial.[55] The toxic effects of IV magnesium sulfate administration mimic hypermagnesemia. The most marked are *hypotension, respiratory arrest,* and *bradycardia.* Transient flushing may also occur.[45] Deep tendon reflexes should be monitored.[40,42,54–56,58]

Hypermagnesemia

Hypermagnesemia is uncommon in the coronary care setting. Renal failure and exogenous magnesium administration are the most frequent causes. Hypermagnesemia occurs in renal failure as a result of decreased excretion and the ingestion of magnesium-containing antacids. Hypermagnesemia may result from excessive magnesium administration in obstetric settings or, more recently, where magnesium is used to prevent hypertension or premature labor.

Increased Mg^{++} levels decrease neuromuscular irritability by inhibiting Ca^{++} transport. Mg^{++} inhibits Ca^{++} transport in the CNS, skeletal muscles (peripheral nervous system), and smooth muscle. Hypermagnesemia may result in CNS depression, respiratory arrest, loss of deep tendon reflexes, and hypotension. The hypotension may be partially due to the inhibition of the vascular slow (Ca^{++}) channels.[45] Mg^{++} also inhibits the cardiac slow channels, resulting in bradycardia.[48]

The ECG effects of hypermagnesemia may be similar to those of hyperkalemia. They include peaking of the T waves and widening of the QRS complex.[30,31,56]

Routine therapy for hypermagnesemia consists of stopping the infusion or correcting the underlying cause. The depressant ef-

Table 4-3. Magnesium imbalances

	↓ Mg++ Hypomagnesemia	↑ Mg++ Hypermagnesemia
Neuromuscular	• Tetany/tremors • Muscle spasms • Hyperreflexia • Paresthesias • Nausea/vomiting • Diarrhea • CNS changes	• Hyporeflexia • Respiratory arrest • Hypotension
Heart	• PVCs/VT/VF • Torsades de pointes • Digitalis toxicity • Supraventricular arrhythmias	• Bradycardia
ECG	• ↑ T wave (early) • ↓ T wave (flat/inverted) • Appearance of U wave • TU fusion • ST depression • Prolonged P–R intervals • QRS widening	• ↑ T wave • QRS widening
Therapy	• IV/IM/Oral Mg++ • ↑ Dietary Mg++	• Stop infusion • Ca++ Cl/gluconate • Fluids and diuretics • Dialysis • Glucose and insulin
Dietary Sources	Meat, seafood, nuts, whole grains, green vegetables, dairy products, chocolate	

fects on muscle may be counteracted with a stimulant such as calcium[58] (e.g., calcium gluconate, 1 g over 3 minutes, or CaCl, 100 to 200 mg every 3 to 5 minutes).[40] If the patient has an adequate urine output, IV fluids plus diuretics may be administered. Dialysis is used in the absence of urine output. Glucose and insulin can also be used to shift Mg++ into the cell.[41,49] Table 4-3 summarizes magnesium imbalances.

SELF-ASSESSMENT

1 A charged particle, or ion, may be loosely referred to clinically as a(n) _____.

Positively charged particles or (cations/anions) are most significant because of their role in (electrical events/acid-base).

electrolyte

cations

electrical events

2 The polarized state is determined primarily by _____. On the single cell ECG or action potential, the polarized state is depicted by phase _____.

Depolarization is determined by _____ influx in fast cells such as the _____ and by _____ influx in slow cells such as the _____ and the _____. On the single cell ECG or action potential, depolarization is illustrated by phase _____.

The $Na^+–K^+$ pump actively pumps Na^+ _____ the cell and K^+ _____ the cell, establishing a _____ gradient for each ion. It requires the electrolyte _____ to break down _____ for energy.

K^+

4

Na^+
Purkinje fibers; Ca^{++}
SA node; AV junction

O

out of
into; concentration
Mg^{++}
ATP

3 Automaticity is a property of (stable/unstable) cells. The resting cell charge of these cells is typically (more/less) negative than that of nonautomatic cells, thus favoring (Na^+/Ca^{++}) channel depolarization.

The property of automaticity is also called phase _____ or spontaneous _____ depolarization. The level of membrane potential at which an action potential is generated is known as the _____. Lowering the threshold allows the cell to generate an impulse (more/less) easily.

unstable

less
Ca^{++}

4
diastolic

threshold

more

4 The two electrolyte imbalances most common in the patient with an acute MI are _____ and _____.

A common cause of hyperkalemia is _____ failure. Increases in serum K^+ also occur in (acidosis/alkalosis). ECG effects include peaking of the _____ wave, widening of the _____, and loss of the _____ wave. These changes are most visible on leads _____. In addition to dialysis, therapy includes _____, _____, _____, and _____.

The most common cause of hypokalemia is _____ therapy. ECG effects include flattening of the _____ wave, appearance of a _____ wave, and _____ fusion.

hypokalemia; hypomagnesemia
renal
acidosis
T; QRS complex

P
V2 to V4
glucose; Ca^{++}; insulin
Kayexalate
diuretic
T
U; T–U

5 Ca^{++} is carried within the blood in _____ forms. It may be bound to _____ or other _____. However, the physiologic effects are produced by the free, or _____, form.

Hypocalcemia may occur in _____ failure, (acidosis/alkalosis), _____ blood, and _____ embolism. The characteristic ECG effect is a prolonged _____. Signs and symptoms include positive _____ and _____ signs. _____ failure may also occur. Therapy includes calcium, _____, and _____ supplementation and _____ binders.,

The most common cause of hypercalcemia is _____. Ther-

three
protein; anions
ionized
renal; alkalosis
stored; fat
ST segment
Chvostek's; Trousseau's
Heart
magnesium; vitamin D
phosphate
cancer

apy includes saline and _____, direct suppression by _____ or _____, inhibition of osteoclast activity by the chemotherapy agent _____ and _____, and binding of calcium with _____ or _____.

diuretics
calcitonin; steroids
mithramycin
biphosphonates
bicarbonate; phosphates

6 The actions of Mg^{++} are like _____ blockade. These actions include (increased/decreased) blood pressure and heart rate and reversal of coronary _____. Inhibited Ca^{++} transport in skeletal muscle can result in _____ depression and decreased deep _____.

calcium channel
decreased
spasm
respiratory
tendon reflexes

Hypomagnesemia typically occurs in the first _____ hours following acute MI due to _____ shifts in response to _____ release. Hypomagnesemia is also associated with an increase in _____ and _____ arrhythmias.

48
intracellular
catecholamine
ventricular; supraventricular

The ECG characteristics of Mg^{++} imbalances (are/are not) as characteristic as those of K^+ and Ca^{++}. However, they most closely mimic the ECG changes of (K^+/Ca^{++}).

are not

K^+

7 The plasma is part of the (intracellular/extracellular) fluid compartment. The concentration of the plasma or serum is measured by the serum _____, which is determined primarily by the cation _____ and the noncharged particles _____ and _____. The concentration of IV solutions is measured by their _____.

extracellular

osmolality
Na^+; glucose
urea
osmolarity

8 Fluids or solutions having the same concentration in relation to each other are referred to as *iso-osmolar* or _____. A solution with a greater isotonic concentration of dissolved particles is referred to as (hypertonic/hypotonic). A solution with a lesser concentration of dissolved particles is referred to as (hypertonic/hypotonic).

isotonic

hypertonic
hypotonic

Clinical states that may result in hypertonicity of the plasma include diabetes insipidus, alcohol intoxication, and _____ _____. With hypertonic plasma, fluid moves (into/out of) the cells, causing them to become (bloated/dehydrated). The amount of fluid in the plasma or vascular compartment is initially (increased/decreased). However, when this fluid is excreted by the kidneys (hypervolemia/hypovolemia) occurs.

diabetes mellitus
out of
dehydrated
increased
hypovolemia

Clinical states that may result in hypotonicity of the plasma include _____ , _____ failure, and the use of _____ agents.

SIADH; liver/congestive heart
diuretic

9 In both hypervolemia and hypovolemia, the plasma osmolality (is hypotonic/is hypertonic/varies). The most common cause of fluid overload (hypervolemia) in the coronary care unit is _____

varies
congestive heart

Table 4-4. Osmolarity and electrolyte content of commonly used crystalloid IV fluids

Solution	Glucose	Na$^+$	Cl$^-$	Other
Isotonic*				
Normal saline (0.9% Na$^+$Cl$^-$)	—	×	×	—
D5W (5% dextrose in water)†	×	—	—	—
D5¼NS (5% dextrose in 0.25% Na$^+$Cl$^-$)	×	×	×	—
RL/LR (ringers lactate/lactated ringers)	—	×	×	K$^+$, Ca^{++}, lactate (HCO$_3^-$)
Ringers	—	×	×	K$^+$, Ca^{++}
Hypertonic				
D5⅓NS (5% dextrose in 0.33% Na$^+$Cl$^-$)	×	×	×	—
D5½NS (5% dextrose in 0.45% Na$^+$Cl$^-$)	×	×	×	—
D5NS (5% dextrose in 0.9% Na$^+$Cl$^-$)	×	×	×	—
D10.2NS (10% dextrose in 0.25 Na$^+$Cl$^-$)	×	×	×	—
3% NS (3% Na$^+$Cl$^-$)	—	×	×	—
Plasmalyte 56 D5W (similar to Normosol M)	×	×	×	K$^+$, Mg^{++}, acetate
Plasmalyte 148 D5W (similar to Normosol R)	×	×	×	K$^+$, Mg^{++}, acetate
Hypotonic				
½NS (0.45% Na$^+$Cl$^-$)	—	×	×	—
Plasmalyte 56 H$_2$O	—	×	×	K$^+$, Mg^{++}, acetate

*Osmolarity within @ 50 mOsm above or below normal serum osmolality.[8,12,31]
†Considered hypotonic by some authorities, since the glucose is metabolized quickly, leaving free water.[10,29]

_____ failure. In this setting the serum Na$^+$ is typically (high/low) because of the release of the hormones _____ (osmoreceptor stimulation) and _____ (pressoreceptor stimulation) in response to a low _____. Stimulation of atrial stretch receptors compensates only partially, causing the release of _____ natriuretic peptide, (ADH/aldosterone) inhibition, and _____ excretion. In this setting, the serum osmolality is (high/low).

> low
> ADH
> aldosterone
> cardiac; output
>
> atrial; aldosterone
> fluid
> low

10 The edema associated with congestive heart failure is due to the excess fluid, hypotonicity, and changes in capillary (pressure/permeability). This edema formation is facilitated by fluid (overload/depletion) and low serum _____.

Edema typically refers to fluid accumulation in the (intracellular/interstitial) space.

> pressure
> overload
> Na$^+$
> interstitial

11 The most common Na$^+$ imbalance in the coronary care unit is (hyponatremia/hypernatremia). This may accompany (fluid overload/fluid depletion/both). Thus, a more accurate method of determining the fluid status is by _____ monitoring.

ECG changes (do/do not) typically occur with serum Na$^+$ imbalances. Symptoms predominantly involve the (central/peripheral) nervous systems. The most serious symptom of hyponatremia is _____.

> hyponatremia
> both
>
> hemodynamic
> do not
> central
> seizures

12 The most common cause of hypovolemia in the patient in a coronary care unit is _____ therapy. As in congestive heart failure, the serum Na^+ is typically (high/low) and (central/peripheral) nervous system symptoms may occur. Additional symptoms are associated with the volume depletion, including signs of (increased/decreased) cardiac output and _____.

    Isotonic (or minimally hypotonic) crystalloid solutions such as _____ and _____ may be used for fluid replacement. In patients with heart disease, D5W is preferred due to the absence of (Na^+/Ca^{++}). Albumin may also be used since it stays in the circulation for (shorter/longer) periods and exerts a _____ osmotic effect. Synthetic plasma expanders acting similar to albumin include _____ and _____.

    Table 4-4 gives the osmolarity and electrolyte content of commonly used crystalloid IV fluids.

diuretic

low; central

decreased
dehydration

D5W
LR/RL NS
Na^+
longer; colloid
dextran
Hespan

REFERENCES/SUGGESTED READINGS
General/sodium imbalances

1. Alspach JG, editor: AACN core curriculum for critical-care nurses, ed 4, Philadelphia, 1991, WB Saunders.
2. Anandi IS et al: Edema of cardiac origin: studies of body water and sodium, renal function, hemodynamic indexes, and plasma hormones in untreated congestive heart failure, Circulation 80(2):299, 1989.
3. Berne RM, Levy MN: Physiology, ed 6, St. Louis, 1992, Mosby–Year Book.
4. Besunder JB, Smith PG: Toxic effects of electrolyte and trace mineral administration in the intensive care unit, Crit Care Clin 7(3):659, 1991.
5. Bigger JT: Electrical activity of the heart. In Hurst JW, Schlant RB, editors: The heart, arteries, and veins, ed 7, New York, 1990, McGraw-Hill.
6. Braunwald E, editor: Heart disease: a textbook of cardiovascular medicine, ed 4, Philadelphia, 1992, JB Lippincott.
7. Chernow Bart, editor: Essentials of critical care pharmacology, Baltimore, 1989, Williams & Wilkins.
8. Cheveny B: Overview of fluid and electrolytes, Nurs Clin North Am 22(4):749, 1987.
9. Civetta J et al: Critical care, Philadelphia, 1988, JB Lippincott.
10. Dawidson I: Fluid resuscitation of shock: current controversies (editorial), Crit Care Med 17(10):1078, 1989.
11. Gasparis L et al: IV solutions: which one's right for your patient, Nursing 19(4):62, 1989.
12. Graves L: Diabetic ketoacidosis and hyperosmolar hyperglycemic nonketotic coma, Crit Care Nurs Q 13(3):50, 1990.
13. Guyton AC: Textbook of medical physiology, ed 8, Philadelphia, 1991, WB Saunders.
14. Innerarity SA: Electrolyte emergencies in the critically ill renal patient, Crit Care Nurs Clin North Am 2:1, 1990.
15. Isley WL: Serum sodium concentration abnormalities, Crit Care Nurs Q 13(3):82, 1990.
16. Levick JR: An introduction to cardiovascular physiology, London, 1991, Butterworths.
17. Lowell JA et al: Postoperative fluid overload: not a benign problem, Crit Care Med 18(7):728, 1990.
18. Marriott HJ, Conover MB: Advanced concepts in arrhythmias, ed 2, St. Louis, 1989, Mosby–Year Book.
19. Martof M: Part I: fluid balance, J Nephrol Nurs 2(1):10, 1985.
20. McAdams R, McClure K: Hypovolemia: when to suspect it, RN, Dec 1986, p 34.
21. Nearman H, Herman M: Toxic effects of colloids in the intensive care unit, Crit Care Clin 7(3):713, 1991.

22. Paradiso C: Hemofiltration: an alternative to dialysis, Heart Lung 18(3):282, 1989.

23. Riggs JE: Neurologic manifestations of fluid and electrolyte disturbances, Neurol Clin 7(3):509, 1989.

24. Shapiro BA et al: Clinical application of respiratory care, ed 3, Chicago, 1985, Year Book Publishers.

25. Sommers M: Rapid fluid resuscitation: how to correct dangerous deficits, Nursing 20(1):52, 1990.

26. Sweetwood HM: Clinical electrocardiography for nurses, Gaithersburg, MD, 1989, Aspen Publications.

27. Valle BA, Lemberg L: Vignettes in coronary care: effective technique of controlling volume in refractory congestive heart failure, Heart Lung 16(6):712, 1987.

28. Weldy NJ: Body fluids and electrolytes: a programmed presentation, ed 6, St. Louis, 1992, Mosby–Year Book.

29. Zipes D, Jalife J: Cardiac electrophysiology: from cell to bedside, Philadelphia, 1990, WB Saunders.

Potassium, calcium, and magnesium imbalances

30. Assessing electrolyte imbalances: a fast reference for these potentially life-threatening abnormalities, Nursing 21(7):32L, 1991.

31. Besunder J, Smith P: Toxic effects of electrolyte and trace mineral administration in the intensive care unit, Crit Care Clin 7:3, 1991.

32. Calloway C: When the problem involves magnesium, calcium, or phosphate, RN 50(5):30, 1987.

33. Calhoun KA: Serum potassium concentration abnormalities, Crit Care Nurs Q 13(3):34, 1990.

34. Ceremuzynski L et al: Threatening arrhythmias in acute myocardial infarction are prevented by intravenous magnesium sulfate, Am Heart J 118(6):1333, 1989.

35. Chernow B et al: Hypomagnesemia in post-op intensive care patients, Chest 95:391, 1989.

36. Davis K, Attie M: Management of severe hypercalcemia, Crit Care Clin 7(1):175, 1991.

37. De Angelis R et al: Hypokalemia, Crit Care Nurse 11(7):71, 1991.

38. Desai TK et al: Prevalence and clinical implications of hypocalcemia in acutely ill patients in a medical intensive care setting, Am J Med 84:209, 1988.

39. Fiaccador E et al: Muscle and serum magnesium in pulmonary intensive care unit patients, Crit Care Med 16(8):751, 1988.

39a. Gettes L: Electrolytes abnormalities underlying lethal and ventricular arrythmias, Circulation 85(Suppl I): I-70, 1992.

40. Graves L: Disorders of calcium, phosphorus, and magnesium, Crit Care Nurs Q 13(3):3, 1990.

40a. Guidelines for cardiopulmonary resuscita- and emergency care: Part III—Adult cardiac life support, JAMA 268(16):2199, 1992.

41. Innerarity SA: Electrolyte emergencies in the critically ill renal patient, Crit Care Nurs Clin North Am 2:1, 1990.

42. Iseri LT: Role of magnesium in cardiac tachyarrhythmias, Am J Cardiol 65(23):47, 1990.

43. Kee J: Potassium imbalance, Nursing 17(9):32, 1987.

44. Lunger DC: Potassium supplementation: how and why? Focus Crit Care 15(5):56, 1988.

45. Magnesium for acute myocardial infarction, Lancet 338(8768):667, 1991.

46. Rasmussen HS et al: Clinical intervention studies on magnesium in myocardial infarction, Magnesium 8(5–6):316, 1989.

47. Riggs JE: Neurologic manifestations of fluid and electrolyte disturbances, Neurol Clin 7(3):509, 1989.

48. Roden DM: Magnesium treatment of ventricular arrhythmias, Am J Cardiol 63(14):43G, 1989.

49. Salem M et al: Hypomagnesemia in critical illness: a common and clinically important problem, Crit Care Clin 7(1):225, 1991.

50. Schuman M, Narins RG: Hypokalemia and cardiovascular disease, Am J Cardiol 65:4E, 1990.

51. Seelig M: Cardiovascular consequences of magnesium deficiency and loss: pathogenesis, prevalence, and manifestations—magnesium and chloride loss in refractory potassium depletion, Am J Cardiol 63(14):4G, 1989.

52. Toto K: When the patient has hyperkalemia, RN 50(4):34, 1987.

53. Toto K: When the patient has hypokalemia, RN 50(3):38, 1987.

54. Underhill S et al: Cardiovascular medications

for cardiac nursing, Philadelphia, 1990, JB Lippincott.

55. Valle G, Lemberg L: Electrolyte imbalances in cardiovascular disease: the forgotten factor, Heart Lung 17(3):324, 1988.

56. Van Hook J: Hypermagnesemia, Crit Care Clin 7(1):155, 1991.

57. Williams ME: Hyperkalemia, Crit Care Clin 7(1):155, 1991.

58. Yarnell RP, Craig MP: Detecting hypomagnesemia: the most overlooked electrolyte imbalance, Nursing 21(7):55, 1991.

59. Zaloga GP: Hypocalcemia in critical illness, Crit Care Clin 7(1):191, 1991.

UNIT 5

Coronary Artery Disease

RELATED SYNDROMES: ACUTE MYOCARDIAL INFARCTION VERSUS ANGINA

Coronary artery disease is manifested by two closely related syndromes—angina and acute myocardial infarction (MI)—as well as by their associated complications. The coronary arteries supply oxygenated blood to the myocardium to meet its metabolic or energy requirements. Since this role is compromised by coronary artery disease, angina and myocardial infarction are considered forms of coronary system failure.

Coronary artery disease includes structural, functional, and metabolic components (Fig. 5-1). The structural coronary changes are the same in both angina and acute MI. Coronary blood supply is diminished and/or interrupted because of a process of coronary narrowing, or *stenosis*, which results in myocardial ischemia.

Three major mechanisms contribute to coronary stenosis: (1) lipid infiltration (atherosclerosis), (2) thrombosis, and (3) coronary spasm. Most cases of acute coronary stenosis or occlusion occur because of atherosclerotic heart disease. Atherosclerosis is characterized by irregular thickening of the intima of the artery, resulting from intimal stress and fatty deposits or lipid infiltration. The thickened area within the intimal lining is also called plaque. Atherosclerosis triggers eventual fibrosis and calcification of the plaque. The roughened atherosclerotic lining can stimulate platelet aggregation and initial clot or *thrombus* formation. Gradual narrowing may occur secondary to progression of atherosclerosis, cracks in the plaque, and platelet aggregation.[91] Sudden rupture or tear in the plaque may also occur. A tear triggers severe platelet aggregation and coronary vasoconstriction or spasm, suddenly and significantly narrowing the lumen. The acute coronary syndromes of unstable angina, MI, and sudden death are thought to be related to these sudden plaque ruptures or tears (Fig. 5-2).[29,91] Fibrin deposition is associated with major tears in the plaque or severe coronary stenosis.[1] Fibrin thrombus formation is often the final event resulting in complete or significant occlusion, usually requiring repeated episodes of thrombus formation.[91] Coronary spasm is common at the site of atherosclerotic lesions[22,34]; it occurs less commonly in the absence of atherosclerotic lesions. Spasm of the coronary arteries is triggered by arterial injury, including plaque rupture and tears; platelet aggregation; and increased sympathetic activity closely related to stress.

Myocardial infarction

Angina and acute MI differ primarily in their functional and metabolic impact. Myocardial infarction (MI) is death, or necrosis, of a section of the cardiac muscle resulting

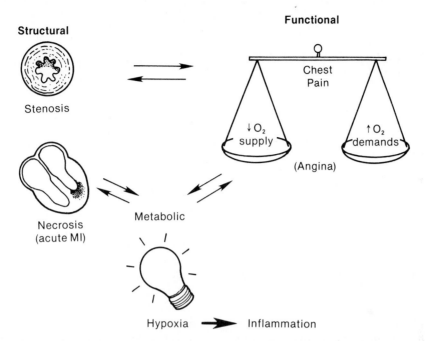

Fig. 5-1 Coronary system failure: structural, functional, and metabolic components. The phases of coronary artery disease or "coronary system failure" form a cycle beginning and ending with structural changes—initially in the coronary arteries and ultimately in the myocardial wall. The relationship between angina and acute MI in this process is illustrated. If uninterrupted, the cycle repeats itself within multiple coronary arteries, adding to the myocardial damage.

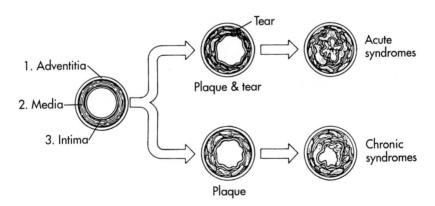

Fig. 5-2 Process of coronary stenosis and occlusion. The three layers of a normal coronary artery *(A)* are illustrated: (1) adventitia, (2) media, and (3) intima. Intimal thickening and atherosclerotic plaque form *(B and C)*, resulting in initial coronary narrowing. Rupture or tear of the plaque *(B)* triggers acute thrombosis, resulting in partial or complete occlusion and their related clinical syndromes. The effects of spasm are not illustrated but occur at any phase.

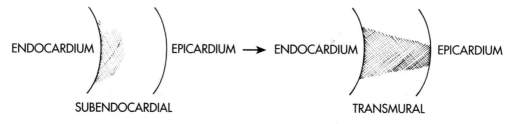

Fig. 5-3   Progression of acute transmural myocardial infarction from subendocardium to epicardium.

from an interrupted or severely diminished supply of oxygenated blood. MI is associated with periods of severe, sustained myocardial hypoxia related typically to coronary occlusion.[91] About 50% of acute MIs occur during sleep or rest, and the other 50% are associated with moderate physical activity and emotional stress.[139] Physical activity and emotional stress cause sympathetic stimulation, which increases blood pressure and predisposes to plaque rupture. Therefore, physical and mental stress are significant acute risk factors for infarction in the patient with existing coronary artery disease.[139]

Most infarctions extend through the entire wall of the heart, from the endocardium to the epicardium, and are thus called *transmural* (Fig. 5-3). Sustained coronary thrombosis has been particularly implicated in transmural MI[22,61] The infarction process, however, begins in and may be limited to the endocardial area.[91] An infarction limited to the en-

docardium and the layer of myocardium adjacent to it is referred to as a *subendocardial* or *nontransmural* infarction (Fig. 5-3). Even in transmural infarction, more damage always occurs in the endocardial area than in the epicardial area. The endocardium has a poorer blood supply than the epicardium and is therefore more vulnerable to a decrease in blood and O_2 supply. Perfusion of the subendocardium is less since the coronary arteries are epicardial vessels with smaller branches feeding the endocardium. In addition, left ventricular filling during diastole exerts pressure against the endocardium, opposing the coronary perfusion of this layer. Other metabolic and unknown factors may also contribute to the subendocardium's vulnerability. Infarctions limited to the subendocardium are more likely to be associated with intermittent occlusion.[61] Angina also typically is associated with involvement of this area.

Angina

In contrast to acute MI, *angina* is a syndrome characterized by chest pain resulting from *transient* myocardial O_2 imbalance and hypoxia. It is *not* usually associated with tissue death. Angina occurs secondary to the same coronary changes that are associated with acute MI. These changes, however, are less severe. Angina can occur either at rest or, more commonly, during exertion. This syndrome is typically triggered by increased

O_2 demands, coronary spasm, or both (Fig. 5-1).

Rest angina is more typically associated with coronary spasm and may occur without atherosclerotic changes. Psychological stress, rather than physical stress, or the effects of cold weather usually trigger rest angina. Smoking and hyperventilation also aggravate rest angina. Cocaine, amphetamines, and some over-the-counter medications aggravate rest angina by causing sympathetic nervous system stimulation.[22,61] Prinzmetal, or "variant," angina is a form of rest angina occurring primarily or exclusively at rest. This form of angina may be associated with transient electrocardiographic (ECG) changes typical of transmural infarction. Prinzmetal angina is often associated with atherosclerotic lesions. Administration of nitrates or calcium channel blocking agents typically relieves the pain of rest angina (see Unit 9). Magnesium may also be beneficial, probably because of its calcium channel blocking effects.[22,61]

Effort, or exertional, angina is more typically associated with increased O_2 demands and "fixed" or permanent atherosclerotic changes. Rest or sublingual nitroglycerin usually rapidly relieves the pain of effort angina. Chronic stable angina is a common form of effort angina associated with episodes recurring over a period of at least 60 days without change in frequency, duration, or precipitating factors.[61]

Acute MI usually does not follow angina. However, one or more episodes of angina, which can act as warning signs, usually precede acute MI. An increase in the frequency, severity, or duration of anginal attacks may indicate that acute MI is imminent. The term *unstable angina* refers to signs and symptoms suggestive of impending infarction. Angina of less than one month onset is considered unstable, especially if precipitated by minimal exertion. Angina at rest, if previously exertional, may also be considered unstable. Terms previously used to describe this type of angina include *crescendo angina, preinfarction angina,* and *acute coronary insufficiency.*[23] Braunwald recently proposed a classification system for unstable angina based on severity (i.e., frequency, time of onset, episodes of rest angina); clinical circumstances (i.e., presence or absence of factors aggravating ischemia such as an infection, thyroid hormones, or anemia); ECG changes; and intensity of therapy required.[23] Most patients with unstable angina either develop acute MI or recover with residual chronic stable angina. These patients require monitoring in a coronary care or a cardiac telemetry unit until their condition stabilizes. They may also be candidates for cardiac catheterization, angioplasty, and/or potential surgical intervention.

Role of collaterals

Collateral vessels linking occluded and patent coronary arteries provide some alternate perfusion to ischemic areas. Gradual development of coronary stenosis promotes the formation of collateral circulation and may naturally occur with aging. Because of these collateral vessels as well as individual variations in O_2 demand and work load tolerance, the degree of stenosis does not always correlate well with the functional or metabolic impact of the disease. The presence of collateral circulation may minimize the detrimental effects of coronary narrowing or occlusion, preventing infarction or minimizing infarction size. Collateral flow may also improve delivery of fibrinolytic agents to a thrombotic lesion. Researchers have reported improved infarct healing with decreased aneurysm formation and increased ejection fractions.[141]

CORONARY ISCHEMIA/REPERFUSION: METABOLIC EFFECTS

The word *metabolism* refers to the chemical processes involving energy release and energy use by the body. Under normal conditions, myocardial cells, unlike other cells in the body, use free fatty acids in preference to glucose as energy (adenosine triphos-

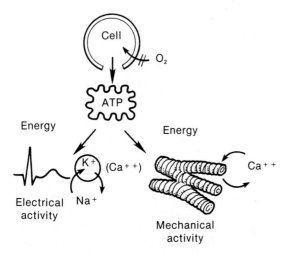

Fig. 5-4   Cardiac electrical and mechanical activity: effects of metabolism, ATP, and hypoxia.

phate, or ATP) sources. (Glucose remains a secondary energy source.) Free fatty acid utilization requires the presence of oxygen. Ischemia inhibits the use of free fatty acids, forcing the heart to rely on glucose. Free fatty acids accumulate as a result of the decreased utilization while glucose utilization increases. These changes may be helpful tracers of ischemia in nuclear diagnostic imaging and can assist in differentiating ischemia from infarction (see Metabolic imaging).

Energy in the form of ATP is required for both electrical and mechanical activity (Fig. 5-4). With ischemia, myocardial hypoxia occurs. In spite of glucose utilization, ATP is depleted with the release of toxins such as lactic acid and free fatty acids. These toxins and others trigger chest pain and arrhythmias. The action of the Na^+–K^+ pump is suppressed because of less available ATP, resulting in intracellular K^+ losses and Na^+ accumulation.[16] (Remember that the Na^+–K^+ pump acts to distribute K^+ back into the cell to maintain a stable polarized state.) With hypoxia, cell membrane permeability also increases, causing further K^+ leakage.[16] These

intracellular K^+ losses result in electrical instability and ventricular arrhythmias. These potassium shifts may also act as tracers of ischemia in nuclear diagnostic imaging.

Because of intracellular Na^+ and water accumulation, intracellular swelling occurs and results in disturbances in mechanical activity in both systole and diastole.[13] This mechanical dysfunction is not necessarily associated with heart failure since the cardiac output may remain unchanged. Systolic changes include asynchronous contraction and wall motion changes, which may be detected with nuclear imaging and echocardiographic techniques. The major diastolic change is a decrease in compliance,[22] which is associated with auscultatory findings (see Unit 8). Hypoxia also acts as a stressor triggering a local inflammatory response that contributes further to edema formation and mechanical dysfunction (see Unit 4 and Stress and Psychological Factors in this unit). Additional toxins released in the presence of inflammation (i.e., histamine, bradykinins, prostaglandins) contribute to the chest pain and electrical instability as well.

Death of tissue (i.e., necrosis or infarction) begins within 20 minutes and is essentially complete within 6 hours.[13,91] Infarction is associated with calcium accumulation inside the cell secondary to ATP depletion. Thus calcium can act as an intracellular tracer for infarction in nuclear diagnostic imaging.

Mechanical dysfunction in the form of wall motion changes can persist up to 1 week even with temporary, reversible ischemia. This phenomenom is referred to as *myocardial "stunning."*[13,17,30,81] Metabolic changes occurring not only during ischemia but also during subsequent reperfusion are thought to be responsible. These changes occur in the presence of therapeutic reperfusion (i.e., thrombolytic therapy, percutaneous transluminal coronary angioplasty [PTCA], coronary bypass surgery) as well as during natural reperfusion (i.e., angina).[13,17,30] Spontaneous reperfusion also occurs in the presence of infarction. When reperfusion occurs within 3 hours, infarction may be limited primarily to the subendocardium with stunning affecting the remainder of the myocardial wall.[17,22]

The metabolic changes associated with myocardial stunning include (1) ATP depletion, (2) myofibril ultrastructure changes, (3) impaired sympathetic response, (4) calcium overload with decreased calcium sensitivity, and (5) oxygen radical release. Myocardial ATP depletion persists for days following severe, reversible ischemia. This change may reflect mitochondrial depletion as well as decreased adenosine diphosphate (ADP) and creatine kinase (CK) isoenzyme activity necessary for ATP formation at contractile protein sites. However, natural and/or artificial restoration of ATP levels does not correlate well with return of myocardial contractility.[17,30,95] Ultrastructural changes such as lengthening of myofibril actin bands, mitochondrial edema and destruction, and damage to the sarcoplastic reticulum (tubular system) occur after 15 minutes of ischemia and can last up to 7 days. Disruption of the collagen matrix and intercalated disks connecting the myocardial cells also occurs.[16,17,30]

Calcium overload and oxygen radical release are the two most popular pathophysiologic theories supporting the changes of myocardial stunning.[16,95] Calcium begins to accumulate inside the cell during severe isch-

emia as well as during infarction as a result of ineffective efflux. Intracellular calcium increases further during reperfusion because of attempts by the Na^+-Ca^{++} exchange system to eliminate the intracellular Na^+ accumulated during the ischemic episode.[17,61,95] This exchange system is ineffective during ischemia because of the effect of acidosis on Ca^{++} uptake and binding. Administration of calcium channel blockers is associated with improved mechanical function when given before the onset of ischemia,[95] presumably by limiting these effects. Calcium overload and impaired sympathetic stimulation can also promote the formation and release of oxygen radicals. Conversely, free radical damage can facilitate Ca^{++} entry and alter the contractile protein responses to calcium.[17,81] Some researchers suggest that calcium fluctuations and high intracellular levels of calcium and free radicals are responsible for the production of reperfusion arrhythmias.[95]

Myocardial dysfunction occurring during chronic ischemia has been called *hibernation*.[22,81] It differs from myocardial stunning since it occurs during rather than after ischemia, is associated with mild to moderate rather than severe ischemia, and is rapidly reversible with no residual ATP, ultrastructure, sympathetic, or O_2 radical changes. Intracellular calcium changes and responsiveness also differ from those reported with stunning.[81]

Oxygen radicals

Oxygen radicals are unstable chemicals containing extra uncombined oxygen electrons. The three most common oxygen radicals are superoxide ($\cdot O_2^-$), hydrogen peroxide (H_2O_2), and hydoxyl ($\cdot OH^-$).[13,16,39] It is not clear if the effects of O_2 and H_2O_2 are direct or indirect since they react with each other in the presence of iron to form the more reactive hydroxyl ($\cdot OH^-$) radical (Haber-Weiss reaction).[17,30,39]

Free O_2 radicals can react with and damage proteins, nucleic acids (DNA), and lipids[16,39] (Fig. 5-5). These changes can produce the sarcolemmic and mitochondrial cell membrane disruption, decreased enzyme activity, and altered contractile protein function associated with myocardial stunning. Reperfusion arrhythmias may also be at least partially caused by oxygen radical release.[39] The hydroxyl radical triggers lipid oxida-

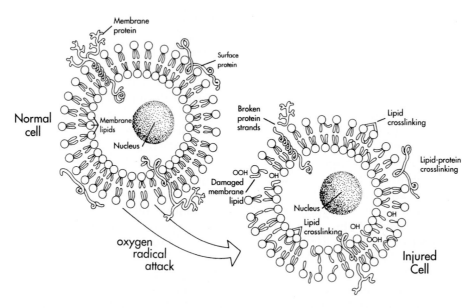

Fig. 5-5 General sites or mechanisms of oxygen radical injury. Oxygen radicals alter and/or destroy lipids and proteins within cell membranes, resulting in impaired membrane permeability, cellular dysfunction, and/or death. Similar intracellular lipid and protein destruction also occurs. (From The Upjohn Co., Kalamazoo, MI, © 1989.)

tion, which generates further O_2 radicals. Oxygen radicals in coronary artery disease are released in response to arachidonic acid secretion triggered by platelet aggregation, lipid oxidation, components of the inflammatory response, and other chemicals.[30]

The body's defenses against O_2 radicals are called *O_2 scavengers*. The primary natural O_2 scavengers are *superoxide dismutase (SOD)*, which converts O_2^- to O_2 and H_2O_2, and *catalase*, which converts H_2O_2 to the more stable O_2 and H_2O.[13,17,30] The effects of stunning are more effectively reversed by catalase rather than SOD, suggesting that hydroxyl or H_2O_2 is more toxic than O_2^-. However, investigators have reported a direct negative inotropic effect of superoxide. Combining both SOD and catalase obtains the best effects.[17]

Inhibition of free radical reactions results

in enhanced recovery of contractility.[17,39] Therapeutic applications are still under investigation and include the pharmacologic administration of the natural scavengers SOD and catalase as well as other commonly used pharmacologic agents. Allopurinol (Zyloprim) acts as a xanthine oxidase inhibitor radical scavengers. Deferoxamine (Desferal), an iron-chelating agent, also acts as a hydroxyl scavenger by inhibiting the interaction of $\cdot O_2^-$ and H_2O_2, which forms $\cdot OH^-$.[30,39] ACE inhibitors with sulfylhydrol components such as captopril (Capoten) inhibit $\cdot O_2^-$ formation.[17] Vitamin E deactivates lipid radicals.[39] N-acetylcysteine (Mucomyst) causes the release of enzymes that can detoxify H_2O_2.[39] Administering these agents prior to or early in reperfusion is associated with the best results. Researchers also have attempted to administer antiserum and monoclonal antibodies to counteract neutrophil activity and to remove neutrophils by filtration.[17] All these investigations are continuing. Trials are also in progress investigating the administration of SOD in conjunction with or just prior to the use of thrombolytics and PTCA.[16]

RELATED COMPLICATIONS

The complications of acute coronary artery disease are both electrical and mechanical. The major electrical complications are arrhythmias, which are associated with the immediate metabolic effects of ischemia and occur in both angina and acute MI. Unit 6 discusses arrhythmias extensively. The major mechanical complications include congestive heart failure (CHF) and cardiogenic shock. Although these can occur in reversible ischemia (i.e., angina) because of the effects of myocardial stunning, they are more typically associated with the more severe, permanent, necrotic changes of acute MI. Unit 8 contains an extensive discussion of CHF, cardiogenic shock, and their related hemodynamic changes.

Miscellaneous mechanical complications associated with acute coronary artery disease include mitral insufficiency, ventricular aneurysm, pericarditis, pulmonary or cerebral embolism, septal or papillary muscle rupture, and free wall rupture. Mitral insufficiency or regurgitation can complicate both angina and acute MI. The other complications are associated only with acute MI. Mitral insufficiency occurs as a result of ischemia or necrosis of the papillary muscles. There is an incidence of between 20% and 50% in acute MI. Mitral insufficiency usually appears within 48 hours[84] and is detected clinically by the presence of a new systolic murmur (see Unit 8). Intermittent murmurs audible only during anginal episodes are compatible with papillary muscle ischemia, while permanent murmurs are compatible with necrosis. Echocardiography can confirm the diagnosis. Both CHF and cardiogenic shock may be potentiated by mitral insufficiency. Therapy focuses on the management of CHF. Surgery with valve replacement or repair is indicated only when regurgitation and CHF are severe.

Ventricular aneurysm is the formation of a sac or pouch due to dilation of the infarcted area. The sac bulges outward during systole, trapping part of the ventricular volume and potentially resulting in or aggravating CHF. An incidence of 20% to 40% follows acute MI.[84] Ventricular aneurysm usually develops after at least 2 weeks following acute MI[19] and may be detected on chest wall palpation or radiographic, echocardiographic, or nuclear imaging studies. Typical ECG changes consist of sustained ST segment elevation without evolution (see ECG changes).[17,61] The major clinical problems associated with ventricular aneurysm include ventricular arrhythmias and CHF. Ventricular arrhythmias may be due to stretching of the surrounding healthy myocardium. Initial therapy concerns the management of ventricular arrhythmias and CHF. Aneurysmectomy is indicated when this treatment is ineffective.

Pericarditis is associated with the necrotic changes of acute MI. Both an immediate and a delayed form of pericarditis complicate acute MI. Each is associated with a different pathophysiologic mechanism. The immediate form usually occurs within the first week after acute MI.[61,129,142,143] It results from the effects of the inflammatory toxins that come into contact with the pericardial sac in transmural MI[84,142,143] and is associated with more extensive anterior wall infarctions.[138] While the immediate form of pericarditis occurs typically from 3 days to 3 weeks after acute myocardial infarction, it may occur within hours in an extensive MI.

The major presenting symptom in both forms of pericarditis is pleuritic chest pain due to friction of the pleura against the inflamed pericardium with respirations (see Patient history). A transient pericardial friction rub may be audible. Atrial arrhythmias commonly occur and may be associated with the larger infarct size.[138] Typical ECG changes are discussed in the section on ECG changes. Significant pericardial effusion and tamponade do not typically develop.[84,138]

The reported incidence of pericarditis (up to 20%) is slightly less than that of either mitral insufficiency or ventricular aneurysm. Therapy consists of antiinflammatory agents such as indomethacin (Indocin) or ASA, positioning, and arrhythmia management. Patients also can receive a single dose of steroids for earlier relief of pain, but more prolonged use may impair healing and predispose to rupture.[61]

A delayed form of pericarditis also occurs. This form is less common, occurs at least 2 weeks after acute MI, and recurs up to 2 years.[84,143] It is associated with an autoimmune inflammatory response to the infarcted tissue. Delayed pericarditis, formerly referred to as Dressler's syndrome, is currently called post–myocardial infarction syndrome (PMIS). The pathophysiology is similar to that responsible for pericarditis after cardiac surgery. Fever, pneumonitis, and pleuritis may also occur. Therapy is the same as with the earlier form.

Both cerebral and pulmonary embolism occur after acute MI, although the incidence is low. Pulmonary embolism occurs secondary to deep vein thrombosis. It is now infrequent because of early ambulation. However, the patient who is hemodynamically unstable or has recurring chest pain and remains immobile for extended periods is at high risk. Peripheral edema due to CHF can also potentiate the risk.[84] Preventive measures in these patients include the prophylactic administration of heparin, use of elastic stockings, and use of compression boots.[61,84] Cerebral and other systemic embolisms occur secondary to thrombus formation on a static left ventricular (LV) wall or on a static, fibrillating left atrial (LA) wall and thus are called *mural* thrombi. Mural thrombi can form within hours of acute MI. The incidence can be as high as 60% with larger anterior wall infarction.[61,84] Detection is by 2D echocardiography. Cerebral embolism secondary to mural thrombi, although rare (approximately 1% to 8%), is a significant complication; anticoagulation can prevent it. Short-term prophylactic therapy is currently recommended for patients with positive echocardiographic findings[22,58,61,143] (see Unit 9) as well as for patients with extensive anterior wall MI.[58] Mural thrombi form within 3 months in about half of the patients with ventricular aneurysm. However, embolization is less likely to occur since the thrombus is protected from intracavitary movements within the aneurysm sac.[22,58] Therefore, anticoagulation in this situation is not indicated.

Septal, papillary muscle, and free wall rupture are rare but serious complications. They occur within 48 hours to 1 week after acute MI.[19,103] Both septal and papillary muscle rupture are detected by the sudden appearance of a loud, palpable systolic murmur. Signs and symptoms of severe CHF or shock develop quickly[19,103] Chest pain may also be present.[19] Ventricular septal rupture occurs almost exclusively in the presence of multivessel disease.[22] Confirmation is an abnormally high O_2 saturation in the right ventricle or pulmonary artery when compared to the right atrium.[19,22,61,143] Echocardiographic findings may also be helpful.[22] Free wall rupture is more common than ventricular septal rupture[19] and presents in its acute form with signs of cardiac tamponade (see Unit 8) or electrical-mechanical dissociation. A subacute, more gradual form also occurs.[19] Free wall rupture occurs more frequently in patients with their first MI. Confirmation is by pericardial tap, echo- cardiographic, or nuclear imaging findings.[22,103,143] Free wall rupture also is more common in patients with anterior wall MI[73,103,143] and in hypertensive women.[19] Early surgical intervention is critical in all forms of rupture.[19,58,103]

RISK FACTORS

The coronary artery disease syndromes— angina and acute MI—occur secondary to coronary artery narrowing or stenosis. Although the exact cause of coronary artery narrowing is unknown, research has identified contributing mechanisms. The three major mechanisms contributing to coronary stenosis are (1) lipid infiltration (atherosclerosis); (2) thrombus formation initially related to platelet aggregation; and (3) spasm of the smooth muscle wall. Factors that precipitate or aggravate any of these processes trigger or accelerate the development of coronary artery disease. They thus may be said to place the patient at risk for the development of coronary heart disease and are called *risk factors*. Living a life-style that controls these risk factors is referred to by the American Heart Association as *prudent heart living*.[62]

Risk factors are grouped into modifiable versus nonmodifiable, or those that can be changed versus those that cannot be changed. The nonmodifiable risk factors include age, sex, race, and family history. Realistic assessment and intervention focus on the many more modifiable risk factors. The three most widely accepted significant risk factors for coronary artery disease are cigarette smoking, hypertension, and elevated blood cholesterol (a lipoprotein).[22,61,62,74] The relative importance of these top three factors is controversial and of little significance, because in any single individual multiple factors probably cause coronary disease. Diabetes also is considered a major risk factor.[62]

Cigarette smoking

Smoking is a particularly significant risk factor because it is avoidable and can be linked to all three mechanisms of coronary stenosis. Smoking increases platelet aggregation and fibrinogen levels[86,149] and can trigger coronary vasoconstriction or spasm by stimulating the sympathetic nervous system.[22] Smoking also alters blood lipoprotein levels. Increased low-density lipoprotein (LDL) and very low-density lipoprotein (VLDL) levels and decreased high-density lipoprotein (HDL) levels have been reported.[22,86,152] Smoking, however, has not been shown to increase atherosclerosis in individuals with normal lipid levels.[86,149] Although risk of both acute MI and sudden cardiac death has been definitely associated with smoking, a similar link has not been shown with incidence of chronic stable angina. This finding suggests a more prominent link with coronary thrombosis.[229] Cigarette smoking has been associated with a significantly higher risk than pipe or cigar smoking.[149]

Moderate smoking doubles the risk of sudden death related to coronary artery disease. The risk is increased 10 times in women who also use contraceptives.[62,74] Quitting smoking results in an immediate risk reduction; 2 years later, the risk is only slightly higher than that of nonsmokers.[62]

Hypertension

Hypertension affects about one in every three adults.[62] It contributes to coronary artery disease primarily by triggering or facilitating lipid infiltration into the vessel lining. Hypertension is associated with increased arterial wall tension, which causes vascular wall changes and increased permeability to even normal levels of circulating lipids, especially cholesterol. This effect is magnified by hyperlipidemia or high blood lipoprotein levels.[22] The damaged vessel lining may also attract platelet aggregation. Hypertension also increases the cardiac work load and can precipitate or aggravate chest pain or heart failure, complicating coronary artery disease.

The risk of a cardiovascular event increases with either systolic or diastolic pressure elevations, whether fixed or labile.[61] This effect is magnified in individuals with high blood cholesterol. In patients with coronary artery disease, elevated diastolic blood pressure is associated with an increased risk of complications.[61] Hypertension is genetically linked. It is more common in men and in blacks. Black women, however, show a slightly higher incidence.[12] No cure exists for primary or essential hypertension (the most common form) since, by definition, no identifiable cause exists. However, essential hypertension is usually controllable. Control of alcohol and sodium intake, weight loss, exercise, and relaxation or biofeedback techniques may correct hypertension without the need for drug therapy.

Cholesterol and triglycerides

Fats or lipids such as cholesterol and triglycerides are carried within the plasma in two forms: free fatty acids bound to albumin and large lipid-protein compounds known as *lipoproteins.* The free fatty acids act as immediate energy sources, whereas the lipoproteins act as backup energy sources and are stored within fat and muscle cells, including those within the coronary artery walls. Lipoproteins are absorbed into the coronary vessel walls and may initiate the process of atherosclerosis, which contributes to the thickening and narrowing of the vessel lumen (Fig. 5-6).

The major fats implicated in coronary artery disease—cholesterol and triglycerides—are carried in lipoprotein compounds in varying proportions. Routine serum cholesterol levels are a reflection of the total cholesterol carried in all these lipoproteins. The total serum cholesterol level is an effective initial screening tool for the risk of coronary artery disease. Genetic and dietary factors primarily determine serum cholesterol levels. Levels of less than 200 mg/dl are optimal.[133,152] As a screening tool, total cholesterol levels should be monitored at least every 5 years in all adults.[133]

Different types of serum lipoproteins can be separated, identified, and measured by electrophoresis. This procedure is also called "cholesterol fractionation." Individuals with total blood cholesterol higher than 240 mg/dl should have a more specific lipoprotein profile performed.[133] The lipoproteins are divided into two major categories: (1) alpha (α) lipoproteins, commonly referred to as HDLs or HDL cholesterol, and (2) beta (β) lipoproteins, commonly called *LDLs,* or *LDL cholesterol.* The cholesterol carried primarily within LDL is absorbed into the coronary vessel wall. LDL levels greater than 160 mg/dl are considered high risk, although a level less than 130 mg/dl is optimal.[133] With existing coronary artery disease or two other risk factors, patients should maintain LDL levels below 130 mg/dl.[133]

Cholesterol is also contained within HDL. The HDL compound absorbs cholesterol and helps to transport it away from the vessel wall and other tissue cells to the liver for excretion. Thus some fats in the form of li-

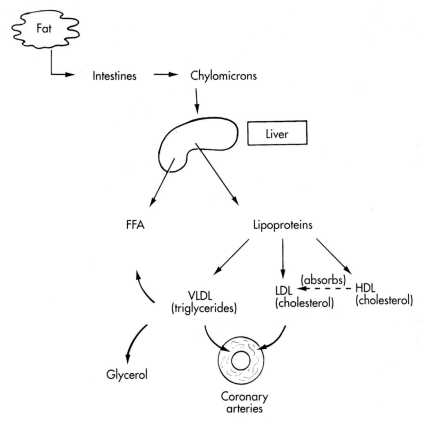

Fig. 5-6 Lipids in coronary artery disease. Fats or lipids are transported from the intestines to the liver as chylomicrons. The liver then breaks these down into circulating free fatty acids and lipoproteins (VLDL, LDL, and HDL), some of which are absorbed into the arterial wall.

poproteins protect against coronary artery disease, whereas others produce the disease. Increased HDL cholesterol levels can help lower serum LDL cholesterol levels, thus protecting against coronary artery disease. These levels may be protective even in the presence of high LDL levels.[73] Assessment of either HDL levels or the serum HDL/LDL ratio is a more accurate reflection of the associated risk of atherosclerotic disease than assessment of the total serum cholesterol or LDL level alone. HDL levels *lower than* 35 mg/dl are considered high risk.[133] The coronary artery risk can be reduced as much as

50% for every 10 mg/dl increase in HDL levels.[73] Decreased HDL levels alone may be a significant risk factor even with normal serum cholesterol levels.[73,152] Therefore, some authorities believe HDL levels should be screened routinely together with the total serum cholesterol.[73] The decreased HDL levels in women after menopause appear to coincide with the increased risk of coronary artery disease at that time.

Serum cholesterol levels between 200 and 239 are typically controlled by diet and should be rechecked annually.[133] Antilipemic drug therapy, although effective, may be associated with significant side effects. Drug therapy is reserved for patients with LDL levels greater than 190 mg/dl when dietary therapy is ineffective or for LDL levels greater than 160 mg/dl if coronary artery disease or other risk factors exist (see Unit 9).[133]

Dietary recommendations by the National Cholesterol Education Expert Panel[133] include limiting total dietary fat content to no more than 30% to facilitate weight loss. Saturated fats, which elevate LDL cholesterol, should be reduced to less than 10%. The remaining fat content should be replaced by polyunsaturated fats such as fish oils and vegetable oils (i.e., corn oil, safflower oil, sunflower seed oil, soybean oil) and monounsaturated fats such as olive oil, canola oil, peanut oil, or high-oleic-acid forms of sunflower seed oil and safflower oil. Foods high in cholesterol and/or saturated fats should be avoided. These foods include egg yolk, whole milk, butter, cheese, bacon, organ meats, red meats, veal, some shellfish such as shrimp, chocolate, coconut, or commercial baked goods. Steaming, baking, broiling, or stir-frying with very little fat is preferred for food preparation. Chicken, turkey, and fish are preferred over red meats and should be prepared without the skin. However, even chicken, turkey, or fish should be limited to 6 ounces per day.[26] Intake of fruits, vegetables, pasta, whole-grain cereals, and breads is encouraged.

Exercise raises HDL levels.[73,133,152] Thus a carefully monitored exercise program is beneficial for the patient with known coronary artery disease and may prevent coronary artery disease in the normal individual. Other measures that can increase HDL levels include weight loss; control of smoking, blood glucose, and triglycerides; increased dietary monounsaturated fats; estrogen administration in menopausal women; mild alcohol consumption (approximately 1 ounce/day); and antilipemics such as niacin (nicotinic acid), gemfibrozil (Lopid), and lovastatin (Mevacor).[73,152] These measures can be initiated at HDL levels below 40 mg/dl in men and below 45 mg/dl in women. Drug therapy can be initiated for individuals with HDL levels below 30 mg/dl in spite of nonpharmacologic efforts or below 35 mg/dl if multiple risk factors are present.[73] Drugs that may lower HDL levels include thiazide and loop diuretics, most beta blockers, and the antilipemic agent probucol (Lorelco). These drugs can be substituted for other antihypertensive or antilipemic agents with either no effect or a positive effect on HDL levels.[73]

Serum triglycerides have also been linked to coronary artery disease. Serum triglycerides are primarily contained within the VLDLs. However, the VLDLs contain small amounts of cholesterol as well, which can be released when these fats are broken down for energy. The role of triglycerides in the production of atherosclerotic disease is not well established. Serum triglycerides alone are a significant risk factor primarily in women.[74,133,152] In men, these lipoproteins are thought to contribute to coronary risk primarily when combined with other risk factors. The role of these lipoproteins may be closely related either to the small amounts of cholesterol carried within them or to their role in fat storage and obesity, which further contribute to hypertension.

Serum triglyceride levels fluctuate throughout the day. Alcohol, glucose consumption, exercise, and stresses such as pregnancy affect them significantly. For accurate levels, instruct the patient to fast for at least 12 hours, abstain from alcohol for at least 16 hours, and avoid any major exercise before the test. Fasting serum levels below 250 mg/dl are associated with little risk of coronary artery disease if the total cholesterol is normal. Levels of 250 to 500 mg/dl are considered borderline and are most commonly related to obesity, diabetes mellitus, or hypothyroidism.[133] Certain drugs such as thiazide diuretics and beta blockers can also elevate triglycerides without an effect on LDL cholesterol.[133]

Triglycerides are the major fat storage form. About 95% of the body's fatty tissue is composed of this lipoprotein. Weight reduction alone can effectively lower serum triglyceride levels. Exercise also can help to lower triglyceride levels. Excessive alcohol intake raises triglyceride levels, and for this reason the patient with coronary artery disease should avoid it. Drug therapy is reserved for patients with familial elevated triglycerides or premature coronary artery disease if diet is ineffective.[133]

Five types of familial elevated blood lipid patterns (hyperlipidemias) have been identified. They are classified according to the type of blood lipid elevated: LDL (cholesterol), VLDL (triglycerides), or chylomicrons. *Chylomicrons* are the form in which fat is transported from the intestines to the liver, where the lipoproteins form (see Fig. 5-6).

Types II and IV are the most common forms of hyperlipidemias. Type II is associated with high cholesterol levels. Type IV is associated with high triglyceride levels. These patterns are typically associated with familial disorders such as diabetes and hypothyroidism. Diabetes may be associated with either type II or type IV hyperlipidemia or both. Hypothyroidism is predominantly associated with type II hyperlipidemia.

Therapy for type II hyperlipidemia consists of diet cholesterol control and/or administration of cholesterol antagonists, such as colestipol (Colestid), cholestyramine (Questran), probucol (Lorelco), or niacin (vitamin B_3). Patients should follow a diet low in total fat content as well as low in saturated fats and cholesterol. Therapy for type IV hyperlipidemia consists of calorie, fat, and alcohol restriction; weight reduction; exercise; and/or triglyceride antagonists, such as clofibrate (Atromid-S). Unit 9 further discusses therapy for hyperlipidemia. The effect of therapy on controlling the severity of coronary artery disease is still controversial. Dietary control is usually preferred over drug therapy, since it is effective and associated with fewer risks.

Diabetes mellitus

Diabetes mellitus aggravates both platelet aggregation and atherosclerosis. Multiple interacting factors probably aggravate atherosclerosis because controlling blood glucose levels alone does not prevent it.[22] However, controlling blood sugar seems to prevent small vessel changes in the retina and kidney.[22] Patients with diabetes mellitus also typically have hypertension and disturbances in serum lipoproteins (increased LDL and VLDL levels and decreased HDL levels). In addition, many diabetic patients are obese. The coronary atherosclerotic effects of diabetes are particularly significant in younger women.[74] For all these reasons, the incidence of both heart failure and coronary artery disease increases in the diabetic patient. Silent MI is also more common in patients with diabetes mellitus.

Contributing factors

Other identified modifiable risk factors for coronary artery disease include lack of exercise, obesity, alcohol intake, menopause, and stress. The American Heart Association classifies these as *contributing factors*.

Lack of exercise is associated with abnormal lipoprotein patterns. Obesity is often associated with both hypertension and abnormal lipoproteins. More recently, studies have identified an increased waist to hip ratio of fat distribution as a more predictive risk factor for coronary artery disease than obesity alone.[22,74,99]

Heavy alcohol intake (more than 2 to 3 drinks per day) has been linked with increased blood pressure, arrhythmias (especially atrial fibrillation), dilated cardiomyopathy, sudden death, and coronary artery disease.[22,61,110] Detrimental lipoprotein effects (increased LDL levels) and increased platelet aggregation also occur with heavy alcohol intake.[152] However, moderate alcohol intake (fewer than two to three drinks per day) is associated with a decrease in coronary artery disease because of a beneficial effect on HDL lipoproteins, platelet aggregation, and fibrinogen levels.[22,99]

Menopause is associated with an increased risk of coronary artery disease due to the onset of abnormal lipoprotein levels (increased LDL or VLDL and decreased HDL).[74,152]

Stress results in the release of sympathetic chemicals, also known as catecholamines. These chemicals can increase platelet aggregation and trigger coronary spasm. Catecholamines can also increase heart rate and blood pressure and predispose to high lipid levels and ventricular arrhythmias.[47,61] Cocaine abuse has been associated with a higher risk of MI as a result of a similar release of sympathetic chemicals. Stress as a risk factor is popularly described in terms of Type A and Type B personalities. The stress-prone personality is the Type A, who typically is competitive, impatient, hostile, easily irritated, and desirous of squeezing the most tasks into the least amount of time. Even typically nonstressful situations may elicit a stress response in these individuals.

Low self-esteem is characteristic.[47] There is an increased incidence of coronary artery disease, high blood pressure and serum cholesterol, anginal episodes, and silent MI in Type A personalities.[22,47] However, researchers report an increased long-term, postinfarction survival rate in Type A personalities when compared with Type B personalities.[22,47,108] The significance of these personality types is still controversial.[61,108]

Occupational triggers of stress in women differ from the triggers for a typical Type A male executive. Females in clerical positions who are married to blue-collar workers and have children are at highest risk for both stress and coronary artery disease. Degree of control may be more significant in women than the stress of the job or roles themselves in predicting coronary artery disease.[71]

Coffee intake and calcium changes have also been recently linked with coronary artery disease.[22] Although the specific link with coronary artery disease is not well established, coffee is associated with increased LDL levels in women and decreased LDL levels in men.[22] Accumulation of calcium in the arterial wall may accelerate the process of atherosclerosis. Preliminary research findings showed that calcium channel blockers inhibit the atherosclerotic process.[122]

Risk factor control is effective in preventing or limiting existing coronary artery disease. "Primary prevention," before clinical symptoms appear, is the most effective in preventing or delaying onset. Prevention after clinical symptoms already exist, "secondary prevention," is a major focus of cardiac rehabilitation. Risk factor control in rehabilitation is probably more effective in limiting the disease, minimizing complications, and maximizing the remaining cardiovascular function.

PATIENT HISTORY

A positive history from a patient who has had an acute MI refers to a description of characteristic *chest pain*. Pain is the presenting symptom in most patients with acute MI and usually follows a characteristic pattern (Table 5-1). Patients, however, may perceive it as discomfort rather than pain because of its pressurelike rather than sharp quality. Patients may also use other terms to describe the pain, such as burning, heaviness, or squeezing.[48,58,123] Patients with acute MI may present with nausea or vomiting, diaphoresis, dyspnea, and apprehension depending on the perceived severity of the pain and the extent of the stress response. Because of vagal stimulation, nausea and vomiting are more common in patients with inferior wall MI.[22,28,68] The reported intensity or severity of the pain varies according to the patient's pain threshold, cultural background, state of denial, and subjective perception.[55,58,123] The blood pressure is typically elevated (see Stress and psychological factors). Pain is composed of a strong emotional as well as physiologic component.[91] Therefore, caregivers should offer emotional support in addition to medication for the relief of pain.

When a patient complains of chest pain, the examiner should assess it within the clinical setting in which it occurs. Because chest pain may be caused by many different conditions, he or she should rule out other causes as soon as possible. In the patient with coronary artery disease the three disorders that most commonly mimic MI are angina pectoris, pericarditis, and pulmonary embolus (Table 5-1). Both pericarditis and, to a lesser extent, pulmonary embolus may occur as a complication of MI. The pain pattern of these disorders is often called *pleuritic* since it is related to respirations and position changes similar to those of other pulmonary causes of chest pain (e.g., pneumonia, pneumothorax).[28,129] A clue may be reluctance to take a deep breath during auscultation. Pleuritic pain is also more typically sharp in quality.[58,129] Pulmonary emboli are typically also accompanied by acute-onset shortness of breath. The pain of pericarditis often radiates to the trapezius area.[129] ECG changes are characteristic and are thus helpful in differentiating this mechanism of chest pain (see ECG Changes). A transient, triphasic pericardial friction rub may be audible.[28,129]

Location, quality, and radiation may be similar in both angina and acute MI since they share a common coronary artery origin.[22] In patients with chronic stable angina, initial comparison with the patient's typical past pain patterns may more easily differentiate MI.[55] Other helpful differentiating characteristics include duration and mode of relief. Radiation to both the ulnar aspects of the left arm and interscapular region of the back is typical of coronary artery disease.[22] When acute onset of dyspnea, dizziness, and/or exhaustion occur as the primary presenting symptoms, they are referred to as angina equivalents.[31,36,58] Pain is triggered by the metabolites of ischemia rather than infarcted tissue. Therefore, pain continuing or recurring for more than 24 hours after acute MI is an ominous sign representing ongoing ischemia and may indicate multivessel disease or infarct extension.

About 20% to 50% of nonfatal MIs are silent or asymptomatic.[22,58] Silent anginal episodes are even more frequent. Silent ischemic episodes occur more often in patients with type II diabetes mellitus. Possible explanations include an increased pain threshold or lesser degrees of affected myocardium.[31,58] Silent MI and/or anginal episodes may be detected by ECG changes, Holter monitoring, exercise testing, or nuclear imaging.

Other cardiovascular causes of chest pain include dissecting aortic aneurysm, aortic

Table 5-1. Differential diagnosis of chest pain

Question	MI pain	Angina	Pericarditis	Pulmonary embolus
Where do you feel the discomfort? (location)	Retrosternal, but may radiate to back, neck, arm, and jaw	Same	Retrosternal or precordial, radiates to back, trapezius, jaw, and arms	Usually over lung fields, to the side and the back
What is the discomfort like? (quality)	Pressure, choking, burning, tightness, viselike, usually *severe*	Similar in description to MI pain	Sharp ache in chest, not necessarily severe but annoying	Similar to pericarditis, except to side and back
How long did it last? (duration)	At least 30 minutes	Relief usually in 15 minutes or less	Continuous; may last for days	Continuous for hours
Did you have any nausea? Did you feel short of breath? Did you feel weak or dizzy? Did you have cold sweats? (accompanying symptoms)	*May have* nausea, dyspnea, weakness, diaphoresis, and dizziness	Usually *not* accompanied by diaphoresis or nausea	Usually *not* accompanied by these symptoms	Accompanied by *acute* shortness of breath, tachycardia, and apprehension (most characteristic—bloody sputum)
Was the pain relieved when you took a deep breath? (effects of respirations)	Not affected by respirations		Increased pain on inspiration	Increased pain on inspiration
Did you feel better when you sat up? (change of position)	Not relieved by change in position	May be only slightly relieved by change in position	Pain decreased on sitting up and increased when on *left* side	Decreased on sitting up
Was the pain relieved by anything?	Usually requires narcotics for relief	Relieved by rest when associated with *exertion*; relieved by nitroglycerin	Continous soreness usually relieved somewhat by ASA or Tylenol	May be relived by narcotics

valve disease, and mitral valve prolapse (see Unit 11). The chest pain of dissecting aneurysm typically radiates to the back, along the pathway of the aorta. A difference between blood pressures in the right and left arms is noted.

Gastrointestinal (GI) causes of chest pain include hiatal hernia,[22] peptic or duodenal ulcer, gallbladder disease, and esophageal spasm.[28] The pain of hiatal hernia is positional (increased when lying flat) and typically occurs an hour after meals. The pain of peptic ulcer is usually localized and may be relieved by medications and/or antacids. Upper GI series and/or endoscopy can confirm the diagnosis of both of these. Esophageal spasm mimics angina most closely since the location may be retrosternal, and it is relieved by nitroglycerin. However, it is often associated with difficulty swallowing and rarely radiates.[22,28]

Chest wall pain can occur with trauma or orthopedic conditions such as costochondritis and muscle spasm. Local tenderness to palpation and with range of motion is characteristic.[28]

NURSING ORDERS: The patient with chest pain

1. Evaluate chest pain according to:
   a. Typical pattern(s) for that patient
   b. Location
   c. Quality (Note specific descriptive terms used and communicate to the staff.[123]) Pain scales (1 to 10 or 1 to 5) help the patient quantify the pain.
   d. Association with respiration and change of position
   e. Accompanying symptoms (shortness of breath, dizziness, cold, clammy skin, nausea or vomiting)
   f. Nonverbal indicators[55] (e.g., grimacing, restlessness, avoidance of eye contact, hands on chest)
2. Obtain vital signs and note alterations in the following:
   a. Blood pressure
   b. Pulse rate
   c. Respiratory rate

Note that an increase in blood pressure is an expected response to pain. Wait until the patient experiences pain relief and take the blood pressure again before administering antihypertensive medications.

3. Obtain a sample ECG tracing in the *inferior, lateral,* and *anteroseptal* monitoring leads. Confirm findings on a standard 12-lead ECG. Analyze the ECG tracing and report the following:
   a. Arrhythmias
   b. Displacement of the ST segment or changes in the T waves
   c. Abnormalities in the QRS morphology
   d. Changes in the polarity of the QRS complex
4. Relieve the patient's pain, a priority for any cardiac patient, as follows:
   a. Promptly administer medication (oxygen, nitroglycerin, morphine).
   b. Place the patient with pericarditis in a high Fowler's position, arms on over-bed table.
   c. Evaluate effectiveness[55] (verbal and nonverbal responses, color, vital signs).
   d. Record mode of relief (rest, administration of nitroglycerin or morphine, ASA, positioning).
5. Prevent further pain by providing rest periods between activities (e.g., bath, visitors).[55]
6. Provide emotional support measures (touch, verbal reassurance, staying with patient).
7. Instruct patient to report lack of relief or return of similar discomfort.
8. Report immediately any chest pain that is:
   a. Different from that which has occurred before
   b. Accompanied by different symptoms
   c. Accompanied by change in the ECG or vital signs
   d. Increasing in frequency or severity or both

DIAGNOSTIC TESTS

Current invasive and noninvasive diagnostic tests detect and evaluate the structural, functional, and metabolic components of coronary artery disease. These tests can also evaluate the electrical and mechanical complications of this disease. The major invasive test is cardiac catheterization, which is considered the standard for detecting structural coronary disease and mechanical dysfunction. Examples of major noninvasive tests are radionuclide studies, echocardiology, and exercise stress testing.

The detection of acute MI requires other diagnostic information readily obtained with the patient at rest. The medical diagnosis of acute MI is based on three major parameters: history, serum enzymes, and ECG changes. Positive results for two of these three indicate a definitive diagnosis of acute MI.

Serum enzymes

Enzymes are proteins that change the speed of chemical reactions. Enzymes are located wherever these chemical reactions take place. The chemical reactions of the body occur in three major sites: (1) within the plasma, (2) within the cells, and (3) within the GI tract. The plasma contains a mixture of the enzymes required for plasma functions such as coagulation, the GI enzymes that are transported by the plasma, and small amounts of the intracellular enzymes that leak out through normal membrane pores. When cellular membrane damage occurs, large amounts of intracellular enzymes are released into the bloodstream and the serum levels of these enzymes increase. Therefore, an elevation in serum enzymes that are primarily intracellular indicates cellular membrane damage.

Characteristic enzymes are present in different types of cells. The major enzymes that exist in high concentrations within cardiac cells are (1) creatine phosphokinase (CPK), now referred to as *creatine kinase* (CK), (2) lactic dehydrogenase (LDH), and (3) serum glutamic-oxaloacetic transaminase (SGOT), now referred to as aspartate aminotransferase (AST).[22,143] With cardiac necrosis, the levels of these enzymes usually become elevated. Cardioversion and defibrillation, cardiac massage, cardiopulmonary bypass, and cardiac surgery can all elevate these enzymes as well.

Each of the cardiac enzymes is also present in other body tissues. CK is found in the tissues of the brain, lung, and skeletal muscle. Increased serum CK levels are highly specific for myocardial injury when abnormalities in the skeletal muscle and brain are ruled out. It is a highly sensitive enzyme; even small amounts of myocardial injury cause it to become elevated.[22] Both LDH and AST may be released from many tissues other than the heart. Therefore, both LDH and AST levels are highly *nonspecific*. Conditions that may elevate the serum levels of both these enzymes include muscle trauma, pulmonary infarction, liver disease, and CHF.

Following MI, the serum levels of the major cardiac enzymes follow a characteristic pattern (Fig. 5-7). However, many normal variants of this pattern occur. For instance, all the enzymes are significantly elevated by the third day, although CK may be back to or approaching normal. The delayed onset and decline of LDH elevation make this enzyme particularly useful in patients who delay reporting the signs of acute MI for a period of days or more than 24 hours before admission.[22]

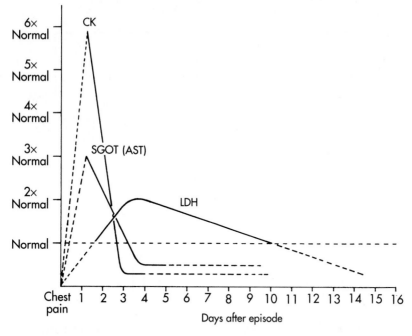

Fig. 5-7   Pattern of enzyme elevation in acute MI.

Isoenzymes

Each of the routinely measured enzymes actually reflects the activity of a group of enzymes that, having only slight molecular differences, influence the same metabolic reactions. The different forms of a particular enzyme are known as its *isoenzymes*. CK has three currently recognized isoenzyme forms. LDH has five. Since AST is highly nonspecific and has no currently recognized isoenzyme forms, AST (SGOT) testing is no longer routine.[22,137,143] Separating total enzyme activity into its components allows for more accurate identification of enzyme elevations indicative of MI. Isoenzymes are currently used in the diagnosis of acute MI. Total CK activity is often evaluated initially. If the total CK activity is elevated, CK isoenzymes are obtained.

CK isoenzymes form three separately colored bands on acetate paper with electrophoresis (Fig. 5-8). The CK contained pri-

marily within skeletal muscle is called *CK₃MM (band)*. This enzyme is released after muscle trauma, during convulsions, after surgical procedures and IV cutdowns, in alcoholic myopathy or shock states, and after intramuscular injections. CK-MM also exists within cardiac muscle and may become elevated after myocardial trauma or infarction.

The CK contained within the brain is called *CK₁BB (band)*. In CNS disorders, it is unusual to see elevations in CK-BB, since it does not cross the blood-brain barrier. CK elevations in these disorders are usually associated with accompanying release from skeletal muscle and are thus of the CK-MM type. CK-BB is also found in the lungs, bladder, bowel, stomach, prostate, and thyroid.[137] CK-BB may be elevated after cardiac arrest because of cerebral ischemia and may be predictive of outcome.[143]

The third CK isoenzyme occurs selectively

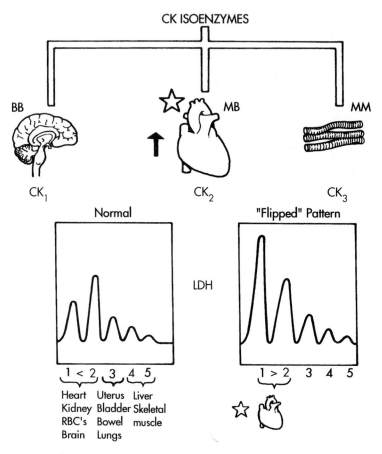

Fig. 5-8 Isoenzyme pattern in acute MI. The starred areas indicate diagnostic findings.

within cardiac muscle. This isoenzyme form is referred to as *CK₂MB (band)*. CK-MB is highly specific and sensitive for myocardial necrosis. Since it is the enzyme of primary interest in acute MI, it may be the only isoenzyme reported. CK-MB levels begin to rise at 3 to 5 hours.[30,137] Since only minimal amounts of this isoenzyme form (3% to 5%) are present in the plasma of normal subjects, any recorded activity over 5% is considered abnormal. CK-MB activity is reported in units as well as in percentage of total CK activity. When reported in units, small CK-MB elevations may be more easily detected. Serial CK-MB results have been correlated with infarct size, arrhythmic complications, ventricular performance, and prognosis. However, elevated CK-MB levels are expected after thrombolytic therapy or PTCA as a result of reperfusion and washout of the area and do not have the same significance.

CK-MB levels are elevated after cardiac surgery and in myocardial trauma, myopathy, and severe myocardial ischemia (i.e., unstable angina)[77,137] as well as in acute MI. Elevated CK-MB levels due to cardiac surgery return to normal rapidly. Therefore, levels elevated significantly longer than 12 to 18 hours are suggestive of acute MI, especially in the presence of new Q waves and a positive technetium-99-pyrophosphate scan.[22,77,143] Any patient with a suspect history and positive CK-MB activity should be given the benefit of the doubt and treated as if he or she had sustained an acute MI.

LDH is another useful cardiac enzyme, with five currently recognized isoenzyme forms (see Fig. 5-8). LDH_1 is the primary LDH isoenzyme contained within the heart.[M6] LDH_1 and LDH_2 are concentrated within the heart, kidneys, and red blood cells. LDH_4 and LDH_5 are concentrated within the liver and skeletal muscle and become elevated in CHF with acute MI. LDH_3 is located in the pancreas, spleen, thyroid and adrenal glands, and white blood cells.[137] Serum LDH_2 activity usually exceeds LDH_1 activity in the normal individual. In acute MI, LDH_1 activity exceeds LDH_2 activity. This pattern is referred to as a *flipped* LDH pattern and may also be reported as an LDH_1/LDH_2 ratio.[22,143] The combination of elevated CPK-MB levels in the serum and a flipped LDH isoenzyme pattern (or LDH_1/LDH_2 ratio greater than 1) is currently diagnostic for acute MI. However, LDH isoenzymes may not be necessary when the CK-MB band is elevated unless the patient is admitted more than 48 hours after the onset of pain.[111] LDH isoenzymes may also be helpful in the patient with bowel infarction, since chest pain may be present and CPK-MB is elevated. However, LDH isoenzymes should remain normal unless the patient has a MI.[77] (The assessment of hydroxybutyrate dehydrogenase [HBD] has been used in the past in some institutions as a rough estimate of both LDH_1 and LDH_2 levels, but it does not reveal the flipped pattern.)

Consider the following points when evaluating serum enzymes: (1) avoid hemolysis of blood specimens; (2) look for the flipped LDH pattern as well as levels of LDH_1 and LDH_2; (3) check CPK-MB activity; and (4) in the presence of CPK-MB activity greater than 5% and a flipped LDH pattern, treat the patient as if he or she had sustained an acute MI.

Isoforms and myoglobin levels

Isoenzymes may be broken down further into isoforms, which have been recently identified. Isoform levels rise as early as 1 hour after acute MI and may allow for earlier diagnosis when faster analysis methods are developed.[22,44] Isoforms are currently recognized only for CK-MM and CK-MB, which are found in the heart. The MM^{31} isoform is located peripherally in the myofibril structures, while MB^{29} is located more centrally in the myocardial cell or sarcomere. Therefore, with myocardial injury MM^{31} is released earlier than MB.[29] The MM^{31}/MM^{23} ratio may also be helpful in differentiating angina from acute MI.[5,105]

Serum myoglobin levels may also detect MI. This intracellular protein is released into the serum with myocardial necrosis earlier than CK. Its value, however, is limited currently since it remains elevated for only a very short time. In addition, it is highly nonspecific since it is also a component of skeletal muscle.[22,51]

ECG changes

The ECG changes of acute MI reflect the effects of pathophysiologic changes on electrical events. Myocardial infarctions are classified as *transmural* or *nontransmural* depending on the thickness of the muscle wall involved. (Remember that the infarction process begins in and may be limited to the subendocardium, resulting in subendocardial or nontransmural infarction.) Completed transmural infarctions, which extend to the epi-

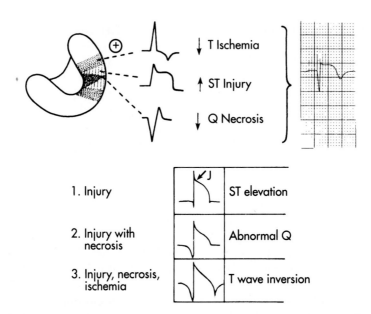

1. Injury		ST elevation
2. Injury with necrosis		Abnormal Q
3. Injury, necrosis, ischemia		T wave inversion

Fig. 5-9   ECG changes and evolution: acute transmural MI. The ECG changes described as ischemia, injury, and necrosis correspond roughly to the pathophysiologic zones of acute MI. The typical sequence of these changes is also described. Remember that J point elevation is synonymous with ST elevation.

cardial wall, are easier to detect on the ECG since the sensing (+) electrode on most of the standard leads reflects the outer or epicardial LV surfaces (see Unit 2). Determining the location of an infarction by ECG patterns enables the nurse to anticipate the types of complications that are likely to occur.

A completed transmural infarction has three zones: a central necrotic core surrounded by a second zone of inflammation and a third border zone of ischemia without inflammation (Fig. 5-9). The earliest clinically detectable change is usually inflammation, which is a manifestation of a local stress response (see Unit 4). ST segment elevation corresponds with this process and thus is the first routinely detected sign of acute transmural MI. By convention, ST segment shifts are referred to as injury. [35,61,132]

The first stage in the ECG evolution of a transmural MI is ST segment elevation in the leads, reflecting the injured epicardial area (Fig. 5-9). The J or "junction" point marking the end of the QRS complex and the beginning of the ST segment serves as a reference point for determining ST elevation or depression. The J point normally occurs on the baseline, level with the beginning of the QRS complex (see Unit 2). An ST segment beginning more than 1 mm above the baseline is considered significantly elevated.[15] J point elevation is synonymous with ST elevation.

The next stage in the ECG evolution of a transmural MI is the appearance of abnormal Q waves, called *necrosis*. Abnormal Q waves indicate electrical death, or the inability to transmit electrical impulses, temporarily or permanently. Although these changes correlate roughly with the necrotic zone, abnormal Q waves do not necessarily indicate that the cells are mechanically dead, because documented Q waves have been known to disappear.[35] Q waves represent depression or loss of forces traveling toward the positive electrode. They may also reflect depolarization of the opposite wall (away from the positive electrode) with the infarcted wall acting like a transparent window.[22,35] Q waves develop within 2 to 9 hours of infarction, thus correlating roughly with the time frame of pathologic death of tissue.[35,87] For this reason they usually are not visible on admission. An abnormal Q wave is one that is wider than 0.04 second and deeper than one fourth of the R wave.[35,59,89] In this stage there is still evidence of myocardial injury because a zone of injury always surrounds an area of necrosis. Loss of R wave amplitude occurs in some individuals instead of or in addition to Q wave formation and is considered a Q wave equivalent.[3,14,35,87,132] Q wave formation may not be visible when the infarcted area is small.

The third stage is *ischemia.* Symmetrical inversion of the T wave denotes electrical ischemia. In this situation, the inversion correlates with physiologic ischemia as well. However, by convention, T wave inversion is referred to as "ischemia," regardless of the situation or cause.[61] Ischemia appears as the injury or inflammation subsides. When Q waves develop, they usually precede T wave inversion.[61] Thus in the typical fully evolved MI, T wave inversion occurs in conjunction with ST elevation and abnormal Q waves (see Fig. 5-9).

In the recovery stage the current of injury subsides rapidly, especially within the first 12 hours,[35,131,132] but the necrosis and ischemia remain (Fig. 5-10). Ischemia may then subside. The only ECG manifestation of infarction that then remains is the abnormal Q wave. In some patients the abnormal Q wave may also subsequently disappear, leaving no ECG evidence of acute MI. Some patients retain ischemic T waves.

The ECG changes described occur in the leads directly reflecting the area of infarction. *Indirect* ECG evidence of myocardial in-

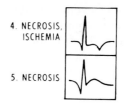

Fig. 5-10   Recovery stages: acute transmural MI.

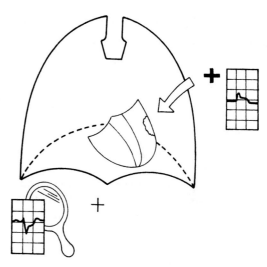

Fig. 5-11   Reciprocal changes in acute transmural infarction. ST segment elevation in the lateral leads (I, aVL) will produce reciprocal ST segment depression in the inferior leads (II, III, aVF) since the injury in acute MI is localized to a single epicardial surface.

jury may be obtained from leads that are *opposite* the injured area—within the same plane (see Unit 2).[61] These changes are referred to as *reciprocal changes* and are a mirror image of the ECG changes recorded directly from the infarction site (Fig. 5-11). Therefore, reciprocal changes to injury or ST segment elevation are manifested on the ECG as ST segment depression. Within the frontal plane, the lateral and inferior surfaces are considered opposite or reciprocal to each other. Within the horizontal plane, the anterior and posterior surfaces are reciprocal. The endocardium and epicardium are also considered reciprocal to each other. Changes within the horizontal plane leads, however, are not consistently considered reciprocal to those within the frontal plane leads.[15,35,61,132]

Since transmural infarction begins in the subendocardial area, subendocardial ischemia, with its corresponding ECG changes, occurs prior to the transmural changes and may be detected in some individuals. Subendocardial ischemia produces local $Na+-K+$ shifts, which cause reciprocal peaked T waves in the epicardial leads reflecting the involved surface. These early ECG changes are called *hyperacute T wave changes*.[35,87] They are usually masked quickly by more significant changes and thus are often missed on the ECG. Increased amplitude of the R wave may also show up initially.[35,132]

Both severe subendocardial ischemia and infarction are associated with inflammation or injury limited to the subendocardial layer. Reciprocal ST segment depression is recorded in the standard leads, most of which reflect the epicardial surface.[89] Q waves do not typically form even in the presence of in-

Q wave versus non–Q wave infarction

Infarctions are also currently classified according to their ECG pattern rather than the extent of myocardial wall involved. This classification system allows easier and more accurate determination of pathologic, prognostic, and therapeutic implications.[3,15,35,151] Thus it continues to grow in popularity. Infarctions that result in Q wave formation on the ECG are called *Q wave infarctions*. Infarctions that do not result in Q wave formation are referred to as *non–Q wave infarctions*. Most Q wave infarctions are transmural.[93,151] However, extensive nontransmural or subendocardial infarction may also result in Q wave formation according to autopsy studies.[3,93] Thus Q wave formation does not require necrosis of the entire thickness of

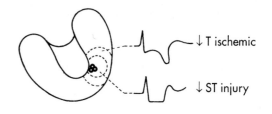

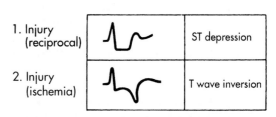

Fig. 5-12 ECG changes and evolution: subendocardial (nontransmural) infarction.

farction. Inverted T waves appear initially and in the process of evolution after the injury subsides, since the ischemic zone extends to the epicardium (Fig. 5-12). Since these same subendocardial changes occur with transient reversible ischemia, both ST depression and T wave inversion are loosely referred to as "ischemic" changes (see Patterns Associated with Angina).

the myocardial wall.[54] Most non–Q wave infarctions are limited to the subendocardium.[151] However, according to autopsy studies, transmural infarction may occur in the absence of Q waves.[3,54,93,131,151] Therefore, accurately determining the myocardial layers involved is difficult from ECG changes alone.[15,35]

Q wave infarctions, as expected by their more frequent transmural involvement, are typically associated with initial peaked T waves followed quickly by ST elevation on most of the standard leads. In contrast, non–Q wave infarctions are most commonly associated with initial T wave inversion and/or reciprocal ST depression.[151] Various ECG patterns, however, may occur, such as

T wave changes alone or ST elevation, which occurs in up to 40% of non−Q wave MIs.[3,14,15,93] Therefore, the ECG changes are less specific and serum enzymes are necessary to validate the presence of infarction. T wave inversion occurs in the evolution of both Q wave and non−Q wave infarctions. Initial ST segment elevation is highly suggestive of eventual Q wave rather than non−Q wave infarction and can serve as a basis for initial therapeutic decisions.

The incidence of Q wave infarctions (50% to 70%)[60,63] is more common than the incidence of non−Q wave infarctions (20% to 90%).[61,75,93] Q wave infarctions are associated with proximal, complete coronary artery occlusion and more extensive infarction as determined by CK-MB levels and autopsy findings.[75,151] Patients are more likely to be hemodynamically unstable on admission, especially if the MI is located in the anterior wall, because of the larger infarction.[151] Non−Q wave infarctions[3,75,93] are associated with smaller infarctions and either incomplete coronary occlusion or complete occlusion with spontaneous reperfusion usually within 72 hours.[3,14,15,54,75,151] Regional wall motion changes may not be present.[145]

The incidence of complications, including reinfarction or infarct extension and mortality, also differs. The highest incidence of reinfarction and infarct extension occurs with non−Q wave infarction, especially after discharge.[3,59,151] Recurrent ischemia or postinfarction angina is also more common in non−Q wave infarction.[3,14,93,145,151] Inadequate collateral circulation may contribute to this difference.[14] The higher incidence of infarction or extension is thought to be the result of completion of an initially incompletely occluded, unstable lesion. Although initial complication and mortality rates for non−Q wave infarctions are lower, long-term mortality after 1 to 2 years is similar to Q wave MIs.[3,93,145] The ECG finding of ST segment depression is particularly associated with high delayed mortality.[14] Patients with non−Q wave infarctions may also have a higher risk of sudden death.[93]

Therapeutic differences exist as well. Beta blockade does not improve survival in patients with non−Q wave infarction.[75,93] However, studies show diltiazem (Cardizem) prevents reinfarction and minimizes postinfarction angina in patients with non−Q wave infarction only.[3,93,151] The effect on mortality is controversial.[75] Patients with acute non−Q wave infarction generally do not receive thrombolytics since they are less likely to have occlusive thrombi.[150] Predischarge exercise testing, preferably together with thallium SPECT imaging, may be beneficial in identifying the patients with non−Q wave infarction at highest risk.[151] Cardiac catheterization with coronary angioplasty is indicated in patients with chest pain at low activity levels.[151]

Transmural anterior wall myocardial infarction

An anterior wall myocardial infarction may be defined as one affecting either the septal, the lateral, or both portions of the anterior surface of the left ventricle. An infarction affecting both the septal and lateral walls may be called either an *extensive anterior wall MI* or *anterolateral MI*.[35,54] Anterior wall MI occurs as a result of *left* coronary artery pathology, most commonly involving a proximal lesion in the anterior descending branch.[35,132] Extensive anterior wall MI is associated with occlusion of the main trunk of the left coronary artery or multivessel disease.

The leads that reflect the electrical activity of both the septal and lateral areas of the left ventricle are the frontal plane leads I and aVL and the horizontal plane leads V1 to V6 (Fig. 5-13). Therefore, extensive anterior wall infarction produces changes in these leads. The ST segment elevation occurs in the V leads and in leads I and aVL. Abnormal Q waves, if they develop, also appear in these leads. Reciprocal ST segment depression occurs in leads II, III, and aVF (Fig. 5-14). The ST segment elevation is often dramatically more significant on lead V2.[132] For this reason, obtain a lead V2 (or MCL2) trace in addition to or instead of V1 (MCL1) in the patient presenting with chest pain. Confirm changes on a standard 12-lead ECG.

Left coronary artery occlusion commonly produces necrosis of large areas of the left ventricular musculature. Therefore, patients with anterior wall MI usually develop *pump*

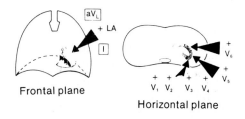

Fig. 5-13 Leads reflecting extensive anterior wall MI.

failure more severe than that accompanying right coronary artery pathology.

The left coronary artery supplies the following structures of intraventricular conduction system: (1) the right bundle branch, (2) the anterosuperior division of the left bundle branch, and (3) the posteroinferior division of the left bundle branch. For this reason, it can be anticipated that interventricular conduction disturbances such as right bundle branch block, left anterior hemiblock, and left posterior hemiblock frequently accompany left coronary artery pathology. Related atrioventricular (AV) blocks such as Mobitz II can also be anticipated (see Unit 1, Unit 7, and Unit 8).

Anteroseptal changes. Anterior wall MI may be limited to the septal portion of the anterior wall. Occlusion of the left anterior descending branch of the left coronary artery produces *anteroseptal wall MI.* Intraventricular conduction disturbances associated with anteroseptal MI include right bundle branch block and left anterior hemiblock. AV blocks such as Mobitz II also accompany anteroseptal MI.

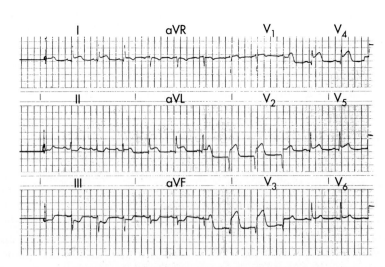

Fig. 5-14 ECG changes in extensive anterior wall MI. This would also be considered a Q wave infarction. Abnormal Q waves are present in leads V2 and V3 in addition to the classic ST segment changes.

The leads that reflect the electrical activity of the anteroseptal wall of the left ventricle are leads V1 through V4 (Fig. 5-15). Note that leads V2 and V3 lie directly over the septum. Therefore, these leads record the most significant changes.[132] There are no posterior positions on the six standard chest leads. Therefore, reciprocal changes reflecting localized anteroseptal injury are usually not seen. Reciprocal changes are more common in inferior wall MI than in anterior wall MI.[132]

Lateral wall changes. Anterior wall MI may also be limited to the lateral portion of the anterior wall. Occlusion of the circumflex branch of the left coronary artery produces infarction in this area. Left posterior hemiblock may occur, but AV block and significant heart failure are unusual. Characteristic ECG changes are recorded in only 50% of patients with circumflex lesions since the infarction may be small or may overlap with the distribution of the right coronary artery.[132]

The leads that reflect the electrical activity of the lateral wall of the left ventricle are leads I and aVL and V4 through V6 (Fig. 5-16). The ST segment elevation occurs in leads I, aVL, and V4 through V6, and the reciprocal changes occur in leads II, III, and aVF—the leads reflecting the inferior wall (Fig. 5-17). ST elevation may also be limited to leads I and aVL.[132] Note that leads V4 through V6 reflect the lower lateral left ven-

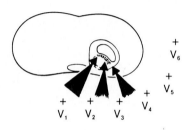

Fig. 5-15 Leads reflecting anteroseptal MI.

tricular surface and leads I and aVL reflect the upper lateral left ventricular surface, which is more directly supplied by the circumflex branch.

NURSING ORDERS: The patient with left coronary artery occlusion

RELATED NURSING DIAGNOSES: Alteration in cardiac output related to arrhythmias; alteration in cardiac output or impaired gas exchange related to CHF or cardiogenic shock
1. Anticipate the development of heart failure.
    a. Check lungs for rales.
    b. Auscultate heart for gallops.
    c. Check fluid balance.
    d. Check wedge readings.
    e. Anticipate sinus tachycardia, rapid atrial arrhythmias.
2. Monitor the patient for the development of intraventricular conduction disturbances and type II or Mobitz II AV blocks.

Transmural inferior wall myocardial infarction

An inferior wall MI can be defined as one affecting the inferior or diaphragmatic surface of the left ventricle. Inferior wall MI occurs as a result of *right* coronary artery pathology. Right coronary artery occlusion commonly causes ischemia to the SA node, the AV junctional tissue, and the parasympathetic (vagal) fibers supplying these structures. As a result of this ischemia, *bradyarrhythmias,* or slow rates, occur. The specific

bradyarrhythmias commonly associated with right coronary artery occlusion are (1) sinus bradycardia and (2) type I or Wenckebach AV block. AV block usually appears within the first 3 days, especially within the first 24 hours, and is associated with larger inferior wall infarction involving the posterior or lateral wall.[35]

The leads that reflect the electrical activity of the inferior wall of the left ventricle are

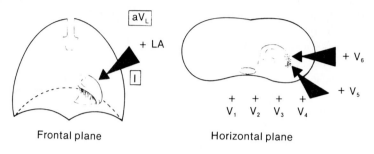

Frontal plane   Horizontal plane

Fig. 5-16 Leads reflecting lateral wall MI.

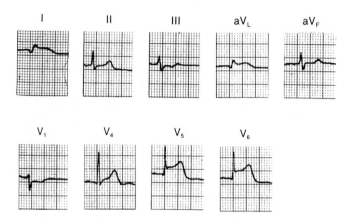

Fig. 5-17 ECG changes reflecting lateral wall MI.

the frontal plane leads II, III, and aVF (Fig. 5-18). ST segment elevation appears in these leads with reciprocal ST depression in leads I and aVL—the leads reflecting the lateral surface (see Fig. 5-20).

Posterior and lateral changes. Inferior wall MI, when extensive, often involves either the posterior wall or lower lateral wall of the left ventricle, or both, in addition to the diaphragmatic surface. Involvement of either the posterior or lower lateral wall (apex) results in changes in the horizontal plane. Involvement of the posterior wall is especially common, occurring in approximately 50% of patients with inferior wall MI.[35] When both the inferior and posterior walls are involved,

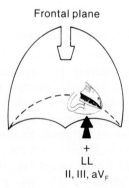

Frontal plane

+
LL
II, III, aV$_F$

Fig. 5-18 Leads reflecting inferior wall MI.

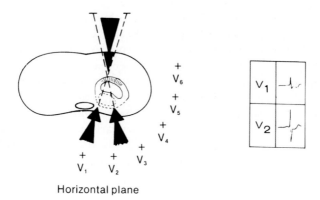

Horizontal plane

Fig. 5-19 Leads reflecting the posterior wall. The ECG changes associated with posterior wall injury and infarction are also illustrated.

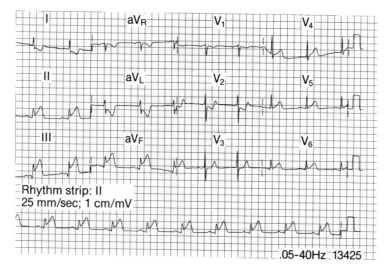

Fig. 5-20 ECG changes in inferoposterior wall MI. The tall R wave in V2 is compatible with abnormal Q wave formation in the posterior wall. Abnormal Q waves are not present in the inferior leads (II, III, and aVF).

the infarction can be described as inferoposterior wall MI. Infarction (Q wave formation) may be limited to the inferior wall with injury extending to the posterior wall. As the infarction evolves, the posterior wall injury often subsides.

No electrodes in a standard 12-lead ECG look directly at the posterior surface of the left ventricle. Therefore, to detect the elec-

trical activity of the posterior wall, the leads located directly opposite this surface are used. These leads are the horizontal plane leads V1 and V2 (Fig. 5-19). Posterior wall injury is thus reflected in leads V1 and V2 by reciprocal ST segment depression (Fig. 5-20). The ST segment depression may extend to V4. It was suggested in the past that this ST segment depression might represent simple reciprocal changes to inferior wall injury. Many experts currently dispute this explanation, however.[15,35,132] ST segment depression in V1 through V4, although less likely, may also be interpreted as ischemic anterior subendocardial injury secondary to coexisting left anterior descending disease.[15,35,132] Current studies do not support this.[15] As the infarction evolves, anterior subendocardial injury is followed by T wave inversion. In contrast, posterior wall injury is followed by reciprocal symmetrically peaked T waves. Regardless of the interpretation, precordial ST segment depression in inferior wall MI is associated with increased complications, including heart failure and increased mortality.[59,132]

Infarction is confirmed by the presence of an abnormal Q wave, which is recorded as an initial negative deflection. In the leads *opposite* an area of necrosis or infarction, a large positive deflection or R wave is recorded instead. Thus in posterior wall infarction, there is an increase in the amplitude of the R waves in V1 and V2.

Less commonly, infarctions may be limited to the posterior wall of the left ventricle. The inferior surface of the left ventricle is that surface resting against the diaphragm. The "true" posterior surface of the left ventricle is that surface lying closer to the atria. Infarctions limited to the posterior wall occur as a result of either left coronary artery or right coronary artery occlusion.[59] The circumflex branch of the left coronary artery is often involved. Anticipated complications are similar to those of lateral wall MI except for the potential for sinus bradycardia.

Lateral wall changes associated with inferior wall MI are recorded in leads V4 through V6 in addition to II, III, and aVF (Fig. 5-21). They are referred to as inferolateral infarction[54] and were formerly described as inferoapical infarction. ST elevation may not appear in leads I and aVL since these leads reflect the upper lateral rather than lower lateral ("apical") wall. The upper lateral wall is supplied by the circumflex branch of the left coronary artery, and the lower lateral wall is supplied in part by the posterior descending branch of the right coronary artery.

Right ventricular infarction. The right coronary artery supplies the right ventricle as well as the left ventricle. Proximal occlusion[132] of the right coronary artery may produce right ventricular infarction together with left ventricular infarction. Logically, right ventricular infarction occurs in combination with inferior wall MI. Right ventricular dysfunction occurs in a large percentage (33% to 52%) of patients with inferior wall MI.[35,59,87,114] No correlation exists with posterior or lateral wall involvement. The detection of right ventricular infarction is important because it is associated with significant hemodynamic compromise in approximately 10% of these patients.[59] Treatment and signs and symptoms vary as well. A pulmonary artery (PA) catheter is indicated (see Unit 8). Signs of RV failure such as neck vein distention are present in the absence of LV failure, indicated by clear breath sounds.[32,87]

The ECG diagnosis of right ventricular infarction is confirmed by obtaining the ECG with *"reversed"* chest leads, that is, V leads obtained on the *right* side of the chest. Leads V3R through V6R are generally recommended,[35,54] although lead V4R is the best single lead[59,87,114] (see Fig. 5-21, *A* and *B*). The ST segment elevation on these leads is transient, typically subsiding within 10 to 24 hours.[59,61,87,132] The ST segment may also be slightly elevated in V1 and V2 with minimal ST changes in II, III, and aVF.[54,87,132] These changes differ from those occurring with anteroseptal MI since the ST segment elevation decreases rather than increases from V1 through V4.[32,132] The diagnosis of right ventricular infarction may also be supported by infarct imaging with techne-

Standard ECG

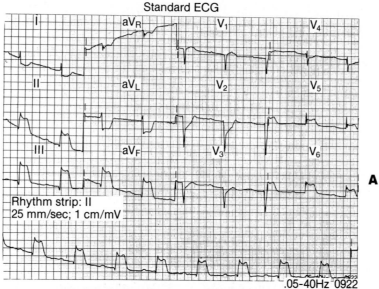

NOTE: The ECG shows ST elevation in leads II, III, aV$_F$, V$_5$, and V$_6$, which suggests acute inferoapical injury/infarction. ST depression in I, aV$_L$ represents a reciprocal change. ST depression in leads V$_1$ and V$_2$ is suggestive of posterior wall injury. Note rhythm is 2° AV block with 2:1 conduction.

Reverse ECG

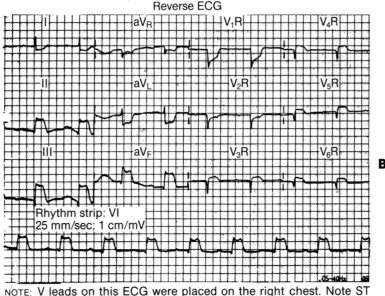

NOTE: V leads on this ECG were placed on the right chest. Note ST elevation in leads V$_3$R through V$_6$R suggestive of right ventricular injury/infarction. The limb leads are positioned normally.

Fig. 5-21 ECG changes in inferolateral wall MI and RV infarction. ST segment changes are compatible with transmural infarction, although abnormal Q waves are not yet present. ST depression in leads V1 and V2 *(A)* is suggestive of posterior wall injury as well.

tium-99m-pyrophosphate, radionuclide angiography (see Nuclear and tomographic imaging), and echocardiography, which can help rule out other disorders with similar hemodynamic patterns.[32,87]

Left ventricular filling and cardiac output are reduced secondary to right ventricular failure. Avoid agents that further decrease left ventricular filling by decreasing either venous return or circulating volume, or use them with caution. These agents include morphine, nitroglycerin, and diuretics. These patients are also more sensitive to decreases in heart rate and become more easily symptomatic with the bradyarrhythmias typically associated with inferior wall MI. Pacing is required more often. Dual-chamber pacing is preferred since maximal cardiac output is obtained[32,59,87] (see Unit 10). Additional modes of therapy include fluid administration, as well as oxygen and dobutamine (Dobutrex), which promote pulmonary vasodilation and decrease the right ventricular (RV) work load.[32,87]

NURSING ORDERS: The patient with right coronary artery occlusion

RELATED NURSING DIAGNOSES: Alteration in cardiac output related to bradyarrhythmias; alteration in cardiac output related to right ventricular failure and decreased left ventricular filling

Pericarditis

Pericarditis represents a more diffuse form of myocardial injury since the pericardium surrounds the entire heart. Pericarditis may not be related to coronary artery disease. However, it may occur with acute MI because the myocardial injury extends to the epicardium, thus triggering an inflammatory response in the pericardium. Since inflammation of the pericardium produces chest pain, pericarditis can complicate the differential diagnosis of acute infarction (see Related Complications and Patient History).

1. Anticipate the following bradyarrhythmias:
   a. Sinus bradycardia
   b. First-degree AV block
   c. Type I or Wenckebach AV block
2. Watch for ventricular or supraventricular tachyarrhythmias that may break through in the presence of slow rates (see Unit 6).
3. Have atropine at the bedside.
4. Be cautious with the administration of depressive drugs such as morphine or with vagal stimulation such as taking rectal temperatures. Monitor patients during these interventions and during bowel movements for the effects of vagal stimulation (bradycardia, dizziness, syncope). Teach not to strain at stool.
5. Monitor for right ventricular infarction within the first 24 hours. Assess patient for distended neck veins in the presence of clear lungs and note ST elevation on leads V1 and V2. If these are present, recommend 16-lead ECG (including V3R through V6R) and infarct imaging.
6. With confirmed right ventricular infarction, use morphine and nitrates with extreme caution. Question the use of diuretics. Anticipate the insertion of a PA catheter and administration of large amounts of fluids, O_2, and dobutamine (Dobutrex).

The ECG changes produced by pericarditis are predictably diffuse. In the presence of pericarditis, ST segment elevation appears in *all* the epicardial leads. Reciprocal ST depression occurs only in the endocardial lead aVR and sometimes leads V1 and aVL, which may also act as endocardial leads depending on the heart's position (Fig. 5-22).[54,61,129] Diffuse T wave inversion occurs as the injury subsides, but unlike infarction patterns these inversions do not occur in conjunction with an elevated ST seg-

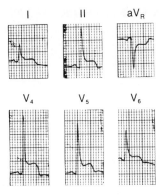

I   II   aV_R

V₄   V₅   V₆

Fig. 5-22 ECG changes in pericarditis.

ment.[54,129] Abnormal Q waves do not occur. When pericarditis complicates acute MI, the location of the MI may become evident later if Q waves develop in the leads reflecting the infarcted surface. Reciprocal ST changes typically associated with infarction are not present. The presence of a positive history and enzymes for acute MI suggests pericarditis with infarction.[129]

Subendocardial infarction

Infarctions confined to the subendocardial layer are classically associated with more subtle symptomatology and ECG changes. These infarctions are usually not associated with Q wave formation and are therefore included under the heading of non–Q wave infarction. The diagnosis is suspected in the presence of sustained ECG changes compatible with subendocardial injury or ischemia. However, due to the absence of Q waves, serum enzyme changes more accurately confirm infarction.

ECG changes associated with subendocardial injury may be localized, or diffuse, depending on the extent of the injury. Injury is typically recorded on the ECG as ST segment elevation. However, most standard leads reflect the epicardial surface. Therefore, in the presence of subendocardial infarction the standard leads reflect and record the opposite or reciprocal change, that is, ST depression. Only the endocardial lead aVR records ST elevation (Fig. 5-23). Note that leads V1 and aVL may also act at times as endocardial leads, depending on the cardiac position, and may thus also record ST elevation.

Diffuse subendocardial injury is detected by noting similar ST changes in normally reciprocal epicardial leads (e.g., leads I and II) and then confirming the change by checking the endocardial lead aVR for ST elevation (see Fig. 5-23). T wave inversion occurs as the infarction evolves. These changes may also occur independently.

Localized subendocardial injury may also occur in patients with symptomatic coronary artery disease. This type of injury is suspected with the following ECG evidence: (1) ST depression on selected epicardial leads; (2) absence of reciprocal changes on the epicardial leads; and (3) ST elevation on leads aVR, V1, or aVL. These local injury changes are far more difficult to recognize and interpret. They may mimic other acute or chronic disease changes, such as the patterns of left ventricular or right ventricular hypertrophy and strain and acute posterior MI.

Patterns associated with angina

Angina may be associated with either transmural or subendocardial ECG changes. Prinzmetal's angina due to coronary spasm is typically associated with transient ST elevation suggestive of transmural injury.[22,35,61] Other forms of angina such as chronic effort

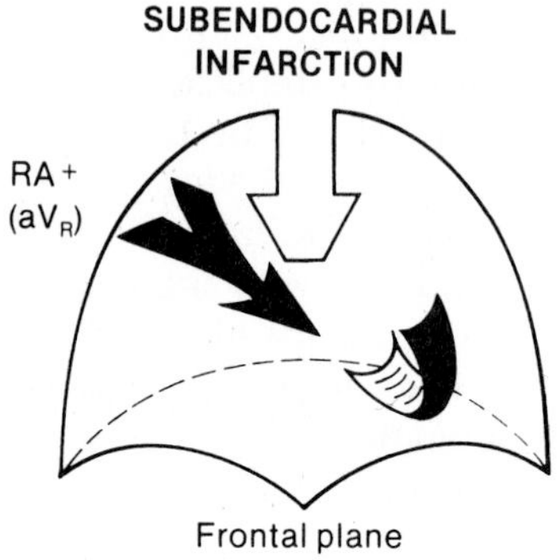

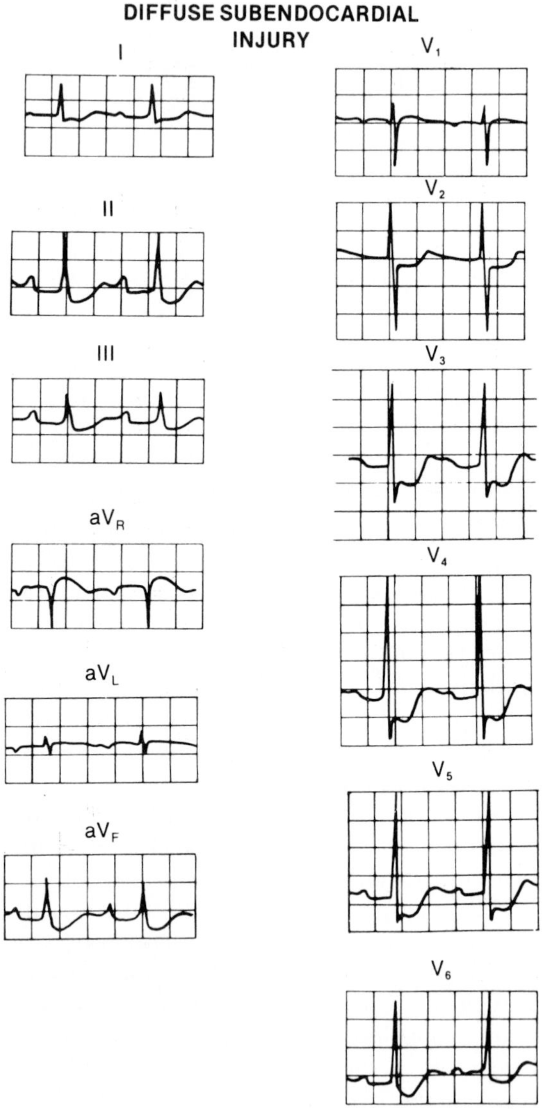

Fig. 5-23 Leads and ECG changes reflecting subendocardial injury. These changes are compatible with subendocardial and non–Q wave infarction in the presence of positive enzymes. Lead aVR is the only lead that directly and consistently reflects the endocardial surface, thus recording ST elevation.

angina and unstable angina are more typically associated with transient subendocardial changes such as inverted T waves or ST depression. Specific patterns of ST depression associated with angina or silent ischemia are discussed further in the section on exercise testing (see Exercise stress (tolerance) testing). Deep T wave inversion in the precordial leads, especially leads V2 and V3, in the patient with unstable angina suggests a proximal significant left anterior descending lesion. This pattern is called Wellens syndrome.[35] It indicates intervention is necessary to prevent extensive anterior wall MI.

Systematic approach

Step 1: Look for injury (ST elevation first, then depression). Look on any leads, but consider each plane separately. In the frontal plane examine limb leads I, II, III, aVR, aVL, and aVF. In the horizontal plane examine chest leads V1 through V6. Note the presence of abnormal Q waves or T wave inversion in leads where you find injury.

Step 2: Determine what surface the lead with ST elevation reflects.

Step 3: Determine if the injury is localized or diffuse by checking for reciprocal changes in the epicardial leads.

Remember that injury localized to a single myocardial surface is compatible with acute transmural MI. Reciprocal changes are recorded in the leads reflecting the opposite surface. The absence of reciprocal changes is compatible with the diffuse injury occurring in either pericarditis or subendocardial ischemia/infarction.

Exercise stress (tolerance) testing

Exercise stress testing is a noninvasive procedure that involves monitoring the cardiovascular electrical and mechanical response to continuous, progressively strenuous, dynamic exercise. The exercise acts as a "stress" or *work load challenge* to the heart to determine normal versus abnormal function and work load capacity. The use of the word *stress* in stress testing can be misleading and disturbing, since it is easily confused with the stress response, which is potentially harmful to the heart and regarded as a risk factor. Alternate terms include exercise *tolerance* testing (ETT), graded exercise testing (GXT),[57] or merely exercise testing.

Exercise testing is used primarily to detect and evaluate the functional impact of coronary artery disease. Unlike cardiac catheterization, exercise testing is unable to localize and evaluate the extent of coronary stenosis. However, it is more effective in determining when diseased coronary arteries are no longer able to meet an individual's increased myocardial oxygen demands without metabolic compromise. Therefore, exercise testing is usually adequate when screening for significant coronary artery disease and initiating appropriate medical therapy. Its recommended use is as a screening tool in men over the age of 40 with two or more risk factors or in high-risk occupations, and in apparently healthy individuals in the coronary age group who want to pursue cardiovascular conditioning programs.[61,96] It may also be useful in men with atypical symptoms such as epicardial distress or in patients with only rest angina.[27] Although exercise testing elicits symptoms such as angina and ST elevation in only 30% of patients with rest an-

Step 4: Determine nursing implications (right coronary artery disease versus left coronary artery disease).

gina, it can identify individuals with significant underlying fixed disease.[27] Continuous ECG (Holter) monitoring can be a helpful adjunct in this population.

Exercise therapy is safer, less expensive, and more easily available than cardiac catheterization and is more effective in predicting prognosis. As a prognostic tool, exercise stress testing predicts mortality and morbidity, especially in patients recovering from acute MI who undergo predischarge testing.[61] It allows evaluation of the immediate and long-term effects of drug therapy, coronary artery bypass surgery, PTCA, and exercise, as well as the progress of the disease. Patients with unstable angina should be pain-free for at least 48 to 72 hours before testing. Although stress testing is primarily a diagnostic and prognostic procedure, other common uses include guiding and evaluating intervention, rehabilitation, and physical conditioning (see Patient Teaching and Cardiac Rehabilitation). It can be used with CHF to assess work load capacity, with symptomatic exercise-induced arrhythmias, and with hypertension to assess blood pressure response to exercise.[57,61,102]

Do not attempt exercise stress testing in patients with bundle branch block or WPW since ST segment distortions are expected. In women, the exercise stress test is not an accurate indicator of coronary artery disease, particularly when relying on ECG changes. Estrogens may produce digitalis-like effects on the ST segment.[96] To improve accuracy, include other parameters such as heart rate response, endurance, and chest pain.[96] For best results combine it with thallium imaging, although breast shadows limit anterior wall signals.[96] In patients who are unable to exercise because of neurologic, vascular, or orthopedic disorders, consider pharmacologic stress testing combined with thallium imaging or echocardiography as an alternative (see Echocardiography/Perfusion and Infarct Imaging).

The two main modes of dynamic exercise used for exercise testing in the United States are the treadmill and bicycle ergometry. Bicycle ergometry is most commonly used in combination with radionuclide angiography because of the patient positioning required. The treadmill is used most commonly in routine stress testing or in combination with thallium radionuclide imaging.

The stages of the exercise stress testing protocols are commonly correlated with various levels of oxygen demands known as *METs*. MET is an abbreviation for *met*abolic equivalent. A MET corresponds to the equivalent of the usual metabolic requirements, or amount of O_2 used per minute, at rest. An increased MET value correlates with increased exercise intensity. The concept of MET is supported by the American Heart Association. METs can also be correlated with calories for diet and weight control.

Treadmill exercise protocols vary according to initial intensity (METs) and amount and timing of exercise increments. Work loads are increased by changes in the treadmill speed, or the grade (incline), or both. The response of the patient at different work loads or *stages* is then evaluated. The Bruce multistage protocol is the most popular treadmill protocol. In this particular protocol, the speed and grade of the treadmill are increased at 3-minute intervals until significant symptoms appear or the patient complains of fatigue. The initial MET level is high at approximately 5 METs.[57] This protocol allows the patient to judge his or her maximal ability to a greater extent than other protocols. It is also the easiest and most efficient to administer.[R6] Other protocols such as the modified Bruce, Naughton, Weber, and Balke-Ware protocols use lower initial MET levels of 1.5 to 2.0 METs and smaller work load increments, increased at shorter 1- to 2-minute intervals; they are useful in patients with CHF with decreased work load capacity[61] or in pre- and postdischarge testing following MI.[57,143]

The normal cardiovascular response to exercise is an increase in heart rate and stroke volume in an attempt to increase cardiac output and O_2 delivery. This response results from sympathetic nervous system stimulation. Normal women have an increased sympathetic response that may produce coronary spasm and distort the stress test results.[96] In early exercise, the heart rate is the primary determinant of cardiac output.[6] The stroke volume is increased because of an increased force of myocardial contraction and increased venous return secondary to mild venoconstriction. Blood pressure increases secondary to increases in cardiac output and arterial vasoconstriction.[6] The greater these compensatory increases in cardiac output and blood pressure, the greater the work load on the heart. This work load is commonly expressed as the product of the heart rate and mean arterial pressure. It is known as the *rate pressure product* (RPP) or *double product*. This product reflects the myocardial O_2 consumption at any given exercise work load.[61,143]

This cardiovascular response to exercise has normal physiologic limits. The ability of the heart rate to increase in response to increased demands for cardiac output is characteristically limited by a unique age-related ceiling on rate. Normal compensatory increases in heart rate do not occur beyond this maximal point, logically referred to as the *maximal predicted heart rate*. Curiously, the stroke volume reaches its normal compensatory limits at about the same time the peak heart rate is reached. Thus further increases in cardiac output are not possible. When these physiologic limits are reached, oxygen demands can no longer be effectively met, and myocardial and systemic hypoxia occur. Extended periods of hypoxia are potentially harmful and life-threatening, and the patient can best prevent them by ceasing exercise at this point or before. *Sustained* exercise *beyond* this point is potentially harmful even in the normal individual and is best avoided. For this reason, suggested target heart rates for conditioning programs in normal individuals are usually 70% to 80% of the maximum predicted heart rate. Conditioning programs after acute MI use more conservative target heart rates (see Patient Teaching and Cardiac Rehabilitation).[61]

Maximum heart rate is commonly estimated by subtracting the patient's age from 220, which is theoretically a newborn's maximum achievable heart rate. A mean deviation of 10 to 12 points is then allowed. For example, a 50-year-old man would have a maximum predicted heart rate of 170 ± 12, or a range of 162 to 182 beats per minute.[143] This method is used in a variety of cardiovascular conditioning programs and during diagnostic stress testing as a normal end point. However, use of maximum heart rates can be misleading since significant individual variances occur and cardioactive medications may affect their attainment.[143]

Multistage exercise stress tests are usually symptom-limited or heart rate–limited. They are classified as maximal or submaximal, depending on whether the patient reaches his or her physiologic limits or stops at an earlier predetermined end point. A submaximal test is terminated when the patient reaches 70% to 80% of the age-predicted maximum heart rate or earlier using other parameters. Some investigators believe that maximal tests provide more accurate information of physical performance capacity.[61] However, submaximal or low-level tests are clearly indicated for selected subsets of patients, such as those tested soon (1 to 3 weeks) after MI or after bypass surgery or those known to have significant coronary artery disease.[57] The low-level predischarge stress test after acute MI may be limited to 5 to 6 METs intensity[57,61] and heart rate less than 120 beats per minute (or 110 beats per minute if on beta blockers).[143] A modified Bruce, Naughton, or Balke-Ware protocol is used.[57,143] The test can provide guidelines for safe activity.[57] A negative test is associated with low 1-year mortality[44] and may have psychological benefits.[57] A positive test can identify those who may need follow-up such as PTCA, antianginal or antiarrhythmic agents, and/or careful monitoring.[57]

A positive stress test is one that must be terminated before the patient achieves predicted maximal or submaximal limits because of signs or symptoms of cardiovascular decompensation. These signs and symptoms reflect metabolic compromise and/or excessive sympathetic stimulation. They include chest pain, ECG changes, blood pressure changes, and life-threatening arrhythmias. Generally, the earlier the signs and symptoms of cardiovascular decompensation become manifest, the more serious the extent of the disease. The patient may also choose to terminate the test based on subjective feelings of fatigue, exhaustion, shortness of breath, or dizziness. The highest work load achieved is called the patient's *exercise* or *functional capacity.*[143]

Chest pain by itself may not necessitate exercise termination unless it is part of a typical anginal syndrome or is accompanied by ST segment changes. Anginal chest pain occurring during stress testing can be useful in predicting the likelihood of subsequent coronary events. Both the heart rate and anginal response may be obscured by antianginal agents such as the beta blockers, calcium channel blockers, and nitrates.

The most common ECG sign of cardiovascular decompensation is ST segment depression. ST depression reflects subendocardial

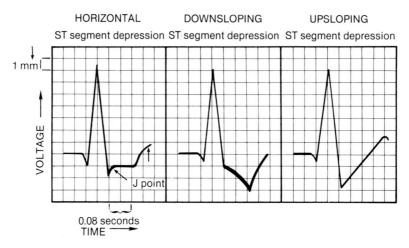

HORIZONTAL DOWNSLOPING UPSLOPING
ST segment depression ST segment depression ST segment depression

1 mm

VOLTAGE ——

J point

0.08 seconds
TIME ——

Fig. 5-24 Positive ECG findings in exercise stress testing. The third example, up-sloping ST segment depression, is the least predictive.

injury secondary to physiologic ischemia (see ECG Changes). T wave changes may also occur but are affected by body position, respirations, and hyperventilation.[61] ST-T waves and rhythm changes should be continuously monitored before, during, and for some time after the test.[143] The stress test is considered positive for myocardial ischemia when the magnitude and configuration of the ST segment fulfill any of the following criteria: (1) 1-mm *flat* ST segment depression lasting for 0.80 second; (2) 1-mm *downsloping* ST segment depression lasting for 0.08 second; or (3) 1.5- to 2.0-mm *upsloping* ST depression lasting for 0.08 second (Fig. 5-24).[61] ST upsloping is the least predictive of the three criteria[143]; ST depression with a downsloping ST segment has the highest predictive value for coronary artery disease. About 75% to 80% of significant ST segment depression appears on leads V4 through V6.[61] However, multilead monitoring is preferred. Lead V4R may be helpful in confirming right coronary artery disease.[61] The test is terminated when ST segment depression is greater than 3

mm.[61,143] Although less common, ST segment elevation of 1 mm for at least 0.08 second has the same significance as ST segment depression. ST segment elevation is more likely to appear on leads correlating with the LV surface and coronary artery involved.[61]

Other factors that produce ST segment shifts or cause ST-T wave abnormalities include drugs such as digitalis, hyperventilation, electrolyte abnormalities, hypertrophy, bundle branch block, and WPW.[61,143] ST segment depression is common in both right and left bundle branch block.[61] As stated, earlier patients with left bundle branch block or WPW should be referred for pharmacologic stress testing in conjunction with nuclear or echocardiographic imaging. Note that digitalis effects on the ST segment are more marked during exercise.[61] Obtain baseline ECG traces in the sitting, standing, or supine position for later comparison. To rule out hyperventilation, obtain a later resting hyperventilation trace and compare it to the exercise ST changes.[61]

Life-threatening arrhythmias may also

serve as a marker of cardiac decompensation. These occur in response to the release of sympathetic chemicals or pH changes.[61,102] Most investigators believe that severe exercise-induced arrhythmias are strongly suggestive of heart disease. They may occur immediately after exercise in the "cool-down" period as well as during exercise.[102] The presence of PVCs alone in apparently healthy individuals during routine testing is of little prognostic significance. PACs are also considered benign. Sustained supraventricular tachycardia is uncommon and has little prognostic significance. However, the test must be terminated. Arrhythmias present before testing even in those with known coronary artery disease may be abolished as the heart rate increases with exercise. The occurrence of bradycardia including AV block is an indication for test termination. Generally, arrhythmias that would require treatment in a coronary care unit (CCU) necessitate termination of the stress test. Of particular concern are the life-threatening ventricular arrhythmias. The stress test may also unmask adverse reactions to antiarrhythmic therapy.[99]

The blood pressure response to exercise is another important marker of cardiovascular decompensation. Most investigators terminate the exercise test when the systolic blood pressure approaches 220 to 250 mm Hg.[61,137] Failure to raise the blood pressure or a sudden drop in blood pressure with dynamic exercise is also a sign of cardiovascular decompensation. Hypotension manifested during exercise, especially at low work loads, is a poor prognostic sign indicative of severe cardiac disease. Dizziness, sudden pallor, or gait disturbances may precede a drop in blood pressure. The cardiac disease may be valvular disease or cardiomyopathy, as well as coronary artery disease.

The results of the exercise stress test can be a useful basis for individualized discharge instructions after MI or after bypass surgery.

They may also guide the individual without known coronary artery disease who is starting out in a cardiovascular conditioning program (see Patient Teaching and Cardiac Rehabilitation).

NURSING ORDERS: Exercise stress testing

RELATED NURSING DIAGNOSES: Alteration in comfort, knowledge deficit, alteration in cardiac output

1. Explain the procedure to the patient and obtain his or her signed consent.
2. Assess the patient with special attention to risk factors, exercise patterns, and presence of abnormal heart or lung sounds.
3. Instruct the patient to fast and avoid stimulants, such as cigarettes or caffeine, 2 to 3 hours before testing.[145,154,155]
4. Have the patient wear nonrestrictive, comfortable clothing and rubber-soled, supportive shoes. Women should wear bras, unless special supportive shirts are available.
5. Instruct the patient to continue all usual medication, unless the physician specifies otherwise.[137,143] Record any cardiac medications, especially digitalis, antiarrhythmics, and antianginal agents.
6. Do not schedule stress testing on the same day as a glucose tolerance test or barium enema. A glucose load may produce ST shifts and thus alter test results. The laxative preparation used with barium enemas may induce hypokalemia, which also produces ST-T abnormalities.
7. Validate the presence and operation of all emergency equipment.
8. Record a baseline ECG, blood pressure, and heart rate immediately before testing.
9. Demonstrate the correct stance and gait for the patient and allow for practice on the treadmill before beginning the test. Instruct the patient not to hold on to the

handrails since functional capacity can be significantly overestimated.[61]

10. Emphasize to the patient the importance of reporting even subtle symptoms that could indicate myocardial ischemia.

11. Assess the patient's heart rate, blood pressure, and ST segment carefully during stress testing, recording rhythm strips at intervals specified by the physician. Correlate the responses with the level of work load and other symptomatology.

12. Observe the patient for subtle signs of exercise intolerance, such as changes in facial expression, gait, respiratory rate, and skin temperature and color; correlate them with the work load.

13. Encourage the patient to continue with the test if he or she exhibits no adverse symptomatology or has not attained the target heart rate.

14. When terminating the test, allow the patient to sit; record the heart rate and blood pressure every 1 to 3 minutes, until they return to baseline.

15. Instruct the patient not to shower for 2 hours after the test to prevent vasomotor alterations that could occur with extremely cold or hot water temperatures.[61,137]

Echocardiography

Echocardiography is considered a form of cardiac imaging since the examiner obtains a picture, or image. Unlike nuclear or radiographic images, an echocardiographic image is obtained by the use of sound waves. Echocardiography involves beaming painless, high-frequency (ultrasonic) sound waves into the chest and recording reflected vibrations, or *echoes*. These sound waves are transmitted, received, and translated into electrical signals on an oscilloscope by a pencil-like device called a *transducer*. A transducer is an instrument capable of translating one form of energy into another form of energy.

The vibrations are reflected by the chest wall and solid structures of the heart. Thus this procedure allows for the examination of the size, shape, and motion of the cardiac structures to detect mechanical dysfunction. A simultaneous ECG trace is recorded for reference only. The major structures visualized are the four cardiac valves, RV and LV walls and chambers, and pericardial sac. Major abnormalities detected include valvular stenosis or insufficiency, septal defects, hypertrophy, aneurysms, mural thrombi, asynchronous or ineffective LV contraction, and pericardial effusion.

Coronary artery disease is detected primarily by the presence of regional wall motion abnormalities or asynchronous LV contraction. Hemodynamically significant coronary artery disease may also be confirmed and quantified from evidence of decreased or ineffective LV contraction. The effectiveness of LV contraction is determined from measurements of ejection fraction. Ejection fraction is the percentage of the diastolic volume that is ejected during systole. Normal ejection fraction is 70%. Ejection fraction can be estimated from changes in the LV chamber diameter during diastole and systole. Echocardiographic determinations are comparable to those obtained during radionuclide angiography. The effectiveness of reperfusion techniques can be confirmed by recovery of wall motion and improved ejection fraction.[6] Atherosclerotic changes in the left main coronary artery produce bright echoes, which may be detected on the echocardiographic image. The clinical significance of these findings, however, is not clear at this time.[6]

Echocardiography may also facilitate the diagnosis of complications after acute MI. Sudden systolic murmurs caused by ventricular septal rupture may be differentiated from those caused by papillary muscle rupture. Echocardiography easily detects the pericardial effusion associated with cardiac tamponade and may allow it to be differentiated from RV infarction, especially in the context of the similar hemodynamic patterns (see Unit 8). Confirmation of the presence or absence of a mural thrombus as well as its morphology and mobility can facilitate the decision whether to anticoagulate after MI.[6,42] Echocardiography may also confirm the presence of ventricular aneurysm.[6]

Echocardiography can be performed with either a narrow-angle or a wide-angle beam. The older narrow-beam method is known as M-mode or motion mode. In the newer, wide-angle method the sound beams sweep like arcs over a broader cross-section of the heart, allowing more of a two-dimensional view. This method, although also a motion mode, is referred to by comparison as two-dimensional (2D) echocardiography. Two-dimensional echocardiography allows for a lifelike view of the cardiac structures, making it easier to detect most of the major abnormalities. The major advantage of M-mode is its ability to detect rapidly occurring changes better, since it more simply and rapidly obtains the pictures. Pericardial effusion may also be more easily seen on an M-mode view.

Recently, specialized contrast agents have been developed to augment the reflected sound waves. These agents can be injected into the coronary arteries during cardiac catheterization to highlight perfused myocardial areas when simultaneous echocardiographic imaging is used.[6,112] This technique can provide information on myocardial perfusion previously not available during cardiac catheterization.

The three latest modalities added to echocardiography include color flow Doppler, stress echocardiography, and transesophageal echocardiography (TEE). In color flow Doppler imaging, sound waves are reflected off the moving red blood cells to provide color-coded information about the direction and velocity of blood flow.[112] This information is most helpful in assessing valvular regurgitation or stenosis, the function of prosthetic heart valves, and septal defects. Color flow imaging may also provide estimates of intracardiac pressures and cardiac output which correlate with invasive measurements and which could be adapted in the future into continuous noninvasive monitoring techniques.[112]

No special patient preparations are required for M-mode, 2-D, or color flow echocardiography. Inform patients that the tests are painless. No sedation is necessary. Do not withhold any drugs, and allow patients to eat and drink normally before the test.

Echocardiographic stress testing can act as an alternative to nuclear imaging in pharmacologic and exercise stress testing. Echocardiographic imaging can be performed immediately after treadmill exercise testing. New wall motion abnormalities are consistent with significant ischemia[6,85] and add to the accuracy of a borderline or nonspecific exercise stress test.[18] Echocardiographic stress testing is also useful in patients with ST segment changes due to left ventricular hypertrophy, bundle branch block, or digitalis.[85] Results are comparable to thallium imaging, less expensive to the patient, and totally noninvasive. In addition, the test involves no radiation exposure.[6]

In patients who are unable to exercise, the practitioner can combine echocardiography with pharmacologic stress testing using either dipyridamole (Persantine) or dobutamine (Dobutrex). Sensitivity for multivessel disease is higher than with single-vessel disease.[104] Ironically, adenosine is neither sensitive nor specific when used in combination with echocardiography, although it is closely related to dipyridamole and is useful as an adjunct to nuclear imaging.[85] Dipyridamole and dobutamine induce ischemia by different mechanisms. Whereas dipyridamole as a vasodilator acts on the coronary supply (see Perfusion and infarct imaging), dobutamine acts on oxygen demands, similar to exercise, by increasing heart rate, contractility, and blood pressure.[85,104] Dosages are administered in a stepwise fashion by increments of 5 mcg/kg/min every 5 minutes up to 20 mcg/kg/min, thus mimicking exercise protocol stages. Results are comparable with either agent. A higher incidence of ventricular arrhythmias occurs with dobutamine, but these usually are not life-threatening.[85,104] However, the pulmonary side effects seen with dipyridamole do not occur. Therefore, dobutamine offers an alternative for those with bronchospastic pulmonary disease. Other reported side effects with dipyridamole, including chest pain, dizziness, and bradycardia, are not associated with dobutamine.

Exercise or pharmacologic echocardiography can be performed immediately before discharge or within 3 weeks after acute MI to determine prognosis. New wall motion abnormalities are associated with an increased risk of a second cardiovascular event.[6,18,85,104] Patient preparation is similar to that for routine exercise testing or dipyrimadole nuclear imaging.

TEE involves the introduction of an esophageal probe via endoscopy. The ultrasound transducer is mounted on the tip. Informed consent is required and the patient should fast for at least 4 hours before the procedure. Local anesthesia is accomplished with lidocaine spray to decrease the gag reflex.[70] Sedation is administered if severe LV dysfunction or lung disease is not present. The patient is asked to swallow as the probe is advanced. Pulse oximetry may be used to monitor for signs of hypoxemia. Secretions are suctioned as indicated. Although patient discomfort is a concern and limiting factor in the awake patient, complications are unusual.[83] Complications are less common than with routine endoscopy since TEE is not attempted in patients with potential esophageal disease. The most common side effect is an increase in systolic blood pressure with initial insertion of the probe.[83] Transient bradycardias and ventricular arrhythmias have been reported. Also, occasional anginal attacks have occurred in patients with severe coronary artery disease.[83]

The major advantages of this technique are the elimination of chest wall interference and intrathoracic distortion and better visualization of posterior structures such as the left atrium and thoracic aorta. The elimination of chest wall interference allows for better-quality pictures, especially in obese patients, patients with obstructive pulmonary disease, and those with other chest wall changes. Primary indications include detection of atrial masses (tumors or thrombi), aortic disease, especially that involving the aortic arch or descending aorta, and vegetations associated with endocarditis. TEE is also useful in evaluating prosthetic valves, atrial septal defects, and mitral regurgitation or valvuloplasty.[83] Two-dimensional and color flow imaging principles are used.

TEE can be used during coronary artery surgery or valve replacement to monitor LV function and volume status. It can provide images without disturbing the surgical procedure. New wall motion abnormalities correlate with myocardial ischemia or infarction more accurately than ECG or PA changes and can identify high-risk patients.[83] Since TEE determines volume status directly from LV dimensions, values are more accurate than those obtained by pulmonary artery wedge pressure, which may be affected by other factors[83] (see Unit 8).

Transesophageal echocardiography has other potential uses in the patient with coronary artery disease. TEE provides clearer images of the proximal portion of the left coronary artery when compared to simple 2D echo. The full length of the left coronary artery and coronary flow has been recently imaged,[83] allowing determination of the extent of coronary stenosis. However, use of TEE for this purpose is not widespread at this time. A major limitation is difficulty in visualizing the right coronary artery.[83] TEE may also detect complications of coronary artery disease such as mitral insufficiency. However, simple 2D echo is usually sufficient.

Cardiac catheterization

Cardiac catheterization is an invasive procedure that involves the introduction of a catheter into the right or left side of the heart and the coronary artery system. Cardiac catheterization employs the concept of *angiography,* which is the visualization of blood flow through the chambers or blood vessels through use of a radiopaque dye or nuclear tracer. Ventriculography is a form of angiography limited to visualization of the ventricles. Coronary arteriography is a form of angiography limited to visualization of the coronary arteries. During cardiac catheterization, both ventriculography and coronary arteriography are commonly performed.

Cardiac catherization can be used to detect and evaluate disorders of cardiac mechanical activity and coronary artery structure. It is primarily a diagnostic procedure, that is also used therapeutically because of its access to the coronary circulation. It is the most accurate diagnostic tool for determining the presence and severity of coronary artery disease and serves as the standard against which all other methods of assessing coronary artery disease are measured.[61] Cardiac catheterization is indicated when a precise diagnosis is critical to the selection of appropriate medical or surgical therapy. It is most commonly used to exclude the presence of surgically treatable disease and/or to define the cardiac anatomy preoperatively. Cardiac catheterization can also be used to assess the effectiveness of medical ther-apy, progress of disease, and graft patency.[8]

Cardiac catheterization should be performed only when similar noninvasive tests cannot provide sufficient diagnostic information to guide therapy. A limitation of cardiac catheterization as a diagnostic tool is its inability to determine the functional significance of varying degrees of stenosis without the concurrent use of pacing or exercise.

Cardiac catheterization allows assessment of both right-sided and left-sided mechanical function. Right-sided heart access is accomplished via the brachiocephalic or femoral vein. A cutdown in the right antecubital area allows for catheter insertion in the brachiocephalic vein. Percutaneous catheter insertion via the femoral vein is currently a more common route of access to the right side of the heart.[136,140] A tubular sheath is commonly advanced over the catheter to facilitate the introduction of a variety of catheters as needed.[61] Passage of the catheter into the superior or inferior vena cava and right heart is facilitated by the use of fluoroscopy and physical maneuvers such as deep breathing, coughing, and position change. A flow-directed, balloon-tipped catheter is most common (see Unit 8).[61,136]

Right-sided heart catheterization allows assessment of right-sided structures and pressures, as well as the presence of intracardiac shunts, pulmonary hypertension, and cardiac output.[136] Ventriculography of the right side of the heart is not done routinely. However, if pressure findings indicate the probability of a structural or functional abnormality, dye is injected at this point and right ventriculography is performed. An RV pacer may be inserted prophylactically after the right-sided heart catheterization in patients at high risk for developing conduction abnormalities during the catheterization procedure.

Left-sided catheterization is accomplished by retrograde insertion of the catheter through an artery into the aorta. The patient receives systemic heparin before insertion of the catheter to reduce the chance of thrombus formation on the catheter tip with subsequent embolization. With left-sided heart catheterization the catheter is inserted into either the brachial artery via cutdown (Sones's technique) or femoral artery via percutaneous route (Judkins's technique). An arterial sheath is also commonly used. The catheter is advanced in a retrograde manner through the aorta, guided by fluoroscopic imaging.

Catheterization of the left ventricle allows pressure measurement, oxygen sampling, and assessment of left-sided structural and functional abnormalities. Ventriculography of the left ventricle is commonly performed to assess such mechanical parameters as regional wall motion abnormalities and ejection fraction (see Unit 8). The left atrium is not routinely catheterized unless pressure abnormalities indicate severe mitral valve disease.

Right and left coronary arteriography (angiography) is accomplished by advancing the catheter into the coronary orifices and injecting a small amount of radiopaque dye. Nitroglycerin may be given sublingually before dye injection to maximize visualization and prevent vessel spasm caused by mechanical catheter irritation. Intracoronary nitroglycerin may also be indicated if severe spasm is induced during the procedure. Other coronary vasodilators, such as the calcium channel blocking agent nifedipine (Procardia),

may also be used before and after catheterization to minimize vessel spasm. In selected patients a provocative test that induces spasm may be employed to ascertain the role of spasm in rest angina. Provocation of coronary artery spasm with ergonovine maleate was formerly used with regularity.[136]

During coronary arteriography, rotating the patient from side to side maximizes visualization of the coronary arteries. The views, or projections, imaged are similar to those used with radionuclide angiography. Having the patient cough after each dye injection can help clear residual dye from the coronary circulation.

Visualization of the coronary arteries allows assessment of the site and severity of stenotic lesions and also general characteristics of the vessels in terms of size, collateral flow, distal runoff, and mass of myocardium served. Cardiac drugs, exercise, and pacing can be used in conjunction with cardiac catheterization to attempt to assess the functional significance of coronary artery stenosis. The stenosis is considered significant regardless of the extent if it triggers angina or other signs of ischemia during times of increased oxygen demand.

Complications occurring during the catheterization procedure are primarily related to catheter manipulation and dye injection. Right-sided catheterization may cause a vasovagal reaction by irritation of nerve endings in the right-sided structures. Arrhythmias may also occur as the catheter is manipulated through the right cardiac chambers. The most common arrhythmias are bradycardia caused by increased vagal tone and ventricular arrhythmias caused by mechanical irritation of the ventricles from catheter manipulation. Left-sided cardiac catheterization may also produce arrhythmias due to mechanical irritation of the ventricles from catheter manipulation. Vessel spasm may complicate coronary arteriography during a left-sided catheterization. Medications such as nitroglycerin and nifedipine are useful in preventing and treating coronary spasm. Systemic heparinization can reduce the risk of cerebral embolization with left-sided catheterization. Rarely, embolization within a coronary artery caused by thrombus or plaque disruption may also complicate this procedure and could result in myocardial infarction.

Sensitivity reactions to the iodine-based radiopaque dye may occur during either right or left ventriculography or coronary arteriography. These reactions may range from a mild urticaria to a severe anaphylactic reaction. With careful screening and premedication before cardiac catheterization, anaphylactic reactions are rare.[24] ECG changes including ST segment elevation or depression, T wave changes, axis shifts, ventricular arrhythmias, and sinus bradycardias occur within 10 to 15 seconds of dye injection. These changes are transient, lasting less than 90 seconds, rarely result in ventricular fibrillation, and are thought to be a direct effect of the dye on the cardiac cells rather than a reflection of ischemia or sensitivity.[24] Renal toxicity can occur, especially in diabetic pa-

tients and patients with a history of renal insufficiency.[24] Newer, recently introduced dyes such as Isovue are associated with fewer allergic reactions and less renal insufficiency.

Patient discomfort or distress, including transient heat sensation, nausea, chest pain,[24] or anxiety, may also complicate the catheterization procedure. However, appropriate precatheterization instruction, premedication, and reassurance during the procedure usually avert or minimize this problem.[92]

Postcatheterization complications are related primarily to access site trauma, which can result in bleeding or ischemia in the involved limb. Close observation for overt bleeding and hematoma formation or expansion at the insertion site is crucial in the first 2 to 4 hours after catheterization. Maintenance of prescribed pressure dressings and/or sandbags and limb immobility is also important. Circulation checks of the involved limb with documentation of pulses, color, temperature, and sensation facilitate detection of any signs of thrombotic or embolic occlusion of a vessel.

Pharmacologic intervention

Cardiac catheterization is also used therapeutically in the management of coronary artery disease. Therapeutic application of cardiac catheterization is directed toward the three major mechanisms of coronary artery stenosis in an attempt to prevent or minimize MI.

Two pharmacologic agents, nitroglycerin and streptokinase, may be injected directly into the coronary circulation when the patient has signs and symptoms of acute infarction. The patient with suspected infarction is taken directly to the catheterization laboratory. After coronary arteriography and documentation of vessel occlusion, nitroglycerin is usually the initial drug infused. Nitroglycerin, a vasodilator, relaxes the smooth mus-

cle of the vessel wall and may reestablish flow by reversing spasm. Failure to reestablish flow after nitroglycerin infusion justifies the use of the more potent thrombolytic agents such as streptokinase or urokinase.

Intracoronary as well as intravenous thrombolytics act to lyse the acute thrombus, which is usually the final event resulting in coronary artery occlusion. The patient receives maximum benefits from intracoronary nitroglycerin or thrombolytics in acute MI when this mode of therapy is instituted within 2 to 4 hours after the onset of acute symptoms. The use of intracoronary streptokinase is rapidly being replaced by the use of IV thrombolytic agents (see Unit 9).

Percutaneous transluminal coronary angioplasty

Another procedure used both acutely and electively to alter the structural changes contributing to coronary stenosis is known as percutaneous transluminal coronary angioplasty, or PTCA. This procedure requires direct access to the coronary circulation and therefore is performed only in the catheterization laboratory.

PTCA is directed toward the atheromatous plaque and involves the controlled compression and disruption of the plaque with a specially designed balloon catheter. Compression is accomplished by introducing the catheter into the coronary artery across the stenotic area and intermittently inflating the balloon. This controlled intimal disruption results in expansion of the arterial lumen and improved coronary artery blood flow (Fig. 5-25).

PTCA is considered an alternative to coronary bypass surgery primarily in the patient with angina or silent ischemia and is often elective. Many institutions have successfully performed both single- and multi-vessel angioplasty. However, patients with single-vessel disease are still considered ideal candidates.[119,127,140] Multiple lesions may be dilated within a single artery or major branch.[119,140] Long-term effectiveness of PTCA compared with coronary bypass surgery is still under investigation, especially in patients with multivessel disease.[119,140]

PTCA is also used to reopen occluded coronary bypass grafts. Higher success rates are reported with internal mammary grafts.[119,140] Patients with both unstable and stable angina are considered candidates, in spite of conflicting reports regarding initial success and complication rates in unstable angina.[119,121,127]

The use of PTCA in the patient with acute MI is controversial.[4,117,119,140] Thrombolysis has advantages over PTCA since it does not require immediate access to a catheterization laboratory and is associated with equal or better survival rates. Initial PTCA offers no advantage over thrombolysis followed by PTCA, and researchers report better long-term survival with thrombolysis alone than with thrombolysis followed by immediate PTCA.[10] The recently completed TIMI2 study results indicate that follow-up PTCA is unnecessary unless the patient has postinfarction angina or a positive exercise stress test.[4,10,44,140] Patients in cardiogenic shock or those in whom thrombolytic therapy is contraindicated may benefit from PTCA.[10,49,140] There is general agreement that PTCA should not be performed in difficult lesions, in lesions with borderline stenosis (50% to 60%), or in arteries other than the infarct-related artery immediately after infarction.[33,44,119]

Because of revised balloon design and steerable guidewires, success rates for PTCA have improved from 67% before 1982 to

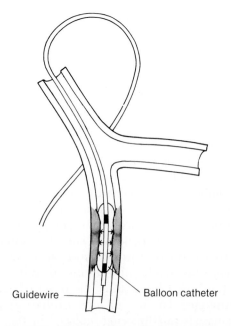

Guidewire ———   ——— Balloon catheter

Fig. 5-25   PTCA balloon dilation catheter.

90% in 1991.[120] Success is measured by a reduction in the obstruction to less than 50% and by the absence of major short-term complications.[8,119,120] Successful angioplasty is no longer affected by female gender, distal location, or configuration of the stenotic lesion.[120] The current primary limiting factors are calcified, noncompressible lesions, thrombosis, complete occlusion, ostial location, and lesions at angulated segments or bifurcations.[119,120] Major contraindications include diffuse disease, long lesions, and lesions in the main trunk of the left coronary artery.[8,119,140]

The patient undergoes coronary arteriography before PTCA, preferably at an earlier date, to define the anatomy, determine the suitability of the lesion for angioplasty, and allow for consultation if necessary.[119] Measuring the drop in pressure across the lesion at this time verifies the extent of the arterial narrowing and allows for subsequent assessment of the results of the angioplasty. The drop in pressure across the lesion is known as the pressure gradient. Generally, the larger the pressure change, or gradient, the more severe the narrowing, or stenosis.

The balloon is inflated gradually at progressively greater pressures for periods no greater than 3 minutes at a time. Chest pain normally occurs during balloon inflation. The patient receives morphine or meperidine (Demerol) if pain is severe or does not subside after deflation.[8]

After angioplasty the gradient across the involved lesion may be reassessed to determine the effects of the procedure. However, with improved catheter design allowing better visualization of residual stenosis, this reassessment is frequently not necessary.[140] A decrease in the pressure gradient should occur with successful angioplasty, indicating increased flow across the stenotic area. Arteriograms of the involved vessels are also performed immediately after angioplasty. These

initial films show a fuzzy appearance at the site of the procedure because of intimal disruption. Follow-up arteriograms several weeks later do not show this fuzzy appearance, since the increased blood flow allows for healing of the endothelial injury.

PTCA is associated with the usual risks and complications of cardiac catheterization as well as its own unique risks. As with routine cardiac catheterization, premedication with vasodilators such as nitroglycerin and calcium channel blockers reduces the risk of coronary artery spasm. The use of antiplatelet agents such as aspirin or dipyridamole (Persantine) or anticoagulants such as heparin reduces the risk of thrombus formation with subsequent embolization (see Unit 9). Effectiveness of heparin is monitored by the activated clotting time (ACT) rather than the partial thromboplastin time (PTT). The ACT is maintained at more than 300 seconds during the angioplasty procedure.[140] The use of prophylactic antiarrhythmic medications reduces the risk of life-threatening ventricular arrhythmias.

Complications unique to PTCA include immediate reocclusion, arterial dissection, and MI. They are more likely to occur in elderly patients (more than 80 years old) and in patients with hypertension or diabetes.[119,140] Vessel closure shortly after balloon removal requires immediate intervention to reestablish coronary blood flow. In the past, abrupt reclosure was managed by emergency coronary artery bypass surgery. Today it is treated with repeat balloon dilation.[119,127,140] Stents or laser therapy may also be used but are still experimental.[127,140] Arterial dissection leading to coronary occlusion and MI may occur during the angioplasty procedure. If this occurs, emergency coronary bypass surgery is required. Stents are also used in some situations to manage acute dissection. Repeat dilation with long inflations at low pressure has also been successful in sealing the tear.[140] Release of thrombogenic factors with plaque compression and disruption may also precipitate MI by promoting thrombus formation, although the administration of antiplatelet agents and anticoagulants decreases this probability.

Late restenosis rates are reported at 25% to 35%.[127,140] Antiplatelet agents may be continued for the first few months after PTCA to reduce the chance of restenosis.[127] The use of laser, atherectomy, or stents in conjunction with PTCA may decrease these rates, but early experimental results have not shown this.[10]. A lower incidence of restenosis occurs in follow-up PTCA.[140]

Patient preparation for PTCA is complex. The patient must be advised of the risks involved and consent to coronary artery bypass surgery should complications occur. A surgical team is on call at the time of the procedure should it be needed. Coronary artery disease screening tests are commonly performed before and after angioplasty.[92]

Nursing care after angioplasty is similar to the nursing care after cardiac catheterization with a few differences. Prompt reporting and treatment of chest pain assume critical importance since they may indicate vessel spasm and/or restenosis. Monitoring patients with chest pain in leads that reflect the coronary artery or arteries involved is a nursing priority. Monitor the right coronary artery in leads II, III, and aVF. Monitor the left coronary artery in lead V2 or MCL2. Also check lead V5 (MCL5) periodically since early subendocardial ischemia is often detected in this lead. A heparin drip may be infused for several hours after angioplasty.[8,127] The arterial and venous sheaths are commonly left in place for at least 3 to 4 hours after the last dose of heparin or until the ACT is less than 170 seconds.[140] The sheaths are usually removed by the physician or specially trained nurse in the CCU or specialized interventional unit. Anticipate bradycardia as they are removed, due to vagal stimulation. Have atropine readily available during the sheath removal. In some institutions PA catheters are inserted and left in place for several hours after angioplasty.

Stents, laser, and atherectomy

Stents, laser, and atherectomy are currently under investigation as adjuncts or alternatives to PTCA.[56,100,140] Stents are expandable tubular wire or steel sheaths that fit over an angioplasty balloon. As the balloon expands, the stent is pressed against the inner vascular linings sealing off some of the intimal disruption and providing support. Within a week the surface of the stent is covered with an initial layer of smooth endothelium.[56] However, complete endothelialization may not occur for weeks to months. For this reason warfarin (Coumadin) therapy is required for several months after stent placement. The stent acts as an internal brace or splint minimizing spasm and dissection. Because of the current design, its use is limited to short lesions in relatively straight vessels. Thrombosis is still a problem because of the foreign material, and closure still occurs.[56,140]

Laser therapy is the use of light energy to generate heat which disrupts and fuses the plaque, providing a smooth channel. It has been used extensively in peripheral vascular disease. Laser energy may be provided via a modified angioplasty catheter with an optical fiber contained within the balloon and the tip extending slightly beyond. Laser therapy may be of benefit in diffuse disease, longer lesions, ostial stenosis, and totally occluded arteries where PTCA guidewires cannot pass.[140] The smooth channel should minimize thrombosis.

Atherectomy catheters use a small rotating blade that cuts the plaque and then traps or vacuums the debris.[92] This mode of therapy shows promise in ostial lesions. Nursing care for all of these procedures is the same as for a patient undergoing PTCA.

NURSING ORDERS: Before cardiac catheterization or PTCA

RELATED NURSING DIAGNOSES: Knowledge deficit, anxiety

1. Verify the patient's understanding of the procedure and obtain his or her informed consent.
2. Remind the patient that food will be withheld before the cardiac catheterization.
3. Assess the patient for history of iodine allergies or previous reactions to radiopaque dyes.
4. Encourage hydration before catheterization to facilitate dye excretion after catheterization and to prevent inaccurate readings caused by hypovolemia.
5. Remind the patient that he or she may feel a transient, hot, flushing sensation[31] or nausea with the dye injection. Remind the patient undergoing PTCA that chest pain is common with balloon inflation, and instruct the patient to report the severity so that he or she can receive medication.
6. Check for recent vital signs and ECG documented in chart record.
7. Document the circulation status of all four extremities, including pulses, temperature, color, and sensation, to serve as a baseline for postcatheterization assessment.
8. Premedicate the patient, and remind the patient to void before catheterization.
9. Continue with usual medications unless otherwise specified.

NURSING ORDERS: After cardiac catheterization or PTCA

RELATED NURSING DIAGNOSES: Potential altered tissue perfusion, hypovolemia, alteration in comfort, knowledge deficit

1. Check dressing and access site, limb pulses, sensation, color, and temperature every 15 minutes × 4, every 30 minutes × 4, every hour × 4, then every 2 to 4 hours. If hematoma occurs at the access site, mark borders clearly, and watch for signs of expansion. If expansion occurs, report to physician.
2. Maintain pressure bags and/or dressings over access sites as prescribed.
3. Check vital signs with each pulse and dressing check. If hypotension occurs, a fluid bolus may be indicated. If you suspect bleeding, check hemoglobin and hematocrit immediately.
4. Instruct patient to remain flat and to avoid bending the involved leg. You can restrain the extremity with a folded, tucked-in sheet as a reminder. However, the patient may elevate the head of the bed 30 degrees for meals.[8]
5. Encourage voiding as soon as possible after catheterization. Monitor urine output, BUN, and creatinine in diabetic patients and patients with a history of renal insufficiency.
6. Watch for signs and symptoms of delayed reactions to the radiopaque dye such as urticaria or hives.
7. Instruct patient not to smoke after catheterization. Nicotine may aggravate coronary artery spasm, especially after vessel manipulation, causing reocclusion.
8. Assess patient for unusual persistent signs and symptoms such as nausea, abdominal pain, or repetitive hypotensive episodes, which may indicate a retroperitoneal bleed.
9. Instruct patient to avoid over-the-counter medications since some contain vasoconstricting agents (e.g., nasal sprays, cold medications).
10. Additional measures after PTCA:
   a. Instruct patient to report chest pain immediately. Monitor in lead V2 for left anterior descending lesions or lead

II/aVF for right coronary lesions.

b. Monitor clotting tests including PTT and ACT while patient is receiving heparin therapy.

c. Monitor neurologic signs (e.g., level of consciousness, pupils) for embolism.

d. Monitor PA wedge pressure, if available. Report high pressures immediately since they could indicate reocclusion. Low pressures could indicate hypovolemia secondary to the effects of the dye (see Unit 8).

e. After pulling of arterial and/or venous sheaths, maintain pressure at access site for at least 15 minutes. You may also use pressure dressings, sandbags, and/or C-clamps to assist in achieving hemostasis.[69] Reinstitute site checks every 15 minutes for the first hour after sheath removal.

f. Before discharge, instruct patient regarding risk factor modification, signs and symptoms of angina, and importance of medication regimen.

Nuclear and tomographic imaging

Nuclear cardiac imaging, or radionuclide, studies are noninvasive methods for assessing cardiac function or myocardial perfusion. These procedures involve the injection of a minimal amount of radioactive material into the circulation. These radioactive chemicals are either bound to blood cells or absorbed by the myocardial cells and are called *radiopharmaceuticals*. Radionuclide substances emit particles in the form of gamma rays that sparkle and flash when reacting with the camera crystals. These *scintillations* can be detected by a special camera, and the picture or image visualized is known as a *scintigraphic* image. Since the camera recording the image usually moves across or around the body at different angles, most of these procedures are also called *scans*.

Similar imaging procedures involving the use of x-rays, magnetic fields, and radiofrequency signals have been more recently introduced for cardiac diagnostic purposes, including coronary artery disease diagnosis. These procedures include computed tomography (CT scan) and magnetic resonance imaging (MRI). MRI uses nuclear principles but uses the body's own hydrogen as a nuclear source (Table 5-2). Although these tests are used extensively in other fields of medicine, their use in coronary artery disease is still evolving.

Radionuclide imaging can be used to study the mechanical function of the heart as well as assess the functional and/or metabolic impact of coronary artery disease. Multiple types of nuclear studies are in common use in coronary artery disease today. These include (1) *perfusion and/or infarct imaging* using thallium, technetium (Tc) 99m compounds, and more recently indium-111 antimyosin; (2) *radionuclide angiography* (also known as gated blood pool studies) using ^{99m}Tc compounds; and (3) *metabolic imaging* using a variety of tracers.

Two primary imaging modes are employed in the different forms of nuclear imaging: planar and tomographic (Table 5-2). In the planar, or earlier, mode, the camera is directed at different angles to obtain single two-dimensional plane views of the heart. In one of the more recently introduced tomographic modes, the camera is rotated around a 180- or 360-degree radius to obtain cross-sectional segmental views. This mode is called *single-photon emission computed tomography (SPECT)* imaging. SPECT provides the advantage of differentiating between myocardial areas supplied by specific coronary artery branches. The tracers used in both SPECT and planar imaging (i.e., thallium, technetium) emit photon waves. Metabolic imaging uses more unstable tracers with

Table 5-2. Nuclear and tomographic imaging

	Nuclear/other	Tracer	Planar (2D)	Tomographic (3D)
Perfusion imaging (cold spot)*	Nuclear (photons)	Thallium-201 Tc-Sesta MIBI (isonitrile) Tc-Teboroxime	Yes	Yes (SPECT)
Infarct imaging (hot spot)	Nuclear (photons)	Technetium-99m-pyrophosphate Indium-III antimyosin	Yes	Yes (SPECT)
Radionuclide angiography* (MUGA) (ERNA)	Nuclear (photons)	Technetium-99m-pyrophosphate	Yes	Yes (SPECT) Experimental
Metabolic imaging*	Nuclear (positrons)	Fluoro-2 deoxyglucose (FDG) C-labeled palmitate C-labeled acetate O-labeled water Rubidium N-labeled ammonia (NH_3)	No	Yes (PET)
Magnetic resonance imaging* (MRI) (NMR)	Nuclear (protons) Radiofrequency waves	Hydrogen Gadolinium DTPA (contrast)	No	Yes
Computed tomography (CT scan)*	X-rays	Iodine-based dye (contrast)	No	Yes
Cardiac catheterization	X-rays	Iodine-based dye (routine)	Yes	No

*These studies may be used in combination with exercise or pharmacologic stress testing.

multiple excess protons that eventually convert into particles referred to as positrons. Tomographic imaging—similar to SPECT imaging but using these tracers—is called *positron emission tomography,* or *PET,* imaging.

Perfusion and infarct imaging uses radioactive myocardial cell tracers in contrast to radionuclide angiography, which uses blood cell tracers. Metabolic imaging uses more specific myocardial cell tracers, which track metabolic processes.

Perfusion and infarct imaging

Perfusion imaging assesses perfusion *indirectly* by recording the effects of changes in coronary perfusion on the myocardial cells. The radioactive cell tracers are absorbed only by the *normal,* well-perfused myocardial cells, providing a contrast between them and ischemic or infarcted tissue. Since the tracer is absorbed only by normal myocardium, the ischemic or infarcted tissue shows up as a blank area (referred to as a "cold spot" or negative image).

Infarct imaging identifies infarcted tissues. In contrast to perfusion imaging, the radioactive cell tracers are absorbed only by the *abnormal* (infarcted) cells, providing a contrast between them and normal cells. Since the tracer is absorbed only by infarcted tissue, this tissue shows up as a "hot spot" or positive image.

Thallium-201 (thallous chloride) is the radioisotope most commonly used in perfusion imaging. The absorption of thallium depends on myocardial blood flow and intracellular potassium shifts. Thallium-201 is a radioactive analog of, or chemical similar to, potassium (K^+) and thus moves as K^+ does into and out of myocardial cells.

In healthy myocardium there is more K^+ inside the cell than outside the cell. In the presence of ischemia, infarction, or both, inactivation of the Na^+–K^+ pump occurs together with alterations in cell membrane permeability. Both these factors contribute to losses of intracellular K^+ in the affected areas only. Since thallium-201 is an analog to K^+, it is not taken up in areas of ischemia or infarction. This results in the blank spot called a *cold spot* or *negative image* (Fig. 5-26).

Thallium-201 scans can be used early in the detection of myocardial ischemia or infarction. They are particularly useful in detecting small infarctions associated with only

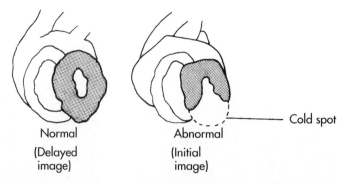

Normal
(Delayed image)

Abnormal
(Initial image)

Cold spot

Fig. 5-26 Thallium-201 imaging. Typical ischemic changes are illustrated. During initial imaging at peak exercise, a thallium perfusion defect or cold spot is evident. The defect is absent in the delayed rest image with restoration of perfusion.

small increases in serum enzymes. Thallium-201 scans are also helpful in detecting ischemia or infarction in patients with abnormal ventricular conduction patterns, such as left bundle branch block, pacer rhythm, and preexcitation, which can mask the classic ECG signs of infarction.

An initial drawback of thallium-201 scans was the inability to distinguish between ischemic and infarcted tissue. This drawback is overcome by obtaining serial images with a usual delay between images of 2 to 4 hours (see Fig. 5-26). This delay allows time for resolution of acute ischemia with filling in of the cold spot image. Any defect remaining on the second image may be assumed to be a permanent metabolic change—most typically necrosis. Any defect resolving or disappearing between the initial and delayed image may be assumed to be a temporary metabolic change or ischemia. Occasionally, the effects of a severe ischemic response may persist long enough that a defect is present on a 3- to 4-hour delayed image. If the physician believes a defect is a possibility, he or she may order a repeat scan in 24 hours to verify the findings.

Multiple projections or views are necessary to localize ischemic and infarcted areas. Commonly used projections are anterior, left anterior oblique, and left lateral (Fig. 5-27).

The anterior view is best for localizing lateral wall abnormalities of the left ventricle. The left anterior oblique view is best for localizing anteroseptal or inferoapical changes. The left lateral projection is best for inferoposterior wall changes. Inferior wall changes are the most difficult to verify because of uptake of thallium-201 by subdiaphragmatic organs.

Thallium-201 imaging has wide application as an adjunct to exercise stress testing. Dynamic exercise increases myocardial oxygen demands, triggering ischemic changes in areas supplied by significantly narrowed coronary arteries. Vasodilators such as dipyridamole (Persantine) or adenosine (Adenocard/Adenoscan) may be used in combination with thallium as alternatives to exercise in patients who are unable to participate in exercise stress testing. These patients include those with orthopedic, neurologic, or peripheral vascular problems. This recently introduced and now commonly used diagnostic alternative to exercise stress testing is called *pharmacologic stress testing*. Similar to exercise testing, these vasodilators trigger ischemic changes in areas supplied by significantly narrowed coronary arteries and in this sense may be said to "stress" the heart. The exact mechanism of action differs, however. While exercise testing acts on oxygen

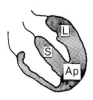 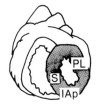 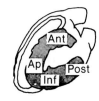

| Anterior
(best for lateral
wall) | LAO (best
for anteroseptal and
inferoapical walls) | Left lateral
(best for
inferoposterior wall) |

Fig. 5-27   Common projections: radionuclide studies. LV surfaces visualized best in each of the common projections are highlighted.

demands, vasodilators act directly on the supply. Since diseased arteries are less responsive to vasodilation, primarily the normal vessels are affected. Perfusion is preferentially distributed to the normal areas, further compromising the blood supply—especially collateral circulation—to marginally ischemic myocardium. This phenomenon is called myocardial "steal syndrome."[147,157] Thallium is also preferentially distributed to the perfused areas, thus accentuating the difference between these normal areas and the ischemic areas on the thallium scan. Pharmacologic stress testing may be used with other isotopes in perfusion imaging, radionuclide angiography, or (MRI). Unlike exercise testing, vasodilators are not used as a separate diagnostic tool.

Thallium-201 exercise or pharmacologic stress testing is indicated to screen for coronary artery disease in high-risk individuals; to assess the functional significance of suspicious or borderline lesions; to verify equivocal or uncertain exercise test results; and to assess the patency of coronary artery bypass grafts or vessels that have undergone previous angioplasty. The use of thallium-201 imaging in conjunction with stress testing increases the accuracy of the stress test results. Negative results no longer require follow-up with cardiac catheterization.[22,156] Dipyrimadole stress testing provides preoperative screening in patients with a history of angina or MI who are scheduled for vascular surgery.[12] If the patient can tolerate it, exercise testing is preferable to pharmacologic stress testing since the blood pressure, heart rate, and work load responses add prognostic significance.[12]

In exercise stress testing, the patient receives an injection of thallium-201 at the peak of exercise, and the patient continues exercising for 1 to 2 minutes to allow the chemical to circulate and be absorbed.[156] The patient then immediately undergoes planar or SPECT imaging to verify the presence or absence of an ischemic response. A delayed redistribution image obtained 2 to 4 hours later serves as a "rest," or baseline, image for comparison. Thallium defects apparent with exercise images that disappear on the delayed image represent an area of myocardium metabolically compromised because of ischemia. Fixed defects are compatible with prior (preexisting) infarction. Late rest imaging after 24 hours following a second thallium dose may detect further viable myocardium in some patients with delayed exercise recovery.[156]

With pharmacologic stress testing, the patient receives dipyridamole (Persantine) over 4 minutes, with the thallium injection about 4 minutes after completion of the infusion. Imaging then begins immediately to verify the presence or absence of an ischemic response.[157] Alternatively, the patient receives adenosine for 3 minutes, then the thallium injection, and the infusion continues for another 3 minutes. Imaging begins immediately after the infusion is completed. In both cases a delayed image obtained 2 to 4 hours later[157] serves as a baseline. Dypyridamole (Persantine) acts by blocking the reabsorption of naturally occuring adenosine, thus increasing the amount available to cellular receptors. Adenosine infusion directly activates these receptors, which in turn may inhibit the slow calcium channels of the vascular smooth muscle cells.[147] Side effects are common, especially with adenosine. Side effects occurring with both adenosine and dipyramidole include shortness of breath, flushing, chest pain, headache, and nausea.[12,37,109] The interaction of adenosine and its receptors may be directly responsible for the production of anginal chest pain since it occurs even in normal individuals given adenosine.[37] ST changes occur less frequently with either dipyridamole or adenosine than in exercise testing even with an abnormal thallium scan.[12,37,157] Conduction abnormalities including transient second-degree and third-degree AV block occur more commonly with adenosine[37] but are quickly reversed without therapy due to adenosine's short half-life (approximately 10 seconds).[37,157] Dosages are comparable to those used to treat PSVT (approximately 0.14 mg/kg or 7 to 14 mg) but are administered more slowly—over a 1-minute period. However, adenosine is best avoided in patients with sick sinus syndrome.[147] Significant bronchospasm is more common with dipyridamole. A history of asthma is considered a relative contraindication. Aminophylline is an antidote to dipyridamole for sustained side effects such as bronchospasm since it blocks adenosine receptor sites.[109,157] Aminophylline should be available whenever dipyridamole is administered.[109]

New technetium-99m compounds introduced as alternatives for thallium in rest or stress imaging include Tc-Sesta MIBI (Cardiolite) and Tc-Teboroxime. Tc-Sesta MIBI produces more distinct images, especially with SPECT imaging.[22,156] It is absorbed in normally perfused areas by passive diffusion into the cells. It then binds to the mitochondria and thus, unlike thallium, is not cleared for several hours. Since no significant redistribution occurs, the ischemic defect may be imaged hours later, long after the ischemia has subsided.[22] Rest images can be obtained initially with a smaller dose or on separate days. A major advantage is that first pass radionuclide angiography can be performed together with the perfusion imaging, allowing for determination of left ventricular ejection fraction.[22] In contrast to Tc-Sesta MIBI, Tc-Teboroxime is absorbed and clears more quickly than thallium and requires serial imaging within 3 to 5 minutes of injection.[22,156] However, the test can be completed more rapidly. Clinical research using Tc-Teboroxime is still limited. Investigators are still determining specific indications for the use of both these tracers.

The use of tomographic rather than the traditional planar techniques for thallium and technetium perfusion imaging provides added diagnostic benefits. The various forms of tomographic imaging offer sequential parallel segmental views in each of the three major planes of the heart itself. Cross-sectional (horizontal plane) views slice along the width or *short axis* of the heart and are also called transverse images. Frontal and sagittal plane views slice along the length or *long axis* of the heart. Frontal plane views are also referred to as horizontal long axis or coronal images, and sagittal plane views are called vertical long axis or oblique sagittal images (Fig. 5-28).

In SPECT imaging, the camera is rotated around a 180- or 360-degree radius to obtain multiple views of each segment at different angles (Fig. 5-28).[22,101] These include short axis views (horizontal plane), horizontal long axis views (frontal plane), and vertical long axis views (sagittal plane). The short axis images are interfaced or superimposed by computer to provide a polar or "bull's-eye" view, which allows for more specific separation of the distribution areas of each major coronary artery branch (Fig. 5-29).[22,61] SPECT imaging more accurately detects perfusion defects than does single planar imaging.[47] Computer filters allow for better contrast and clearer images. Although this method of obtaining nuclear images is most commonly used in perfusion imaging with thallium, it can be used with other tracers as well in perfusion imaging, infarct imaging, or, more recently, radionuclide angiography. Images can be obtained at rest or in combination with exercise and/or pharmacologic stress testing.

Infarct imaging currently uses either technetium-99m-pyrophosphate or indium-11 antimyosin antibodies as tracers. Unlike thallium-201, technetium-99m-pyrophosphate and indium-11 are taken up by infarcted tissue. Thus these tracers provide a contrast between normal and infarcted tissue, result-

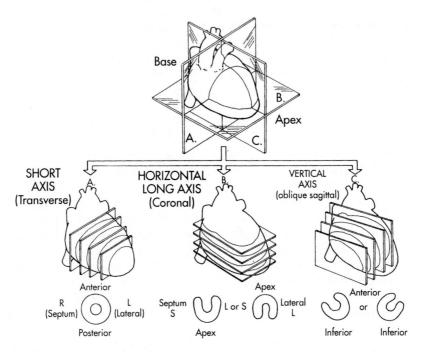

Fig. 5-28 Nuclear tomographic imaging. Parallel segmental views are obtained in each of the three major planes of the heart: *(A)* short axis, *(B)* horizontal long axis, and *(C)* vertical long axis. Corresponding LV images are shown below the view of each plane.

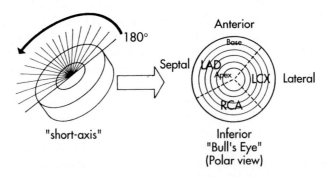

Fig. 5-29 SPECT imaging. Short axis views are interfaced to obtain the typical "bull's-eye" picture, which allows for designation of areas perfused by the major coronary branches.

ing in what has been called a hot spot or positive image. Major uses of this form of imaging are to detect infarction when ECG and enzyme data are unclear or when a new MI is suspected in an area of old infarction.

When infarct imaging is used in conjuction with SPECT imaging, infarction size can also be estimated.[150]

The major mechanism by which technetium-99m-pyrophosphate is taken up by infarcted tissue is binding with calcium. Absorption of this chemical is thus dependent on deposition of significant calcium wastes within the mitochondria of infarcted tissue. This process occurs about 8 to 12 hours after MI and is associated with irreversible myocardial cell death, or necrosis. The maximum sensitivity is 24 to 72 hours after MI since the calcium in necrotic tissue is eventually reabsorbed. The chemical's usefulness is limited since in most cases the diagnosis of MI is complete via ECG and enzyme values by the time a pyrophosphate scan is positive. Technetium-99m-pyrophosphate also binds readily with calcium complexes in the bone matrix of the overlying ribs and sternum (Fig. 5-30). Thus interpreting test results may be difficult, especially in inferior wall MI, if the infarcted surface is aligned with an overlying rib. Technetium-99m-pyrophosphate imaging is probably most useful in assessing intraoperative damage after bypass surgery. In this situation differentiating chest wall pain from coronary chest pain is particularly difficult because the serum enzymes may be elevated as a result of surgery alone. Technetium-99m-pyrophosphate imaging can be useful in validating successful reperfusion since it is usually positive within 1 hour in this situation.[150] It may also be helpful in patients who delay reporting atypical chest pain and in patients with left bundle branch block.[150]

Monoclonal antibodies specific for cardiac myosin have been more recently developed and can be labeled with either ^{99m}Tc or, more commonly, indium-11. These highlight infarcted cells by binding to irreversibly damaged myocytes in a manner similar to

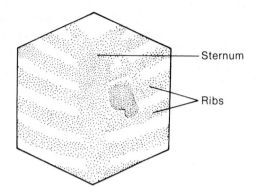

Fig. 5-30 Technetium-99m-pyrophosphate infarct imaging. ^{99m}Tc-pyrophosphate is absorbed by bony structures, sternum, ribs, and infarcted tissues.

the binding of digoxin immune Fab (Digibind) to digitalis (see Unit 10).[64] The major side effect is low-grade fever (lower than 101° F) which could also be attributed to the MI.[64] Images are positive at 24 hours and up to 2 weeks after acute MI.[64] In contrast to technetium-99m-pyrophosphate imaging, this type of scanning normally images the blood pool and liver rather than the skeletal structures. Detection of necrosis is equally or more accurate than by ECG changes. Faint uptake is characteristic of inferoposterior infarction.[64] An indium scan may also be positive in unstable angina, indicating focal necrosis, and is predictive of future cardiac events.[156] Indications appear similar to those for technetium-99m-pyrophosphate scans but are still under investigation.[22,150] Indium may also be helpful in detecting myocarditis and rejection in cardiac transplant patients.[22,150]

Radionuclide angiography

Radionuclide angiography provides a noninvasive means of assessing cardiac mechanical function. These gated blood pool scans are also referred to as multigated acquisition (MUGA) studies or equilibrium radionuclide angiography (ERNA). Angiography is a picture or image of the blood flow through a vessel or the heart. With radionuclide angiography, an image, or picture, of the blood flow through the heart is obtained by labeling the blood cells with the radioactive chemical technetium. Labeling of the blood pool is most commonly done within the body (in vivo) by first injecting stannous pyrophosphate and then, 30 minutes later, injecting technetium-99m-pertechnetate to complete the labeling. The properties of this radionuclide are such that it remains evenly mixed for several hours after injection.

As the labeled blood cells, or blood pool, circulate, radioactive particles are emitted from the blood cells. These particles, which sparkle and flash, are known as scintillations. They can be detected by a special camera and the picture visualized is known as a scintographic image. Although planar imaging is currently used, SPECT imaging may be added in the future.

Radionuclide angiography is accomplished by placing the patient in a supine position beneath the camera and obtaining multiple serial images as the radioactive blood pool circulates through the heart. These images are synchronized with the phase of the cardiac cycle (systole and diastole) via the electrocardiogram. The ECG serves as the physiologic trigger that interfaces the scintillation data with the cardiac cycle. Each cardiac cycle is actually divided into many intervals or gates at which multiple images are obtained and are then computer analyzed and displayed as an endless-loop movie so that the beating heart can be visualized (Fig. 5-31).[22]

Radioactivity in the cardiac chambers with systole and diastole reflects ventricular volume. Measurement of systolic and diastolic dimension becomes possible when images of radioactivity are recorded. Parameters most commonly analyzed with gated flood pool scans are right and left ventricular wall motion and ejection fraction.[22,150] Gated blood pool studies can also measure ventricular size, ventricular volumes, septal thickness, septal motion, and valve regurgitation.

Detection of wall motion abnormalities allows identification of possible ischemic or infarcted areas but does not allow for differentiation between the two unless exercise scans are used as comparison. Wall motion analysis also may detect aneurysms. Terms commonly used to describe wall motion changes include hypokinetic (decreased motion), hyperkinetic (increased motion), akinetic (without motion), and dyskinetic (asynchronous motion).

Ejection fraction is the percentage of dia-

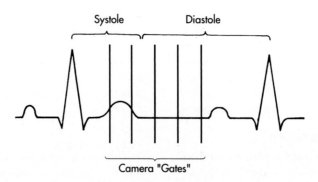

Fig. 5-31 Gated imaging in radionuclide angiography. Pictures are obtained at different time intervals or "gates" during systole and diastole using the ECG complex as a guide.

stolic volume ejected with each systolic event. It serves as another parameter to evaluate mechanical performance (see Unit 8). Comparison of systolic and diastolic images can be used to estimate ejection fraction abnormalities. Ejection fraction may be more accurately calculated by measuring radioactivity emitted by the blood pool with systole and diastole.[156] Good correlations have been reported between the left ventricular ejection fraction determined by radionuclide techniques and by contrast left ventriculography (cardiac catheterization). Ejection fractions can be useful in determining prognosis in patients with MI or after cardiac arrest.[22]

The patient can be exercised during the gated blood pool scan to assess mechanical function with exercise. The bicycle ergometer is used for this procedure. The patient is placed at a 45-degree angle for comfort, and assess parameters normally monitored during stress testing, such as heart rate, blood pressure and ECG changes, and other signs and symptoms. A physician, nurse, and emergency equipment should be on hand during this procedure as with any form of stress testing. Gated blood pool images obtained at rest and exercise can be displayed side by side as endless-loop movies.

A variation of this technique uses nonimaging probes and miniaturized equipment that the patient can wear, similar to the ECG Holter monitoring system. This system allows the patient to be monitored during routine activities or over a period of hours in the intensive care unit (ICU).[156] It is called the ambulatory ventricular function monitor, or VEST.[22,156]

Comparison of wall motion and ejection fractions during exercise and rest allows for further evaluation of the functional consequences of cardiac disease. The normal re-

sponse to dynamic exercise is to raise the ejection fraction. Failure to increase the ejection fraction with exercise is a sign of severe mechanical dysfunction and is associated with poor prognosis.[22] A new regional wall motion abnormality induced with exercise is a very specific indicator of the presence of coronary artery disease.

First-pass radionuclide scans are similar to gated blood pool scans in that a radionuclide is injected intravenously and traced as it passes through the heart and great vessels. However, unlike gated studies, which record multiple images, first-pass scans show only the initial pass of the isotope through the cardiac chambers. If another image is required, the isotope must be reinjected. The test may be performed separately or as the first step of a combination of first-pass and gated pool studies. However, combined studies are not commonly done, since gated pool studies alone are adequate tests of left ventricular function. Parameters of both right and left ventricular mechanical function, such as ejection fraction and wall motion, can also be evaluated with a first-pass scan. The time it takes the radionuclide to move, or transit, from the right side of the heart through the lungs to the left side also allows for evaluation of many cardiac structural and functional abnormalities. A delay in tracer movement, or transit time, may be the result of factors such as shunting,[22] changes in cardiac output, chamber size, and pulmonary blood volume. The best use of first-pass studies is to assess right ventricular function.[156] A right anterior oblique projection allows for clear separation of right-sided and left-sided structures. First-pass studies can be performed at rest or with exercise using bicycle ergometry.

Metabolic imaging

Metabolic imaging uses unstable nuclear tracers, called positrons, and tomographic im-

aging to trace metabolic changes. This form of imaging is more commonly referred to as positron-emission tomography, or PET, imaging. The most frequently used tracers are fluoro-2 deoxyglucose (FDG), which acts as a tracer of glucose metabolism, C-labeled palmitate, which acts as a tracer of free fatty acid metabolism, and C-labeled acetate, which acts as a tracer of O_2 consumption.[22,121] Myocardial blood flow (perfusion) may be simultaneously imaged with any one of these using rubidium, O-labeled water, or N-labeled ammonia (NH_3).[121,124,156] Under normal conditions, myocardial cells use free fatty acids in preference to glucose as their primary energy source. During ischemia, free fatty acids use is inhibited, forcing the heart to rely on its secondary energy source, glucose. Thus glucose utilization increases. If the blood flow is critically reduced, however, glucose transport is limited and stores are rapidly exhausted. When myocardial blood flow is imaged during ischemia with rubidium or N-labeled ammonia followed immediately by imaging with glucose tracers (FDG), uptake of the perfusion tracer decreases in the ischemic areas and uptake of the glucose tracer increases in the same areas.[22,150] This phenomenon is called a blood-flow metabolism mismatch[121] and may occur in the absence of ECG changes. An abnormal blood-flow metabolism match is indicative of necrosis. The mismatch pattern is obtained as long as the blood flow is not reduced to less than 40%.[121] Contractility may be impaired in these areas with the patient at rest as detected from other imaging studies, suggesting chronic ischemic *hibernating* myocardium (see Metabolic Changes).

Perfusion and/or glucose PET imaging can be combined with exercise or pharmacologic stress testing.[121,124] Simultaneous C-palmitate and FDG imaging during ischemia results in increased FDG uptake due to increased glucose use with decreased C-palmitate due to decreased FFA use.[22,150] After an acute ischemic episode, the abnormal changes in glucose and free fatty acids may persist for up to 1 week, supporting the concept of myocardial *stunning*[121] (see Metabolic Changes). PET imaging thus identifies myocardial viability and can help to differentiate stunned or hibernating myocardium from infarction.[22,121] It is significantly more sensitive in identifying viability than either planar or SPECT thallium imaging.[22] PET imaging is also helpful in identifying viable areas after acute MI and determining response to therapy. Unfortunately, the cost of the system is a major limiting factor.

Computed tomography (CT) and magnetic resonance imaging (MRI)

Both the CT scan and MRI use tomographic principles. Unlike perfusion, infarct, or PET imaging, but similar to echocardiography, CT and MRI show other surrounding solid structures within the chest wall in each slice or segment (Fig. 6-26). Images can be gated to the cardiac cycle similar to radionuclide angiography to obtain a picture referred to as cine or ultrafast (rapid) CT or cine MRI. Both rapid CT and MRI provide more accurate assessment of LV function than radionuclide angiography as a result of the more precise definition of endocardial and epicardial outlines.[22] They may be more accurate than echocardiography because of the more direct parallel or perpendicular angles obtained.[22] They can determine LV volume, ejection fraction, wall motion abnormalities, LV wall thickness, and infarct size. Both of these tests as well as echocardiograms image calcification in proximal portions of the coronary arteries, document patency of bypass grafts in asymptomatic patients, determine great vessel morphology, and detect pericardial effusion.[22]

The CT scan uses tomographic principles in conjunction with radiographic (x-ray) techniques. Image intensity is dependent on the density of the tissue.[22] The planes of the body rather than those of the heart itself are used. A single frontal plane (coronal) view may look very much like a simple chest radiograph since the chest radiograph is an example of planar imaging using these same planes. The major differences are the provision of multiple segmental, sequential images with the incorporation of tomographic principles and the optional use of iodine-based dyes as contrast similar to those used in cardiac catheterization (see Table 5-2).

MRI uses the naturally occurring hydrogen within body water as a nuclear source within a magnetic field, while intermittently introducing radiofrequency (RF) waves.[101] The magnetic field aligns the H^+ atoms. The RF waves are then introduced, exciting and realigning the H^+ atoms and causing them to vibrate. As they realign, a signal is produced that is translated by computer into a visual image. This process is also referred to as *nuclear magnetic resonance* (NMR) imaging. The realignment characteristics of different tissues provide a contrast between them and the blood flow. The cardiac chambers and great vessels are outlined. The contrast between solid and soft tissues is clearer than that obtained with a CT scan even without the use of a radioisotope or contrast agent. Specific MRI contrast agents such as gadolinium DTPA are available but are not critical and are not associated with the side effects and allergic reactions of iodine-based dyes.[101] Infarcted tissues may be differentiated from normal myocardium by increased signal intensity as early as 30 minutes after coronary occlusion,[156] LV wall thinning, and hypokinesis.[64,150] MRI can also evaluate valvular anatomy and function, although echocardiographic measures are still preferred.

For MRI the patient lies on a stretcherlike bed, which is introduced into a circular tunnel. Sedation is required both to decrease the psychological effects of being enclosed and to decrease patient movement, which may distort the image. Instruct the patient to anticipate intermittent humming or thumping noises.[101] These are caused by the radiofrequency waves. Remove all metal objects, including hearing aids, jewelry, hairpins, keys, and cosmetics (some have metallic bases).[101] Ask the patient about surgical clips, bullets, prostheses, or shrapnel since these may distort the image. The test, however, is not contraindicated unless the patient has a pacemaker, certain aneurysm clips, or metallic ear implants.[101]

NURSING ORDERS: Radionuclide and tomographic angiography

RELATED NURSING DIAGNOSES: Anxiety, knowledge deficit, alteration in comfort

1. Check with physician before the test about whether any cardiac medications should be withheld 24 hours before the test.
2. Record factors affecting K^+ shifts that may distort thallium results such as pH shifts and administration of drugs such as diuretics, dopamine, epinephrine, or laxatives.
3. Do not schedule barium enemas or glucose tolerance tests with thallium-201 imaging.
4. Do not schedule nuclear tests closely together.
5. If perfusion or infarct imaging is positive, care for the patient as an acute cardiac patient.
6. With exercise imaging:
   a. Instruct patient that he or she will receive nothing by mouth after midnight if test is in early morning or after a light breakfast if test is later.
   b. Instruct patient not to smoke or drink caffeinated drinks for at least 2 hours before the test and not to shower for at least 1 hour after the test.
   c. Explain the purpose of serial images.

Patients are usually allowed only non-dairy liquids between the initial image and the 2- to 4-hour delayed image, to prevent energy substrates from altering the test results. If the initial image is negative, the physician usually cancels the repeat scan. If both initial and 2- to 4-hour delayed scans are positive, some physicians may order a repeat scan 24 hours later to validate those findings.

    d. During the test, the nurse and physician should remain with the patient.

    e. Prepare the patient for isotope injection at peak exercise and rapid transfer for imaging.

7. With pharmacologic stress testing:

    a. Assess patient for wheezing before and during the test.

    b. Report history of asthma and use of aminophylline derivative or caffeine to physician.

    c. Have aminophylline readily available.

    d. Instruct patient to report chest discomfort or shortness of breath, assuring the patient that these are usually transient.

    e. Observe for transient AV block.

8. With MRI:

    a. Instruct patient about procedure, including humming or thumping sound, importance of being still, enclosed area, sedation, and availability of personnel in room although not visible.

    b. Remove all metal objects and explain to patient.

Other diagnostic tests

Another routinely used noninvasive test reflecting mechanical dysfunction is the chest radiograph. It is considered a form of cardiac imaging. Electrical dysfunction can be evaluated by invasive electrophysiologic studies, including His bundle studies, or by noninvasive methods, such as vectorcardiography or Holter monitoring, in addition to the already discussed 12-lead ECGs and exercise stress testing.

Electrocardiographic monitoring and/or invasive testing provide information related to either rhythm disturbances (arrhythmias) or changes in the ECG pattern (QRS–ST-T wave complex). This information can facilitate the detection of, evaluation of, and follow-up therapy for these disorders. Invasive ECG testing is most extensively indicated in patients with rhythm disturbances, such as those with (1) unexplained palpitations or syncope; (2) exercise-related palpitations; (3) documented life-threatening arrhythmias; (4) implanted pacemakers; or (5) complex ventricular arrhythmias in chronic coronary artery disease.

Although chronic ventricular and supraventricular arrhythmias are common in the general population, both at rest and during exercise, certain patterns are more suggestive of coronary artery disease, especially in patients in high-risk categories (see Exercise Stress (Tolerance) Testing). Arrhythmias occurring in coronary artery disease—especially ventricular—are generally more serious and require more careful monitoring and treatment. Arrhythmias have also been implicated in sudden death in patients with noncoronary cardiac syndromes, such as mitral prolapse, idiopathic hypertrophic subaortic stenosis (IHSS), and Wolff-Parkinson-White (WPW) syndrome.

Rhythm disturbances are best detected and monitored initially by noninvasive means such as telemetry, Holter monitoring, or stress testing. Transtelephonic ECG transmission is also useful and very popular in patients with implanted pacemakers. Continuous 24-hour ECG recording, or Holter monitoring, is the most sensitive method of detecting the frequency and character of arrhythmias whether at rest or correlated with various forms of activity or symptoms. Invasive electrophysiologic testing should be reserved for the follow-up evaluation of more complex, hard-to-control arrhythmias.

STRESS AND PSYCHOLOGICAL FACTORS

Many of the presenting symptoms associated with acute MI represent a manifestation of the stress response. Prolonged excessive stress is also a long-term risk factor for coronary artery disease. The concept of stress is based on the theory of *patterned* physiologic responses to factors that upset either physiologic or psychological balance.[143] These responses may be triggered by a variety of factors (stimuli). The response is *nonspecific,* that is, not characteristically associated with a certain type of stimulus, and is dependent on the individual's perception of the situation as a threat.[88,143] Factors potentially triggering a stress response are called *stressors.*

Minimal, short-term stress can provide health challenges that make life more interesting and satisfying. However, severe or long-term stress can trigger potentially harmful stress responses, or *distress.* Unfortunately, the latter is more common. Harmful stress responses are typically triggered when normal compensatory mechanisms have been exceeded or exhausted.

Patterned, nonspecific responses are either *local* (inflammation) or *systemic.* The local response, often called the *local adaptation syndrome* (LAS), is discussed in Unit 4. The systemic response was first described by Selye, who referred to it as the *general adaptation syndrome.* This response occurs in three stages: (1) the alarm *reaction,* (2) the stage of *resistance,* and (3) the stage of *exhaustion.* The alarm reaction signals the cerebral cortex and hypothalamus to trigger a dual autonomic and adrenocortical response. Balance is restored during the stage of resistance. When balance cannot be restored, the stage of exhaustion is reached.

Let us consider the *alarm reaction* in more detail. In the alarm reaction, signals are first transmitted to the cerebral cortex and hypothalamus. The hypothalamus is in direct communication with the pituitary gland and is the site of origin of the autonomic nervous system (Fig. 5-32). The autonomic nervous system is composed of the sympathetic and parasympathetic nervous systems.

The initial response to acute stress is stimulation of the sympathetic nervous system. The response to sympathetic stimulation is dual: (1) increased discharge of sympathetic nerve fiber endings throughout the body and (2) stimulation of the adrenal medulla to release hormones that act as chemical *mediators* for sympathetic activity (see Unit 9). These chemicals are also referred to as catecholamines because of their common catechol rings. The key end organs of sympathetic stimulation are the heart, blood vessels, lungs, and liver. During sympathetic stimulation, heart rate and contractility increase. Thus cardiac output increases. The cardiac output may exceed the amount necessary for meeting O_2 demands at the expense of an increase in myocardial work and O_2 consumption. In response to sympathetic stimulation, the blood vessels of the skin, kidneys, and GI tract constrict. The vascular resistance and blood pressure thus increase, placing an even greater work load on the heart. Platelet aggregation increases, predisposing to thrombus formation.[88] Coronary spasm may also be triggered. Ischemia may become more pronounced, resulting in recurring angina or extension of the infarcted area. Arrhythmias may also occur because of the direct effects of the sympathetic chemicals. Catecholamine levels peak in the early morning, coinciding with the peak incidence of acute MI.[88]

Also in response to sympathetic stimulation, the bronchioles of the lungs dilate, providing a beneficial effect. The liver is stimulated to convert glycogen stores into free glucose to meet extra energy demands. This process is known as glycolysis. However, at the same time, the action of insulin is inhibited, which produces the paradox of an increase in blood glucose with cellular starvation. In borderline diabetes this change may produce more severe, labile hyperglycemia with its accompanying side effects. For this reason, diabetic patients are often given regular insulin therapy in the period immediately after an MI.

During the alarm reaction, stress signals from the hypothalamus also stimulate both the anterior and posterior pituitary gland to cause the release of specific hormones (see Fig. 5-32). Stimulation of the posterior pituitary causes the release of antidiurectic hormone, or ADH (vasopressin), resulting in the reabsorption of water and increased circulating blood volume. Stimulation of the anterior pituitary gland causes the release of adrenocorticotropic hormone (ACTH), which in turn stimulates the adrenal *cortex* to release the glucocorticoid *cortisone* and the mineral corticoid *aldosterone*. Cortisone acts to increase the blood glucose level from protein and fat breakdown (gluconeogenesis). Cortisone also decreases local inflammatory responses by a variety of mechanisms, such as stabilization of cell membranes, lysosomes, and mitochondria; inhibition of histamine release; decreased capillary permeability; and decreased migration of platelets, anti-

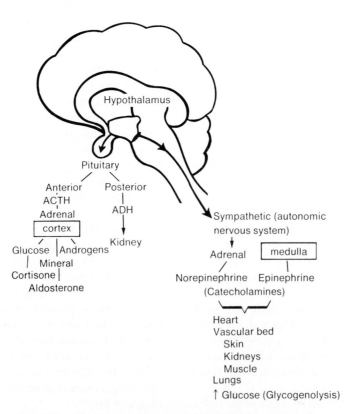

Fig. 5-32 Physiologic characteristics of the stress response.

bodies, and white blood cells. Alterations in the blood cells may also occur, including increased red blood cells and hemoglobin, and increased neutrophils with decreased levels of other white blood cells and platelets. The effects of aldosterone include increased absorption of Na^+ and water with increased excretion of K^+. Gastric and duodenal ulcers also occur in response to the cortisone release during stress.

Stressors may be either physiologic or psychological. Pain is a key stressor in the acute phase of MI. As mentioned, this key stressor has both physiologic and psychological components. Pain—especially chest pain—represents a threat to both physiologic and psychological integrity. Sudden sensations of severe chest discomfort accompany feelings of instability, helplessness, and impending death. In response to pain, the patient with acute MI experiences stimulation of the sympathetic nervous system. Blood pressure, heart rate, and serum glucose levels elevate. Myocardial O_2 consumption increases. Arrhythmias may occur because of the effects of the chemicals epinephrine and norepinephrine. If the pain is severe, nausea, vomiting, and diaphoresis may occur. Therefore, one of the highest priorities in the care of the patient who has acute MI is the immediate relief of chest pain. An elevated blood pressure in the presence of chest pain is most likely caused by a stress response. The patient should not receive antihypertensives unless the elevated blood pressure persists after the pain is relieved.

Psychological stress has been correlated with ischemic changes on ambulatory ECG (Holter) monitoring, thallium scans, PET scans, and radionuclide angiography.[72,78,88] Decreased ejection fractions occur during mental stress as well as during physical exercise in the absence of chest pain or ECG changes.[72] A high degree of stress after acute MI has been correlated with significantly higher mortality.[78,88]

In addition to influencing the complications and prognosis of coronary artery disease, psychological stress has been well recognized for some time as a coronary risk factor (see Risk Factors). The Type A personality traits, although controversial, have been associated with negative stress responses. These traits include hurriedness, competitiveness, and attempting multiple tasks within short time frames. Research studies have shown hostility to be the most significant negative response.[88]

In nursing care of patients with either angina or acute MI or after coronary artery bypass surgery or PTCA, incorporate methods of dealing with stress. Assess patients for nervousness, excessive worrying, hostility, pessimism, lack of family support, and the need to repeatedly retell the events surrounding the infarction.[66,135] Teach patients to examine their own reactions to specific stressful situations, reduce negative "self-talk" and hostility reactions, and choose alternative behavior or coping mechanisms. They can reflect on their physiologic responses, immediate thoughts, and feelings. Teach relaxation techniques, which can be helpful even in recurring anginal pain. These techniques include taking a deep breath; focusing on a word, image, or prayer; meditation; yoga; and progressive muscle relaxation.[88] These methods may be used initially with patients in the coronary care unit.

Regular relaxation periods assist in the long-term managment of stress and can be incorporated into progressive care and rehabilitation settings. Instruction can include tapes, pamphlets, more formal classes, and group sessions. Key elements for regular relaxation include quiet, comfortable surroundings, a regular time and location, and no interruptions. Other stress management techniques useful to the patient with coronary artery disease include the support of family, friends, and other patients and refocusing of problems such as physical limitations and life-style changes into opportunities.[88] Regular rest periods, meals, vacations, hobbies, and exercise are also important.

In addition to physiologic responses, psychological stress may produce a syndrome of nonspecific subjective reactions as well as objective reactions and defense mechanisms. Denial, anxiety, hostility, anger, and depression are all common reactions in the patient with an acute MI. They are associated with the grieving process.[82] Potential related nursing diagnoses include anxiety, alteration in coping mechanisms, knowledge deficit, and powerlessness.

The reported incidence of anxiety and depression after discharge in patients with acute MI ranges from 20% to 80% and is higher in women than men.[38] Depression becomes more pronounced after discharge and is manifested by apathy, insomnia, appetite changes, and negative self-image.[66] Signs of depression may persist up to 6 to 8 weeks in approximately 15% of these patients but usually resolve within 6 months.[38,41] The degree of physical limitation (pain, shortness of breath) influences the extent of depression.[38,66] Encouraging the patient to verbalize is important. Patient teaching regarding infarction, expected recovery, and limitations is helpful in clearing misconceptions and relieving anxiety. Counseling regarding feelings, reactions, and coping mechanisms is also beneficial even in the first few days after infarction.[135]

Short-acting tranquilizers, usually benzodiazepines such as alprazolam (Xanax), may be prescribed for anxiety or depression on a short-term basis. Xanax can lower catecholamine levels and, unlike other tranquilizers, has no cardiovascular side effects and will not potentiate depression.[41] Caution the patient not to stop Xanax or other short-acting benzodiazepines suddenly since sei-

zures can occur.[41] Barbiturates may be used up to 6 weeks after acute MI for nightmares associated with rapid eye movements. Tricyclic antidepressants such as imipramine (Tofranil) and amitriptyline (Elavil) are not recommended prior to 6 weeks after acute MI or in patients with bundle branch block due to cardiovascular side effects such as QRS and ST-T wave changes, arrhythmias, and decreased contractility. Patients who develop psychosis may receive haloperidol (Haldol) since it has few cardiovascular side effects.[41]

The patient's initial response to chest pain is denial, followed by anxiety, then denial again as the chest pain subsides.[116] Denial reduces anxiety and may thus be protective in the period immediately following MI.[20,38,82,116] Denial becomes unhealthy in later phases or when it causes the patient to delay or disregard therapy.[20,82,116] Assess the patient for both verbal and nonverbal signs of denial.[116] These signs include excessive calm, cheerfulness, or use of humor, attempting to do too much too soon, superficial conversation, noncompliance, testing staff by asking the same questions, and avoiding information about heart attacks.[78,116]

In a small, recent study of 14 patients, the stage of denial, referred to as "defending oneself," lasted up to 7 days.[66] Some patients allowed themselves to be passively cared for while "distancing themselves" from the situation.[66] Strategies used in the adjustment phase after MI center on regaining control. They include facing mortality and imagined limitations, seeking explanations, learning to recognize body signals, comparing oneself with others, and accepting real limitations. Women were uncomfortable allowing themselves to be cared for, rather than providing care, and were reluctant to relinquish household tasks. In contrast, men enjoyed family attention but had difficulty relinquishing their work roles.

In the initial days after acute MI, avoid reinforcing denial without necessarily confronting the patient, especially if the patient is compliant with treatment.[20] Allow the patient as much independence and control as possible. Introduce information about MI gradually.[66,116] Measure positive adjustment or adaptation by return to work, life-style changes, and resolution of anxiety or depression.[82]

Spouses experience similar or greater anxiety, depression, and distress up to 1 year after their spouse's infarction.[82] Fear of recurrence and death coupled with a sense of responsibility as the primary caregiver contribute to these feelings.[63] The spouse becomes overprotective, generating marital conflict, which in turn affects the patient's outcome.[82] In the acute phase, primary needs are for information, visiting, and emotional support. Simple explanations of procedures, patient status, and prognosis; flexible visiting hours; nurse-family conferences; and consistent caregivers are helpful in reducing the anxiety of the spouse and other family members. In the chronic phase, separate support groups for spouses, especially females, can be effective.[82]

NURSING MANAGEMENT

Nursing management of the patient with coronary artery disease reflects the nursing process. A comprehensive assessment leads to the formation of nursing diagnoses, which determine the focus of daily nursing care and assist in priority setting. The assessment data base should include key history, physical, and psychosocial findings. The cardiovascular history includes a history of chest pain patterns, risk factors, family history, significant cardiovascular events, presenting symptoms, immediate events leading to admission, and past medications and diagnostic tests. Key physical assessment data include routine vital signs; rhythm; lung sounds; heart sounds; mentation (orientation, level of consciousness); skin color, moisture, and temperature; and quality of peripheral pulses. A complete psychosocial history is critical to the cardiac rehabilitation process and should include past activity and stress patterns, knowledge of coronary artery disease and risk factor control, educational level, occupational and recreational activities, and characteristics of the home environment. Assessment of family interactions is also important. Minimal initial psychosocial information consists of identification of spouse, key family members, significant others, and health care surrogates and the presence of advance directives. Major patient and family concerns as well as verbal and nonverbal expressions of anxiety should also be identified. Ongoing psychosocial assessment parameters are addressed in the section of this chapter on stress and psychological factors.

Nurses are obligated to support the medical diagnostic and therapeutic processes while establishing their own focus. Nurses can also use the medical diagnosis or the medical diagnostic tools to guide their assessment processes. They should review progress notes and current medical orders, including medications and diagnostic tests, as part of the assessment data base. The medical and nursing diagnostic processes should ideally complement each other, becoming interdependent rather than isolated, independent processes.

Standards of care based on the most commonly seen nursing diagnoses can be developed, referenced, and incorporated into practice (Table 5-3). These standards include patient outcomes and are adapted as necessary to reflect individual patient differences.

Nursing standards of care can serve as resources in the development of collaborative

Table 5-3. Standard of care: the patient with an acute MI

Patient problems	Expected outcomes	Nursing action

1. Alteration in comfort: chest pain related to:
 	
—Metabolic changes in ischemic areas (usually within first 24 hours)
—Angina associated with other diseased vessels
—Extension of infarction or new infarction (usually if after first 24 hours)
—Postresuscitation trauma
—Pulmonary emboli
—Pericarditis
	1. Reports onset of new chest pain to nursing staff
	
	2. Reports symptoms suggestive of coronary ischemia that may not be readily identified as pain:
	  —Burning
	  —Pressure
	  —Numbness in upper extremities
	  —Other:_____
	
	3. Expresses relief of pain following medication
	
	4. Expresses at least partial relief of pain following positioning and/or medication
	
	5. Blood pressure and/or heart rate will return to baseline following the relief of pain
	(Circle appropriate outcome or outcomes.)
		1. Immediately obtain tracing from monitoring leads reflecting multiple surfaces—at least lead I (lateral), lead II (inferior), lead V_1 or MCL_1, and MCL_2 (anterior). *Report and document:*
		  —Displacement of ST segment
		  —T wave peaking or inversion
		  —Changes in QRS morphology (width and polarity)
		  —Arrhythmias associated with pain *or* occurring immediately before it
		Later, compare any suspected change with former tracing and verify by obtaining a standard 12-lead ECG record.
		
		2. Obtain vital signs and document any alterations in:
		  —Blood pressure ($\uparrow$ or $\downarrow$)
		  —Pulse rate ($\uparrow$ or $\downarrow$)
		  —Respiratory rate ( )
		  —PAEDP (wedge pressure).
		If blood pressure is elevated, wait until pain is relieved and take blood pressure again. Auscultate for presence of S_4 gallop.
		
		3. Evaluate chest pain quickly according to:
		  —Location
		  —Quality
		  —Duration
		  —Precipitating factor, such as activity, meals, visitors, expressed anxiety, change in routines, or multiple procedures

—Effects of respirations, change of position, movement of extremities, or local pressure.

Note accompanying symptoms: shortness of breath, dizziness, nausea or vomiting, or cold, clammy skin.

4. Medicate *promptly* with:
   —Nitroglycerin gr.___
   —Morphine sulfate___ may repeat × 1___
   —Other _____.
   (Circle as per physician order.)
   Document mode of relief with dosage.
   Document other modes of relief, i.e., sitting up, antacids, rest.
5. Consider effects of drugs that may ↑ demand for O_2 (digitalis).
6. Provide for O_2 administration.
7. Instruct patient to report any new pain.
8. Instruct patient to report signs and symptoms that may indicate coronary ischemia and not be recognized as pain.
9. Look for nonverbal communication of pain.
10. Explain intended effects of pain medication.
11. Reassure patient that pain will subside.
12. Ask patient what makes him or her the most comfortable.
13. Monitor serum enzymes and isoenzymes.

2. Alteration in cardiac output: arrhythmia related to:
   —Ischemic ventricular areas

1. Absence of ventricular fibrillation (VF)
2. Immediate correction of VF
3. VR <100

1. ECG observation and documentation:
   —Monitor rhythm continuously.
   —Document rhythm interpretation with trace at least every 2–4 hours.

Continued.

Table 5-3. Standard of care: the patient with an acute MI—cont'd

Patient problems	Expected outcomes	Nursing action

—Hypoxemia and hypoxia
—K+ or Mg+
—Acidosis or alkalosis
—Stress
—Heart failure
—Drug toxicity
—Pericarditis
—Conduction defects associated with specific location of MI
—Metabolic changes associated with reperfusion
	4. Absence of sustained symptomatic bradycardia
	5. Demonstrates hemodynamic stability during arrhythmias as evidenced by absence of:
	  —Diaphoresis
	  —Respiratory depression
	  —Altered mental status
	  —Cool skin temperature
	  —Hypotension
	(Circle one or more outcomes.)
		—Obtain direct ECG record of any arrhythmia and memory record for previous precipitating changes.
		—Note changes in lead or size/gain in rhythm tracing.
		2. Arrhythmia prevention:
		  —Monitor blood gases.
		  —Monitor serum electrolytes.
		  —Maintain supplementary O_2.
		  —Watch for signs of CHF (see problem 3).
		  —Reduce psychological stressors (see problem 4).
		  —Keep environments calm.
		  —Monitor free fatty acid levels.
		  —Substitute caffeine-free coffee.
		3. Keep atropine and lidocaine (Xylocaine) at bedside.
		4. When arrhythmia occurs, document and report any of the following symptoms:
		  —Dizziness or altered levels of consciousness
		  —Cold clammy skin
		  —Rales, S_3 gallop
		  —Changes in rate or character of respirations.
		5. Maintain patient IV.
		6. Make sure cardioverter or defibrillator is in working order.
		7. Have equipment for emergency pacemaker insertion available.
		8. In the presence of VF follow ACLS protocol, open airway, confirm absence of pulse, then defibrillate (for indicated intervention with specific arrhythmias see Units 7 and 10).

3. Impaired gas exchange/activity intolerance related to:
   — Heart failure
   — Cardiogenic shock

1. Respiratory rate < ___
2. Absence of use of accessory muscles on inspiration or expiration
3. Lungs clear
4. Heart rate <100
5. Absence of S_3 gallop
6. Absence of PACs
7. Skin warm and dry
8. Blood pressure > ___ but < ___
9. Urine output) ___
10. Absence of serious hemodynamic imbalance as indicated by:

1. Elevate head of bed.
2. Monitor vital signs at least every 2 hours first 24 hours, then every 4 hours or as ordered.
3. Auscultate heart and lungs with each set of vital signs, and note abnormal respiratory pattern.
4. Decrease O_2 demands:
   — Assisting with activities of daily living
   — Bedside commode
   — Scheduled rest periods
   — Refraining from performing nonessential procedures
   — Maintaining comfortable room temperature.

clinical practice guidelines/critical paths for case management of cardiac patients. The most common, high-priority nursing diagnoses identified in the patient with acute MI are (1) alteration in comfort: chest pain, and (2) alteration in cardiac output: arrhythmias. Chest pain is usually related to metabolic changes, and arrhythmias are related to changes in the electrical structures. Problems associated with congestive heart failure and shock are also common and significant. These problems may be described jointly by the diagnostic clusters: alterations in cardiac output, impaired gas exchange: oxygenation, or activity intolerance. The authors' personal bias is to focus on impaired oxygenation in the ICU or CCU setting where various measures of oxygenation are available and activity intolerance in progressive care and outpatient settings. Congestive heart failure and shock are related to changes in the mechanical structures of the heart and are forms of cardiovascular system failure. The patient with acute MI may have multiple psychosocial diagnoses (see Stress and Psychological Factors). Depression is one of the most common. Planning and implementation should take into consideration at least these potential patient problems. Patient teaching and discharge planning are incorporated into the rehabilitation process.

The patient with angina may have diagnoses similar to the above. Congestive heart failure can occur in these patients as a result of the effects of stunning or hibernation (see Metabolic Changes). Other potential concerns include sleep pattern disturbances, alteration in comfort: nausea and vomiting, and fluid and electrolyte imbalances.

PATIENT TEACHING AND CARDIAC REHABILITATION

Cardiac rehabilitation is the process of restoring, developing, and maintaining the cardiac patient's physical, psychological, and social capacities within the limitations of the disease process. Patient and family teaching is the cornerstone of cardiac rehabilitation. The emphasis is on risk factor modification, activity and exercise, and counseling and emotional support for the purpose of reducing symptoms and complications, improving prognosis, and promoting psychosocial adjustment. Major indications for cardiac rehabilitation in coronary artery disease are acute MI, coronary bypass surgery, and PTCA. Protocols for bypass surgery and acute MI are similar, although patients progress more rapidly after bypass surgery. The focus of this discussion is acute MI.

Cardiac rehabilitation after acute MI is typically divided into either three or four phases.[57,65,90,143,144] Phase I most commonly refers to the inpatient phase and begins with admission to the CCU. Phase II usually refers to the outpatient phase immediately after discharge.[33,57,61,65,90] Its exact duration can vary from 2 weeks to 2 to 4 months. Phase III is the late recovery or initial postconvalescent phase lasting up to 6 months. Phase IV is the maintenance phase, which continues for the rest of the patient's life with minimal supervision. Phases III and IV can be combined.[90,143] King and Froelicher use phases I and II to describe the inpatient phase, limiting phase I to the stay in the CCU. They use phases III and IV to describe the major outpatient phases.[143]

Patient and family teaching begins during phase I. In the CCU, the nurse can provide simple explanations regarding diagnostic tests and activity levels. The nurse can also offer more complete information on the telemetry or progressive care unit incorporating group as well as individual sessions. Coordination of inpatient and outpatient programs can facilitate continuity and follow-up.[154] Both formal and informal patient and family education programs discuss similar information such as anatomy and physiology, signs and symptoms to report, risk factors, diet, medications, activity and exercise, stress management, coping with depression and anxiety, life-style changes at home and work, and sexual activity.[21,40,52,154] Patients are most concerned about risk factor modification.[40,154] Management issues such as exercise, medications, and what to do for chest pain, shortness of breath, or palpitations are also rated high as concerns by patients. Patients tend to consider anatomy and physiology content, including why symptoms occur, less important. However, results of studies in this area conflict.[40,154] Research supports the idea that patients retain information provided during inpatient programs, particularly regarding activity and smoking, even in the presence of anxiety or denial.[40,52] Acknowledging the patient's difficulty in accepting the diagnosis is a helpful approach when teaching the patient in denial.

Try to incorporate teaching into routine care activities such as administering medications or assisting with meals and activities.[52] Short 15-minute sessions can be as effective as longer sessions. Use basic language regardless of the educational level. Incorporate adult learning principles, including identifying the need to learn, providing choices, incorporating past experiences, and encouraging active participation.[154] Self-learning audiovisual presentations such as videotapes, audiotapes, and slide or tape programs can be as effective as live explanations.[40] Consider making videotapes available on closed circuit TV. Display instructional posters in halls and patient and family lounges.[154] Provide written information such as pamphlets or discharge instructions for the patient and the family to take home. However, make sure that reading materials do not exceed comprehension levels.[40] Assess the patient and family for information already known, major concerns, nonverbal expressions of anxiety or confusion, and preferred learning methods.[52] Group participation can facilitate learning and verbalization of patient and/or family concerns.[21]

The frequency and often the quality of sexual activity decrease in 50% to 60% of patients after MI. The nursing role includes giving permission to discuss the subject, dispelling myths, and providing written guidelines.[122] Include the patient's partner(s) whenever possible.

Provide a quiet environment and open with general statements such as, "Many patients have questions and concerns about sexual activity after a heart attack." Initially encourage the patient's partner to use less threatening expressions of affection such as touching or holding hands even while the patient is still in the ICU or CCU, and provide time for them alone together. Use nonjudgmental language. For instance, a mistress is better referred to as the "other sexual partner."

Most patients can safely resume sexual activity 4 to 8 weeks after an infarction.[20] Energy expenditure is comparable to climbing one to two flights of stairs.[65,144] Advise the patient to avoid sex when tired, during times of stress such as after an argument, after heavy meals, in very hot or cold places, or within 3 hours of alcohol consumption. No particular position is supported by research, although many physicians think the patient-on-top position is less stressful.[122] Premedication with agents such as nitroglycerin may be prescribed and should be discussed with the physician. Have the patient report symptoms, including chest pain during or after sex, rapid heart or respiratory rate lasting more than 15 to 30 minutes after orgasm, sleeplessness, and fatigue continuing the next day.[20] Offer written information in the form of pamphlets to encourage patient independence, ensure consistency of information, and save nursing time. However, use pamphlets as an adjunct to counseling. They should not stand alone.

The success of cardiac rehabilitation is often measured by the ability to return to work as well as by resolution of depression or anxiety.[21] Return to work is affected by psychological adjustment as well as activity and exercise levels. About 90% of patients with their first MI return to work, usually within 60 to 70 days. However, 20% of these have left their work after 1 year.[126] Quantity and quality of work also often decline. Patients with the most difficulty returning to work include blue collar workers with physically demanding jobs, men over age 55, patients with previous work problems, and those with significant depression or lack of family support. Women are also less likely to return to work than men. These patients need more extensive rehabilitation services.[126] Results of exercise radionuclide or echocardiographyic studies have not been correlated with return to work.[126] Exercise training assists in increasing work capacity and decreasing psychological impairment.

Role of activity and exercise

Exercise training increases the amount of work that the patient can do at a given heart rate and blood pressure, largely as a result of increases in skeletal muscle O_2 extraction.[1,21,46,61] Thus exercise conserves myocardial O_2 consumption and prevents ischemic ECG changes and symptoms. In addition, activity and exercise can decrease weakness, depression, and anxiety, enhance self-esteem, promote sleep, and improve sexuality. Exercise facilitates return to work both by increased work capacity and by psychological benefits. Risk factor profiles (blood pressure, lipids, weight, stress) improve. Complications such as reinfarction can also be reduced, therefore improving prognosis.

Dynamic or *isotonic* exercise is preferred over static or *isometric* exercise for initial conditioning since the latter is associated with less myocardial work. Leg exercises are preferred over arm exercises for similar reasons.[1] Isotonic exercises produce alternating contraction of flexor and extensor muscles, resulting in joint movement. Examples include walking, bicycling, swimming, and running. Isometric exercises generate muscle tension without shortening or joint movement.[1,65,143] They are associated with significant increases in both systolic and diastolic blood pressure.[61] Examples include pushing, pulling, lifting, and carrying. Because many recreational and occupational activities require both isometric and strenuous arm exercise, these can be introduced in the intermediate and late phases of rehabilitation.

The central nursing diagnosis for this component of the rehabilitation process is potential and actual activity intolerance. Related factors include decreased cardiac output with reduced ejection fractions, pulmonary congestion, previous inactivity, depression, and increased skeletal muscle and myocardial O_2 demands. Obtain a history of previous activity patterns, recreational and occupational activities, and attitudes toward exercise early in phase I.

Phase I

Phase I goals focus on activities of daily living (ADL) and progressive increases in low-intensity exercise. Active mobilization begins the day after infarction if chest pain has subsided and no significant arrhythmias or shortness of breath exists.[1,46,57] The resting heart rate should be greater than 50 and less than 100 beats per minute. The resting blood pressure should be greater than 90/50 mm Hg and less than 150/90 mm Hg.[65] Stop activity at any time if the heart rate reaches 120 to 130 beats per minute or exceeds 20 beats over the resting heart rate.[52,57,65,90,143] Heart rate is one of the major components of the rate-pressure product or double product, which in turn is a reflection of the individual patient's myocardial work load tolerance.

Limit activity in the first few days after MI to self-care, upper and lower extremity range of motion (ROM) exercises, use of bedside commode, and sitting in a chair, at an intensity of 1 to 2 METs.[21,57,61,65] Remember that a MET corresponds to the equivalent of the usual metabolic requirement at rest. With today's shorter lengths of stay, the sequence of activity is accelerated. Omit ROM exercises if the patient is actively moving his or her extremities in other ways. Discourage isometric activity, especially that using the upper extremities. Increase activity later to walking down the hall and step and stair climbing at an intensity of 3 to 5 METs, preceded by warm-up bending and stretching exercises.[52,57,65,144] Assess blood pressure and heart rate before and after each activity. Interrupt activity not only when heart rate limits are met but also when any of the following signs and symptoms appear: an increase in systolic blood pressure to 180 to 220 mm Hg or in diastolic blood pressure to 110 mm Hg, a drop in systolic blood pressure greater than 10 mm Hg, new significant ventricular arrhythmias, bradycardia or AV block greater than second degree, angina, bundle branch block, new ST changes, or fatigue.[57,61,65,90] These symptom limits are identical to those used in exercise testing (see Exercise stress [tolerance] testing).

A predischarge low-level (3 to 5 METs) exercise test may be performed at the end of phase I to identify high-risk individuals, the need for further therapy, and discharge activities.[46,52,65] This exercise test may also be done within 1 to 2 weeks after discharge, before beginning phase II. Special protocols can be used (see Exercise stress [tolerance] testing). Energy expenditures of routine household, occupational, and recreational activities are classified according to METs; discuss these with the patient before discharge. In general, have the patient avoid activities exceeding 5 METs immediately after discharge. Most routine household activities, such as cooking, making beds, and washing clothes, and mild recreational activities, such as horseback riding, bowling, and playing golf, fall below the 5-MET level.[61] Examples of activities requiring greater than 5 METs include mowing the lawn, climbing more than two flights of stairs, jogging 5 or more miles per hour, shoveling, and lifting items weighing more than 20 pounds. Instruct patients recovering from an acute MI to avoid such activities immediately after discharge.

Phase II

Begin phase II exercise training about 2 weeks after discharge on an outpatient basis[46,52] and focus on cardiovascular conditioning or fitness. True conditioning requires at least three exercise sessions per week, each of 20 to 30 minutes duration.[65,143] Precede these sessions with a 3 to 5 minute warm-up period, and follow with a 3 to 5 minute cool-down period that includes stretching and bending exercises (calisthenics). The warm-up period allows the cardiovascular system to adapt gradually rather than abruptly to the increased oxygen demands associated with exercise and also prevents musculoskeletal injury. The cool-down or gradual tapering off of exercise allows the body to adapt to the oxygen debt incurred and prevents pooling of blood in the extremities and the development of symptomatic hypotension. Walking and cycling are the major forms of exercise appropriate to this phase. Arm exercises, using arm ergometry or rowing machines, and isometric exercises are added, under supervision, to meet occupational and recreational goals.[20]

Intensity is limited in this phase by using the Borg perceived exertion scale and the Karvaren heart rate reserve method for determining target heart rate.[21,46,143] Determine the heart rate reserve by subtracting the resting heart rate from the peak heart rate on the discharge exercise stress test. Then add 40% to 70% of this value to the resting heart rate to determine the target heart rate. The rate of improvement is highest in the first 3 months, but improvement can continue up to 6 months or more.[21] At 6 to 8 weeks, perform a repeat exercise test to help evaluate improvement and readiness to return to work.[65,143] Inpatient ADL and outpatient phase II exercise programs are contraindicated in patients with ejection fractions below 20%.[46] These programs can be delayed for 3 months to 1 year but can still be implemented in patients with ejection fractions above 20% but below 30%. Patients with ejection fractions greater than these can participate as usual and benefit in spite of mild congestive heart failure.[46] Phase II programs are usually more costly to the patient than either phase I or III programs. Each session can cost $20 to $50 and is only partially covered by insurance.[21]

Phases III and IV

During phases III and IV, increase heart rate limits and perceived exertion limits. At the end of phase III, functional capacity should be at least 8 METs.[21,61,65,143] Then the patient is assigned an independent exercise program to follow. Discuss general guidelines for independent exercise with the patient during these and earlier phases. Instruct the patient to avoid hot showers or saunas, smoking, and alcohol before and after exercise. Also instruct the patient to avoid competitive sports, catching up of missed exercise sessions, exercising in hot weather or while wearing heavy clothes, and exercising within 24 hours of a heavy meal or caffeine intake.[65] These recommendations are similar to the guidelines given for sexual activity, which is a form of exercise.

SELF-ASSESSMENT

1 The two major syndromes of coronary artery disease are _____ and _____ _____. Unlike angina, infarction is associated with _____ of tissue.

angina; myocardial infarction
death

Mechanisms of coronary stenosis in both angina and MI are (1) _____, (2) _____, and (3) _____.

lipid infiltration; spasm; thrombosis

2 Mr. Jones is admitted to the coronary care unit with crushing retrosternal pressure of 2 hours duration, unrelated to respirations or position changes, and radiating to the interscapular area of the back. The pressure was unrelieved by nitroglycerin.

This presenting history is most typical of _____ _____. Relief of pain is a priority to provide patient comfort and to minimize the stress response, which produces an (increase/decrease) in blood pressure as part of the _____ reaction.

myocardial infarction

increase
alarm

3 The following 12-lead ECG changes were recorded (Fig. 5-33):

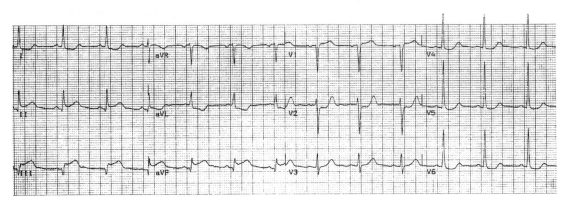

Fig. 5-33   Practice trace

These changes may be diagnosed as (inferior wall MI/anterior wall MI). Changes in the chest leads may be described as (posterior/lateral). The nurse knows that the (right/left) coronary artery is involved and should anticipate (tachycardia/bradycardia) involving the _____ (conduction structures).

inferior wall MI
posterior
right
bradycardia
SA and AV node

Mr. Jones later develops neck vein distention in the presence of clear lungs. The nurse should suspect _____ and validate it on leads _____. Therapy is usually (volume/diuretics).

RV infarction
V3R–V6R; volume

ST segment shifts are described as (injury/necrosis/ischemia). ST segment elevation in leads V1 through V6, I, and aVL is diagnosed as _____ _____.

injury

anterior/lateral or extensive anterior wall MI

4 If no further ECG changes occur, the pattern in Fig. 5-33 would be compatible with (Q wave/non–Q wave) infarction. This infarction is most likely to be (transmural/subendocardial).

Q wave
transmural

Recurrent ischemia and postinfarction angina after discharge are more commonly associated with (Q wave/non–Q wave) infarction. They are most effectively prevented by the use of (beta blockers/diltiazem). These infarctions are also associated with (complete/incomplete) occlusion and generally (are/are not) treated with thrombolytic agents.

non–Q wave
diltiazem
incomplete
are not

5 The enyzme pattern most diagnostic for acute MI is the combination of elevated CPK (MM/MB) levels and a _____ LDH isoenzyme pattern in which LDH1 is (greater than/less than) LDH2.

MB; flipped
greater than

The presence of necrosis is best confirmed from (ECG changes/serum enzymes).

serum enzymes

6 The major electrical complications of acute MI are _____. The major mechanical complications are

arrhythmias

_____ and _____. These may be represented by the priority nursing diagnoses: alteration in _____ _____ and impaired _____ exchange or _____ intolerance.

CHF; shock
cardiac output
gas; activity

The two most common psychological reactions to acute MI are _____ and _____.

denial; depression

The three most common miscellaneous complications are mitral insufficiency, ventricular _____, and _____. Mitral insufficiency occurs as a result of _____ muscle ischemia or necrosis and is detected by the presence of a new _____ murmur. Its presence is usually confirmed by (echocardiography/nuclear imaging).

aneurysm; pericarditis
papillary
systolic
echocardiography

Pericarditis presents with _____ chest pain, _____ arrhythmias, pericardial friction _____, and ST (elevation/depression) on all leads except _____ and sometimes_____ and _____.

pleuritic; atrial
rub; elevation
aVR
V1; aVL

7 Activity following acute MI while the patient is in the hospital is focused on _____ and low-intensity exercise such as sitting in a chair or _____. This period is called phase _____ cardiac rehabilitation. The patient is instructed to avoid active (arm/leg) and (isometric/isotonic) exercises. Activity in this phase is interrupted if the heart rate exceeds _____ beats per minute or _____ beats over the resting heart rate.

ADL
walking; I
arm
isometric
120 to 130; 20

About 90% of patients with their first MI return to work within _____ days. Sexual activity can usually be resumed at _____ weeks.

60 to 70
4 to 8

8 The top three risk factors for coronary artery disease are _____, _____, and elevated blood _____. Mr. Jones's total cholesterol level is 260 mg/dl with an LDL level of 140 mg/dl and an HDL level of 30 mg/dl. According to recommendations by the National Cholesterol Education Expert Panel, he would be best treated with (drug therapy/diet).

smoking; hypertension
cholesterol

diet

The most common method of raising HDL levels is _____.

exercise

9 Necrosis begins within _____ minutes of occlusion and is complete within _____ hours. Thrombolytic therapy initiated within this time frame can allow for reperfusion and limit infarct size. These agents are effective in acute transmural, Q wave infarction since obstruction is usually due to a sudden _____ _____, which triggers _____ formation.

20
6

tear, plaque rupture
clot

Reversible wall motion changes can be present on radionuclide angiography and echocardiography, with symptoms of mild CHF up to 1 week. These changes are compatible with myocardial _____, which is a(n) (electrical/mechanical) phenomenon. The metabolic changes impli-

stunning
mechanical

cated in myocardial stunning include _____ overload and oxygen _____ release.

10 PTCA is performed during cardiac_____ and is
considered an alternative to coronary artery bypass surgery, primarily in
patients with (angina/MI).

    Progressive balloon inflation is normally associated with
_____ _____. Other complications unique to PTCA
include _____, arterial dissection, and
_____. Reocclusion and vascular spasm may be detected
by the recurrence of _____ _____ after the procedure, or high PA _____ pressure, if available. Other nursing responsibilities in caring for the patient undergoing PTCA or diagnostic
cardiac catheterization include inspection of the access site for
_____ formation or overt _____, and checking
_____ distal to the insertion site every 30 minutes for 3 to 4
hours. The patient should also be observed for _____
(dye reaction) and _____ output.

11 Perfusion imaging uses _____ and _____
compounds as nuclear tracers to detect myocardial _____ or infarction and (may/may not) be combined with exercise testing. An initial
blank spot filled in on a second delayed image is characteristic of
(ischemia/infarction).

    PET imaging allows for simultaneous comparison of perfusion
changes with _____ changes, especially glucose and
_____ utilization. Infarction can be differentiated from
reversible mechanical dysfunction due to sustained metabolic changes,
also referred to as _____.

    SPECT imaging is a form of (planar/tomographic) imaging that can be
used in (perfusion imaging/infarct imaging/radionuclide angiography/all
of these). Its major advantage is in more clearly differentiating between
myocardial areas supplied by specific coronary _____.

12 Exercise testing is used as both a _____ (screening)
and _____ tool. Exercise testing is also used to evaluate
functional capacity and guide exercise after acute MI in (phase I/phase II)
cardiac rehabilitation programs.

    Exercise testing is often inaccurate in (men/women), patients with
_____ block, and patients on medications such
as _____. Abnormal responses include _____
(ECG) changes, significant increases and decreases in _____
_____, and life-threatening _____.

13 Echocardiography may be combined with _____ testing, of-
fering a (more/less) costly alternative to perfusion or metabolic (PET) im-

calcium
radical

catheterization

angina

chest pain
reocclusion
infarction
chest pain
wedge

hematoma; bleeding
pulses
urticaria
urine

thallium; technetium 99
ischemia
may

ischemia

metabolic
free fatty acid

stunning
tomographic
all of these

branches

diagnostic
prognostic
phase II

women
bundle branch
digitalis; ST
blood pressure
arrhythmias

exercise
less

aging. Ischemic areas are detected by wall _____ abnormalities that resolve on delayed images. This parameter is also used as an indicator of ischemia in (infarction imaging/radionuclide angiography).

motion

radionuclide angiography

Ejection fraction may also be determined from either echocardiography or _____ angiography and acts as an accurate indicator of (electrical/mechanical) dysfunction.

radionuclide

mechanical

14 Pharmacologic agents that can be used as an alternative to exercise in combination with either nuclear imaging or echocardiographic imaging include _____, _____, and _____. These agents can be used in patients in whom exercise testing may be inaccurate or in patients with orthopedic, peripheral vascular, or _____ problems who are unable to exercise.

dipyridamole; adenosine, dobutamine

neurologic

Dipyridamole (Persantine) and adenosine trigger ischemic changes by affecting myocardial (blood supply/oxygen demands). Bronchospasm is reversed by administration of _____. Dobutamine (Dobutrex) mimics exercise more closely, triggering ischemia by affecting myocardial (blood supply/oxygen demands).

blood supply

aminophylline

oxygen demands

REFERENCES AND SUGGESTED READINGS

1. Alpert JS, Ripple JM: Manual of cardiovascular diagnosis and therapy, ed 2, Boston, 1988, Little, Brown.
2. Altice NF et al: Interventions to facilitate pain management in myocardial infarction, J Cardiovasc Nurs 3(4):49, 1989.
3. Andre-Fouet X et al: "Non–Q wave," alias "nontransmural" myocardial infarction: a specific entity, Am Heart J 117(4):892, 1989.
4. Antman EM et al: Acute MI management in the 1990's, Hosp Pract [Off] 25(7):65, 1990.
5. Apple FS: Diagnostic use of CK-MM and CK-MB isoforms for detecting myocardial infarction, Clin Lab Med 9(4):643, 1989.
6. Armstrong WF: Echocardiography in coronary artery disease, Progr Cardiovasc Dis 30:267, Jan–Feb 1988.
7. See Reference 104a.
8. Barbiere CC: PTCA: treating the tough cases, RN 52(2):38, 1991.
9. Barzilai B et al: Prognostic significance of mitral regurgitation in acute myocardial infarction. The MILIS study group, Am J Cardiol 65(18):1169, 1990.
10. Beauchamp G, Vacek JL, Robuck W: Management comparison for acute myocardial infarction: direct angioplasty versus sequential thrombolysis-angioplasty, Am Heart J 12(2):237, 1990.
11. Becker DM: Debunking the cholesterol myth: scientific support from epidemiologic studies and clinical trials, J Cardiovasc Nurs 5(2):v, 1991.
12. Beller GA: Dipyridamole thallium-201 scintigraphy: an excellent alternative to exercise scintigraphy, J Am Coll Cardiol 14(7):1642, 1989.
13. Black L et al: Reperfusion and reperfusion injury in acute myocardial infarction, Heart Lung 19(3):274, 1990.
14. Boden WE et al: ST segment shifts are poor predictors of subsequent Q wave evolution in acute myocardial infarction: a natural history if early non-Q wave infarction, Circulation 79(3):538, 1989.
15. Boden WE et al: Diagnostic significance of precordial ST segment depression, Am J Cardiol 63(5):358, 1989.
16. Bodwell W: Ischemia, reperfusion, and reperfusion injury: role of oxygen free radicals and oxygen free radical scavengers, J Cardiovasc Nurs 4(1):25, 1989.
17. Bolli R: Mechanism of myocardial "stunning," Circulation 82(3):723, 1990.

18. Bolognese L et al: Stress testing in the period after infarction, Ciruclation 83(5):III-34, 1991.
19. Bolooki H: Surgical treatment of complications of acute myocardial infarction, JAMA 263(9):1237, 1990.
20. Boykoff SL: Strategies for sexual counseling of patients following a myocardial infarction, Dimens Crit Care Nurs 8(6):368, 1989.
21. Brandenburg RO et al: Cardiology: fundamentals and practice, vol 2, Chicago, 1987, Year Book.
22. Braunwald E, editor: Heart disease: a textbook of cardiovascular medicine, ed 4, Philadelphia, 1992, WB Saunders.
23. Braunwald E: Unstable angina. A classification, Circulation 80:410, 1989.
24. Brogan WC, Hillis LD, Lange RA: Contrast agents for cardiac catheterization: conceptions and misconceptions, Am Heart J 122(4Pt1):1129, 1991.
25. Burek KA et al: Exercise capacity in patients 3 days after acute, uncomplicated myocardial infarction, Heart Lung 18(6):575, 1989.
26. Burke LE: Dietary management of hyperlipidemia, J Cardiovasc Nurs 5(2):23, 1991.
27. Castello R et al: The value of exercise testing in patients with coronary artery spasm, Am Heart J 119(2Pt):259, 1990.
28. Chambers CE, Leaman DM: Management of acute chest pain syndrome, Crit Care Clin 5(3):415, 1989.
29. Chesebro JH et al: Pathogenesis of thrombosis in unstable angina, Am J Cardiol 68(7):2B, 1991.
30. Chisholm B: Stunned myocardium, Focus on Critical Care 17(6):458, 1990.
31. Chyun D, Ford CF, Yursha-Johnston M: Silent myocardial ischemia, Focus on Critical Care 18(4):295, 1991.
32. Clawson P: Right ventricular infarction: how to recognize hidden cardiac damage, Nursing 20(3):34, 1990.
33. Cohen LS: Managing patients after myocardial infarction, Hosp Pract [Off] 25(3):49, 1990.
34. Collins P, Fox KM: Pathophysiology of angina, Lancet 1:94, 1990.
35. Conover MB: Understanding electrocardiography: arrhythmias and the 12 lead ECG, ed 6, St. Louis, 1992, Mosby Year Book.
36. Cook DG, Shaper AG: Breathlessness, angina pectoris and coronary artery disease, Am J Cardiol 63:921, 1989.
37. Coyne EP et al: Thallium-201 scintigraphy after intravenous infusion of adenosine compared with exercise thallium testing in the diagnosis of coronary artery disease, J Am Coll Cardiol 17(6):1289, 1991.
38. Cronin SN: Psychosocial adjustment to coronary artery disease: current knowledge and future direction, J Cardiovasc Nurs 5(1):13, 1990.
39. Dart RC: oxygen free radicals and myocardial reperfusion injury, Ann Emerg Med 17(1):53, 1988.
40. Duryee R: The efficacy of inpatient education after myocardial infarction, Heart Lung 2(3):217, 1992.
41. Eliot RS: Stress and the heart: mechanisms, measurements, and management, Mount Kisco, NY, 1988, Futura Publishing.
42. Ezekowitz MD et al: Should patients with large anterior wall myocardial infarction have echocardiography to identify left ventricular thrombus and should they be anticoagulated? Cardiovasc Clin 21(1):105, 1990.
43. Fatzinger D et al: Myths and facts about myocardial infarction, Nursing 19(3):93, 1989.
44. Fisch C et al: ACC/AHA guidelines for the early management of patients with acute myocardial infarction, Circulation 82(2):664, 1990.
45. Fisher EH et al: Transesophageal echocardiography: procedures and clinical application, J Am Coll Cardiol 18(5):1333, 1991.
46. Folta A et al: Exercise and functional capacity after myocardial infarction, Image J Nurs Stand 21(4):215, 1989.
47. Friedman M: Type A behavior: its diagnosis, cardiovascular relation and the effects of its modification on recurrence of coronary artery disease, Am J Cardiol 64:12c, 1989.
48. Gaston-Johansson F et al: Myocardial infarction pain: systematic description and analysis, Intensive Care Nursing 7(1):3, 1991.

49. Gawlinski A: Nursing care after AMI: a comprehensive review, Crit Care Nurs Q 12(2):64, 1989.

50. Gibbons RJ et al: Non-invasive identification of severe coronary artery disease using exercise radionuclide angiography, J Am Coll Cardiol 11:28, Jan 1988.

51. Gibler WB: Myoglobin as a early indicator of acute myocardial infarction, Ann Intern Med 16(8):851, 1987.

52. Gleeson B: After myocardial infarction. How to teach a patient in denial, Nursing 21(5):1991.

53. Graeber CM et al: Alterations in serum creatine kinase and lactate dehydrogenase: association with abdominal aortic surgery, myocardial infarction, and bowel necrosis, Chest 97(3):521, 1990.

54. Grauer K: A practical guide to ECG interpretation, St. Louis, 1992, Mosby Year Book.

55. Guyton-Simmons J, Mattoon M: Analysis of strategies in the management of coronary patients' pain, Dimens Crit Care Nurs 10(1):21, 1991.

56. Halfman-Franey M et al: Using stents in the coronary circulation: nursing perspectives, Focus on Critical Care 18(2):132, 1991.

57. Hall LK, Meyer GC, editors: Cardiac rehabilitation: exercise testing and prescription (vol II), Champaign, IL, 1988, Life Enhancement Publications.

58. Halperin JL, Fuster V: Left ventricular thrombi and cerebral embolism, N Engl J Med 320:392, 1989.

59. Hanisch PJ: Identification and treatment of acute myocardial infarction by electrocardiographic site classification, Focus on Crit Care 18(6):480, 1991.

60. Higgins CB: Nuclear magnetic resonance (NMR) imaging in ischemic heart disease, J Am Coll Cardiol 15(1):150, 1990.

61. Hurst WJ, Sclant RB, editors: The heart, arteries, and veins, ed 6, New York, 1990, McGraw-Hill.

62. Instructors's manual for basic life support, Dallas, 1990, American Heart Association.

63. Johnson JL et al: Regaining control: the process of adjustment after myocardial infarction, Heart Lung 19(2):126, 1990.

64. Johnson LL et al: Antimyosin imaging in acute transmural myocardial infarctions: results of a multicenter clinical trial, J Am Coll Cardiol 13:27, 1989.

65. Karam C: A practical guide to cardiac rehabilitation, Rockville, MD, 1989, Aspen Publications.

66. Keckeisen ME, Nyomathic AM: Coping and adjustment to illness in the acute myocardial infarction patient, J Cardiovasc Nurs 5(1):25, 1990.

67. Kittrell K et al: Promoting sleep for the patient with a myocardial infarction, Crit Care Nurse 9(3):44, 1989.

68. Kittrell K et al: Managing the myocardial infarction patient experiencing nausea and vomiting, Dimens Crit Care Nurs 7(6):340, 1988.

69. Kloner RA et al: Deleterious effects of oxygen radicals in ischemia/reperfusion. Resolved and unresolved issues, Circulation 80(5):1115, 1989.

70. Kuecherer H, Edmond L: Role of transesophageal echocardiography in diagnosis and management of cardiovascular disease, Cardiol Clin 8(2):377, 1990.

71. LaRosa JH: Women, work and health: employment as a risk factor for coronary heart disease, Am J Obstet Gynecol 6(158):1597, 1988.

72. La Veau PJ et al: Cardiac dysfunction during mental stress, Am Heart J 118:1, 1989.

73. Lavie CJ et al: High-density lipoprotein cholesterol. Recommendations for routine testing and treatment, Postgrad Med 87(7):36, 1990.

74. Leaf DA: Women and coronary artery disease. Gender confers no immunity, Postgrad Med 87(7):55, 1990; 17(7):1, 1990.

75. Lewis PS: Clinical implication of non−Q wave (subendocardial) myocardial infarctions, Focus Crit Care 19(1):29, 1992.

76. Linden B: Unit-based phase I cardiac rehabilitation program for patients with myocardial infarction, Focus Crit Care 17(1):15, 1990.

77. Lott JA, Stang JM: Differential diagnosis of patients with abnormal serum creatine kinase isoenzymes, Clin Lab Med 9(4):627, 1989.

78. Lowery BJ: Psychological stress, denial and myocardial infarction, Image J Nurs Sch 23(1):51, 1991.
79. Lucchesi BR: Myocardial ischemia, reperfusion and free radical injury, Am J Cardiol 65(19):14I, 1990.
80. Maddahi J et al: Quantitative single photon emission computed thallium-201 tomography for detection and localization of coronary artery disease: optimization and prospective validation of a new technique, J Am Coll Cardiol 14:1689, 1989.
81. Marban E: Myocardial stunning and hibernation: the physiology behind the colloquialisms, Circulation 83:631, 1991.
82. Marsden C et al: Different perspectives: the effect of heart disease on patients and spouses, AACN Clin Issues in Crit Care Nurs 2(2):285, 1991.
83. Matsuzaki M, Toma Y, Kusukawa R: Clinical applications of transesophageal echocardiography, Circulation 82(3):709, 1990.
84. Mayberry-Toth B et al: Complications associated with acute myocardial infarction, Crit Care Nurs Q 12(2):49, 1989.
85. Mazeika PK et al: Pharmacologic stress echocardiography in the evaluation of coronary artery disease, Postgrad Med J 67(suppl 1): S21, 1991.
86. McGill HC Jr: The cardiovascular pathology of smoking, Am Heart J 115(1):250, 1988.
87. McMillan JY, Little-Longeway CD: Right ventricular infarction, Focus Crit Care 18(2)157, 1991.
88. Medich C et al: Psychophysiologic control mechanisms in ischemic heart disease: the mind-heart connection, J Cardiovasc Nurs 5(4):10, 1991.
89. Menzel LK: The electrocardiogram during myocardial infarction, AACN Clin Issues in Crit Care Nurs 3(1):190, 1992.
90. Messin R: Myocardial infarction rehabilitation in 1990. Role of the general practitioner, cardiologist and paramedical team, Acta Cardiol 45(2):95, 1990.
91. Misinski M: Pathophysiology of acute myocardial infarction: a rationale for thrombolytic therapy, Heart Lung 17(6):743, 1988.
92. Monroe D: Patient teaching for x-ray and other diagnostics, Cardiac Catheterization 54(2):44, 1991.
93. O'Brien TX et al: Q-wave myocardial infarction: incidence, pathophysiology, and clinical course compared with non−Q wave infarction, Clin Cardiol 12(suppl 3):3−9, 1989.
94. O'Connor GT et al: An overview of randomized trials of rehabilitation with exercise after myocardial infarction, Circulation 80: 234, 1989.
95. Opie LH: Reperfusion injury and its pharmacologic modification, Circulation 80(4): 1049, 1989.
96. Osbaken MD: Exercise stress testing in women: diagnostic dilemma, Cardiovasc Clin 19(3):187, 1989.
97. Pappas PJ et al: Ventricular free-wall rupture after myocardial infarction, Chest 99(892), 1991.
98. Pechan MK: Test your knowledge of coronary artery disease and myocardial infarction, Nursing 18(11):106, 1988.
99. Peiris A et al: Adiposity, fat distribution, and cardiovascular risk, Ann Intern Med 110:867, 1989.
100. Pepine CJ, Hill JA, Lambert CR: Therapeutic cardiac catheterization, Part 2, Mod Concepts CV Dis 59(7):37, 1990.
101. Philipp TA: Diagnostic imaging in the 1990's, Spectrum 1(5):10, 1991.
102. Podrid PJ et al: The role of exercise testing in the evaluation of arrhythmias, Am J Cardiol 62(12):24H, 1988.
103. Pohjola-Sintonen S et al: Ventricular septal and free wall rupture complicating acute myocardial infarction: experience in the Multicenter Investigation of Limitation of Infarct Size, Am Heart J 117:809, 1989.
104. Previtali M et al: Dobutamine versus dipyridamole echocardiography in coronary artery disease, Circulation 83(suppl III):27, 1991.
104a. Proulx R et al: Detection of right ventricular myocardial infarction in patients with inferior wall myocardial infarction, Crit Care Nurs 12(5):50, 1992.
105. Puleo PR et al: Early diagnosis of acute myocardial infarction based on assay for subforms of creatine kinase−MB, Circulation 82(30):759, 1990.
106. Quinless F: Myocardial infarction, Nursing 20(10):60, 1990.

107. Quinones-Baldrich W, Caswell D: Reperfusion injury, Crit Care Nurs Clin North Am 3(3):525, 1991.

108. Raglan DR, Brand RJ: Type A behavior and mortality from coronary heart disease, N Engl J Med 318:65, 1988.

109. Ranhosky A et al: The safety of intravenous dipyridamole thallium myocardial perfusion imaging, Circulation 81:1205, 1990.

110. Regan TJ: Alcohol and the cardiovascular system, JAMA 264:377, 1990.

111. Reis GJ et al: Usefulness of lactate dehydrogenase and lactate dehydrogenase isoenzymes for diagnosis of acute myocardial infarction, Am J Cardiol 61:754, 1988.

112. Reynolds T: Noninvasive hemodynamic assessment of intracardiac pressures and assessment of ventricular function with cardiac Doppler, Crit Care Nurs Clinics North Am 1(3):629, 1989.

113. Ritchie JL, Cerqueira MD: Single photon emission computed tomography (SPECT): 1989 and beyond, J Am Coll Cardiol 14(7):1700, 1989.

114. Robalino BD et al: Electrocardiographic manifestations of right ventricular infarction, Am Heart J 118(1):138, 1989.

115. Roberts R: Enzymatic diagnosis of acute myocardial infarction, Chest 93(suppl 1):3S, 1988.

116. Robinson KR: Denial in myocardial infarction patients, Crit Care Nurs 10(5):138, 1990.

117. Ross AM: Role of angioplasty in myocardial infarction management strategies: a review, Heart Lung 19(6):604, 1990.

118. Ross AM: Myocardial infarction: rationale for therapy in 1989, Clin Cardiol 12(suppl 3):10, 1989.

119. Ryan TJ et al: American College of Cardiology/American Heart Association Task Force Report: guidelines for percutaneous transluminal coronary angioplasty, J Am Coll Cardiol 12:529, 1988.

120. Savage MP et al: Clinical and angiographic determinants of primary coronary angioplasty success, J Am Coll Cardiol 17(1):22, 1991.

121. Schelbert HR, Buxton D: Insights into coronary artery disease gained from metabolic imaging, Circulation 78:496, 1988.

122. Schneider JR: Should patients with myocardial infarction receive caffeinated coffee? Focus Crit Care 15(1):52, 1988.

123. Schneider AC: Unreported chest pain in a coronary care unit, Focus Crit Care 14(5): 21, 1987.

124. Schultz SU, Foley CR, Gordon DG: Preparing your patient for a cardiac P.E.T. scan, Nursing 21(9):63, 1991.

125. Severi S, Michelassi C: Prognostic impact of stress testing in coronary artery disease, Circulation 83(5):III-82, 1991.

126. Shanfield SB: Return to work after an acute myocardial infarction: a review, Heart Lung 19(2):109, 1990.

127. Sipperly ME: Expanding role of coronary angioplasty: current implications, limitations, and nursing considerations, Heart Lung 18(5):507, 1989.

128. Soufer R, Zaret BL: Positron emission tomography and the quantitative assessment of regional myocardial blood flow (editorial), J Am Coll Cardiol 15:128, 1990.

129. Spodick D: Pericarditis, pericardial effusion, cardiac tamponade, and constriction, Crit Care Clin 5(3):455, 1989.

130. Steinberg D, Pearson TA, Kuller LH: Alcohol and atherosclerosis, Ann Intern Med 114:967, 1991.

131. Sweetwood HM: Clinical electrocardiography for nurses, ed 2, Gaithersburg, MD, 1989, Aspen Publications.

132. Sweitzer P: The electrocardiographic diagnosis of acute myocardial infarction in the thrombolytic era, Am Heart J 119(3):642, 1990.

133. The Expert Panel: Report of the National Cholesterol Education Program Expert Panel on detection, evaluation, and treatment of high blood cholesterol in adults, Arch Intern Med 148:36, 1988.

134. Thompson C: The nursing assessment of the patient with cardiac pain in the coronary care unit, Intensive Care Nurs 5:147, 1989.

135. Thompson DR et al: Effect of counseling on anxiety and depression in coronary patients, Intensive Care Nurs 5(2):52, 1989.

136. Tilkian AG, Daily EK: Cardiovascular procedures: diagnostic techniques and therapeutic procedures, St. Louis, 1986, CV Mosby.

137. Tilkian SM, Conover MB, Tilkian AG: Clinical implications of laboratory tests, ed 4, St. Louis, 1987, CV Mosby.

138. Toffler GH et al: Pericarditis in acute myocardial infarction, Am Heart J 117:86, 1989.

139. Tofler GH et al: Analysis of possible triggers of acute myocardial infarction (The MILIS Study), Am J Cardiol 66:22, 1990.

140. Topol EJ: Textbook of interventional cardiology, Philadelphia, 1990, WB Saunders.

141. Topol J, Ellis SG: Coronary collaterals revisited: accessory pathway to myocardial preservation during infarction, Circulation 83(3): 1084, 1991.

142. Turk M: Acute pericarditis in the post-myocardial infarction patient, Crit Care Nurs Q 12(3):34, 1989.

143. Underhill SL et al: Cardiac nursing, ed 2, Philadelphia, 1989, JB Lippincott.

144. Valle BK et al: Cardiovascular rehabilitation update, Heart Lung 20(3):312, 1991.

145. Valle BK et al: Non−Q wave versus non-transmural infarction, Heart Lung 19(2): 208, 1990.

146. Valle BK et al: Nonthrombolytic therapy for acute myocardial infarction, Heart Lung 18(5):535, 1989.

147. Verani MS et al: Diagnosis of coronary artery disease by controlled vasodilation with adenosine and thallium-201 scintigraphy in patients unable to exercise, Circulation 82:80, 1990.

148. Wade CR et al: Reperfusion injury and lipid peroxidation, Lancet 335(8703):1464; Comment on: Lancet 335(8692):741, 1990.

149. Wilhemsen L: Coronary heart disease: epidemiology of smoking and intervention studies of smoking, Am Heart J 115(1):242, 1988.

150. Willerson JT: Radionuclide assessment and diagnosis of acute myocardial infarction, Chest 93(1):7S, 1988.

151. Willerson JT, Buja LM: Q-wave versus non−Q wave myocardial infarction, Cardiovasc Clin 20(1):183, 1989.

152. Wilson PWF: High-density lipoprotein, low-density lipoprotein and coronary artery disease, Am J Cardiol 66(6):7A, 1990.

153. Wingate S: Acute effects of exercise on the cardiovascular system, J Cardiovasc Nurs 5(4):27, 1991.

154. Wingate S: Post-MI patients' perception of their learning needs, Dimens Crit Care Nurs 9(2):112, 1990.

155. Yusuf S et al: Routine medical management of acute myocardial infarction. Lessons from overviews of recent randomized controlled trials, Circulation 82(suppl 3):117, 1990.

156. Zaret BL, Wackers FJ: Established and developing nuclear cardiology techniques, Mod Concepts CV Dis (Part I) 60(7):31, (Part II) 60(8):43, 1991.

157. Zhu YY et al: Dipyridamole perfusion scintigraphy: the experience with its application in one hundred seventy patients with known or suspected unstable angina, Am Heart J 121:33, 1991.

Electrical Complications in Coronary Artery Disease: Arrhythmias

---

OVERVIEW

When there are disturbances in the heart's electrical activity, arrhythmias occur. Arrhythmias, then, are manifestations of abnormal electrical activity. They may also be referred to as *dysrhythmias*. Abnormal electrical activity is usually indicated by a sudden change in the rhythm (i.e., a pause, irregular beat, or change in rate and/or pattern). Arrhythmias are considered *ectopic* when they originate outside the sinoatrial (SA) node.

Tachyarrhythmias

Ectopic arrhythmias typically result in tachyarrhythmias and may be either ventricular or supraventricular in origin. Tachyarrhythmias or *tachycardias* are defined as rhythms with ventricular rates exceeding 100 beats per minute.[52,53] Ectopic supraventricular arrhythmias originate above the ventricles in the atria or AV junction.

Tachyarrhythmias may result from either altered automaticity, triggered activity, or altered conduction.[1,8,14,28,33,36,44] The clinical factors identified as *altering automaticity* in a patient with acute myocardial infarction can be grouped into three categories: (1) lack of oxygen (hypoxia), (2) chemical toxicity, and (3) stretch. Figure 6-1 provides a more complete list of factors grouped under these three major headings.[36,57] The clinical factors that alter conduction and result in tachyarrhythmias are essentially the same, with the addition of surgical incisions or areas of myocardial edema and scar tissue.[54] Disturbances in conduction produce ectopic impulses and tachyarrhythmias by the process known as *reentry* (see Mechanisms of Tachyarrhythmic Formation). Clinical factors that can generate tachyarrhythmias due to triggered activity include ischemia, reperfusion, stress, digitalis toxicity, and prolonged Q–T syndromes (see Unit 11).[14,33,36,44,53]

Bradyarrhythmias

Bradyarrhythmias or *bradycardias* are usually associated with ventricular rates of less than 60 beats per minute.[52,53] Bradyarrhythmias occur when automaticity, conduction, or both are depressed. When conduction is depressed, the transmission of an impulse may be delayed or blocked in any structure of the conduction system. Clinical factors identified as depressing automaticity and conduction include (1) ischemia or infarction of the conduction structures, (2) electrolyte imbalances (increased K^+, Ca^{++}, Mg^{++}), (3)

(Automaticity and reentry)

1. Hypoxia

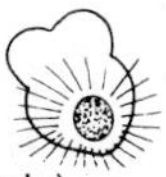

    A. Local ischemia
    B. Systemic (O_2/blood supply)
    C. Metabolic needs (O_2 demands)

2. Toxicity

    A. Drugs/stress/hormones
    B. Lytes
    C. Acid/base

3. Stretch

    A. CHF
    B. Aneurysms

Fig. 6-1 Clinical factors producing arrhythmias. Factors producing either altered automaticity or reentry are listed. Local ischemia occurs in the ventricles in acute myocardial infarction. Systemic hypoxia may occur in shock or respiratory disorders. Electrolyte imbalances typically associated with arrhythmias are low potassium and magnesium. Any acid-base imbalance—acidosis or alkalosis—may predispose to arrhythmias.

drug toxicity, and (4) parasympathetic stimulation such as that associated with Valsalva maneuvers (rectal stimulation, carotid sinus pressure) or increased intracranial pressure.

CLINICALLY SIGNIFICANT ARRHYTHMIAS

Arrhythmias can be grouped according to clinical significance into either *acutely* life-threatening or *potentially* life-threatening. Acutely life-threatening arrhythmias indicate an actual cardiac arrest and are therefore associated with absence of a pulse (Fig. 6-2). They include cardiac standstill or asystole, ventricular fibrillation (VF), and ventricular tachycardia (VT). VT may or may not indicate a cardiac arrest, depending on the individual patient response. Initial therapy for this arrhythmia varies accordingly.

Cardiac arrest may also be associated with electromechanical dissociation (EMD), a form of pulseless electrical activity (PEA). EMD refers to the absence of a pulse in the presence of normal electrical activity. It can occur in severe congestive heart failure (CHF), hypovolemia, cardiac tamponade, tension pneumothorax, hypoxemia, acidosis, pulmonary embolism, and any form of severe shock.[10,52]

Potentially life-threatening arrhythmias either are associated with significant symptoms or signify impending cardiac arrest (Fig. 6-3). Arrhythmias become potentially life-threatening under three conditions: (1) when they originate in the ventricles, (2) when they result in a critically slow ventricular rate, and (3) when they result in a critically fast ventricular rate. Therefore, the three most significant types of arrhythmias are ventricular tachyarrhythmias, supraventricular tachyarrhythmias, and bradyarrhythmias.

Ventricular arrhythmias are clinically significant because they may result in ventricular tachycardia or ventricular fibrillation. VT is clinically significant because it may cause a symptomatic fall in cardiac output or cardiac arrest, or it may lead to ventricular fibrillation, another form of cardiac arrest. Initial therapy in the management of ventricular arrhythmias focuses on depressing ventricular automaticity or interrupting ectopic activity in the ventricles. Subsequent therapy attempts to correct the underlying causes.

Bradyarrhythmias are clinically significant when (1) they result in asymptomatic fall in cardiac output or (2) they allow for the breakthrough of dangerous tachyarrhythmias. Bradyarrhythmias may cause a fall in

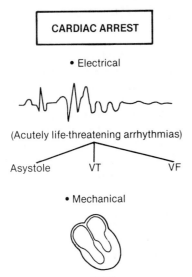

CARDIAC ARREST

• Electrical

(Acutely life-threatening arrhythmias)

Asystole   VT   VF

• Mechanical

(EMD)

Fig. 6-2 Electrical and mechanical disorders associated with cardiac arrest.

cardiac output because cardiac output = stroke volume × heart rate. The following symptoms reflect a significant fall in cardiac output: (1) hypotension, (2) cold, clammy skin, (3) sensorium changes, including decreased level of consciousness, (4) chest pain, (5) shortness of breath, (6) left ventricular failure, (7) ventricular ectopy, and (8) a fall in urine output.[23] Initial therapy in the management of bradyarrhythmias, whether ventricular or supraventricular in origin, focuses on accelerating the ventricular rate.

Supraventricular tachyarrhythmias are clinically significant when they result in a symptomatic fall in cardiac output or compromise cardiac function. Tachyarrhythmias may decrease cardiac output by shortening ventricular filling time during diastole. Because the coronary arteries receive their blood supply during diastole, coronary blood flow may be reduced. The workload of the heart is also increased, predisposing to heart failure. Initial therapy in the management of fast supraventricular arrhythmias attempts

to decrease the ventricular rate. Subsequent therapy may be directed toward depressing atrial automaticity and correcting the underlying cause.

NURSING ORDERS: The patient with a life-threatening arrhythmia

RELATED NURSING DIAGNOSES: Alteration in cardiac output, impaired tissue perfusion

1. Anticipate and be prepared for bradyarrhythmias and ventricular arrhythmias in the first 24 to 48 hours after acute MI.
   a. In anticipation of bradyarrhythmias, have atropine, dopamine (Intropin), epinephrine (Adrenalin), and isoproterenol (Isuprel) available. Also have available a transcutaneous pacemaker and equipment for transvenous pacemaker insertion, as well as resuscitative equipment.
   b. In anticipation of ventricular tachyarrhythmias, have lidocaine (Xylocaine), procainamide (Pronestyl), bretylium (Bretylol), magnesium sulfate, and equipment for cardioversion and defibrillation available.
2. In anticipation of supraventricular tachyarrhythmias, have IV verapamil (Isoptin/Calan), adenosine (Adenocard), diltiazem (Cardizem), esmolol (Brevibloc), and digitalis available as well as equipment for cardioversion.
3. Make certain the patient has a patent IV at all times. If life-threatening arrhythmias occur, immediately begin IV therapy.
4. Monitor for the effects of drugs, electrolyte imbalances, hypoxic states, and any changes in the QRS morphology with a standard 12-lead ECG. Consider low Mg^{++} levels as well as low K^+ levels in repetitive VF.
5. When a significant arrhythmia occurs, immediately assess the patient's response to determine if the patient is symptomatic. Report[23]:
   —Changes in sensorium (e.g., confusion,

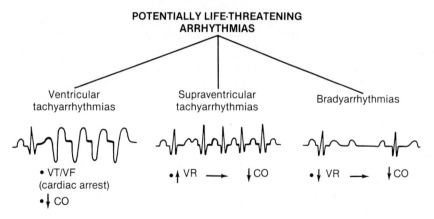

POTENTIALLY LIFE-THREATENING
ARRHYTHMIAS

Ventricular
tachyarrhythmias

Supraventricular
tachyarrhythmias

Bradyarrhythmias

• VT/VF
(cardiac arrest)

• ↓ CO

• ↑ VR ⟶ ↓ CO

• ↓ VR ⟶ ↓ CO

Fig. 6-3 Potentially life-threatening arrhythmias. These arrhythmias are significant because they may be associated with significant symptoms or signify impending cardiac arrest. Symptoms are usually the result of a fall in cardiac output.

decreased level of consciousness, seizures)
— Changes in skin color and temperature
— Chest pain
— Hypotension
— Left ventricular failure (crackles, increased respiratory rate, shortness of breath, gallops)
— Ventricular ectopy
— Decrease in urinary output
6. Record on an ECG trace an example of any new arrhythmia. If possible, record the initiating factor.
7. Institute therapy for ventricular and symptomatic arrhythmias according to American Heart Association standards. (For more specific information, refer to the Nursing Orders for ventricular arrhythmias, supraventricular arrhythmias, and blocks. Also refer to the related drug therapy in Unit 9.)

MECHANISMS OF TACHYARRHYTHMIA FORMATION
Altered automaticity

Automaticity is the ability of certain areas of the heart to initiate electrical impulses. Altered automaticity includes both enhanced normal automaticity and abnormal automaticity. The areas of the heart that normally have the property of automaticity are the SA node, the atrioventricular (AV) junctional tissue, and the ventricular conduction system. Automatic cells are electrically unstable cells that can depolarize spontaneously. The specific electrical characteristics of both stable and unstable (automatic) cells are described in Unit 4. Automaticity in the SA node and the AV node is Ca^{++} dependent. Automaticity in the ventricular Purkinje fibers is Na^+ dependent. These areas may produce tachyarrhythmias when their normal automaticity is enhanced by the previously mentioned clinical factors. Normal automaticity is suppressed at sinus rates and with overdrive pacing.[1,14,28,36]

Tachyarrhythmias may also be produced by abnormal automaticity, which occurs in severely depressed pacemaker or myocardial cells.[14,28,36,44] Myocardial cells in the atria and ventricles do not normally possess the property of automaticity. With clinical factors such as ischemia or electrolyte imbalance, these cells become less negative in the resting state. Their depolarization becomes Ca^{++} dependent. They are more difficult to suppress with overdrive pacing or Na^+-de-

Triggered activity

Triggered activity refers to ectopic impulses that are initiated or triggered by immediately preceding normally depolarized impulses. These ectopic impulses are called *afterdepolarizations* and occur independent of reentry circuits.[8,14,36] Impulses generated during repolarization of the preceding impulse are referred to as early afterdepolarizations (EADs), while impulses generated after full repolarization of the preceding impulse are referred to as delayed afterdepolarizations (DADs).[8,14,28,33,44]

EADs occur secondary to prolonged repolarization and reduction in the outward movement of K^+. Premature inward movements of Na^+ and Ca^{++} are thus facilitated with reversal of the repolarization process.[8,33,44] Factors such as hypoxia and sympathetic chemicals have produced EADs experimentally.[8] EADs, however, are produced clinically primarily by factors that prolong the Q–T interval such as quinidine, procainamide (Pronestyl), potassium and magnesium imbalance, and slow heart rates or long R–R cycles.[8,14,28,36] EADs are effectively treated by overdrive pacing, which increases the heart rate by shortening the Q–T inter-

Reentry

Local disturbances in conduction may produce ectopic impulses and tachyarrhythmias by the process known as *reentry*. Reentry is defined as the ability of an impulse to reexcite some region of the heart through which it has already passed. Reentry usually occurs when an impulse deviates around a circular conduction pathway, forming a loop, (Fig. 6-4).

pendent antiarrhythmic therapy such as lidocaine (Xylocaine).[36,44] Myocardial cells, however, are difficult to clearly differentiate clinically at this time.[8,33] Some cases of accelerated idioventricular rhythm that emerge at adequate sinus rates may be examples.[8,36]

val, and by magnesium.[8,14] The classic example is torsades de pointes[8,28,33] (see Unit 11).

Delayed afterdepolarizations (DADs) are associated with Ca^{++} overload secondary to reperfusion, sympathetic stimulation, and suppression of the $Na^+–K^+$ pump, which in turn influences Ca^{++} exchange.[14,33,36,44] Some of the excess Ca^{++} stored within the tubular system is released into the myocardium, directly generating an inward positive charge or indirectly opening Na^+ channels. The $Na^+–K^+$ pump may be suppressed secondary to ischemia or the effects of digitalis. Researchers believe at least some of the arrhythmias of digitalis toxicity, such as ventricular bigeminy, are related to DADs.[14,28] Treatment of DADs includes K^+ supplementation, which acts to stimulate the $Na^+–K^+$ pump. Beta (sympathetic) blockade and Ca^{++} channel blockade are also effective.[2,28,33,36] Traditional antiarrhythmic therapy with Na^+ channel blockers may be effective as well.[8,14] Fast heart rates favor the development of DADs as a result of compromised diastolic Ca^{++} removal.[14,28,33,44] Increases in heart rate due to fever, exercise, or stress should be avoided.

Three conditions are necessary for reentry to occur: (1) a potential conduction circuit, or circular conduction pathway, (2) a block within part of the circuit, and (3) delayed conduction within the remainder of the circuit.[1,36,52,57] Many small potential circuits (microcircuits) normally exist within the conduction system. These circuits are classically noted within the AV node and in atrial and

CONDITIONS REQUIRED FOR REENTRY

1. A potential [circuit]

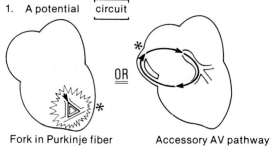

Fork in Purkinje fiber   Accessory AV pathway

2. [Unidirectional block] within the conduction circuit

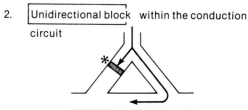

3. [Delayed conduction] within the circuit

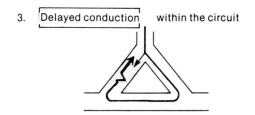

Fig. 6-4   Three major prerequisites for reentry.

REENTRY CIRCUIT (MICRO)

AV node   **Purkinje fibers**

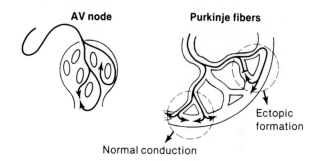

Ectopic formation

Normal conduction

Fig. 6-5   Potential microcircuits for reentry.

REENTRY CIRCUIT (MACRO)

AV node   **Kent pathway (WPW)**

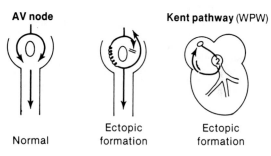

Normal   Ectopic formation   Ectopic formation

Fig. 6-6   Potential macrocircuits for reentry.

ventricular conduction tissue where terminal Purkinje fibers attach to cardiac muscle (Fig. 6-5).[1,36,53,57] Macrocircuits, or larger circular paths, may also form. These circuits are at least partially composed of cardiac conduction tissue. Examples include circuits formed by congenital accessory pathways or by the AV node microcircuits *functionally* grouped into two major pathways (Fig. 6-6).[1,2,14,36,53] Recent evidence from electrophysiologic studies supports the existence of two separate pathways leading to a common AV node.[63] The macrocircuits are thought to play a major role in potentially life-threatening arrhythmias that are not necessarily associated with acute myocardial infarction (MI), including the supraventricular tachyarrhyth-

mias. Microcircuits within the ventricle play a more significant role in acute MI.

Normally, the impulse travels through the conduction fibers in an even and synchronous manner and collides with itself in the potential circuits (see Figs. 6-4 and 6-5). Ischemia, however, can affect selected portions of these conduction fibers, depressing conduction or converting fast cells to slow or hypopolarized cells.[36,53] Slow cells recover slowly from previous impulses since they have extended refractory periods. Thus they may not conduct new approaching impulses.

An impulse entering a circuit that is altered in this way may be blocked anterogradely in one arm of or at one point in the circular path (see Fig. 6-6). When an impulse is blocked in one direction through a pathway, *unidirectional block* is said to exist. When unidirectional block occurs, the electrical impulse detours away from the blocked area. The impulse subsequently deviates around the circular conduction pathway, forming a loop. Impulse transmission is then nonuniform, or asynchronous. The impulse enters the ischemic area in a retrograde direction and is conducted through this tissue slowly, since ischemic (slow) cells have prolonged refractory periods. If tissue surrounding the previously blocked area has recovered excitability, the emerging impulse reenters this adjacent tissue. As a result, the *original* impulse reexcites or depolarizes an area through which it has previously passed. A normal impulse, in this way, may result in the generation of an ectopic impulse (Fig. 6-7). If the reentrant impulse exits early in repolarization, when the disparity in recovery is still pronounced, the impulse may recycle within the circuit, producing a *chain reaction response* or sustained tachyarrhythmia. This response may disintegrate further into chaotic electrical activity and corresponds with the effects of the vulnerable period of the heart. Microcircuits in the ventricles are probably more complex than simple conduction forks, having a weblike or meshlike appearance with several entry and exit points.[36]

Alternate reentry models do not require preexisting anatomic conduction circuits. Instead, a circuit forms during impulse transmission. The impulse wave front is blocked as it approaches an island of abnormally refractory tissue; it then circles around one or both ends and reactivates the initial site via the center or opposite end.[33] Reflection involves adjacent parallel pathways. The impulse is blocked in a portion of one of the pathways, is conducted slowly via the other pathway, and returns in the opposite direc-

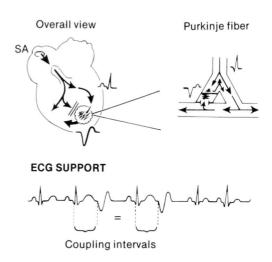

Overall view   Purkinje fiber

SA

ECG SUPPORT

Coupling intervals

Fig. 6-7   Reentrant ventricular arrhythmias. The relationship to the normal impulse is illustrated with its corresponding ECG support. The mechanism by which a tachyarrhythmia may be produced and sustained is illustrated within the Purkinje fiber example.

tion through the previously refractory segment.[14,36,44]

The formation of a reentrant ectopic impulse is closely related to the conduction of the preceding impulse. Thus the ectopic impulse occurs at a fixed distance from the original impulse. This fixed interval is known as the *coupling interval* (see Fig. 6-7). When ectopic beats of the same focus occur at fixed coupling intervals, their mechanism of origin is more likely reentry.[1,57]

Ectopic impulses generated as a result of reentry are usually precipitated by fast rates, which limit recovery time.[36] Ectopic impulses caused by enhanced normal automaticity are typically abolished in the presence of fast rates and facilitated by the presence of slow rates. However, some forms of triggered activity are also precipitated by fast heart rates and may thus be difficult to differentiate from reentry.[2,14,33,44] Reentrant tachycardias are characteristically *initiated* by single electrical stimuli and are *interrupted* by delivery of single electrical stimuli that break the circuit.[1,44] Sustained ventricular tachycardia is most commonly caused by reentry.[2,14,45,52,54] Reentrant supraventricular tachycardias us-ing circuits within the AV node are also common.[63] In these rhythms, vagal maneuvers or drugs that block the AV node typically interrupt the circuit and convert the rhythm.

Role of signal-averaged electrocardiography

Sustained ventricular tachyarrhythmias are most commonly due to reentry, which occurs secondary to delayed conduction. A recently introduced ultrasensitive mode of ECG monitoring detects delayed, disorganized conduction within the ventricular myocardium and/or conduction fibers by analyzing the QRS complex. Because electrical changes secondary to depolarization occur later in these areas than in the normal myocardium, these changes are called *late potentials;* they register late within or immediately after the surface QRS complex.[8,14,59,62] Although these signals may be detected on endocardial electrograms, the voltage is usually too small to be easily detected and differentiated by a routine surface ECG. However, signals obtained from hundreds of QRS complexes may be superimposed, or averaged, to eliminate random electrical activity or artifact and may then be magnified.[8,28,43,59] This process, called *signal-averaged electrocardiography,* allows detection of the low-amplitude late potentials. Signals are obtained from three different leads, reflecting the major body planes and providing three-dimensional information.[14,28,59,62]

Late potentials are considered present when the QRS complex duration is long, predominantly due to terminal, low-amplitude components. Electrophysiologic studies have correlated late potentials with inducible VT and a three to five times greater risk for sudden death.[28,62] Signal-averaged electrocardiography is a useful screening tool for those at risk for the development of VT and sudden arrhythmic death from 72 hours to 1 year after acute MI.[59] This test may also be useful in evaluating potentially malignant ventricular arrhythmias in selected patients without coronary artery disease and in evaluating the effectiveness of ablation or surgical resection for arrhythmia control.[59] The test is not valid in patients with baseline QRS complex abnormalities such as bundle branch block.[62]

Performing signal-averaged electrocardiography at the bedside requires minimal equipment and takes approximately 10 to 20 minutes.[59,62] It is becoming increasingly popular. The nurse should instruct the patient to lie quietly, as with an ordinary cardiogram. Other nursing responsibilities include proper skin preparation, identification of potential candidates, and disconnection of unnecessary equipment that might generate artifact.[59]

SYSTEMATIC APPROACH TO ARRHYTHMIA INTERPRETATION

When interpreting abnormal as well as normal rhythms, we suggest the following systematic approach:

1. Analyze the QRS complex (rule out ventricular arrhythmias).
2. Analyze the P wave (rule out supraventricular arrhythmias).
3. Analyze the P–R interval (rule out AV blocks).

We have previously mentioned some of the practical advantages (see Unit 2). Other authors support this approach as well.[4,35,46]

Analysis of the *QRS complex* initially may enable the practitioner to ascertain, often immediately, whether the ventricular rate is fast or slow and whether the origin of an impulse is *supraventricular* or *ventricular,* thus establishing the primary clinical significance. The clinical significance of ventricular versus supraventricular rhythms differs greatly, particularly in tachyarrhythmias. Treatment of most supraventricular impulses, however, is the same initially, regardless of their more specific origin. The practitioner often can begin critical initial therapy based on the QRS findings alone.

Analysis of the *P wave,* including calculation of the atrial rate, can aid in the differential diagnosis of supraventricular rhythms. As stated, supraventricular rhythms refer to those rhythms originating above the ventricles. The structures above the ventricular that can initiate impulses are the SA node,

the atria, and the AV-junctional tissue. Thus, analysis of the P wave can help differentiate between sinus rhythms and ectopic supraventricular arrhythmias—*atrial* or *junctional (nodal) rhythms.* Analysis of the P wave is also helpful in confirming *sinus arrest,* or *SA block.*

Analysis of the *P–R interval* provides information about the relationship between the atria and the ventricles and aids in the diagnosis of atrioventricular blocks. The practitioner first determines the origin of the rhythm. Next, he or she determines the discharge sequence—rate or timing of the impulse—and finally the conduction sequence. This approach may be used consistently in the interpretation of both normal and abnormal rhythms and allows for simultaneous priority setting.

VENTRICULAR ARRHYTHMIAS

A ventricular arrhythmia is defined as one or more electrical impulses originating somewhere in the ventricles (i.e., in the Purkinje fiber, muscle, or bundle branches). Ventricular arrhythmias have their most significant effect on the QRS complex. Impulses arising within the ventricles are not transmitted through the normal rapid ventricular conduction pathways. Instead, they travel directly through the ventricular muscle. As a result, ventricular depolarization occurs more slowly and in a different direction than the impulses originating above the ventricles. Thus ventricular impulses *usually* produce QRS complexes that are wide (>0.12 to 0.14 second).[14,27,34,36,46,55] A more important characteristic of ventricular impulses is that they produce QRS complexes that change or are different in shape from the patient's normal complexes.[34]

In our experience, relying on width alone as a diagnostic criterion is impractical and may lead to misinterpretation for various reasons. First, slight changes in width may

not be as clearly visible as the changing QRS shape. Premature ventricular complexes, which occur in hearts with minimal disease, normal size, and ejection fractions greater than 40%, are more likely to appear narrow.[14,39] Second, the change in width may be more evident in some leads than in others (Fig. 6-8).[39] Third, ventricular impulses arising high in the ventricular conduction system[14] and those producing ventricular fusion also result in narrower QRS complexes. Therefore, QRS complexes in ventricular ectopic beats may or may not be obviously wide. In a study of wide QRS tachycardia, supported by invasive electrophysiologic studies, 59% of ectopic ventricular rhythms had QRS complexes wider than 0.14 second.[55] In the remaining 41%—still a significant number—the QRS complexes were narrower than 0.14 second. Supraventricular ectopy in preexisting bundle branch block produces QRS complexes wider than 0.14 second.[14,35,55] In these cases, however, the QRS complex does not change from the pat-

Lead I

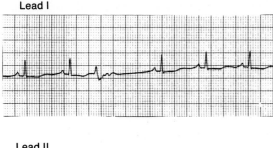

Lead II

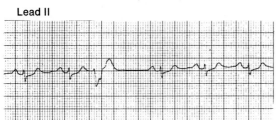

Lead V₁

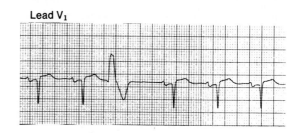

Fig. 6-8   Width of ventricular ectopic beats—effects of different leads. These tracings were obtained simultaneously. The abnormal width is clearly visible in leads II and V1 in this patient, but it is easy to miss in lead I. The change in the QRS pattern is clearly visible, however, regardless of the lead.

tern in sinus rhythm. For these many reasons, we prefer to place more significance on a change or difference in the QRS pattern rather than on width alone.

Ventricular tachyarrhythmias and ventricular bradyarrhythmias differ according to causes, mechanisms, and clinical significance. The ventricular tachyarrhythmias are discussed initially here and in the following sections since their immediate clinical significance is usually greater. The ventricular bradyarrhythmias are then discussed as a group.

The ventricular tachyarrhythmias are ventricular tachycardia and ventricular fibrillation, which is a form of cardiac arrest. These tachyarrhythmias begin with single ventricular ectopic impulses, referred to as premature ventricular complexes (PVCs). Premature ventricular impulses and ventricular tachyarrhythmias may be caused by any of the clinical factors that can alter automaticity or conduction, or produce triggered activity

(see Tachyarrhythmias). The clinical significance of ventricular arrhythmias varies depending on the clinical setting. Ventricular arrhythmias are more likely to result in ventricular fibrillation (cardiac arrest) or symptomatic changes in cardiac output in the patient immediately after acute MI, and they require more aggressive treatment in this setting. The American Heart Association recommends similar guidelines for any patient who has recently undergone cardiac arrest.[52] It is also well recognized, however, that many ventricular arrhythmias are chronic and may not be life-threatening. Signal-averaged electrocardiography holds promise in helping to differentiate noninvasively which patients are at highest risk for significant ventricular tachyarrhythmias.

Therapy for ventricular tachyarrhythmias focuses on suppressing or interrupting the ventricular instability and correcting the underlying causes. The most common forms of intervention are pharmacologic and electrical. The primary mode of pharmacologic intervention is antiarrhythmic therapy (see Unit 9). Intravenous antiarrhythmics commonly used in the management of ventricular arrhythmias include lidocaine (Xylocaine), procainamide (Pronestyl), and bretylium (Bretylol). Magnesium is also used. Electrical intervention includes cardioversion, defibrillation, catheter ablation, and pacemakers (see Unit 10). Selected cases receive surgical intervention, primarily at referral centers.

Ventricular bradyarrhythmias include ventricular escape beats, idioventricular rhythm, and accelerated idioventricular rhythm. In contrast to the ventricular tachyarrhythmias, these rhythms usually occur secondary to depressed conduction and slow heart rates. They are usually compensatory and do not result in cardiac arrest unless suppressed. They require either no therapy or, in symptomatic patients, an increase in the underlying heart rate with atropine sulfate, epinephrine (Adrenalin), isoproterenol (Isuprel), or a pacemaker.

Premature ventricular complexes

An early sign of abnormal electrical activity in the ventricles is the appearance of single ventricular ectopic beats known as *premature ventricular complexes*.[14,52,53] PVCs are also known as premature ventricular contractions, ventricular premature beats, ventricular extrasystoles, and premature ventricular depolarizations.[3,28,34,51] Premature or early beats are beats that occur before the next expected normal impulse. They produce QRS complexes occurring before the next expected normal QRS complex (Fig. 6-9). Since the origin is ventricular, the complexes are different, although they may not be obviously wide.

PVCs that arise from the same focus (place) in the ventricles have the same QRS shape or morphology and are called *unifocal PVCs* (Fig. 6-10). Unifocal PVCs occurring more frequently than six per minute are considered potentially significant. PVCs that arise from different areas or foci in the ventricles have QRS complex shapes that are different from each other as well as different from the normal complexes. These PVCs are called *multifocal* or *multiformed* (Fig. 6-10).[14,29,52,58] They may represent multiple exit sites from a single focus rather than true multiple foci and are more likely to progress to ventricular tachycardia.[29]

PVCs may increase in frequency to the point that they occur every other beat and

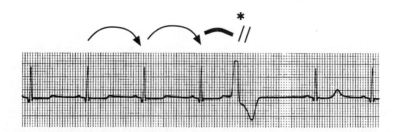

Fig. 6-9 Timing of premature QRS complexes. The premature impulse may also be considered ventricular in origin because the QRS complex changes. It is wider and differently shaped than the normal complexes. The rhythm is completely interpreted as normal sinus rhythm with one PVC.

alternate with the normal beats, forming groups of two. This rhythm is referred to as *ventricular bigeminy* (Fig. 6-11). The PVCs may be either unifocal or multifocal. This pattern indicates PVCs more frequent than 6 per minute. The term *ventricular trigeminy* is most commonly used to describe two sinus beats followed by one PVC, forming groups of three.[8,14]

A single PVC may be significant if it fires early enough to land on the T wave of the preceding beat (Fig. 6-12). This period is considered the heart's vulnerable period. A single stimulus in this period may produce a chain reaction response, leading to ventricular fibrillation. This type of PVC is also referred to as "close coupled" or the "R on T" phenomenon.[14,52]

Unifocal:

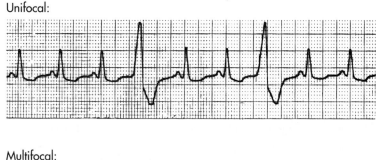

Multifocal:

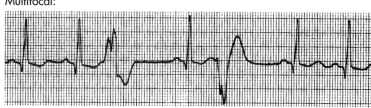

Fig. 6-10   Comparison of unifocal and multifocal (multiformed) PVCs.

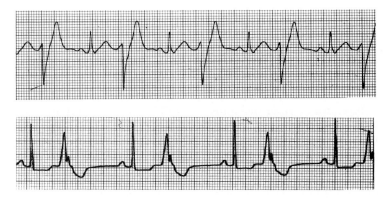

Fig. 6-11   Sinus rhythm with ventricular bigeminy. In these examples, the PVCs are unifocal.

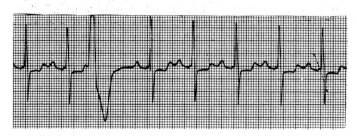

Fig. 6-12   Sinus rhythm with a PVC on the T wave.

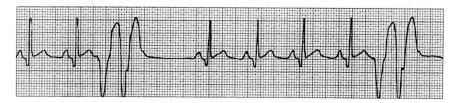

Fig. 6-13   Sinus rhythm with two consecutive (paired) PVCs. These PVCs are potentially significant and may require therapy since their ventricular rate is greater than 100.

PVCs firing consecutively allow estimation of the ventricular rate of the ectopic focus. Two consecutive PVCs with a ventricular rate greater than 100 are precursors to ventricular tachycardia (Fig. 6-13). They are therefore considered more clinically significant than single PVCs. These PVCs are also referred to as paired, couplets, back to back, or simply two in a row.[14,34,52,53,58]

PVCs may be preceded by nonpremature P waves[14,34,46,53] and may or may not have a pause. Both these phenomena are closely related. PVCs primarily depolarize the ventricles and, in at least 50% of the cases, do not conduct retrogradely into the atria.[14] Therefore, they do not interrupt or reset the sinus (P wave) cycle. The QRS complex of a PVC often occurs before the next sinus P wave, obscuring it and preventing its conduction since the ventricles are then refractory. A pause occurs in the ventricular rhythm until the next sinus beat fires. The P to P interval remains regular and can be measured

through the PVC. Therefore, the distance between the beats before and after the PVC, including the pause, is equal to two sinus or normal P wave cycles, and it is called a *full compensatory pause* (Fig. 6-14).[14,52] The full compensatory pause does not reliably differentiate ventricular ectopy from atrial ectopy since atrial ectopy may produce a similar pattern if it does not reset the SA node.[14,20] In addition, when PVCs are retrogradely conducted to the atria, as in slow sinus rates, they can reset the SA node and a full compensatory pause may not be present.[14,52]

When PVCs are only slightly premature, the P wave is not obscured by the ectopic QRS complex and may be visible immediately preceding it. These PVCs are referred to as *end-diastolic* PVCs or simply PVCs. Only the QRS complex is early or premature; the P waves are not premature. Therefore, the P–P interval remains regular. Regular P waves are consistent with an underlying, uninterrupted sinus rhythm (Fig. 6-15). PVCs

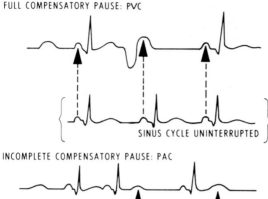

FULL COMPENSATORY PAUSE: PVC

SINUS CYCLE UNINTERRUPTED

INCOMPLETE COMPENSATORY PAUSE: PAC

SINUS CYCLE RESET

Fig. 6-14   The full compensatory pause in PVCs.

preceded by nonpremature P waves are much more common than the literature would suggest and are an excellent area for further nursing research. These PVCs are often considered benign, but do not assume this until you see consecutive beats from the same focus (see Fig. 6-15). Note that when PVCs are only slightly early, no obvious pause occurs. Therefore, PVCs can be preceded by nonpremature P waves and may or may not have a pause. The common denominator between both the compensatory pause and the presence of a P wave is the uninterrupted sinus rhythm or regular P–P interval. The presence of a nonpremature P wave preceding an abnormal QRS complex *will* reliably differentiate between ventricular and nonventricular or atrial ectopy (see Premature Atrial Complexes and Unit 7). When P waves are visible preceding a different QRS complex, measurement of the P to P (P–P) interval is crucial for accurate diagnosis.

With significantly premature PVCs, the si-

nus P wave may follow the ectopic QRS complex at a sufficient distance to allow the ventricles to recover and immediately conduct this sinus P wave. Thus these PVCs are followed by a very slight pause. Because the PVC appears between two consecutively conducted sinus beats without a noticeable pause, this beat is called an *interpolated* PVC (Fig. 6-16). It is distinctly different from the slightly early PVC where a second sinus P wave precedes the ectopic QRS complex. Slow sinus rates further facilitate the occurrence of interpolated PVCs.

Interpolated PVCs have the same clinical significance as noninterpolated PVCs. They appear different on the ECG only because of the timing of the ectopic beat relative to the underlying P wave cycle. The P wave following an interpolated PVC is typically conducted with a prolonged P–R interval (see Fig. 6-16). This altered conduction occurs as a result of AV node refractoriness caused by retrograde penetration by the PVC. Prolongation of the P–R interval may help differentiate an interpolated PVC from artifact.

Let us summarize the key diagnostic criteria for PVCs and review which PVCs are considered potentially significant. The following criteria are diagnostic for PVCs: The QRS complex is different, premature, and may be preceded by a nonpremature P wave. The QRS complex may or may not be obviously wide, and there may or may not be a pause. Traditionally, PVCs are considered potentially clinically significant when they (1) are more frequent than six per minute, (2) fire on the T wave, (3) appear multifocal or multiformed, or (4) fire as two or more consecutive PVCs with a ventricular rate greater than 100.[3,12,52] Therapy may be indicated for any of these types of PVCs, and indications vary greatly from institution to institution and clinical setting to clinical setting.[34] The initial drug of choice is lidocaine (Xylocaine). Disputes currently surround the use of prophylactic lidocaine.[23] Some physi-

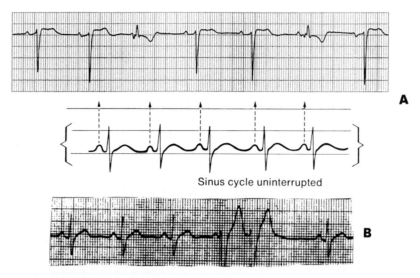

Fig. 6-15 PVCs preceded by P waves. *A*, The P waves are not premature, indicating a sinus origin. Since the PVCs are only slightly premature, there is no obvious pause. However, these PVCs are not always benign, as indicated by the two consecutive PVCs from the same focus in trace *B* with a ventricular rate greater than 100.

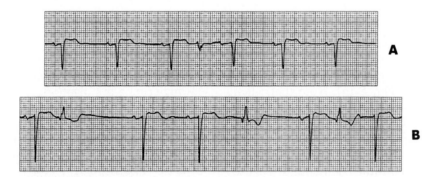

Fig. 6-16 Sinus bradycardia with an interpolated PVC *(A)*. Note the uninterrupted sinus rhythm (P–P interval). In trace *B*, PVCs from the same focus appear first with a distinct pause, then with a slight pause, and finally interpolated.

cians treat only symptomatic ventricular arrhythmias even in acute MI.[14] See the Nursing Orders for American Heart Association recommendations.

Ventricular tachycardia

When three or more consecutive PVCs occur at a ventricular rate greater than 100 beats per minute, the arrhythmia is labeled ventricular tachycardia.[12,14,27,34,52,53,58] Because two consecutive PVCs with a ventricular rate greater than 100 beats per minute

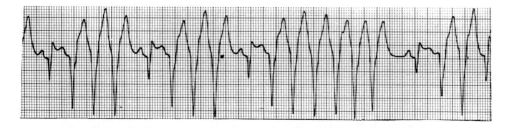

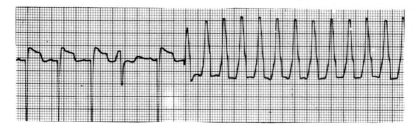

Fig. 6-17 Ventricular tachycardia. The upper trace is an example of short runs of nonsustained VT. The VT in the lower trace may be labeled sustained if it continues for 30 seconds.

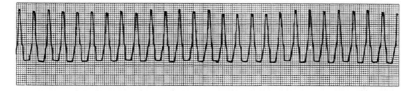

Fig. 6-18 Sustained VT. This rhythm is also called wide QRS tachycardia.

may rapidly lead to VT, their significance is equally ominous. VT may occur in short bursts, converting spontaneously, may continue until interrupted, or may progress to VF. VT that continues for more than 30 seconds is labeled *sustained* VT (Fig. 6-17).[3,12,14,27,28,58] Sustained VT occurring after the acute phase of MI is associated with ejection fractions of less than 40%.[54]

Sustained VT may be difficult to differentiate from a supraventricular tachycardia with bundle branch block when the underlying rhythm is not available for comparison. Analysis of P waves is difficult since they are often hidden in the presence of a tachycardia. This rhythm is commonly called wide

QRS tachycardia (Fig. 6-18). Wide QRS tachycardias present one of the most challenging diagnostic dilemmas for the coronary and critical care practitioner. Multilead assessment is essential for the differential diagnosis (see Unit 7). The practitioner initially should approach this rhythm as VT since it is the most common and most immediately life-threatening cause.[22,55]

VT, especially if sustained, is a malignant arrhythmia and frequently deteriorates into VF. VT may present with or without a pulse and requires different treatment in each case. Pulseless VT is treated like VF. When a pulse is present, anticipate treatment of the rhythm with lidocaine (Xylocaine), procainamide (Pronestyl), and bretylium tosylate (Bretylol), or cardioversion (see Nursing Orders: Actual or potential ventricular tachyarrhythmias). Symptoms of a fall in cardiac output may occur secondary to the fast heart rate and loss of atrial kick. The absence of symptoms, however, does not eliminate the possibility of VT, since some patients are asymptomatic in this rhythm.[23,27]

Bradycardias may potentiate ventricular tachyarrhythmias. If VT appears with a slow heart rate, initial or subsequent therapy is directed toward accelerating the underlying bradycardia. With possible increased intracranial pressure, attempt hyperventilation before other measures to restore the heart rate.

If VT persists after following acute MI, consider diagnostic follow-up with electro-physiologic studies,[27] Holter monitoring, or exercise testing. Further therapy such as oral antiarrhythmic therapy, an implantable cardioverter defibrillator, catheter ablation, or surgery may be necessary. Surgery for VT includes resection of the involved area or ventriculotomy, which involves isolation of the arrhythmic focus via an incision through most of the myocardial wall.[8,21,28] Catheter ablation of ventricular arrhythmias is associated with serious complications and a success rate of only 25% to 50%.[8,64] Therefore, this mode of therapy is more common in the management of supraventricular arrhythmias (see Ectopic Supraventricular Arrhythmias).[63] VT arising in the right ventricle is associated with higher success rates.[28]

Ventricular fibrillation

In VF the electrical activity is so rapid it becomes chaotic and the pattern disintegrates. The complexes no longer have distinct QRS–T wave morphology and are uneven in height. The electrical activity is so disintegrated in this arrhythmia that the heart cannot receive a distinct signal to pump and quivers ineffectually. As a result, there is no pulse and no cardiac output, and clinical death occurs. VF is a form of cardiac arrest, although spontaneous conversion does occur infrequently.

VF is divided into two types according to the size of the fibrillatory waves: *coarse* and *fine* (Fig. 6-19). In coarse VF the waves are of large amplitude. Coarse VF implies that the fibrillation is of recent onset in a stronger heart and that electrical intervention will usually abolish the arrhythmia.[52] If coarse VF is not terminated immediately, the heart becomes anoxic and depressed. The fibrillatory waves then become fine. Pharmacologic intervention, cardiac compression, and ventilation are then necessary before this arrhyth-mia will respond to electrical therapy. For simplicity, however, American Heart Association treatment guidelines combine the treatment of these two forms of VF into one appoach.[23,52]

Ventricular flutter (Fig. 6-19, *C*) differs from coarse VF in that the complexes remain regular or equal in height and thus have not fully disintegrated. The QRS–T complexes, however, have lost the more distinct shape still visible in VT. Ventricular flutter's ventricular rate is usually about 300 beats per minute. Its clinical significance is identical to that of coarse VF. In fact, this intermediate stage between VT and VF does not commonly occur, especially for sustained periods.

Indicated therapy for VF is defibrillation. CPR, however, is performed until a defibrillator is available.[23] See the Nursing Orders for subsequent action recommended by the American Heart Association. Since this rhythm is mimicked by artifact, always check the patient's pulse before defibrillating. Di-

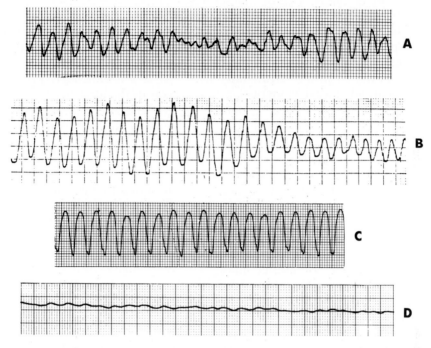

Fig. 6-19 *A* and *B*, Coarse ventricular fibrillation. *C*, Ventricular flutter. *D*, Fine ventricular fibrillation.

agnostic follow-up and long-term therapy for recurrent VF are the same as those for recurrent VT.

NURSING ORDERS: The patient with an actual or potential ventricular tachyarrhythmia

RELATED NURSING DIAGNOSES: Alteration in cardiac output, anxiety, knowledge deficit

1. Assess the patient for the following PVCs[52]:
   a. on the T wave
   b. more than six per minute
   c. multifocal (multiformed)
   d. two or more consecutive PVCs (with a ventricular rate greater than 100 beats per minute)
2. In an acute MI, notify the physician if orders are unavailable for therapy for these PVCs. Anticipate medication of these PVCs with lidocaine boluses, followed by continuous infusion (see Unit 9, Table 9-5). If lidocaine (Xylocaine) is ineffective, the patient may receive procainamide (Pronestyl).[23,52] Assess the patient for potentiating factors (see no. 3). Remember that in some institutions, the patient may not receive medication for these.
3. In situations other than an acute MI, assess the patient for treatable causes such as hypoxemia; K^+ or Mg^{++} imbalances; drug toxicity, including digoxin, aminophylline, and dopamine; CHF; or stress. Collaborate with the physician prior to medication. Therapy may be directed to some of the causes or may be limited to either nonsustained or sustained VT.
4. Assess for accompanying bradyarrhythmias and report.
5. If ventricular fibrillation occurs, confirm

225

that no pulse is present first, administer a precordial blow if witnessed, and initiate basic life support. Defibrillate three times at 200, 300, and 360 J as soon as a defibrillator is available. If unsuccessful, intubate the patient, administer epinephrine, then administer lidocaine (Xylocaine), followed by bretylium tosylate (Bretylol) boluses, magnesium sulfate, and procainamide (Pronestyl), if necessary. Attempt to defibrillate after each dose of medication.[23] Administer lidocaine (Xylocaine) after successful defibrillation; an infusion is recommended for at least 24 hours.[52]

6. If sustained VT occurs, check the patient's pulse. If pulse is absent, treat as VF. If pulse is present, administer lidocaine (Xylocaine) followed by procainamide (Pronestyl) and bretylium tosylate (Bretylol) if VT recurs. The American Heart Association recommends using cardioversion initially in the unstable or symptomatic patient if the ventricular rate is greater than 150 beats per minute.[23] Sedation with diazepam (Valium), midazolam (Versed), or a short-acting barbiturate with or without analgesia is recommended prior to cardioversion in the alert patient. Administer oxygen and attach pulse oximetry.[23] Have a manual resuscitation bag and suction equipment immediately available.

7. Reassure the patient and family that single PVCs are expected following MI and are often treated merely as a precaution. If significant ventricular arrhythmias persist, instruct the patient and family regarding predisposing factors, follow-up diagnostic procedures, and side effects of oral antiarrhythmic therapy. With recurring sustained VT or VF, instruct the family or significant others in basic life support measures. If the patient is to have an implantable cardioverter-defibrillator inserted, give more extensive instruction (see Unit 10).

Ventricular escape beats, idioventricular rhythm, and accelerated idioventricular rhythm

Ventricular bradyarrhythmias may occur secondary to depressed conduction and slow heart rates or long pauses. When a single ventricular ectopic impulse occurs after the next expected normal beat has failed to occur, this impulse is called a ventricular *escape* beat. The QRS complex is different because of the ectopic ventricular origin. This complex occurs after a pause longer than the normal RR cycle (Fig. 6-20).

When the ventricles assume control of the rhythm at the inherent ventricular rate of 20 to 40 beats per minute, the rhythm is referred to as an *idioventricular rhythm* (Fig. 6-21). Therefore, this rhythm is diagnosed by the presence of three or more consecutive ventricular impulses, occurring at a ventricular rate of 20 to 40 beats per minute. Idioventricular rhythm is clinically significant because (1) it is slow and may cause a symptomatic fall in cardiac output and (2) it may allow for the breakthrough of dangerous tachyarrhythmias. This rhythm should *never* be suppressed with lidocaine (Xylocaine).

A ventricular rhythm with a rate greater than 40 beats per minute but less than 100 beats per minute is known as an *accelerated idioventricular rhythm* (AIVR).[2,34,53] The exact

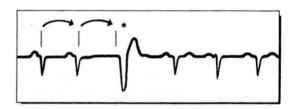

Fig. 6-20 Sinus rhythm with a ventricular escape beat.

rates vary slightly from reference to reference.[14,27,34,51] AIVR is characteristically initiated by a slightly premature (end-diastolic) ventricular ectopic beat, a ventricular escape beat, or a fusion beat, and appears when the sinus rate slows (Fig. 6-22). This rhythm is diagnosed by the presence of three or more consecutive ventricular impulses with a ventricular rate greater than 40 but less than 100 beats per minute.

Fusion beats

Depolarization of the same chamber of the heart by two or more simultaneous impulses may result in a blending or fusing of these impulses within the chamber. The resulting beat is known as a *fusion beat*.[36] When a ven-

Therapy for these three rhythms is the same as for any other bradyarrhythmia. They require no therapy unless the patient is symptomatic. In this case, direct initial therapy toward accelerating the underlying ventricular rate with atropine sulfate. Do not suppress these rhythms with lidocaine unless the ventricular rate accelerates above 100.

tricular ectopic focus discharges at the same time or slightly before a supraventricular impulse enters the ventricles, a fusion beat can occur. The ventricles will be partially depolarized by the supraventricular impulse and

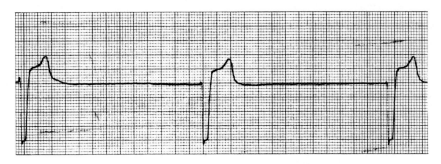

Fig. 6-21   Idioventricular rhythm.

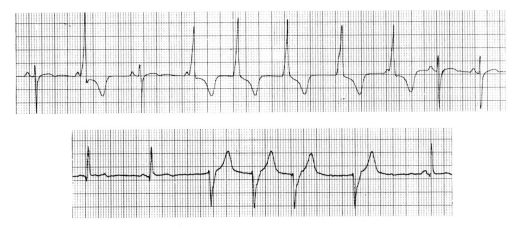

Fig. 6-22   Sinus rhythm with accelerated idioventricular rhythm (AIVR).

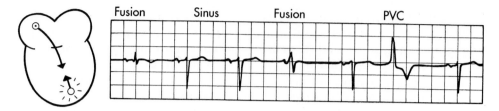

Fig. 6-23 Fusion beats. Sinus rhythm with one clearly premature ventricular ectopic beat and two fusion beats. The configuration of the fusion complexes is intermediate or a "blend" between that of the PVC and the sinus beats.

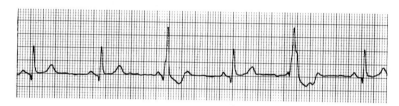

Fig. 6-24 Sinus rhythm with one PVC and a ventricular fusion beat. The fusion beat is formed by a sinus beat with an end-diastolic PVC.

partially depolarized by the ectopic ventricular impulse (Fig. 6-24). The resulting QRS complex will appear as a blend, or fusion, of the two contributing impulses in both contour and duration. This discussion is limited to *ventricular* fusion beats—by far the most common form. The clinical significance of a fusion beat is that an ectopic ventricular focus is attempting to control the ventricles. Consecutive ventricular beats may occur, resulting in either AIVR or VT. For this reason, single fusion beats are treated like PVCs until their consecutive rate is established and they are confirmed to be benign. They occur commonly in AIVR since the ectopic rate is usually close to the sinus rate.

The first step in the identification of fusion beats is to establish the probability that fusion could occur. To determine this probability, evaluate the timing of the ectopic QRS complex relative to the underlying R to R (R–R) cycle. The changing QRS complex may appear slightly earlier, slightly later, or exactly on time with the normal QRS complex cycle. The presence of a sinus P wave preceding the ectopic QRS complex can also indicate the probability that fusion could occur. A sinus P wave with a short P–R interval indicates the probability of a sinus impulse's attempt to enter the ventricles at approximately the same time. However, neither the presence of a sinus P wave nor a short P–R interval confirms the existence of fusion, since these characteristics are also consistent with end-diastolic PVCs.

A diagnosis of fusion beats can be made only when ECG evidence shows that at least two distinct foci are attempting to control the ventricles and have blended together. Therefore, the second step in the identification of fusion beats is to identify the QRS complex of each distinct focus in its naturally occurring form and then determine if the ectopic QRS configuration is a blend of these in contour and duration.[36] The QRS complex of a fusion beat is partially formed by the patient's supraventricular impulse. Therefore, the QRS complex of a fusion

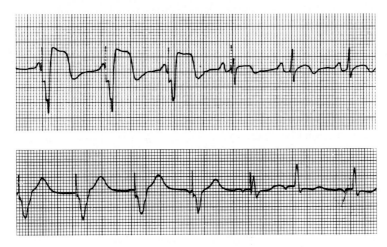

Fig. 6-25 Sinus rhythm with pacemaker fusion beats. The fusion beats are formed by sinus beats with a single-chamber ventricular pacemaker.

beat typically will appear partially narrow. However, fusion complexes will appear different from the normal QRS complex because of a concurrent ventricular impulse. These beats may appear multifocal upon initial comparison with the nonfused form of the same ectopic focus (Fig. 6-24). True multifocal beats, however, are more typically *both* distinctly early PVCs.

Common examples of ventricular fusion beats are a sinus beat with an end-diastolic PVC or AIVR (Fig. 6-24) and a sinus beat with ventricular pacemaker beats (Fig. 6-25). Expect fusion beats when the artificial pacemaker rate is close to the sinus rate. They are considered part of normal pacemaker function and are not clinically significant (see Unit 10). In wide QRS tachycardias, fusion beats may help confirm the presence of a ventricular ectopic focus. They may thus aid in distinquishing VT from supraventricular tachycardia with preexisting bundle branch block or aberrant conduction (see Unit 7).

ECTOPIC SUPRAVENTRICULAR ARRHYTHMIAS

An ectopic supraventricular arrhythmia is an impulse originating above the ventricles but outside of the SA node. This impulse therefore originates in either the atria or the AV junctional tissue. Supraventricular impulses are usually transmitted through the normal conduction pathways to the ventricles. Therefore, supraventicular impulses usually produce a narrow, unchanging QRS complex. The presence of a narrow, unchanging QRS complex can be an initial guide to determining that the impulse is supraventricular, but it does not differentiate between an atrial or a junctional focus. P wave changes provide information for the differential diagnosis of the ectopic supraventricular arrhythmias. Atrial ectopic impulses produce P waves that are premature, resulting in an irregular P–P interval, or a P wave rate greater than 150. In junctional or nodal impulses, the P wave either is not visible preceding the QRS complex or is inverted (on lead II) with a short P–R interval. If the underlying rhythm is not available and the rate is too fast to determine if P waves are present, the rhythm is simply called supraventricular tachycardia, or SVT (Fig. 6-26).[40,52]

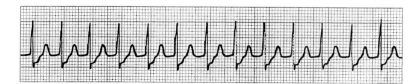

Fig. 6-26 Supraventricular tachycardia. In the absence of an underlying rhythm, P waves cannot be differentiated from T waves. Therefore, the specific supraventricular origin cannot be determined.

Most ectopic supraventricular arrhythmias predispose to tachyarrhythmias since a fast atrial rate may result in a fast ventricular rate. The supraventricular tachyarrhythmias are atrial tachycardia, atrial flutter, atrial fibrillation, and junctional (nodal) tachycardia. The atrial tachyarrhythmias begin with single atrial ectopic impulses, called premature atrial complexes (PACs). When the ventricular response is fast, supraventricular arrhythmias may result in a symptomatic fall in cardiac output. In addition, the myocardial work load increases and the coronary blood supply decreases.

Initial therapy focuses on controlling the ventricular rate. Supraventricular arrhythmias are diagnosed by the P wave but are treated initially by the ventricular (QRS) response. Subsequent therapy is directed towards correcting the underlying cause, suppressing the atrial instability, and conversion to sinus rhythm. Intervention may be pharmacologic, electrical, or surgical. The American Heart Association currently recommends verapamil (Isoptin/Calan) and adenosine (Adenocard) as initial drugs for the control of ventricular rate in rapid supraventricular tachycardias.[23] Intravenous diltiazem (Cardizem) is recommended when these are ineffective or a more sustained effect is needed. Although esmolol (Brevibloc), propanolol (Inderal), and metoprolol (Lopressor) may be used, they are less popular at this time (see Unit 9). Additional modes of acute therapy include vagal stimulation by Valsalva maneuvers, stimulation of the gag reflex, squatting, carotid sinus pressure, and coughing.[23] (Coughing may interrupt a supraventricular tachyarrhythmia.) Treatment of underlying heart failure is particularly critical in patients with acute MI since it is the most common cause of supraventricular arrhythmias in acute MI.[7] Electrical intervention includes cardioversion, catheter ablation, and pacemakers (see Unit 10). Surgical intervention is also used, primarily at referral centers.

Premature atrial complexes

Atrial arrhythmias are a manifestation of abnormal electrical activity in the atria. They are most commonly caused by hypoxemia, atrial distention due to CHF or valve disease, stress, pericarditis, SA node disease, mitral valve prolapse, and Wolff-Parkinson-White syndrome. The last two are not typically associated with coronary artery disease and are discussed further in Unit 11. Pulmonary disease is commonly associated with atrial arrhythmias secondary to either hypoxemia or right ventricular failure. Hyperthyroidism, smoking, fatigue, caffeine, and alcoholic cardiomyopathy also predispose patients to atrial arrhythmias.[40,48]

Premature atrial beats are an early sign of abnormal electrical activity in the atria. They may originate anywhere in the atria outside of the SA node. They appear on the ECG as *early P waves*. The P waves of premature

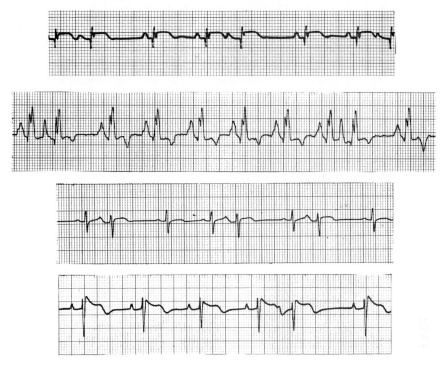

Fig. 6-27 Sinus rhythm with PACs. In the second trace, the underlying sinus rhythm has a wide QRS complex, probably due to a bundle branch block. In the premature beats, the QRS complexes, although wide, are the same shape, indicating a supraventricular origin. Large, upright, premature P waves are visible preceding these complexes.

atrial beats occur before the next expected P wave when compared with the underlying P to P cycle. They disrupt the regularity of the P–P interval. A single premature atrial impulse is called a *premature atrial complex* (PAC).[14,48] PACs are also known as *premature atrial contractions, atrial extrasystoles, atrial ectopic beats, or premature atrial depolarizations.*[40] The ectopic P wave may appear different from the P wave of the sinus impulse. This difference, however, is often slight and may be difficult to detect on isolated monitoring leads.

When a premature atrial impulse reaches the ventricles, it is usually uniformly conducted through the normal bundle branch system. The premature P wave of a PAC is therefore usually followed by a normal QRS complex, which is narrow or the same as that of the basic rhythm, or both (Fig. 6-27). The normal sinus impulse occurs after a pause. The premature QRS complex is usually noticed initially since it results in a change in the rhythm. The premature P waves precede these QRS complexes. Premature P waves are often buried on the T wave of the previous beat, distorting its configuration. The T wave configuration of that beat should be compared with that of the patient's usual T waves. P waves are small forces and may be best seen when the amplitude, or gain, is increased. Both normal and ectopic P waves usually are best seen on either lead II or V1 (MCL1).

P

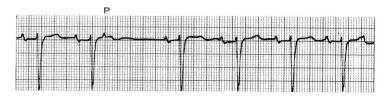

Fig. 6-28   Sinus rhythm with a nonconducted PAC.

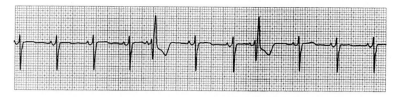

Fig. 6-29   Sinus rhythm with aberrantly conducted PAC.

If a premature atrial impulse is significantly premature, when it reaches the ventricles, the bundle branch system may still be completely refractory. The premature atrial impulse is not conducted at all and is called a *nonconducted* or *"blocked" PAC.*[13,34,46,48] The premature P wave is not followed by a QRS complex (Fig. 6-28). The major change in the rhythm will be a sudden pause. The early P wave will distort the T wave at the beginning of the pause. Nonconducted PACs are the most common cause of sudden pauses.

If a premature atrial impulse finds only one of the bundle branches refractory, the impulse will be blocked in that branch and will be conducted with delay in a different direction, using the other bundle branches. This deviation from the normal conduction pathway is called *aberrant conduction.* A wider QRS complex, conducted differently or *aberrantly,* follows the premature P wave (Fig. 6-29). A PAC conducted in this manner is referred to as an *aberrantly conducted PAC.* These beats are easily mistaken for PVCs or, unfortunately, vice versa. PVCs may also be preceded by P waves, but, in contrast to PACs, the P waves are not premature. A

changing QRS complex should be considered ventricular in origin, unless there is clear evidence to the contrary such as a *premature P wave.* Characteristic QRS patterns supporting aberrant conduction are discussed in Unit 7. PACs may be conducted in all of these three ways in a given patient (Fig. 6-30). The criterion common to all of these PACs is the premature P wave.

PACs may be conducted with normal or long P–R intervals. P–R intervals that are longer than normal occur because the ectopic atrial impulse finds the AV node partially refractory.[53] Following a PAC, an incomplete compensatory pause may occur because the ectopic atrial impulse penetrates the SA node and resets the sinus cycle. However, PACS do not consistently reset the SA node. Therefore, the presence of an incomplete versus a complete or full compensatory pause does not reliably differentiate PACs from PVCs (see Premature ventricular complexes).

PACs are clinically significant because they may indicate an underlying problem such as CHF or hypoxemia, and they may be precursors to more serious atrial arrhythmias. A PAC that falls during the vulnerable period

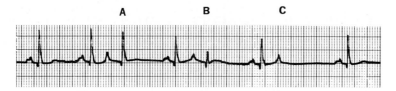

Fig. 6-30 Sinus rhythm with a normally conducted PAC *(A)*, an aberrantly conducted PAC *(B)*, and a nonconducted PAC *(C)*.

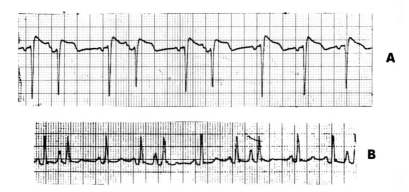

Fig. 6-31 Sinus rhythm with atrial bigeminy *(A)* and atrial trigeminy *(B)*.

of the *atria* may produce atrial flutter or fibrillation. Treat frequent PACs the same, whether normally conducted, nonconducted, or aberrantly conducted. Initial therapy is directed towards correcting the underlying causes. If this is ineffective, digitalis may be initiated to prevent tachyarrhythmias.

PACs may increase in frequency until they begin to occur every other beat in a *bigeminal*

Atrial tachycardia

PACs may continue to increase in frequency until they begin to occur consecutively. When three or more PACs occur in a row, the arrhythmia is called atrial tachycardia. Since this arrhythmia appears and disappears suddenly, it is commonly known as *paroxysmal atrial tachycardia,* or PAT. In atrial tachycardia (PAT), the atrial rate may range from 150 to 250 beats per minute. Specific rate ranges vary in different references.[40]

pattern (Fig. 6-31). In atrial bigeminy, the second beat is usually the ectopic impulse, while the beat after the pause is the sinus impulse. Obtaining the underlying rhythm can more clearly demonstrate this. The resulting P–P interval is irregular. The term *atrial trigeminy* is most commonly used to describe groups of three beats, composed of two sinus beats followed by one PAC (Fig. 6-31).

Characteristically the atrial rate is in the lower range—usually about 150 beats per minute (Fig. 6-32). The atrial rate can be calculated by measuring the P wave rate, or it can be estimated to be approximately 150 when P waves are separated by two large boxes on the ECG graph. At an atrial rate of 150, if the AV node is functioning normally, every atrial impulse should be conducted to the ventricles. Therefore, the ventricular

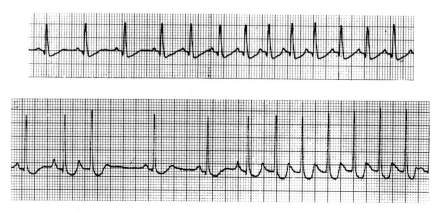

Fig. 6-32   Sinus rhythm with paroxysmal atrial tachycardia (PAT).

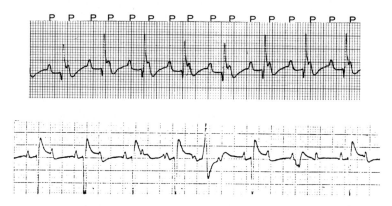

Fig. 6-33   PAT with block secondary to digitalis toxicity. P waves at an atrial rate of 150 are not all followed by QRS complexes. In the second trace, two other signs of digitalis toxicity are present. The shorter P–P intervals on either side of the R wave are characteristic. Multifocal PVCs are also present, typical of the arrhythmias of digitalis toxicity, which occur in twos.[14]

rate will be the same as the atrial rate. When P waves at a rate of 150 are not conducted to the ventricles, the rhythm is referred to as a PAT with block and is a sign of digitalis toxicity (Fig. 6-33). In patients with chronic lung disease, atrial tachycardia is often multifocal, resulting in ectopic P waves of three or more different shapes.[13,14,31,53]

Atrial tachycardia is differentiated from sinus tachycardia at a rate of 150 by the sudden change in the rhythm. When sinus tachycardia reaches or exceeds an atrial and ventricular rate of 150, it does so gradually, usually accompanying an increase in activity or fever. The response to vagal stimulation can also help differentiate between these two rhythms. In sinus tachycardia, the heart rate gradually slows, whereas in atrial tachycardia, the rhythm is interrupted with sudden conversion to sinus rhythm.

Atrial tachycardia is a form of supraventricular tachycardia. When the underlying rhythm is unavailable, differentiating P waves from T waves is difficult. This rhythm

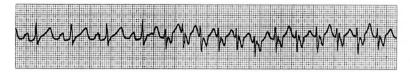

Fig. 6-34   Paroxysmal supraventricular tachycardia (PSVT) secondary to AV node reentry.

is best labeled supraventricular tachycardia, or SVT, even though the ventricular rate of 150 is consistent with atrial tachycardia (see Fig. 6-26). With a history of sudden onset, this narrow QRS tachycardia may also be referred as *paroxysmal* supraventricular tachycardia, or PSVT.[14,52] However, when ectopic P waves occur at a P wave rate of 150, the origin of the SVT is clearly atrial tachycardia and should be labeled as such.

In the absence of clear P waves during the tachycardia, what may appear to be PAT is often a more complex form of PSVT, triggered by a PAC but involving a reentry circuit in the AV node.[13,14,34] The triggering PAC usually has a prolonged P–R, signifying AV node penetration and unmasking of the reentry circuit. Inverted P waves, indicating retrograde conduction to the atria, are typically present in the tachycardia but are usually difficult to see (Fig. 6-34).

Emergency cardioversion is currently recommended for tachyarrhythmias with a ventricular rate greater than 150 in the unstable patient presenting with symptoms of chest pain, hypotension, or CHF.[23,31,52] An initial dose of adenosine (Adenocard) may be administered in the normotensive patient.[23]

Intravenous administration of adenosine or verapamil (Isoptin/Calan) usually rapidly controls the ventricular rate of PSVT or PAT. Adenosine is the current initial drug of choice in the patient whose blood pressure remains stable (Unit 9).[11,23] Verapamil is indicated, in the normotensive patient, for recurrent PSVT or PSVT unresponsive to adenosine. These drugs act on the AV node, interrupting the reentry circuit and, if effec-

tive, typically converting most forms of PSVT to sinus rhythm. Carotid sinus pressure and vagal maneuvers such as coughing, breath holding, stimulation of the gag reflex, squatting, or performing a Valsalva maneuver have similar effects and may be attempted prior to drug therapy.[23] Diltiazem (Cardizem), beta blockers such as esmolol (Brevibloc), and digitalis have similar effects and may be used if both adenosine and verapamil are ineffective. The delayed onset of action of digitalis as well as its ineffectiveness in the presence of increased sympathetic stimulation limits its current use in the acute setting.[19,47]

Long-term management of PSVT and PAT includes the administration of digitalis, oral antiarrhythmics such as quinidine sulfate (quinidine) and procainamide (Pronestyl), and oral verapamil (Isoptin/Calan). Recurrent supraventricular tachyarrhythmias refractory to drug therapy may be treated with pacemakers, catheter ablation, or surgery. Catheter ablation may be more effective and associated with fewer risks than antitachycardia pacing.[63]

Catheter ablation is becoming increasingly popular.[63] Ablation involves the partial or complete destruction of the AV node, or the accessory pathways involved in Wolff-Parkinson-White syndrome (see Unit 11), by the use of electrical or photo (laser) energy.[8,28,63,65] This energy may be delivered via a transvenous catheter. The safest and most common form of electrical energy used today is alternating current (AC) in the form of radiofrequency waves.[63,64,65] After electrophysiologic studies that locate the critical arrhythmia pathways, the electrical energy is applied for 30 to 90 seconds.[63] The heat generated destroys the tissue. Side effects include nausea and vomiting, hypotension, pleuritic chest pain, coronary artery spasm, torsades de pointes, and cardiac tamponade.[63-65] Nursing care is similar to that for the patient undergoing cardiac catheterization. Success rates are 90% or higher in patients with accessory pathways.[28,65] Ectopic beats may persist but do not trigger tachycardia.

Surgery for supraventricular tachyarrhythmias involves dissection and disconnection of accessory pathways, isolation of the atrial focus, or destruction of part or all of the AV node–His bundle and surrounding tissues (surgical ablation).[21,28] Because of the current success rate, lesser expense, and reduced patient discomfort with catheter ablation, however, surgery is rarely indicated.[8,64] When the AV node is completely destroyed by either catheter or surgical ablation, a pacemaker is inserted, and the patient becomes pacemaker dependent.

Atrial flutter

An increase in the atrial rate leads to an arrhythmia known as *atrial flutter*. In atrial flutter, the atrial rate usually falls between 250 and 350 beats per minute. Characteristically, the atrial rate is in the middle of this range: 300 beats per minute.[53] The atrial rate can be estimated to be 300 when P waves are separated by approximately one large box on the ECG graph. The atria are discharging impulses so rapidly that even a healthy AV node is unable to transmit all the impulses. Part of the physiologic function of the AV node is to protect the ventricles from rapid atrial rhythms. The ventricular rate may be either regular or irregular (Fig. 6-35).

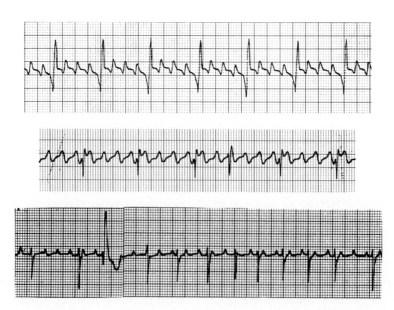

Fig. 6-35 Atrial flutter. In the beginning of the bottom trace on lead V1, the P wave rate of 300 is clearly visible in spite of the absence of the typical sawtooth pattern.

In atrial flutter, the atria are initiating impulses so rapidly that this arrhythmia may assume a sawtooth appearance on certain leads. The characteristic sawtooth appearance is most clearly visible on leads II, III, and aVF. P waves may also be clearly identified in lead V1 in the absence of a sawtooth appearance (Fig. 6-36).[14] Note that the characteristic sawtooth pattern is not necessary for the diagnosis of atrial flutter when P waves are clearly visible at an atrial rate of 300.

With a healthy AV node, two-to-one conduction in atrial flutter is common. Every other impulse is conducted to the ventricles. Thus the ventricular rate is half of the atrial rate, or approximately 150 beats per minute. The rhythm is described as atrial flutter with two-to-one conduction (Fig. 6-37). Detection of this arrhythmia is difficult because P waves may be hidden in the T waves or QRS complexes. Initial diagnosis of the rhythm may be supraventricular tachycardia or PSVT. Always include atrial flutter with two-to-one conduction in the differential diagnosis of a supraventricular tachycardia with a ventricular response of 150. An extra P wave may be found halfway between more clearly visible P waves if anticipated and searched for carefully.

Begin immediate therapy for atrial flutter when the ventricular rate is rapid (>150) and the patient is symptomatic or has acute coronary artery disease.[23] Determining the ventricular response is essential. The initial modes of therapy are similar to those for atrial tachycardia or PSVT (other forms of supraventricular tachycardia), although the response and preferred agents differ. Cardioversion is indicated in the unstable patient.[23] Drug therapy is attempted initially or following ineffective cardioversion in the patient who is not hypotensive.

In response to drug therapy acting at the AV node, the ventricular rate decreases but the rhythm does not convert to sinus. Reentry circuits, if involved, are located within the atria rather than at the AV node and thus are not directly affected by these modes of therapy. Verapamil and diltiazem are preferable to the very short acting adenosine in atrial flutter and fibrillation.[23] (An irregular ventricular response is suggestive of these rhythms rather than PSVT.) The use of digitalis is indicated when a more gradual decrease in ventricular rate is acceptable and is

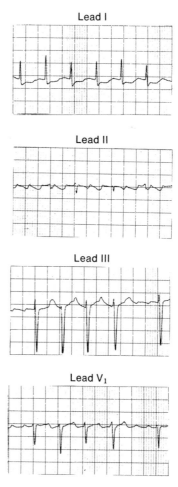

Fig. 6-36 Atrial flutter on different leads. The sawtooth pattern is visible on lead II, although it is not the best monitoring lead due to the small QRS complex. P waves are clearly visible in lead V1.

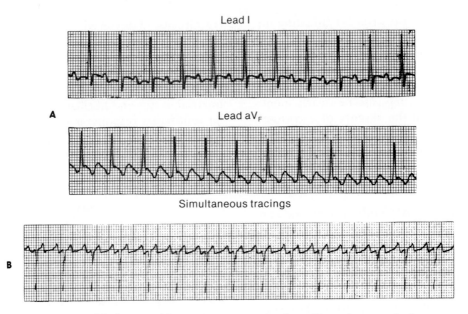

Lead I

A

Lead aV$_F$

Simultaneous tracings

B

Fig. 6-37 Atrial flutter with two-to-one conduction. Note the ventricular rate within a small box of 150.

most effective in patients with left ventricular failure.

Ventricular responses between 60 and 100 usually do not require immediate treatment. If the ventricular response is slow instead of the expected, more typical, fast ventricular response and the patient is symptomatic, increase the ventricular rate with atropine. Therefore, this atrial arrhythmia is truly diagnosed by the P wave and treated at least initially by the QRS response.

Since the signals fire too rapidly in atrial flutter, effective atrial contraction does not occur, resulting in atrial stasis. After several

Atrial fibrillation

If the rate of impulse discharge from the atria becomes faster, the arrhythmia known as *atrial fibrillation* may occur. With this rapid atrial rate, the shape or morphology of the P waves begins to deteriorate. A distinct, regular P wave and P wave rate no longer are identifiable. The ventricular response is typically rapid, limited only by the refractori-

days, clots may accumulate within the static atrial walls, placing the patient at risk for arterial embolization.[53] Echocardiographic studies can detect the presence of this mural thrombus, and the patient may receive prophylactic anticoagulation. Do not perform cardioversion in chronic atrial flutter because of the risk of dislodging emboli when sinus rhythm and atrial contraction are restored. In recent onset atrial flutter, as in atrial fibrillation, anticipate pharmacologic or electric cardioversion (see Atrial fibrillation). Use prophylactic anticoagulation a few weeks prior to and following cardioversion.

ness of the AV node. In atrial fibrillation, the AV node is bombarded with impulses. The AV node selects and conducts impulses randomly. Therefore, the ventricular response is irregular (Fig. 6-38). Atrial fibrillation is the most commonly occurring sustained supraventricular arrhythmia.[15,18,19,31]

Atrial fibrillation may be paroxysmal (in-

238

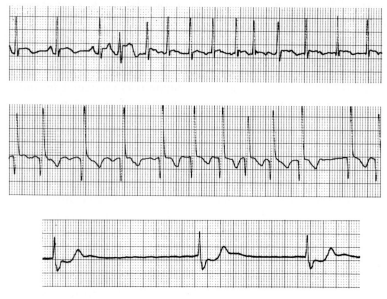

Fig. 6-38 Atrial fibrillation. In the top two examples the ventricular response is typically fast, whereas in the last example the ventricular response is slow.

termittent), acute but persistent and chronic.[7,31,47] In acute MI, atrial fibrillation correlates with the severity of left ventricular dysfunction[7,14,22] and, according to at least one study, is usually paroxysmal.[7] Therefore, management of heart failure is key in treating or preventing atrial fibrillation. Another common cause in acute MI is pericarditis.[14] Although frequent PACs are common, the incidence of atrial fibrillation is less than in other situations. In contrast, atrial flutter is more common in coronary artery disease.[23]

Immediate therapy is indicated when the ventricular rate is rapid (>150) and the patient is symptomatic. Direct treatment toward slowing the ventricular rate to relieve symptoms and hemodynamic compromise (heart failure and hypotension).[23,43,52] Perform electrical cardioversion in the "unstable" (symptomatic) patient.[23,52] As in atrial flutter, verapamil or diltiazem may be administered initially or following ineffective cardioversion in the normotensive patient.

Diltiazem may be preferable since it has weaker negative inotropic effects, does not interact with digitalis or class IA agents, and is associated with only a mild drop in blood pressure.[18] Use boluses, followed by continuous infusion, for up to 48 hours. Intravenous beta blockers such as esmolol (Brevibloc) are effective, but esmolol is associated with significant hypotension during infusion.[18] The calcium channel blockers and beta blockers act on the AV node to decrease the ventricular response but do not convert the rhythm to sinus. As in atrial flutter, reentry circuits, if involved, are located within the atria rather than the AV node and are thus not affected. If the ventricular rate in atrial fibrillation is atypically slow and the patient is symptomatic, therapy is directed toward increasing the ventricular rate.

Ultimate conversion to and maintenance of sinus rhythm is preferred to decrease the risk of thrombus formation and prevent arterial embolism, especially cerebral.[42,43] The highest number of embolic episodes occur in patients at the onset of atrial fibrillation.[42,43] Paroxysmal atrial fibrillation is associated with fewer emboli than chronic atrial fibrillation, however.[42] Patients at highest risk are those with rheumatic heart disease, previous MI, uncontrolled hyperthyroidism, and prosthetic valves.[14,42,43]

Elective cardioversion may be accomplished pharmacologically as well as electrically through the use of class IA, IC, or III antiarrhythmic agents.[43] The class IA agents, especially quinidine, have been used for years for this purpose. Quinidine may cause acceleration of the ventricular rate as a result of an initial vagolytic response and is best administered in conjunction with digitalis, verapamil, or beta blockers.[14] The newest class IC agent propafenone (Rhythmol) has fewer significant side effects than the other IC agents and may offer an alternative to the class IA agents when intolerance occurs.[43]

Mural thrombi begin to develop within the first week of elective cardioversion. Cardioversion after that time may trigger embolization. Widely accepted practice is to administer anticoagulation prophylactically a few weeks prior to and following elective cardioversion.[14,23,43] Potential contraindications to elective electric cardioversion include a large left atrium (>5.5 cm), a mural thrombus, digitalis toxicity, a recent meal, and a history of sick sinus syndrome or recurrent atrial fibrillation.[43]

Do not attempt cardioversion in atrial fibrillation of more than 6 months to 1 year duration.[31,43] Allow patients to remain in atrial fibrillation when (1) it is of longer than 6 months to 1 year duration, (2) it is unresponsive to cardioversion, or (3) it recurs frequently following cardioversion.[43] In these situations recommended treatment is long-term anticoagulation with warfarin (Coumadin).[14,42,43] The ventricular rate is controlled

with calcium channel blockers, beta blockers, or digitalis.

The efficacy of digitalis in both acute and chronic atrial fibrillation has been recently challenged.[18,19,23,47] Because the action of digitalis is mediated by the parasympathetic nervous system, it is less effective when arrhythmias are related to increased sympathetic activity.[19,47] This action is the major limitation, although digitalis is also difficult to titrate, has significant toxic effects, and interacts with verapamil and quinidine.[18] In paroxysmal atrial fibrillation, digitalis is not effective in preventing episodes or controlling the ventricular rate, and may extend the length of the episodes.[19,47] Nor has digitalis proved effective in preventing postoperative atrial fibrillation in cardiopulmonary patients.[46] In chronic atrial fibrillation, although digitalis controls resting heart rates, the effects on heart rates during exercise are much less, limiting exercise tolerance.[19,47] However, the combination of digitalis with calcium channel blockers or beta blockers is more effective on exercise heart rates than either one alone.[19,47]

The ineffectiveness of digitalis in patients with paroxysmal atrial fibrillation, following cardiopulmonary surgery, or during exercise may be explained by the increased sympathetic activity associated with each of these. Digitalis may also be ineffective in arrhythmias related to fever, hypoxia, or blood loss where sympathetic activity similarly increases.[19] Digitalis does not convert acute atrial fibrillation and may take some time to decrease the ventricular rate. Digitalis is also contraindicated in patients with Wolff-Parkinson-White syndrome and hypertrophic myopathy with outflow obstruction (see Unit 11).

Because of its beneficial effects on contractility, digitalis is effective and continues to be indicated for all forms of atrial fibrillation associated with significant left ventricular failure.[19,47] In left ventricular failure, digitalis is preferred over calcium channel blockers or beta blockers. Digitalis may also be beneficial in patients with chronic atrial fibrillation and a sedentary life-style, in combination with calcium channel blockade or beta blockade in active patients, or for more gradual rate control in patients with acute atrial fibrillation.[19,47]

Both catheter ablation and surgical intervention in atrial flutter and fibrillation are reserved for symptomatic cases unresponsive to other modes of therapy.[43] Catheter ablation for atrial flutter or fibrillation requires complete destruction of the AV node, resulting in a junctional response of 40 to 70 beats per minute. Pacemaker implantation may be necessary.[28,63] The atria continue to fibrillate, thus maintaining the risk of embolization and the loss of atrial contribution to cardiac output.

Junctional or nodal arrhythmias

Junctional, or nodal, arrhythmias originate in the AV junctional tissue. Junctional arrhythmias are therefore supraventricular. The QRS complex is typically narrow and unchanging, consistent with its supraventricular origin. It is the P wave characteristics that differentiate these arrhythmias from most of the atrial arrhythmias. When a junctional arrhythmia occurs, the atria are depolarized in a reverse direction. This phenomenon is known as retrograde atrial depolarization. Retrograde depolarization of the atria results in inversion of the P wave. (The P wave in lead II is negative.) The inverted P wave may be visible either before or after the QRS complex, depending on whether the AV junction activates the atria or ventricles initially.[9] If the P wave appears in front of the QRS complex, the P–R interval will be *short* (<0.12 second or shorter than the patient's normal P–R interval) since activation of the atria only *slightly* precedes activa-

The maze procedure is the most recently developed surgical intervention for atrial flutter, paroxysmal atrial fibrillation or chronic atrial fibrillation.[15,43,49] This procedure is designed to prevent or interrupt the multiple atrial reentry circuits characteristic of atrial fibrillation. The surgeon makes incisions and draws sutures throughout the atria, creating a maze of pathways with the SA node at one end and the AV node at the other. An impulse originating in one area is unable to form a circuit returning to the same area without crossing suture lines. Thus sinus rhythm and atrial contraction are restored. The procedure maximizes hemodynamics and eliminates the risk of thromboembolism. Earlier procedures involved isolating either the left atrium or a corridor of tissue between the atria and ventricles.[15,43] Parts of the atria continued to fibrillate.

tion of the ventricles (Fig. 6-39). In leads where P wave inversion may be normal, such as lead V1, suspect a junctional arrhythmia with a preceding P wave in the presence of this short P–R interval and confirm it, if necessary, on lead II.

If the atria are depolarized at the same time as the ventricles, the P wave may become hidden within the QRS complex. The ventricular response will remain regular, thus distinguishing this rhythm from atrial fibrillation in which P waves are also not clearly visible preceding the QRS complex but the ventricular response is irregular (Fig. 6-40). In summary, P waves in a junctional or nodal arrhythmia may be either absent or inverted preceding the QRS complex. If the P wave is inverted, the P–R interval should also be short. In both junctional rhythms and fine atrial fibrillation, the P waves are not clearly visible. Therefore, an additional criterion is necessary to differentiate be-

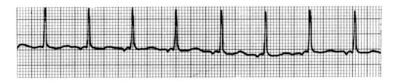

Fig. 6-39   Junctional (nodal) rhythm.

Junctional arrhythmia

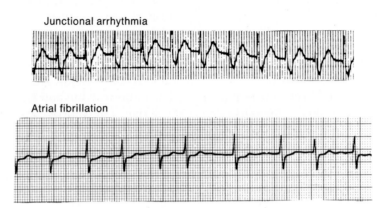

Atrial fibrillation

Fig. 6-40   Junctional arrhythmia compared with fine atrial fibrillation. The major distinguishing characteristic is the irregular R–R (QRS) interval in atrial fibrillation and the regular R–R (QRS) interval in the junctional arrhythmia.

tween them. In a junctional rhythm, the ventricular rhythm and R–R interval remain regular, whereas in atrial fibrillation, the ventricular rhythm and R–R interval are irregular.

The three major categories of junctional arrhythmias are caused by three independent mechanisms. Their therapy also differs. Single premature beats that originate in the AV junctional tissue are known as *premature junctional contractions* (PJCs) or *premature nodal contractions* (PNCs). PJCs do not necessarily progress to junctional tachycardia. Their exact mechanism and cause are unknown. PJCs thus are usually not clinically significant and occur less frequently than PACs. The following are characteristics of PJCs: (1) the QRS complexes are early, or premature, and (2) if a P wave is associated with the premature beat, it will be inverted

with a short P–R interval (Fig. 6-41). The P wave may not be visible at all preceding the ectopic QRS complex.

When the normal pacemaker in the SA node is depressed, the AV junctional tissue may assume control of the rhythm at a rate usually between 40 and 60 beats per minute. All other previously discussed characteristics of a junctional arrhythmia are present. Clinical causes include digitalis and inferior wall MI. The resulting rhythm is called *junctional (nodal) rhythm* (Fig. 6-42). Usually no therapy is indicated. If symptomatic from the slow ventricular rate and/or the loss of atrial kick, the patient can receive atropine. He or she can receive epinephrine, dopamine, or isoproterenol if atropine is ineffective and a transcutaneous pacemaker is unavailable.[9,23]

When automaticity is enhanced in the AV junctional tissue, the AV node may again

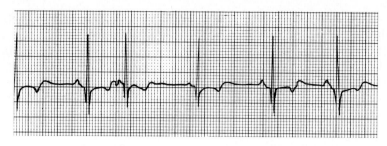

Fig. 6-41   Sinus rhythm with a single PJC (PNC).

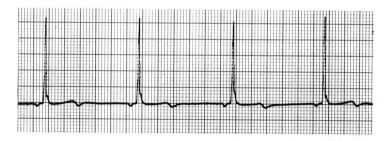

Fig. 6-42   Junctional (nodal) rhythm.

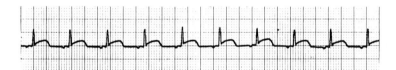

Fig. 6-43   Junctional (nodal) tachycardia.

control the rhythm. When that occurs and the ventricular rate is greater than 100 beats per minute, the arrhythmia is known as *junctional* or *nodal tachycardia* (Fig. 6-43). Junctional tachycardia is frequently associated with increased automaticity secondary to digitalis toxicity. Reentry circuits also have been implicated. A junctional rhythm with a ventricular rate exceeding 60 but less than 100 beats per minute may be referred to as an accelerated junctional rhythm.[9,14] Exact rate limits of junctional tachycardia and accelerated junctional rhythm vary from reference to reference. Accelerated junctional rhythm is a manifestation of enhanced automaticity but is often facilitated by depressed automaticity in the SA node, as in junctional rhythm.

NURSING ORDERS: The patient with a supraventricular arrhythmia

RELATED NURSING DIAGNOSES: Alteration in cardiac output, impaired gas exchange, impaired tissue perfusion, anxiety, knowledge deficit (patient/family)

1. Notify physician of frequent PACs or intermittent atrial arrhythmias, together with signs and symptoms of heart failure or hypoxemia.

2. Assess for and report the following signs of heart failure:
   —crackles (rales) or S3 gallop
   —decreased urine output
   —underlying sinus tachycardia
   —elevated wedge pressure if pulmonary artery (PA) catheter is in place
   Also check intake and output, serum Na^+, and urine lytes for signs of Na^+ and fluid retention.
3. Assess for and report the following signs of hypoxemia:
   —shortness of breath or other signs of respiratory distress
   —SaO_2 less than 92% if on pulse oximeter
   —PaO_2 less than 60 mm Hg; SaO_2 less than 90% on arterial blood gases (ABG).
4. In the patient with of signs of hypoxemia:
   —Position for optimal chest expansion.
   —Replace O_2 mask or prongs if removed by patient or family.
   —Increase O_2 supply or substitute with other mode of O_2 therapy if the respiratory pattern is variable.
5. In the patient with a sustained supraventricular arrhythmia, determine the ventricular rate and assess patient response.
   —Is the patient experiencing chest pain?
   —Check blood pressure, level of consciousness, skin color, and temperature.
   —Assess for new onset of heart failure.
   —Attach pulse oximeter and determine SaO_2. Provide O_2 as needed.
6. If ventricular rate is greater than 150 and symptoms are present (patient considered unstable), the American Heart Association recommends immediate cardioversion.[2] Anticipate sedation. Obtain manual resuscitation bag, suction equipment, and cardioverter. If the patient is not hypotensive, consider giving an initial trial of adenosine or verapamil (see Units 7 and 8).

7. In the patient with PAT or PSVT (regular rhythm):
   —Have patient cough, hold breath, or perform a Valsalva maneuver.
   —Notify physician.
   —Anticipate adenosine order or carotid sinus pressure by physician. Check patient for carotid bruit prior to carotid sinus pressure and report to physician if present.[23]
   —For recurrent PSVT, anticipate IV verapamil, diltiazem, or beta blockers such as esmolol.
   —Obtain order for maintenance digitalis, beta blockade, or calcium channel blockade.
8. In the patient wth atrial flutter or fibrillation (irregular rhythm):
   —With fast ventricular rate, anticipate IV verapamil, diltiazem, or beta blockers such as esmolol or digitalis for gradual rate reduction.
   —Anticipate maintenance digitalis especially in patients with heart failure.
   —A ventricular rate of 60 to 100 requires no immediate therapy. Notify physician if onset is new. Anticipate elective pharmacologic or electrical cardioversion with prophylactic anticoagulation unless duration is greater than 6 months to 1 year.
9. Note if arrhythmias could be stress related.
   —Watch for nonverbal as well as verbal expressions of anxiety.
   —Is any event (e.g., family or staff visits) associated with the arrhythmias?
10. Consider other causes. Does the patient have evidence of pericarditis? Could drug therapy (isoproterenol, dopamine, theophylline, inhaled $beta_2$ agents) be associated with the arrhythmias?
11. Collaborate with physician for anticoagulation in chronic atrial flutter and fibrillation especially in the presence of mural thrombi.

12. Instruct the patient and family regarding predisposing factors, modes of self-treatment, follow-up diagnostic or therapeutic procedures (such as catheter ablation), and side effects of medications.
13. Does the patient have coronary artery disease? Consider more aggressive rate control.
14. If there is PAT with block, junctional tachycardia, or very slow ventricular rate, consider digitalis toxicity. Check serum digitalis and other patient symptoms (see Unit 9).
15. In the patient with a junctional rhythm:
    —Check for patient symptoms.
    —If patient is symptomatic, notify physician and anticipate atropine.
    —If patient is asymptomatic, no treatment is necessary; continue to observe.[9]

HEART BLOCKS

A heart block is defined as a delay or block within the heart's conduction system. Blocks occur either at the SA node or within the atrioventricular conduction system. Blocks at the SA node level include SA block and sinus arrest. Blocks between the atria and the ventricles or within the AV conduction system are called AV blocks.

SA BLOCK AND SINUS ARREST

In SA block, the sinus impulse is formed and released but fails to reach the atria. In sinus arrest or sinus pause, the SA node is suppressed so that the impulse never forms. In both SA block and sinus arrest, the atria are not activated. Therefore, neither a P wave nor a QRS complex appears, unless escape beats occur. A sudden long pause results. SA block is a manifestation of depressed conduction between the SA node and the atria. The rhythm of the SA node is not interrupted. Therefore, the pause in the rhythm is usually equal to a multiple of the original P–P cycle (Fig. 6-44). In sinus arrest, the automaticity of the SA node is suppressed, and the rate and rhythm are reset. Unlike in SA block, the pause in the rhythm associated with a sinus arrest is of no predictable length (Fig. 6-44).[14,53]

Both SA block and sinus arrest may be due to drug toxicity, inferior wall MI, or chronic conduction system disease. They are potentially clinically significant because they may result in a slow ventricular rate and cause a symptomatic fall in cardiac output. Initial therapy in the symptomatic patient focuses on increasing the ventricular rate with atropine sulfate, transcutaneous pacing, dopamine (Intropin), epinephrine (Adrenalin), and/or isoproterenol (Isuprel). Temporary transvenous and permanent pacing may be necessary if this arrhythmia continues for extended periods or recurs. Asymptomatic patients do not require any intervention.

AV block

AV block is a block in the conduction system between the atria and ventricles, either at the AV node or within the bundle branch system. The block occurs after atrial depolarization but before ventricular depolarization. Therefore, the major ECG characteristic is a change in the P–R interval. In AV blocks either the P–R interval is too long or changing, a P wave occurs without a QRS complex, or there is a combination of these changes. Causes of AV block include myocardial infarction, cardiomyopathy, cardiac surgery, drug therapy, and chronic conduction system disease. AV blocks are immedi-

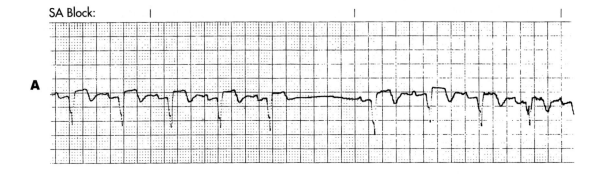

SA Block:

A

Sinus Arrest:

B

Fig. 6-44 *A,* SA block and, *B,* sinus arrest.

ately clinically significant when they result in a symptomatic slow ventricular rate.

AV blocks are classified according to the degree of pathologic severity and the site of the block. The classification according to degree (first, second, and third) is based on ECG analysis. However, the resulting ventricular rate, not the degree of pathologic severity, ultimately determines the clinical significance. Initial therapy focuses on increasing the ventricular rate with atropine sulfate (Atropine), transcutaneous pacing, dopamine (Intropin), epinephrine (Adrenalin), or isoproterenol (Isuprel), in that order.[23] Subsequent clinical significance depends on the site of the block and helps determine whether temporary transvenous or permanent pacing is indicated.

AV blocks are classified according to site as either above or below the His bundle. AV blocks that occur above the bundle of His at the AV node are generally more benign, more responsive to atropine, and, when associated with acute MI, typically transient.

AV blocks that occur below the bundle of His within the bundle branch system are generally more malignant and respond poorly to atropine, requiring dopamine, epinephrine, or isoproterenol when transcutaneous pacing is unavailable.[23] When associated with acute MI, blocks within the bundle branch system are chronic and recurring.

Complete analysis of an AV block includes an assessment and description of the atrial rate. The atrial rate at which the block develops can indicate the severity of the conduction system disease.[25,35] A fast sinus rate may predispose to AV block in an ischemic conduction system. Subsequent therapy in this case may include treatment of the causes of sinus tachycardia such as fever. When AV block occurs in the context of an atrial arrhythmia, the atrial arrhythmia is considered the primary abnormality. The AV block may be due to the intended effects of drug therapy or to refractoriness of the AV node secondary to the atrial rate.[35,36] Conduction system disease may not be present.

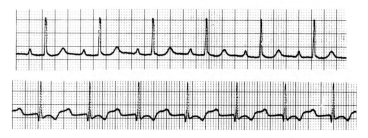

Fig. 6-45 Sinus rhythm with first-degree AV block.

First-degree AV block

In first-degree AV block all impulses are conducted, but with delay. Therefore, the diagnosis of first-degree AV block is made when the P–R interval is prolonged (>0.20 second) (Fig. 6-45). First-degree AV block may occur as a result of pathology either above or below the His bundle.[8,16,36,52] To determine the location, analyze the rhythm within the clinical setting in which it occurs.

Second-degree AV block

In second-degree AV block, some impulses are conducted while others are not. Atrial depolarization occurs normally, originating in the SA node, but ventricular depolarization does not always follow.[46] Therefore, in second-degree AV block, some P waves will not be followed by a QRS complex, giving the appearance of a "dropped" QRS.

In second-degree AV block the ventricular response may be regular or irregular. Initially the ventricular response is irregular, indicating only occasional dropped beats. At this stage, the second-degree AV block is referred to by ECG pattern as either Wenckebach (Mobitz I) or Mobitz II, depending on the characteristics of the preceding P–R interval. Second-degree AV block may be classified as type I or type II depending on the location of the block above or below the bundle of His.[14,16,35,36,52,53]

Wenckebach is diagnosed when a dropped QRS complex is preceded by progressive prolongation of the P–R interval (Fig. 6-46). The progressive prolongation eventually causes the P wave to fall within the refractory period of the ventricles and become blocked. Small increments in the P–R interval may be difficult to detect, especially if they occur over a long series of beats.[8,30] Other characteristics of second-degree AV block, Wenckebach (Mobitz I), are (1) constant P to P (P–P) intervals with a P wave rate less than 150 (indicating its sinus origin) and (2) irregular, sometimes decreasing, R–R intervals.

Wenckebach is considered a form of type I AV block, which is associated with a block at the AV node above the bundle of His.[14,16,35,52,53] Type I second-degree AV block was initially recognized by its Wenckebach pattern.[8,30] Many clinicians continue to use the two terms (Wenckebach and type I) interchangeably.[8,52,53] Since the AV node is primarily supplied by the right coronary artery, blocks that occur at the AV node are usually associated with right coronary artery pathology or inferior wall MI.[8,14,16,53] Wenckebach blocks are also typical of digitalis toxicity, which affects the AV node. Wenckebach block is clinically significant because (1) it may result in a slow ventricular

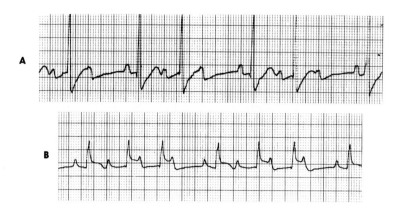

Fig. 6-46 Second-degree AV block, Wenckebach (Mobitz I, type I). The complete interpretation in *A* is sinus rhythm with second-degree AV block, Wenckebach. The complete interpretation in *B* is sinus tachycardia with second-degree AV block, Wenckebach. Note that the P–P intervals remain regular in both, whereas the R–R intervals are irregular.

rate, causing a symptomatic fall in cardiac output, and (2) it may be the precursor of more severe AV block. If the ventricular rate falls and the patient becomes symptomatic, this rhythm is usually responsive to atropine. Wenckebach, however, is typically benign and transient, requiring no therapy. Pacing rarely is necessary.[8,53]

AV block in inferior wall MI is thought to be due, in part, to stimulation of vagal fibers in the area of the AV node secondary to ischemia.[5,6] Results of the recent TIMI II trial that examined heart block in patients receiving thrombolytic therapy suggest that heart block is a marker of increased infarction size and mortality in inferior wall MI.[5,6,38] AV block in inferior wall MI is usually transient. It typically occurs and is resolved within the first 3 days, although some studies have reported it up to 7 days.[5,16,50] Early onset block (within 24 hours) is associated with increased vagal tone and is responsive to atropine.[16,37,50] Late onset AV block (after 24 hours) is less responsive to atropine, however, and is thought to occur secondary to a local rise in extracellular potassium or localized edema that remains for up

to 3 days.[5,37,50] Patients experience similar mortality rates with both forms.[50]

Mobitz II is diagnosed when a dropped QRS complex is not preceded by P–R prolongation. The P–R interval remains fixed, and the dropped beat occurs without warning (Fig. 6-47). Other characteristics of second-degree AV block, Mobitz II, include (1) regular P–P interval with a P wave rate under 150 (consistent with a sinus origin) and (2) irregular R–R intervals. The P wave characteristics occur in all AV blocks and do not help differentiate between them. An accompanying irregular R–R interval occurs only in second-degree AV block and indicates either Wenckebach (Mobitz I) or Mobitz II. The P–R interval is the major distinguishing characteristic between these two.[14,28,35,36,46,53]

Mobitz II is considered a form of type II second-degree AV block, which is associated with pathology within or below the bundle of His, usually in the bundle branch system.[14,28,35,36,46,53] Because the bundle branches are primarily supplied by the left coronary artery, blocks that occur within the bundle branch system usually are associated

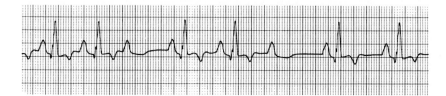

Fig. 6-47 Second-degree AV block, Mobitz II (type II). The complete interpretation is sinus rhythm with second-degree AV block, Mobitz II. Note that in this form of second-degree AV block, similar to Wenckebach, the P–P intervals are regular and the R–R intervals are irregular. The major characteristic differentiating this rhythm from Wenckebach is the constant P–R interval prior to the dropped or missing QRS complex.

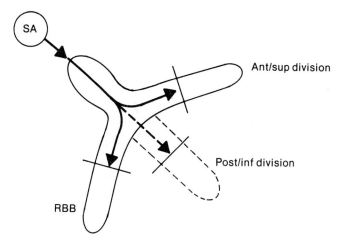

Fig. 6-48 Intermittent trifascicular block producing Mobitz II.

with left coronary artery pathology or extensive anterior wall MI.[53]

The bundle branch system is composed of three fascicles: the right bundle branch, the anterosuperior division of the left bundle branch, and the posteroinferior division of the left bundle branch. Mobitz II second-degree AV block usually occurs as a result of intermittent trifascicular block and is preceded by bifascicular block (Fig. 6-48). The most common forms of bifascicular block in anterior wall MI are right bundle branch block and a block in the anterosuperior division of the left bundle branch (left anterior hemiblock). The presence of right bundle branch block is detected by characteristic changes on lead V1, while the presence of left anterior hemiblock is detected by left axis deviation (see Unit 7). New Mobitz II and bundle branch blocks (right, left, alternating, or bifascicular) in acute anterior wall MI are indications for prophylactic transvenous pacing, regardless of patient symptoms.[16,23,28,45] Atropine should be avoided since it acts primarily on the SA and AV nodes, above the bundle of His.[14,23,36] An increase in the block may occur secondary to increases in the atrial rate, without an in-

Table 6-1. Second-degree AV blocks

Wenckebach	Mobitz
Lesion at AV node: supra-Hisian (type I)	Lesion in bundle branch system: infra-Hisian (type II)
Associated with inferior wall MI, digitalis toxicity, chronic lesion of conduction system	Associated with anterior wall MI, chronic lesions of conduction system
Described as ischemic, reversible, and transient in nature	Described as necrotic in nature
Dropped QRS complex preceded by progressive prolongation of the P–R interval (irregular R–R)	Dropped QRS complex preceded by fixed P–R interval (irregular R–R)
Regular P–P intervals	Regular P–P intervals
P wave rate <150	P wave rate <150
Can progress to 2:1	Can progress to 2:1
Usually responds well to atropine	Responds better to dopamine, epinephrine, or isoproterenol
May require temporary pacing in symptomatic patients	Requires temporary and permanent pacing in acute MI

crease in the ventricular rate. In the symptomatic patient, initial transcutaneous pacing is used instead.[23] Table 6-1 summarizes and compares Wenckebach (Mobitz I) and Mobitz II according to typical site within the conduction system, related MI, pathophysiology, ECG criteria, and usual therapy.

As second-degree AV block progresses in severity, 2:1 conduction occurs with only every other P wave conducted. In those P waves that are followed by QRS complexes, a constant, although sometimes long, P–R interval indicates conduction is normal in those beats (Fig. 6-49).

Second-degree AV block with 2:1 conduction may be the end result of either Wenckebach (Mobitz I) or Mobitz II, reflecting *either* a type I or type II mechanism.[8,14,16,34–36,52,53] Without a recording of the block's onset, determining whether it represents a type I or type II mechanism may be difficult. However, a 2:1 second-degree AV block, type I, is usually associated with narrow QRS complexes, compatible with a block within the AV node.[8,14,16,20,28,34-36] Previous episodes of classic Wenckebach in the same patient are common. Type I AV block also is more likely to occur with inferior wall MI. In contrast, type II 2:1 second-degree AV block is usually associated with a wide QRS complex, suggesting bundle branch block (see Fig. 6-49).[8,14,35,36] Intra-Hisian block also may complicate the interpretation of 2:1 second-degree AV block.[14,20,28] When in doubt, it is best and always accurate to refer to the rhythm as merely second-degree AV block with 2:1 conduction.

When two or more consecutive P waves are not conducted, the block may be referred to as *high-grade* or *advanced* second-degree AV block.[8,14] The ECG pattern reflects conduction ratios of 3:1, 4:1, and so on, or varying ratios, still with constant P–R intervals.[16,35,36,46,53] The block may involve either a type I or type II mechanism.[16,36,53]

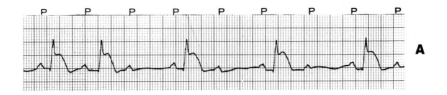

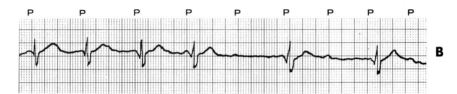

Fig. 6-49 Sinus rhythm with second-degree AV block and 2 to 1 conduction. In trace A the 2 to 1 conduction (last three beats) is the end result of Wenckebach (Mobitz I, type I). In trace B the 2 to 1 conduction (last three beats) is the end result of Mobitz II (type II). Once 2 to 1 conduction is established, the P–P interval, R–R interval, and P–R interval are constant in both. If the onset of the rhythm were not available, the only distinquishing characteristic between the type I and type II mechanisms would be the narrow QRS complexes in type I *(A)* and the wide QRS complexes in type II *(B)*.

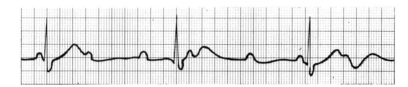

Fig. 6-50 Sinus rhythm with third-degree (complete) AV block.

Third-degree AV block

The pathology involved in AV block can continue to progress in severity until *all* sinus impulses are blocked. When this occurs, the AV block is known as *third-degree*, or complete, AV block. Although QRS complexes follow some P waves, no fixed relationship exists between the atria and ventricles, as indicated by a varying P–R interval (Fig. 6-50). As in the other forms of AV block, the P–P intervals remain regular and the P wave rate is under 150, consistent with a sinus origin.

Like second-degree AV block, third-degree AV block may occur at the AV node or within the bundle branch system. When third-degree AV block occurs at the AV node, the ventricles usually are under the control of the bundle of His (junctional tissue). The ventricular response is idiojunctional, as indicated by a narrow QRS complex and a ventricular rate between 40 and 60 beats per minute.[12,46,52] This form of third-degree AV block typically occurs in inferior wall MI. Some authorities question the

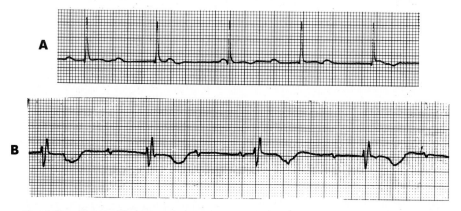

Fig. 6-51 Comparison of third-degree AV block with an idiojunctional response *(A)* and third-degree AV block with an idioventricular response *(B)*. The first example may not reflect a true form of complete heart block since the ventricular rate is 60.

existence of true complete AV block when the ventricular rate is more than 40 to 45 beats per minute.[16,35,36,53]

When third-degree AV block occurs within the bundle branch system, the ventricles usually control the rhythm. The ventricular response is idioventricular, as indicated by a wide QRS complex and a ventricular rate between 20 and 40 beats per minute. Complete heart block secondary to chronic conduction system disease is usually associated with a block within the bundle branch system.[14,28,36] This form of third-degree AV block also typically occurs in anterior wall MI.

The regular QRS complexes of third-degree AV block mimic second-degree AV block with 2:1 conduction or some forms of high-grade (advanced) second-degree AV block. In second-degree AV block, however, the identifiable P–R intervals are constant, whereas in third-degree AV block the P–R intervals vary.

Third-degree, or complete, AV block is clinically significant when it is associated with a symptomatic fall in cardiac output. Third-degree AV block with an idiojunctional re-sponse is less likely to cause a fall in cardiac output than third-degree AV block with an idioventricular response since the ventricular response is usually faster and more stable.[16,52] Initial therapy in third-degree block, as in all AV blocks, is directed towards increasing the ventricular rate if the patient is symptomatic with pacing, dopamine, epinephrine, or isoproterenol. In third-degree block with wide QRS complexes (idioventricular response), initial transcutaneous pacing is used.[23] Atropine is not administered, since it is less likely to increase the ventricular rate and may potentiate the block by increasing the atrial rate.[36]

NURSING ORDERS: The patient with a bradyarrhythmia due to sinus arrest, SA block, or AV block

RELATED NURSING DIAGNOSES: Alteration in cardiac output, impaired tissue perfusion, knowledge deficit

1. Determine the ventricular response.
2. Report new onset AV block to physician.
3. Assess patient for symptoms (chest pain, hypotension, shortness of breath, PVCs, change in mental status).
4. If patient is symptomatic:

—Anticipate atropine, transcutaneous pacing, dopamine, epinephrine, or isoproterenol.

—In patients with type II second-degree AV block or third-degree block with wide QRS complexes, omit atropine and use initial transcutanous pacing instead.

5. Determine whether the patient is receiving any medications that suppress AV node conduction (e.g., verapamil, diltiazem, beta blockers, digitalis, amiodarone).

6. In the patient with inferior wall MI:
   —Watch for the development of first-degree AV block; type I second-degree AV block, Wenckebach, 2:1, or advanced with narrow complexes; and third-degree AV block with idiojunctional response.
   —If patient is asymptomatic, continue to observe.

7. In the patient with anterior wall MI:
   —Monitor lead V1 pattern for the development of right bundle branch block (see Unit 7).
   —Monitor leads I, aVF, and II for the development of left anterior hemiblock (see Unit 7).
   —In the presence of Mobitz II, new right or left bundle branch block, alternating bundle branch block, bifascicular block, or third-degree AV block with idioventricular response, notify physician immediately and prepare for prophylactic transvenous pacing even in the asymptomatic patient.[23,28] Anticipate probable pacemaker implantation[28] (see Unit 10).
   —In anticipation of AV block, have an external pacemaker or epinephrine drip immediately available.

8. Instruct patient and family regarding follow-up diagnostic tests, transvenous pacing, and/or pacemaker implantation if necessary.

AV DISSOCIATION

AV dissociation is a general term that can describe any cardiac arrhythmia in which the atria and ventricles beat independently.[14,35,36,41] Both the P–P intervals and the R–R intervals remain regular. However, the P–R interval varies. Examples of arrhythmias exhibiting AV dissociation include (1) ventricular tachycardia (Fig. 6-52), (2) junctional rhythm or tachycardia (some forms), and (3) third-degree or complete heart block. Ventricular pacing also results in AV dissociation since the atria, for the most part, are unaffected.

AV dissociation occurs by two major mechanisms: usurpation or default.[8,37,53] Usurpation involves the acceleration of a junctional or ventricular pacemaker so that it fires faster than the sinus node. Default involves slowing or blocking the sinus impulses, allowing junctional or ventricular escape rhythms to control the ventricles while the SA node maintains control of the atria.

AV dissociation is a description, not a diagnosis, encompassing many different arrhythmias of grossly varying clinical significance.[8,13,14,37] If the term is used at all, a more complete interpretation is necessary (e.g., AV dissociation due to ventricular tachycardia or AV dissociation due to complete heart block).[8]

In junctional rhythms, AV dissociation typically occurs when the AV junction fires only slightly faster than the SA node secondary to either usurpation or default. The AV junction is unable to activate the atria, which have already been depolarized by the SA node. Since atrial and ventricular rates are almost the same, this arrhythmia is called *iso-*

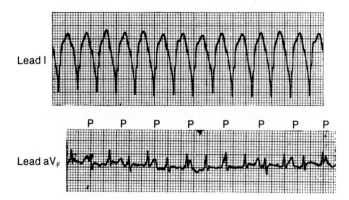

Lead I

Lead aVF

Fig. 6-52 AV dissociation due to ventricular tachycardia. Simultaneous tracings in leads I and aVF are provided. The dissociation between the P waves and QRS complexes is more noticeable in lead aVF.

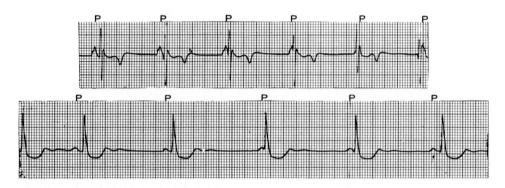

Fig. 6-53 Isorhythmic AV dissociation due to a junctional rhythm.

rhythmic AV dissociation. The P waves remain upright, rather than inverted, and appear to march into and past the QRS complex, forming a characteristic pattern (Fig. 6-53).[41] Isorhythmic AV dissociation with a junctional pacemaker has the same clinical significance as any other junctional rhythm. The arrhythmia terminates when the SA node accelerates and again controls the entire heart. If therapy is necessary, in the symptomatic patient, the drug of choice is atropine. Although the term is used most commonly to describe junctional rhythms, isorhythmic AV dissociation also occurs

in ventricular rhythms such as accelerated idioventricular rhythm or ventricular pacing.[41]

Clinical signs may aid in the diagnosis of AV dissociation. When the atria and ventricles beat independently, atrial and ventricular depolarization and contraction may randomly coincide. Reflux of blood into the superior vena cava occurs when the atria attempt to empty their contents against closed AV valves. This reflux appears as an accentuation of normal neck vein pulsations. These accentuated atrial waves are known as *cannon waves.* These large intermittent pulsations are easily visible on inspection of the neck.[8]

Another clinical sign indicative of a dissociated rhythm is varying intensity of the first heart sound (S1).[8] The intensity of the S1 is related to the timing of ventricular systole. If ventricular systole occurs when the valves are widely open, a loud sound is produced. Short P–R intervals are associated with widely opened AV valves and loud first heart sounds, and long P–R intervals are associated with soft first heart sounds. Since the P–R intervals vary in AV dissociation, the intensity of the S1 also varies (see Unit 8).

ASYSTOLE, PULSELESS ELECTRICAL ACTIVITY, AND ELECTROMECHANICAL DISSOCIATION

Ventricular asystole and electromechanical dissociation (EMD) are both forms of cardiac arrest since no pulse is present. Their ECG patterns, mechanisms, and intervention differ, however.

The term *asystole* usually refers to ventricular asystole or the absence of ventricular electrical activity. QRS complexes are absent, although P waves may or may not be present.[36,52] Ventricular fibrillation may appear like asystole in selected leads. Confirmation of the ECG pattern on at least two leads is necessary. Asystole may occur spontaneously or may be the end result of ventricular fibrillation, EMD, sinus arrest, SA block, or AV block.

Therapy for asystole begins with CPR and intubation. Confirm the ECG pattern on another lead to rule out ventricular fibrillation. Do not attempt defibrillation unless you confirm ventricular fibrillation, since parasympathetic discharge occurs, inhibiting the return of electrical activity.[23] Transcutaneous pacing may be helpful if initiation is early. If pacing is ineffective or not available, administer epinephrine (Adrenalin) IV push, followed by atropine. Atropine can be effective when the mechanism of asystole is increased parasympathetic tone.[23]

Electromechanical dissociation refers to the presence of normal electrical activity without mechanical activity. Clinical manifestations are a normal ECG without a pulse. A recently proposed, broader term, *pulseless electrical activity* (PEA), includes arrhythmias such as idioventricular rhythms with similar causes and intervention where the pulse may also be absent.[23] Both EMD and PEA may result from depressed contractility, obstruction, decreased preload, or decreased afterload. The most common cause is hypovolemia.[23] Other specific causes include extensive MI, cardiac tamponade, tension pneumothorax, massive pulmonary embolism, hypoxemia, acidosis, hyperkalemia, hypothermia, sepsis, and anaphylactic shock.[10,23,52] Suspect pneumothorax, pulmonary embolism, or tamponade in the patient with distended neck veins.[52] Partial or complete absence of breath sounds can confirm pneumothorax. For other clinical signs of tamponade, refer to Unit 8. Suspect hypovolemia in the trauma patient with flat neck veins. Investigators also have reported PEA or EMD as a toxic effect of calcium channel blockade.[10,23] The use of calcium is avoided except in hyperkalemia or calcium channel blockade.[10]

Treatment of EMD is directed towards restoring and maintaining mechanical activity until a correctable cause can be identified. Maximize ventilation and oxygenation initially by basic CPR, intubation, and delivery of 100% O_2. Carry out specific interventions as indicated (volume, needle aspiration, chest tube insertion, thrombolytics). Administer sodium bicarbonate for hyperkalemia or preexisting acidosis. If there is no response, administer epinephrine (Adrenalin) IV push or via the endotracheal tube. If bradycardia occurs, administer atropine.[23]

SELF-ASSESSMENT

1 The mechanisms of both supraventricular and ventricular tachyarrhythmias include altered _____,

_____ activity, and altered _____. Altered conduction involves activation of _____ circuits. Afterdepolarizations are forms of (automaticity/triggered activity). Areas of altered conduction that potentially could lead to reentrant arrhythmias are detected by _____ electrocardiography.

Clinical causes of altered automaticity or conduction include hypoxia and _____ toxicity secondary to _____, drugs, _____, and acid-base imbalance.

automaticity

triggered; conduction

reentry

triggered activity

signal-averaged

chemical; stress, electrolytes

2 Tachycardias are defined as rhythms with ventricular rates greater than _____ beats per minute. Bradycardias are defined as rhythms with ventricular rates less than _____ beats per minute.

100

60

3 The most common arrhythmias occurring within the first few hours of acute MI are (ventricular/supraventricular) arrhythmias.

ventricular

The remainder of the self-assessment consists of ECG traces. Determine the interpretation and immediate intervention, then refer to the authors' interpretation immediately following each trace.

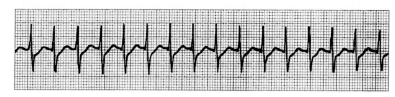

Fig. 6-54   Trace 1.

INTERPRETATION:

INTERVENTION:

TRACE 1

QRS COMPLEX:
- *Contour/appearance:* Narrow and unchanging
- *Rate/regularity:* 150, regular

P WAVE:
- *Appearance:* No clear P wave precedes the QRS complexes.
- *Rate/regularity:* NA

P–R INTERVAL: Cannot be obtained in the absence of clear P waves

INTERPRETATION: Supraventricular tachycardia/paroxysmal supraventricular tachycardia (PSVT)

IMMEDIATE INTERVENTION: Assess patient for symptoms. Report to physician immediately. If symptomatic, anticipate cardioversion or adenosine (PSVT) if normotensive. Encourage vagal maneuvers such as coughing or breath holding.

COMMENTS: The narrow, unchanging QRS complex signifies the rhythm is supraventricular. In the absence of an underlying rhythm, when the QRS complexes are this close together, differentiating between T waves and P waves is difficult. Therefore, the exact supraventricular origin is difficult to determine. At a ventricular rate of 150, the rhythm may be sinus tachycardia, atrial tachycardia, or atrial flutter with 2 to 1 conduction. The ventricular rate of 150 makes junctional tachycardia less likely, depending on the upper rate limits used. Atrial tachycardia is differentiated from sinus tachycardia by the sudden change in the rhythm, which in this case needs further clinical investigation.

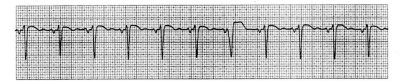

Fig. 6-55   Trace 2.

INTERPRETATION:

INTERVENTION:

TRACE 2 This trace shows one abnormal impulse (beat 7 from the left), designated by the sudden change in QRS morphology.

QRS COMPLEX: (beat 7)
- *Contour/appearance:* Changing or different in morphology when compared to those in the underlying normal rhythm (slightly wider with no initial positive deflection)
- *Rate/regularity:* Only slightly premature, not noticeably irregular

P WAVE: (beat 7)
- *Appearance:* A clear P wave precedes the different QRS complex.
- *Rate/regularity:* The P–P interval is regular (not premature) at a rate equal to the underlying sinus rate.

P–R INTERVAL: Shorter in beat 7 than in the normal beats, but not critical to the interpretation

INTERPRETATION: Normal sinus rhythm with one PVC

IMMEDIATE INTERVENTION: No immediate intervention is indicated. Observe for increased frequency and possible underlying causes.

COMMENTS: A changing QRS complex indicates ectopic ventricular origin unless there is clear evidence to the contrary such as a *premature* P wave. A nonpremature preceding P wave is characteristic of PVCs that are only slightly premature. These PVCs are sometimes called *end-diastolic.*

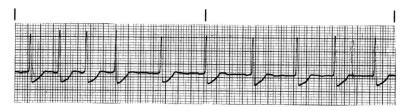

Fig. 6-56   Trace 3.

INTERPRETATION:

INTERVENTION:

TRACE 3

QRS COMPLEX:
- *Contour/appearance:* Narrow and unchanging
- *Rate/regularity:* Approximately 110, irregular

P WAVE:
- *Appearance:* Not visible preceding the QRS
- *Rate/regularity:* NA

P–R INTERVAL: Cannot be obtained in the absence of clear P waves

INTERPRETATION: Atrial fibrillation

IMMEDIATE INTERVENTION: No immediate urgent intervention is indicated since the rhythm is supraventricular and the ventricular rate is only slightly fast. Report to physician. Anticipate digitalis to control the ventricular rate. Assess patient for potential causes and intolerance secondary to loss of atrial contraction.

COMMENTS: The narrow, unchanging QRS complex signifies the rhythm is supraventricular. Since no P waves are visible preceding the QRS complexes, the rhythm cannot be sinus and must be either atrial fibrillation or junctional. The irregularity of the QRS complexes rules out junctional.

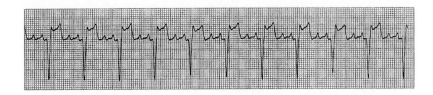

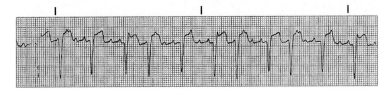

Fig. 6-57   Trace 4.

INTERPRETATION:

INTERVENTION:

TRACE 4

QRS COMPLEX:
- *Contour/appearance:* Narrow and unchanging
- *Rate/regularity:* Varies from regular R–R at rate of 80 (top trace) to irregular R–R at rate of approximately 100 (bottom trace)

P WAVE:
- *Appearance:* Many P waves clearly visible preceding the QRS complexes
- *Rate/regularity:* P–P interval regular at rate of approximately 300

P–R INTERVAL: Not critical to interpretation

INTERPRETATION: Atrial flutter with a ventricular response of 80 to 100

IMMEDIATE INTERVENTION: No immediate intervention is indicated since the ventricular reponse is not rapid. Report to physician if new onset. Assess patient for underlying causes or symptoms secondary to loss of effective atrial contraction.

COMMENTS: The narrow, unchanging QRS complex signifies the rhythm is supraventricular. The P wave rate of 300 confirms that the rhythm is atrial flutter regardless of the absence of the typical sawtooth pattern on this lead. Note that in atrial flutter the QRS complex can be either regular or irregular.

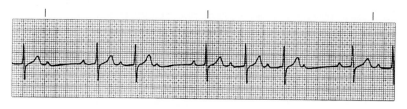

Fig. 6-58 Trace 5.

INTERPRETATION:

INTERVENTION:

TRACE 5

QRS COMPLEX:
- *Contour/appearance:* Narrow and unchanging
- *Rate/regularity:* R–R irregular at rate of approximately 60 (using 6-second indicators)

P WAVE:
- *Appearance:* Clearly visible preceding each QRS complex
- *Rate/regularity:* Rate 85, P–P regular

P–R INTERVAL: Some P waves not followed by QRS complexes, P–R interval changes, with gradually prolonged intervals before the dropped beat

INTERPRETATION: Sinus rhythm with second-degree AV block, Wenckebach (Mobitz I, type I)

IMMEDIATE INTERVENTION: Immediate intervention usually is not indicated at a ventricular rate of 60 unless the patient is symptomatic. However, symptoms do not typically occur at this rate. Report to physician if new in onset. Continue to observe for progression of block and further decreases in ventricular rate.

COMMENTS: The narrow, unchanging QRS complex signifies the rhythm is supraventricular. Visible, upright, regular P waves at a rate less than 150 indicate that the origin of the P waves is sinus. Since some of these normal P waves are not followed by QRS complexes, the arrhythmia is an AV block, second degree or greater. However, irregular R–R intervals appear only in second-degree AV block, Wenckebach (Mobitz I), or Mobitz II. The progressive P–R prolongation before the dropped beat confirms that the arrhythmia is Wenckebach. This pattern may be mimicked by atrial bigeminy (PACs). However, the P waves will be premature.

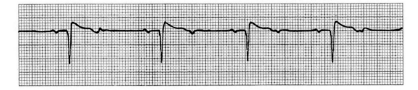

Fig. 6-59   Trace 6.

INTERPRETATION:

INTERVENTION:

TRACE 6

QRS COMPLEX:
- *Contour/appearance:* Narrow and unchanging
- *Rate/regularity:* Rate 43, R–R regular

P WAVE:
- *Appearance:* Clearly visible preceding each QRS complex, biphasic
- *Rate/regularity:* Rate 90, P–P regular

P–R INTERVAL: Some P waves not followed by QRS complexes, P–R interval constant in those P waves that are followed by QRS complexes

INTERPRETATION: Sinus rhythm with second-degree AV block, 2 to 1 conduction, and a ventricular rate of 43 (most likely type I)

IMMEDIATE INTERVENTION: At a ventricular rate of 43 the patient is likely to be symptomatic. Assess the patient and report to physician immediately. In the symptomatic patient, anticipate atropine administration followed by transcutaneous pacing if ineffective. If pacing is not immediately available, anticipate administration of dopamine and epinephrine infusion. In the asymptomatic patient, no immediate therapy is indicated.

COMMENTS: The narrow, unchanging QRS complexes indicate the rhythm is supraventricular. Visible, regular P waves at a rate less than 150 indicate that the origin of the P waves is sinus. Biphasic P waves commonly appear in lead V1 and are considered normal. The negative QRS complexes suggest that this is a lead V1, although it is not labeled. Since some of these normal P waves are not followed by QRS complexes, the arrhythmia is an AV block, second degree or greater. The regular R–R intervals may occur in both second-degree and third-degree AV blocks. However, the constant P–R intervals confirm that the rhythm is second-degree AV block. The narrow QRS complexes suggest a type I (AV node) mechanism.

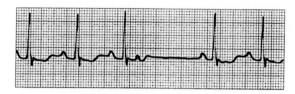

Fig. 6-60   Trace 7.

INTERPRETATION:

INTERVENTION:

TRACE 7 The major abnormality is the pause.

QRS COMPLEX:
- *Contour/appearance:* None present in the pause
- *Rate/regularity:* NA

P WAVE:
- *Appearance:* Not visible at expected time
- *Rate/regularity:* P–P irregular (premature P)

P–R INTERVAL: No QRS complex follows the premature P wave. The P–R interval is slightly long (0.22 second) in the sinus beats.

INTERPRETATION: Sinus rhythm with borderline first-degree AV block and one nonconducted PAC

IMMEDIATE INTERVENTION: No immediate action is indicated. Observe for increased frequency and evaluate potential causes.

COMMENTS: The premature P wave confirms the presence of a PAC, one of the most common causes of pauses. The QRS is absent secondary to refractoriness rather than pathology within the conduction system. Always examine the T wave at the beginning of a sudden pause and compare it with the T waves of the sinus beats, for the possibility of a concealed premature P wave. This pattern is mimicked by second-degree AV block, Mobitz II, and SA block or sinus arrest. However, in Mobitz II the P waves are regular, and in SA block and sinus arrest there is no P wave at all.

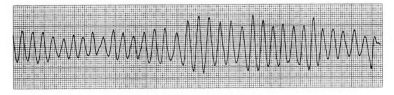

Fig. 6-61   Trace 8.

INTERPRETATION:

INTERVENTION:

TRACE 8

QRS COMPLEX:
- *Contour/appearance:* QRS-T wave complexes cannot be clearly identified, deflections uneven in height ("disintegrated")
- *Rate/regularity:* NA

P WAVE:
- *Appearance:* NA
- *Rate/regularity:* NA

P—R INTERVAL: NA

INTERPRETATION: Ventricular fibrillation (coarse)

IMMEDIATE INTERVENTION: Confirm the absence of pulse. Begin CPR and obtain defibrillator. Defibrillate, then anticipate administration of epinephrine, lidocaine, bretylium, magnesium, and/or procainamide.

COMMENTS: When you find no clear QRS-T complexes, stop the interpretation process. Begin intervention for ventricular fibrillation immediately. The absence of a pulse rules out artifact.

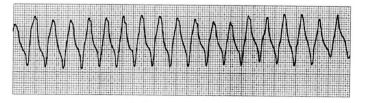

Fig. 6-62   Trace 9.

INTERPRETATION:

INTERVENTION:

TRACE 9

QRS COMPLEX:
- *Contour/appearance:* QRS-T wave complexes clearly visible, wide, even in height
- *Rate/regularity:* Rate 210, R–R irregular

P WAVE:
- *Appearance:* Not visible
- *Rate/regularity:* NA

P–R INTERVAL: NA

INTERPRETATION: Wide QRS tachycardia—rule out ventricular tachycardia

IMMEDIATE INTERVENTION: Confirm the absence of a pulse. If no pulse, treat as ventricular fibrillation. In a patient with a pulse, notify physician immediately. If symptomatic, consider cardioversion and administration of lidocaine. Take subsequent action to differentiate from other less common causes of wide QRS tachycardia (see Unit 7).

COMMENTS: These beats are likely to be ventricular in origin (PVCs) since the QRS complexes are wide. Without the underlying rhythm, however, it is impossible to determine whether they are different in morphology from the patient's sinus complexes, a more characteristic finding. Three or more consecutive PVCs at a ventricular rate greater than 100 are considered ventricular tachycardia. Although other mechanisms of wide QRS tachycardia occur, ventricular tachycardia (VT) is the most common and most immediately life-threatening. Therefore, initially consider this rhythm ventricular and treat it as such.[23] If it continues for longer than 30 seconds, consider it sustained VT.

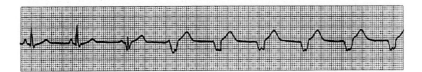

Fig. 6-63   Trace 10.

TRACE 10 Beats 1 and 2 from the left are normal. The abnormal beats are beats 3 to 9.

QRS COMPLEX (beats 3 to 9)
- *Contour/appearance:* Different, changing (wider, different direction). The shape of the complex in beat 3 is a blend of the complex of the normal beats (1, 2) and the totally abnormal beats (4 to 9).
- *Rate/regularity:* Rate of 72 in beats 4 to 9, R–R regular, beat 3 occurs after a pause longer than the normal R–R cycle

P WAVE (beats 3 to 9)
- *Appearance:* Visible only in beat 3 preceding the QRS complex
- *Rate/regularity:* Rate of 69, P–P regular

P–R INTERVAL: Shorter than normal in beat 3

INTERPRETATION: Sinus rhythm with a run of accelerated idioventricular rhythm (AIVR), beginning with a fused ventricular escape beat

IMMEDIATE INTERVENTION: Assess patient. If patient is asymptomatic, no therapy is indicated. If patient is symptomatic, treat with atropine. Report to physician if new in onset.

COMMENTS: Three or more consecutive ventricular ectopic beats at a rate of 40 to 100 is referred to as AIVR. If the ventricular rate accelerates beyond 100, label and treat it as ventricular tachycardia. The initial beat in AIVR is usually a slightly premature ventricular complex or a ventricular escape beat. Either can fuse with the complex of the sinus beat as in this case.

OVERVIEW: ARRHYTHMIAS IN ACUTE MI

```
┌─────────────────────────────┐
│   Acutely life threatening  │
└─────────────────────────────┘
        (cardiac arrest)
      /        |        \
  Asystole     VT        VF
```

	Asystole	VT	VF
Pharmacological intervention	• Epinephrine • Atropine	• Lidocaine • Procainamide • Bretylium	• Lidocaine • Bretylium • Magnesium sulfate • Procainamide
Electrical intervention	Pacemaker	• Cardioversion • Defibrillation	• Defibrillation
Other	←	• Precordial blow • Cardiac massage with ventilation	→

```
┌─────────────────────────────┐
│ Potentially life threatening │
└─────────────────────────────┘
      /        |        \
```

	Ventricular tachyarrhythmias	Supraventricular tachyarrhythmias	Bradyarrhythmias
Major problem	Electrical instability	Ventricular rate ↑	Ventricular rate ↓
Pharmacological intervention	*Antiarrhythmics	• Adenosine • Ca++ blockage • Parasympathetic stimulation • β sympathetic blockade	• Parasympathetic blockade • β sympathetic stimulation
Electrical intervention	Cardioversion pacemaker	Cardioversion pacemaker	Pacemaker
Other	Precordial blow	• Valsalva maneuvers • Carotid massage • Cough	———

Fig. 6-64 Management of acutely life-threatening and potentially life-threatening arrhythmias: overview.

Table 6-2. Summary of arrhythmia categories (ECG criteria/clinical significance)

Rhythm	Significance	ECG	Treatment
Tachyarrhythmias: ventricular			
Premature ventricular contractions (PVCs)	May lead to: —Ventricular tachycardia (see VT), or —Ventricular fibrillation (cardiac arrest)	QRS: "different" (i.e., changing) and premature —May be preceded by nonpremature P wave —May or may not have a pause —May or may not be obviously wide	Acute:—Lidocaine (Xylocaine) —Procainamide (Pronestyl) —> 6/min —On T wave ("close coupled") —Multifocal —2 or more consecutive (VR > 100)* Long-term: —Quinidine —Procainamide (Pronestyl) —Disopyramide (Norpace) —Propranolol (Inderal) (PO)
Ventricular tachycardia (VT)	May ↓ CO or indicate a form of cardiac arrest, or lead to ventricular fibrillation (cardiac arrest)	QRS: "different" (i.e., changing) —3 or more consecutive beats —VR > 100	Acute: —Lidocaine (Xylocaine) —Procainamide (Pronestyl) —Bretylium (Bretylol) —Cardioversion NOTE: Without pulse treat as VF. Long-term: (see PVCs) Also pacemakers implantable cardioverter-defibrillator, surgery
Ventricular fibrillation (VF)	Cardiac arrest	QRS: "disintegrated" —No distinct QRS/T complexes —Wave of uneven height (coarse) —May appear as wavy baseline only mimicking asystole (fine)	Acute: —Check pulse —Precordial blow —CPR —Defibrillation —Intubation —Epinephrine (Adrenalin) —Lidocaine (Xylocaine) —Bretylium (Bretylol) —Magnesium sulfate —Procainamide (Pronestyl) Long-term: (see PVCs/VT)

Continued.

Table 6-2. Summary of arrhythmia categories (ECG criteria/clinical significance)—cont'd

Rhythm	Significance	ECG	Treatment
Tachyarrhythmias: supraventricular (ectopic)			
Premature atrial contractions (PACs) •Normally conducted •Non-conducted •Aberrantly conducted	May lead to: —Other sustained atrial arrhythmias with rapid VR and ↓ CO —Often indicate CHF or hypoxemia	P wave: premature (irregular pp)	Acute: None Long-term: —Digitalis —Verapamil (PO) —Propranolol (Inderal) (PO) —Quinidine —Procainamide (Pronestyl) —Treat Cause
Atrial tachycardia (PAT)	↑ VR (↓ CO)	P wave rate: 150–250 (typically: 150)	Acute: —Adenosine —Verapamil (IV) —Diltiazem (IV) —Esmolol —Cardioversion —Digitalis —Valsalva maneuver —Carotid sinus pressure Long-term: (see PACs), also catheter ablation, surgery
Atrial flutter	↑ VR (↓ CO)	P wave rate: 250–350 (average: 300)	Acute: (see PAT, starting with verapamil) Long-term: (see PACs), also catheter ablation surgery
Atrial fibrillation	↑ VR (↓ CO)	P wave: "disintegrated" —No distinct visible P waves —QRS complexes: irregular	Acute: (see PAT, starting with verapamil) Long-term: (see PACs), also catheter ablation, surgery
Premature junctional contractions (PJCs)	Usually of no clinical significance	P wave: not visible, or if visible, inverted on lead II with short P–R	Acute: None Long-term: None
Junctional tachycardia (JT)	↑ VR (↓ CO) R/O digitalis toxicity	P wave: not visible, or if visible, inverted on lead II with short P–R —QRS complexes (regular) —VR > 100	Acute: —Diphenylhydantoin (Dilantin) —Propranolol (Inderal) (avoid digitalis and verapamil, unless diagnosis unclear, i.e., "SVT")

Bradyarrhythmias: AV blocks

First-degree AV block	↓ VR (↑ CO) —Block in AV node or bundle branches	P–R interval: prolonged (>0.20 sec)	Acute (if symptomatic only): —Atropine —Pacemaker (transcutaneous) —Dopamine (Intropin) —Epinephrine (Adrenalin) —Isoproterenol (Isuprel) —Pacemaker (transvenous)
Second-degree AV block	↓ VR (↓ CO)	P–R interval: Some P waves not followed by QRSs	Acute (if symptomatic only): —Atropine —Pacemaker (transcutaneous) —Dopamine (Intropin) —Epinephrine (Adrenalin) —Isoproterenol (Isuprel) —Pacemaker (transvenous)
—Fixed ratio (example: "2 to 1")	Block in AV node or bundle branches	—R–R regular —constant P–R in those P's followed by QRS complex	Long-term: Pacemaker (permanent)
—Wenckebach (Mobitz I)	Block in AV node (usually)	—R–R irregular —"4 p's": previous, progressive, PR, prolongation	
—Mobitz II	—Block in bundle branches (usually) —May result in sudden asystole	—R–R irregular —No previous progressive P–R change	
Third-degree AV block	↓ VR (↓ CO), or —asystole (especially if in bundle branches)	P–R interval: —Some P waves not followed by QRS —R–R regular —Varying P–R in those P's followed by QRS complexes	Acute: (see second-degree AV block) Long-term: (see second-degree AV block)

Continued.

Table 6-2. Summary of arrhythmia categories (ECG criteria/clinical significance)—cont'd

Rhythm	Significance	ECG	Treatment
Bradyarrhythmias: other			
SA block	↓ VR (↓ CO)	P wave: absent (pause = multiples of original P wave cycles)	Acute (if symptomatic only): —Atropine —Pacemaker (transthoracic) —Dopamine (Intropin) —Epinephrine (Adrenalin) —Isoproterenol (Isuprel) —Pacemaker (transvenous) Long-term: Pacemaker (permanent)
Escape beats (ventricular)	Compensatory, prevent ↓ VR (↓ CO)	QRS: "different" (i.e., changing) timing: after the next expected natural QRS has not appeared	Acute: None, or support with atropine DO NOT SUPPRESS.
Idioventricular rhythm	↓ VR (↓ CO)	QRS: "different" (i.e., changing) —3 or more consecutive beats —VR < 40	Acute: —Atropine —Pacemaker (transcutaneous) —Dopamine (Intropin) —Epinephrine (Adrenalin) —Isoproterenol (Isuprel) —Pacemaker (transvenous) Long-term: Pacemaker (permanent) DO NOT SUPPRESS.
Accelerated idioventricular rhythm (AIVR)	↓ VR (↓ CO)	QRS: "different" (i.e., changing) —3 or more consecutive beats —VR > 40 < 100	Acute: None or support with atropine
Junctional rhythm	↓ VR (↓ CO)	QRS: normal P wave: not visible, or if visible, inverted on lead II with short PR —VR < 100	Acute (if symptomatic only): —Atropine —Pacemaker (transthoracic) —Isoproterenol (Isuprel) —Pacemaker (transvenous)

Table 6-3. Arrhythmia recognition matrix

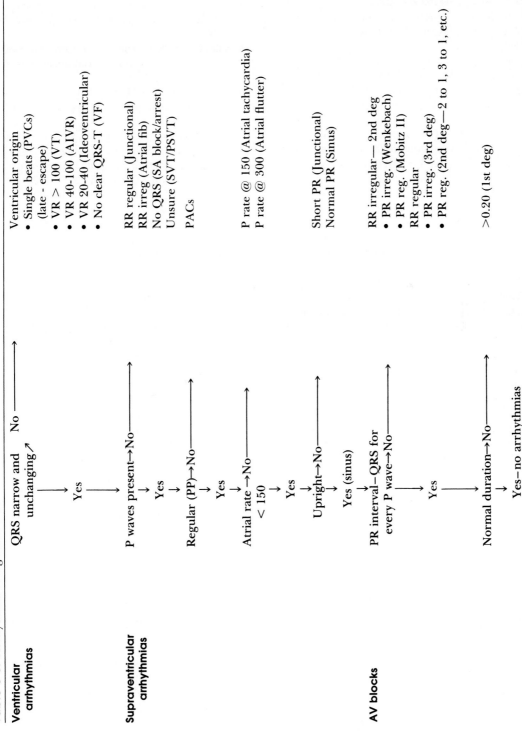

Ventricular arrhythmias

QRS narrow and unchanging —No——→ Ventricular origin
- Single beats (PVCs) (late - escape)
- VR > 100 (VT)
- VR 40-100 (AIVR)
- VR 20-40 (Ideoventricular)
- No clear QRS-T (VF)

↓ Yes

Supraventricular arrhythmias

P waves present→No——→ RR regular (Junctional)
RR irreg (Atrial fib)
No QRS (SA block/arrest)
Unsure (SVT/PSVT)

↓ Yes → PACs

Regular (PP)→No——→ P rate @ 150 (Atrial tachycardia)
P rate @ 300 (Atrial flutter)

↓ Yes

Atrial rate →No——→ Short PR (Junctional)
< 150   Normal PR (Sinus)

↓ Yes

Upright→No——→

↓ Yes (sinus)

AV blocks

PR interval–QRS for every P wave→No——→ RR irregular— 2nd deg
- PR irreg. (Wenkebach)
- PR reg. (Mobitz II)

RR regular
- PR irreg. (3rd deg)
- PR reg. (2nd deg—2 to 1, 3 to 1, etc.)

↓ Yes

Normal duration→No——→ >0.20 (1st deg)

↓ Yes– no arrhythmias

(Courtesy Linda Kisner, R.N.,for suggesting this diagram.)

REFERENCES/SUGGESTED READINGS

1. Abraham T: Arrhythmogenic mechanisms, AACN Clin Issues Crit Care Nurs 3:157, 1992.
2. Akhtar M et al: Mechanisms of clinical tachycardias, Am J Cardiol 61(suppl):9, 1988.
3. Alpert JS, Rippe JM: Manual of cardiovascular diagnosis and therapy, ed 3, Boston, 1988, Little, Brown.
4. Andrews LK: ECG rhythms made easier with algorithms, Am J Nurs 89(3):365, 1989.
5. Berger PB, Ryan TJ: Inferior myocardial infarction. High risk subgroups, Circulation 81:401, 1990.
6. Berger PB, et al: Incidence and prognostic implication of heart block complicating IWMI treated with thrombolytics—results of TIMI II, J Am Coll Cardiol 20(3):533, 1992.
7. Berisso MZ et al: Frequency, characteristics and significance of supraventricular tachyarrhythmias detected by 24-hour electrocardiographic recording in the late hospital phase of acute myocardial infarction, Am J Cardiol 65:106, 1990.
8. Braunwald E, editor: Heart disease: a textbook of cardiovascular medicine, ed 4, Philadelphia, 1992, WB Saunders.
9. Catalano JT: AV nodal arrhythmias, Crit Care Nurs 10(6):76, 1990.
10. Charlap S et al: Electromechanical dissociation. Diagnosis, pathophysiology, and management, Am Heart J 118:355, 1989.
11. Chronister C: Clinical management of supraventricular tachycardia with adenosine, Am J Crit Care 2(1):41, 1993.
12. Chou T: Electrocardiography in practice, ed 3, Philadelphia, 1991, WB Saunders.
13. Chung EK: Cardiac emergency care, ed 4, Philadelphia, 1991, Lea & Febiger.
14. Conover MB: Understanding electrocardiography, ed. 6, St. Louis, 1992, Mosby–Year Book.
15. Cox JL et al: Successful surgical treatment of atrial fibrillation. Review and clinical update, JAMA 226(14):1976, 1991.
16. Cross JA: Atrioventricular block, AACN Clin Issues Crit Care Nurs 3(1):166, 1992.
17. Domenico JM: Cardiac arrest following myocardial infarction, J Cardiovasc Nurs 4(2):56, 1990.
18. Ellenbogen KA: Role of calcium antagonists for heart rate control in atrial fibrillation, Am J Cardiol 69:36B, 1992.
19. Falk RH, Leavitt JI: Digoxin for atrial fibrillation, a drug whose time has gone, Ann Intern Med 114(7):573, 1991.
20. Fisch C: Electrocardiography of arrhythmias, Philadelphia, 1990, Lea & Febiger.
21. Gallagher JJ et al: Surgical treatment of arrhythmias, Am J Cardiol 61:27A, 1988.
22. Goldberg RJ et al: Impact of atrial fibrillation on the inhospital and long-term survival of patients with acute myocardial infarction: a community-wide perspective, Am Heart J 119:996, 1990.
23. Guidelines for cardiopulmonary resuscitation and emergency cardiac care, Part III. Adult cardiac life support, JAMA 268(16):2199, 1992.
24. Henry SB: Clinical decision making of critical care nurses managing computer-simulated tachydysrhythmias, Heart and Lung 20(5 Pt 1):469, 1991.
25. Jensen GV et al: Prognosis of late versus early ventricular fibrillation in acute myocardial infarction, Am J Cardiol 66(1):10, 1990.
26. Kahn JK: Anticoagulant therapy for atrial fibrillation, Postgrad Med 92(3):119, 1992.
27. Kastor JA: Ventricular tachycardia, Clin Cardiol 12:586, 1989.
28. Kay GN, Bubien RS: Clinical management of cardiac arrhythmias, Gaithersburg, MD, 1991, Aspen Publications.
29. Kessler KM et al: Multiform ventricular complexes: a transitional arrhythmia form? Am Heart J 118(3):441, 1989.
30. Lange HW: Prevalence and clinical correlates of non-Wenckebach, narrow-complex second-degree atrioventricular block detected by ambulatory ECG, Am Heart J 115:(1 Pt 1):114, 1988.
31. Lazarus M, Nolasco V, Luckett C: Cardiac arrhythmia. Diagnosis and treatment, Crit Care Nurs 8(7):57, 1988.
32. Lazzara R, Scherlag BJ: Generation of ar-

rhythmias in myocardial ischemia and infarction, Am J Cardiol 61:21A, 1988.

33. Lazzara R: Electrophysiological mechanisms for ventricular arrhythmias, Clin Cardiol 11:III1, 1988.

34. Lounsbury P, Frye SJ: Cardiac rhythm disorders: a nursing process approach, ed 2, St. Louis, 1992, Mosby–Year Book.

35. Marriott HJL: Practical electrocardiography, ed 8, Baltimore, 1988, William & Wilkins.

36. Marriott HJL, Conover MH: Advanced concepts in arrhythmias, ed 2, St. Louis, 1989, CV Mosby.

37. Marriott HJL, Myerburg RJ: Recognition of cardiac arrhythmias and conduction disturbances. In Hurst JL, Schlant RC, editors: The heart: arteries and veins, ed 7, New York, 1990, McGraw-Hill.

38. Mavric Z et al: Prognostic significance of complete atrioventricular block in patients with acute inferior myocardial infarction with and without right ventricular involvement, Am Heart J 119:823, 1990.

39. Moulton KP, Medcalf T, Lazzara T: Premature ventricular complex morphology: a marker for left ventricular structure and function, Circulation 81:1245, 1990.

40. Ordonez RV: Monitoring the patient with supraventricular dysrhythmias, Nurs Clin North Am 22:49, 1987.

41. Patel A et al: Isorhythmic atrioventricular dissociation revisited, Am Heart J 124(3):823, 1992.

42. Peterson P: Thromboembolic complications of atrial fibrillation and their prevention: a review, Am J Cardiol 65:24C, 1990. Fibrillation: reassessing the role of drug therapy and approach to the high risk patient, J Am Coll Cardiol 16(3):532, 1990.

43. Repique LJ, Shah SN, Marais MB: Atrial fibrillation 1992. Management strategies in flux, Chest 101(4):1095, 1992.

44. Rosen MR: Mechanisms for arrhythmias, Am J Cardiol 61:2A, 1988.

45. Rosenfeld LE: Bradyarrhythmias, abnormalities of conduction and indications for pacing in acute myocardial infarction, Cardiol Clin 6:49, 1988.

46. Rowlands DJ: Clinical electrocardiography, Philadelphia, 1991, JB Lippincott.

47. Sarter BH, Marchlinski PE: Redefining the role of digoxin in the treatment of atrial fibrillation, Am J Cardiol 69:716, 1992.

48. Snowberger P: Premature atrial contractions, RN 27:38, 1991.

49. Sorenson LM et al: The maze procedure: a new treatment for atrial fibrillation, AACN Clin Isssues Crit Care Nurs 3(1):209, 1992.

50. Suguira T et al: Factors associated with late onset of advanced atrioventricular block in acute Q wave inferior infarction, Am Heart J 119(5):1008, 1990.

51. Sweetwood H: Clinical electrocardiography for nurses, ed 2, Gaithersburg, MD, 1989, Aspen Publications.

52. Textbook of advanced cardiac life support, ed 2, Dallas, 1990, American Heart Association.

53. Underhill SL et al: Cardiac nursing, ed 2, Philadelphia, 1989, JB Lippincott.

54. Weiss JN et al: Ventricular arrhythmias in ischemic heart disease, Ann Intern Med 114:784, 1991.

55. Wellens HJ: Diagnosis of ventricular tachycardia from the 12-lead electrocardiogram, Cardiol Clin 5(3):511, 1987.

56. Wellens HJ: Approach to nonsustained ventricular tachycardia after myocardial infarction, Circulation 82(2):633, 1990.

57. Weller DM, Noone J: Mechanisms of arrhythmias: enhanced automaticity and reentry, Crit Care Nurs 9(5):42, 1989.

58. Zolna CJ, Miller RK, editors: Treatment of ventricular arrhythmias, Whippany, NJ, 1991, Knoll Pharmaceuticals.

Signal-averaged electrocardiography

59. Lansdown LM: Signal-averaged electrocardiograms, Heart Lung 19(4):329, 1990.

60. Moser DK et al: Signal-averaged electrocardiography, Crit Care Nurs Q 14(2):30, 1991.

61. Rotche RM et al: Signal-averaged electrocardiography. Promising tool for predicting sudden cardiac death. Postgrad Med 87(5):123, 1990.

62. Schactman M et al: Signal-averaged electrocardiography: a new technique for determining which patients may be at risk for sudden cardiac death, Focus Crit Care 18(3):202, 1991.

Catheter ablation

63. Moulton L et al: Radiofrequency catheter ablation for supraventricular tachycardia, Heart Lung 22(1):3, 1993.
64. Scheinman MM: Catheter ablation: present role and projected impact on health care for patients with cardiac arrhythmia, Circulation 83(5):1489, 1991.
65. Scheinman MM et al: Catheter ablation for cardiac arrhythmias: personnel and facilities. NASPE Policy Statement, Journal of Arrhythmia Management, Spring 1992.

Intraventricular Conduction Disturbances

OVERVIEW

The components of the intraventricular conduction system are best viewed initially in the *horizontal plane*. The two main components are the right bundle branch (RBB) and the main left bundle branch (LBB). The main left branch divides further into two major branches: the *anterior* division and the *posterior* division. (When viewed in the frontal plane, the anterior division is also superior and the posterior division is also inferior.) Ultimately, then, there are three major branches within the intraventricular conduction system (Fig. 7-1). Each of these branches may also be called a *fascicle*.

The term *bundle branch block* refers to a block in one of the two main bundle branches. Therefore, the two forms of bundle branch block are *right bundle branch block* (RBBB) and *left bundle branch block* (LBBB). Blocks that occur in half of the left bundle branch are called *hemiblocks*. The two forms of hemiblock are blocks in either the anterosuperior division or the posteroinferior division. A block in the anterosuperior division is known as *left anterior hemiblock* (LAH). A block in the posteroinferior division is known as *left posterior hemiblock* (LPH).

A block in any one of the three major branches, or fascicles, of the bundle branch system is referred to as a *monofascicular block*. A block in two fascicles is called *bifascicular block*. The most common bifascicular blocks are the combinations of RBBB with left anterior hemiblock, or RBBB with left posterior hemiblock. A block in all three fascicles is referred to as *trifascicular block*. Trifascicular block results in AV block, most typically Mobitz II or greater. Bifascicular block with first-degree AV block may also be a form of early trifascicular block. Recognition of the earlier patterns of bundle branch block or hemiblock allows the nurse to anticipate these serious forms of AV block and to facilitate therapeutic intervention.

When either of the two main bundle branches is blocked, the primary changes in ventricular activation are directed either to the right or to the left. For this reason, bundle branch blocks are most clearly diagnosed by changes in the horizontal plane (chest) leads V1 and V6, where the positive electrode is located either to the right or to the left of the chest.[14] Hemiblocks do not produce significant changes in these leads, however, since the unaffected division is still part of the left ventricular conduction system. The primary changes in ventricular activation are directed superiorly or inferiorly. For this reason, hemiblocks are diagnosed instead by changes in the frontal plane axis or limb leads.[6]

Blocks within the intraventricular conduction system may be *chronic* or *acute* and intermittent (temporary) or sustained (per-

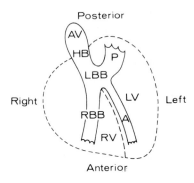

Fig. 7-1 The intraventricular conduction system: horizontal plane view.

manent). Chronic conduction system blocks occur because of calcification and sclerosis of the conduction system, congenital heart disease, cardiomyopathy, congestive heart failure, and left ventricular hypertrophy.[6,20] The incidence in the general population is low (6% to 7%), but they occur more commonly in men.[20] There is no evidence that asymptomatic patients need extensive follow-up.[20] Acute conduction system blocks are associated with coronary artery disease, valvular disease, or surgical trauma. Researchers have recently linked exercise-induced hemiblock with coronary artery disease, although the association with complete bundle branch block is less definite.[21] Patients may not tolerate AV blocks secondary to bundle branch block well since the ventricular response is slow and unreliable.

Intraventricular conduction defects associated with temporary changes in refractoriness are called *aberrant conduction* and occur most commonly with premature supraventricular beats or supraventricular tachycardias. The QRS complex is distorted, making the resulting patterns difficult to distinquish from the more significant ventricular ectopy.

RIGHT BUNDLE BRANCH BLOCK

The right bundle branch and the anterosuperior division of the left bundle exist in a common portion of the septum for a short segment. Then the right bundle emerges as a thin, single fascicle. The anterior two thirds of the right bundle branch is supplied by the anterior descending branch of the left coronary artery. It can thus be anticipated that acute RBBB will occur most frequently in anterior rather than inferior wall MI. However, the incidence is only 3.7% in acute MI.[9] The development of acute RBBB is associated with an increase in hospital and 1-year mortality rates.[25] The cause of death is usually congestive heart failure or ventricular fibrillation. Only 15% of patients with acute RBBB progress to third-degree AV block.[25]

The most distinct, characteristic changes in RBBB are visible on lead V1 (MCL1). Normal ventricular activation occurs predominantly toward the left, resulting in a negative (inverted) complex in lead V1 (see Unit 2). The first part of the ventricles activated normally, as well as in RBBB, is the septum.[9,13,14] Septal depolarization occurs from left to right using the left bundle branch. A corresponding small r wave appears in lead V1. A small q wave may also be present in lead V6. Subsequent ventricular activation occurs through the left bundle branch to the left for a short time, then predominately toward the right in order to activate the right ventricle (Fig. 7-2).[2,9,13] The major terminal ventricular forces travel toward the positive electrode of V1, thus resulting in a predominantly positive (upright) complex in lead V1. The direction of the QRS complex is completely opposite that of the normal complex and is therefore distinctly different.

In RBBB the left ventricle is activated nor-

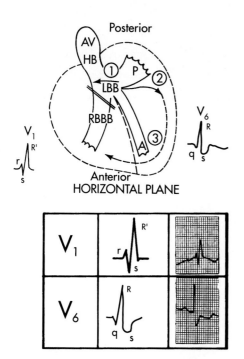

Fig. 7-2 Right bundle branch block (RBBB). The sequence of activation and corresponding ECG pattern in leads V1 and V6 are illustrated.

mally, but the right ventricle is activated with delay, resulting in a wide QRS complex (0.12 second or greater).[13,14,36] More specifically, this delay occurs in the last portion of the QRS complex and is called *terminal delay*. The changes appearing on lead V6 are limited primarily to terminal delay (slurring and widening of the S wave) and are easy to overlook.[14,31] At a glance, the QRS complex may appear essentially normal (Fig. 7-2). Terminal delay may appear on any lead. However, the pattern in lead V1 is easier to identify since it represents a complete change in the QRS direction as well as the delay. Changes in repolarization occur secondary to the changes in depolarization, resulting in an inverted T wave in lead V1.[2,9,14,31]

The most typical QRS complex in lead V1 has an rSR′ pattern described as *triphasic* because of its three deflections. Ideally, the triphasic pattern should also be present on lead V6 with a qRs configuration. However, as in the normal ECG, the small q wave in lead V6 is often not visible. Atypical RBBB patterns in lead V1 are also common.[9,14] Since the r and s waves in lead V1 are small, in selected patients they may not be clearly visible, resulting in an upright, but atypically monophasic pattern (Fig. 7-3). If the septal forces are lost, as in anteroseptal myocardial infarction (MI), the small r wave in lead V1 will not be present. The QRS complex will then assume a biphasic qR configuration.[9,14] Both the monophasic and biphasic variants may make it difficult to differentiate RBBB from ventricular ectopy (see Wide QRS Tachycardia). In these patterns, characteristic V6 changes are helpful in confirming that these patterns are "RBBB equivalents" (Fig. 7-3).[14]

Another helpful clue in diagnosing a bundle branch block is a preceding related sinus P wave (see Unit 2). This clue is particularly helpful in the presence of atypical patterns on V1 (Fig. 8-7). The differential diagnosis of upright wide complexes on V1 includes not only RBBB but also LV ectopy and Wolff-Parkinson-White syndrome (see Unit 11). Since atypical RBBB patterns on V1 are common, RBBB is best confirmed on lead V1 by upright and wide QRS complexes in the presence of sinus rhythm (normal related P waves with normal P–R intervals). An essentially normal complex on lead V6 (except for terminal delay) is an additional helpful characteristic. RBBB does not significantly affect the frontal plane axis.[26]

In incomplete RBBB, the width of the QRS complex is 0.10 to 0.12 seconds.[14,26] The triphasic pattern or terminal R wave is present in lead V1, but the QRS complex may not be predominantly upright.

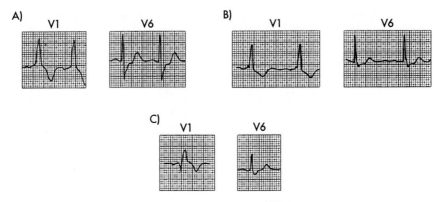

Fig. 7-3 Atypical RBBB patterns: normal variants. In lead V1, monophasic patterns are present in traces A and B. A biphasic (QR) pattern is present in trace C as a result of anteroseptal infarction. Note in all three examples an essentially normal complex in V6. Closer examination of the complexes in V6 reveals the presence of terminal delay.

LEFT BUNDLE BRANCH BLOCK

The main left bundle branch emerges from the bundle of His and lies against the septum. The main left bundle has a dual blood supply from both the right and left coronary arteries.[27] For this reason LBBB can occur in either inferior wall or anterior wall MI. The incidence in acute MI is slightly higher than with RBBB (5.2%), but it is associated with only half the risk of developing CHB.[9] LBBB, however, is associated with a higher cardiovascular mortality than RBBB.[2] LBBB is also caused by sclerosis or calcification of the conduction system, congestive heart failure, and left ventricular hypertrophy.

In left bundle branch block, the most distinct QRS complex changes are visible on lead V6 (MCL6). Normal ventricular activation occurs predominantly toward the left, resulting in a positive (upright) complex in lead V6 (see Unit 2). In LBBB, the ventricles are activated in the same direction through the right bundle branch. However, activation of the left ventricle occurs with delay, resulting in a wide QRS complex (0.12 second or greater) (Fig. 7-4). Unlike in RBBB, the de-lay occurs in the middle portion of the QRS complex. Notching of the QRS complex may or may not be present. As with RBBB, repolarization changes occur secondary to the depolarization changes. The pattern looks distinctly different from the normal pattern on lead V6, although the medial delay may be visible on any lead.

In LBBB, initial septal depolarization no longer occurs through the left bundle branch. Instead, the septum is activated from left to right together with the other portions of the ventricles. Therefore, the small septal r wave normally visible on V1 typically disappears . However, a small, narrow r wave (0.03 second or less) is present in about 30% to 45% of patients with LBBB (Fig. 7-4).[9,14] Investigators believe this r wave is due to possible disease in the septal branches of the right bundle branch with initial activation of the free wall of the right ventricle[9,25] Initial activation of the right ventricle is rapid. In lead V1, this activation is reflected by a rapid downslope in the QRS complex (0.06 second or less from the beginning of the complex to the peak negative de-

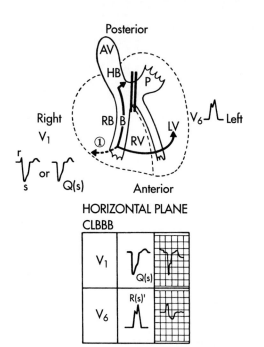

Fig. 7-4 Left bundle branch block (LBBB). The sequence of activation and corresponding ECG patterns in leads V1 and V6 are illustrated. An initial R wave may be present in V1 as a result of initial activation of the RV free wall (1). Notching may not be present in either V1 or V6.

flection).[18] The resulting wide, negative complex in lead V1 is not distinctly different from the normal V1 complex. The specific characteristics, however, are helpful in differentiating this pattern from ventricular ectopy. Incomplete LBBB, diagnosed by a QRS width of 0.10 to 0.12 seconds with slurring of the complex, is more subtle than incomplete RBBB and is not clinically significant.[2,14,31]

LBBB may be accompanied by left axis deviation, although the significance is unclear.[26] The cause is not always known, but possible explanations include incomplete LBBB with left anterior hemiblock (LAH), incomplete left posterior hemiblock (LPH) with LAH, thoracic wall deformities, and pulmonary disease.[6]

AXIS DEVIATION

The ventricular axis, defined as the summation ventricular force, is reflected on the ECG as the QRS complex (see Unit 2). Since the left ventricle has more electrical forces than the right ventricle, the normal ventricular axis in the adult is usually shifted toward the left (Fig. 7-5).

The ventricular axis of the heart is considered the major axis. It is usually determined from the QRS pattern on the frontal plane or limb leads. Leads I and aVF form quadrants that, when superimposed over the heart, serve as guides outlining the normal as well as potentially abnormal axis ranges (Fig. 7-6). If the electrical axis lies within the lower left quadrant, the axis is normal

(NA). If the ventricular forces deviate toward the lower right quadrant, the diagnosis is right axis deviation (RAD). If the ventricular forces deviate toward the upper left quadrant, the diagnosis is left axis deviation (LAD). LAD is further divided into normal and abnormal left axis. Abnormal left axis deviation (ALAD) occurs when the axis is shifted far to the left and superior. If the heart's electrical forces deviate toward the upper right quadrant, the axis is considered to be indeterminate axis deviation (IAD).[6,14,19] (This quadrant is also referred to as right superior, northwest, or "no man's land.") The usual cause of this deviation is a combination of RAD and ALAD mecha-

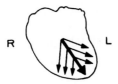

Fig. 7-5 The normal ventricular axis: contributing factors.

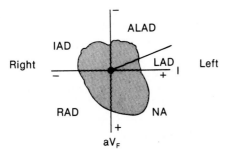

Fig. 7-6 Designation of axis quadrants using leads I and aVF.

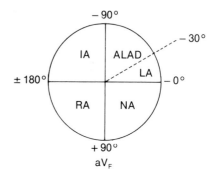

Fig. 7-7 Assignment of degrees to axis ranges.

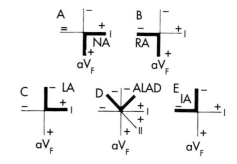

Fig. 7-8 Quadrant method of estimating the ventricular axis. The analysis of the QRS pattern in lead II is critical only in the presence of left axis (LA).

nisms[6] or ventricular ectopy (see Wide QRS Tachycardia).

The coordinates of these quadrants may be joined by a circle, and degrees assigned to them as reference points (Fig. 7-7). Normal axis lies between O and +90 degrees. Right axis lies between +90 and +180 degrees. Some references consider RAD significant only when it is greater than +110 to +120 degrees.[9,31] Left axis lies between O and −90 degrees. Abnormal left axis lies between −30 and −90 degrees.[6,9,14] Indeterminate axis lies between −90 and −180 degrees. Assignment of exact degrees is not critical in determining patient management.[14] It is more important to assess the QRS morphology, generally identify the presence of axis deviation, and determine the mechanism.

The quadrant method of estimating axis is the method we have preferred for many years. It is fast, logical, easy to learn, and sufficiently accurate.[11,14,19] The axis is within normal limits when the net ventricular

forces travel toward the positive electrodes of both leads I and aVF (Fig. 7-8). The corresponding QRS complexes are predominantly positive in both leads I and aVF. Determining that an axis is within normal limits confirms that it lies between 0 and +90 de-

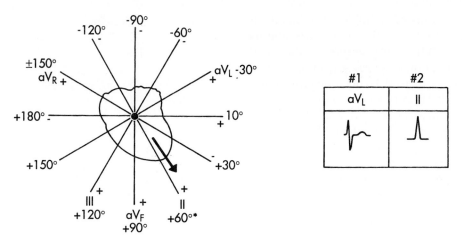

Fig. 7-9   Determining the electrical axis by selecting the equiphasic complex.

grees. A more specific estimate may be helpful in detecting significant shifts within the normal axis range. If the complexes in both leads I and aVF are equally positive, the axis lies halfway between 0 and +90, or at +45 degrees. If the complex is more positive in lead I, estimate it to be closer to 0 and adjust it according to whether it is slightly or significantly more positive.[14]

The quadrant method can also be useful in determining axis deviation. When the QRS complex is predominantly positive in lead aVF and negative in lead I, the axis is shifted to the right. When the QRS complex is positive in lead I and negative in lead aVF, the axis is shifted to the left. When diagnosing abnormal left axis, consider the QRS morphology in lead II as well as in leads I

and aVF.[14] When the axis is abnormal left, the QRS complex is positive in lead I and negative in leads II and aVF (see Fig. 7-8). When the axis is indeterminate, the QRS complex is negative in both leads I and aVF.

Another popular and more exact method of determining the electrical axis involves selecting the lead with the most equiphasic complex.[9,19] Next select the lead perpendicular to this lead in the hexaxial reference system (e.g., I and aVF, II and aVL, III and aVR). Examine the morphology of the QRS complex on this perpendicular lead to determine whether the forces are directed toward the negative or positive electrode of this lead. Then assign the corresponding degrees (Fig. 7-9).[9,31]

Left anterior hemiblock

A block of the anterosuperior division of the left bundle branch is known as left anterior hemiblock. The anterosuperior division is usually supplied by the left anterior descending branch of the left coronary artery. Thus the anterosuperior division is most commonly involved in infarctions of the anterior wall of the heart. LAH is the most commonly reported intraventricular conduc-

tion defect in acute MI (4.2% to 12.6%) and has the lowest mortality rate.[9] The anterosuperior division of the left bundle appears to be the most vulnerable structure of the intraventricular conduction system. This vulnerability is caused by (1) its anatomic location in the hemodynamically turbulent area, (2) its thinness and length, and (3) its singular blood supply from the LAD.[6,9,27]

ECG diagnosis of hemiblocks is based on axis shifts. In LAH, the axis shifts abnormally to the left. The presence of abnormal left axis deviation is diagnosed by a positive QRS complex in lead I and a negative complex in leads II and aVF (−30 degrees).[6,9,14] Many clinicians require an axis of −40 degrees or greater to confirm LAH.[2,9,13,31] These clinicians may choose other leads such as III or aVR as reference points. The width of the QRS complex is normal because activation of both ventricles continues to occur simultaneously rather than separately as in RBBB and LBBB.[13]

Leads I, aVF, and II are derived in the frontal plane. Therefore, to understand the mechanism of axis shifts produced by hemiblocks, the intraventricular conduction system must be visualized in the frontal plane (Fig. 7-10). Note that in the frontal plane the anterosuperior division of the left bundle lies superiorly.

When the anterosuperior division of the left bundle branch is blocked (LAH), the left ventricle is activated through the posteroinferior division. Because activation occurs through this posteroinferior division, the initial force in LAH shifts inferiorly and to the right. This initial force produces a small r wave in leads II and aVF and a small q wave in lead I (Fig. 7-10).[2,6,9,13] The main forces then shift superiorly and to the left. These forces produce deep S waves in leads II and aVF and a large R wave in lead I. Because the main forces shift superiorly and to the left, the axis shifts to abnormal left.

The practitioner must differentiate ALAD secondary to LAH from other causes of ALAD. Other causes include hyperkalemia, emphysema, Wolff-Parkinson-White syndrome, right ventricular (RV) apical pacing, ventricular ectopic rhythms, and extensive inferior wall MI.[6,19,31] Pregnancy, ascites, and other causes of abdominal distention can also cause ALAD, but physical findings can quickly rule these out.[19,31] Since ALAD

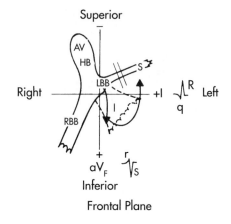

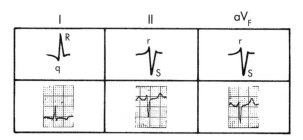

Fig. 7-10 Left anterior hemiblock (LAH). The sequence of activation and corresponding ECG pattern in leads I, aVF, and II are illustrated. Note that within the frontal plane, the anterior division of the left bundle branch lies superiorly.

occurs from forces shifted superiorly as well as to the left, left ventricular (LV) hypertrophy does not produce these changes.[6] The pattern of hyperkalemia mimics that of LAH since the mechanism is hemiblock secondary to K$^+$ changes. In the absence of a typical history and peaked T waves in V2 to V4, this cause may be ruled out (see Unit 4). Consider chronic obstructive pulmonary disease (COPD) primarily with a positive history, p pulmonale or peaked P waves in leads II and V1, and low voltage.[6] Without a typical history of tachycardia or the presence of a pacemaker, Wolff-Parkinson-White syndrome and apical pacing can be easily ruled out. The remaining main differential diag-

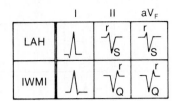

Fig. 7-11 Comparison of ALAD due to LAH and inferior wall MI. Note major differences in leads II and aVF.

nosis is between LAH and inferior wall MI.

In inferior wall MI, the QRS complexes in leads II and aVF are negative secondary to a large Q wave, compatible with extensive necrosis (see Unit 5). The normal forces are shifted away from the necrotic inferior surface. The resulting complete QRS configuration is Qr. This configuration is distinctly different from the rS configuration produced by LAH (Fig. 7-11).

IAD may occur with LAH plus right ventricular hypertrophy (RVH). IAD may also occur from the combination of LAH and extensive lateral wall MI.[6] The complexes are negative in leads II and aVF secondary to LAH. The complex in lead I is negative secondary to the lateral wall involvement and abnormal Q wave formation.

Left posterior hemiblock

A block of the posteroinferior division of the left bundle branch is known as left posterior hemiblock, according to its initial anatomic description. The posteroinferior division of the left bundle branch is supplied by both the right and left coronary arteries.[9] This division is the least vulnerable structure of the intraventricular system. This fact is attributed to its (1) anatomic location in a hemodynamically nonturbulent area, (2) thickness and length, and (3) dual blood supply.[9,14,27]

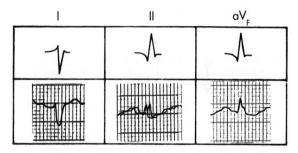

Fig. 7-12 Left posterior hemiblock (LPH). The sequence of activation and corresponding ECG pattern in leads I, aVF, and II are illustrated. Note that within the frontal plane, the posterior division of the left bundle branch lies inferiorly.

In LPH, the axis shifts abnormally to the right. Diagnosis of RAD is by a positive QRS complex in lead aVF and a negative complex in lead I. In the frontal plane, the posteroinferior division lies inferiorly (Fig. 7-12).

When the posteroinferior division of the left bundle branch is blocked (LPH), the left ventricle is activated through the anterosuperior division. Because activation occurs through the anterosuperior division, the initial forces in LPH shift superiorly and to the left. This initial force produces a small r wave in lead I and a small q wave in lead aVF (Fig. 7-12).[2,6] The main forces then shift inferiorly and to the right. These forces produce deep S waves in lead I and a large R wave in aVF. Because the main forces shift inferiorly and to the right, in LPH the axis shifts to the right. The changes in LPH are a mirror image of the changes in LAH.

The practitioner must differentiate RAD secondary to LPH from other causes of RAD. Other causes include RVH, hyperkalemia, emphysema, Wolff-Parkinson-White syndrome, slender build, ventricular ectopy, and extensive lateral wall MI.[6,11,19] Changes on the V leads can differentiate RVH from LPH. Forces in RVH travel toward the positive electrode of V1, producing an upright complex. Unlike in RBB, the normal conduction pathways are still used and the complex remains narrow. The pattern of hyperkalemia can mimic that of LPH as well as that of LAH since the mechanism is hemiblock secondary to K$^+$ changes. In the absence of a typical history and peaked T waves in V2 to V4, this cause may be ruled out (see Unit 4). Consider chronic obstructive lung disease such as emphysema with a

	I	aV$_F$	II
LPH	r / S		
LWMI	r / Q		

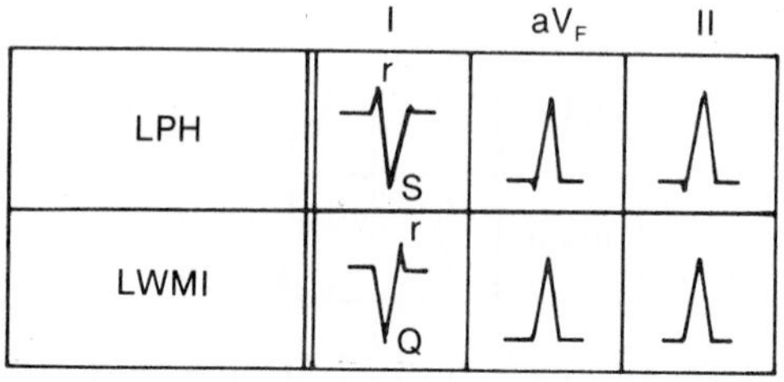

Fig. 7-13 Comparison of RAD due to LPH and lateral wall MI. Note major differences in lead I.

positive history, p pulmonale or peaked P waves in leads II and V1, and low voltage. Without a typical history of tachycardia, Wolff-Parkinson-White syndrome can easily be ruled out. The remaining differential diagnosis is between LPH and lateral wall MI.

In lateral wall MI, the QRS complex in lead I is negative secondary to a large Q wave, compatible with extensive necrosis (see Unit 5). The normal forces shift away from the necrotic lateral surface. The resulting complete QRS configuration is Qr. This configuration is distinctly different from the rS configuration produced by LPH (Fig. 7-13).

BIFASCICULAR BLOCK

Bundle branch blocks and hemiblocks are clinically significant because they are the precursors of symptomatic type II or Mobitz II atrioventricular (AV) blocks (see Unit 6). A block that occurs in one fascicle may also be called monofascicular block. Examples of monofascicular blocks are RBBB, LAH, and LPH. A block that occurs in two fascicles is known as a bifascicular block. Examples of bifascicular blocks are RBBB plus LAH and RBBB plus LPH.

Bifascicular block is a precursor of trifascicular block, or block in all three fascicles. Trifascicular block occurs when the right bundle branch and anterior and posterior

divisions of the left bundle branch are blocked simultaneously. Trifascicular block may be transient or permanent. Mobitz II is an example of transient or intermittent trifascicular block. It is a form of type II AV block which refers to second-degree AV block occurring within the bundle branch system (see Unit 6). Transient or permanent complete heart block may also occur with an idioventricular response or asystole depending on the reliability of ventricular escape pacemaker sites. Even with reliable ventricular response, complete heart block secondary to bundle branch block is frequently symptomatic since the ventricular rate is slow. Bifascicular block with first degree AV block (in the third fascicle) is also a form of trifascicular block.[2,9,13]

Trifascicular block may occur secondary to either acute or chronic changes in the bundle branch system. Acute trifascicular block is less likely to have a reliable, well-tolerated ventricular response. Although acute trifascicular block may occur after open heart surgery, the most common cause is anterior wall MI.

Symptomatic trifascicular (AV) block in anterior wall MI usually is preceded by the development of bifascicular block (RBBB plus LAH or LPH). Nurses who can diagnose bundle branch blocks and hemiblocks can anticipate the development of this AV block and are better prepared. The most common bifascicular block in anterior wall MI is RBBB plus LAH. These two fascicles are thin and have a common blood supply— the LAD branch of the left coronary artery.[9,27] RBBB is most easily diagnosed initially by a change in the QRS morphology in lead V1. LAH is diagnosed initially by the development of ALAD, which is detected best on leads aVF and II. Therefore, with anterior wall MI, if no fascicular blocks are present, monitor the patient on either lead II or V1.[11] We recommend lead V1, with frequent assessment of lead II, because the development of RBBB in spite of some blood supply from the right coronary artery may indicate a more significant change. In the presence of RBBB, observe the patient for the development of LAH. Therefore, monitor the patient on lead II. RBBB with LPH is less common but is associated with a greater risk of complete heart block and higher mortality.[9,27] Diagnose LPH by the development of RAD, which is detected best in lead I.

If bifascicular block develops, notify the physician immediately. Either new bifascicular block or Mobitz II in acute anterior wall MI is an indication for at least a temporary pacemaker.[11,14,15] Until the physician arrives, be prepared to use a transcutaneous pacemaker or epinephrine infusion. Note that atropine is not effective in AV block secondary to bundle branch block and may actually increase the severity secondary to selective increases in the atrial rate (see Unit 6).

AV block secondary to bilateral bundle branch block (RBBB plus LBBB) may develop in patients with preexisting left bundle branch block and anterior wall MI. Alternating RBBB and LBBB has similar significance.[11,27] The physician may insert a prophylactic pacemaker or wait for signs of trifascicular block such as Mobitz II. Bilateral bundle branch block may also occur in these patients during insertion of a pulmonary artery (PA) catheter since the right bundle branch may be traumatized.[27] However, a standby transcutaneous pacer may suffice.

NURSING ORDERS: The patient with acute anterior wall MI and bundle branch block, hemiblock, or bifascicular block (Fig. 7-14).

RELATED NURSING DIAGNOSES: Alteration in cardiac output related to bradycardia; anxiety; knowledge deficit

1. If no fascicular blocks are present, monitor the patient on lead II or MCL1 (V1), periodically checking the other lead for changes.

2. In the presence of RBBB, monitor the patient on lead II for the development of LAH.[11]

3. In the presence of LPH or LAH, monitor the patient on lead V1 for the development of RBBB.

4. In the presence of bifascicular block:
   —Notify the physician immediately.
   —Prepare for prophylactic pacemaker insertion.
   —Obtain a transcutaneous pacemaker if available and place at bedside or prepare standby epinephrine infusion.

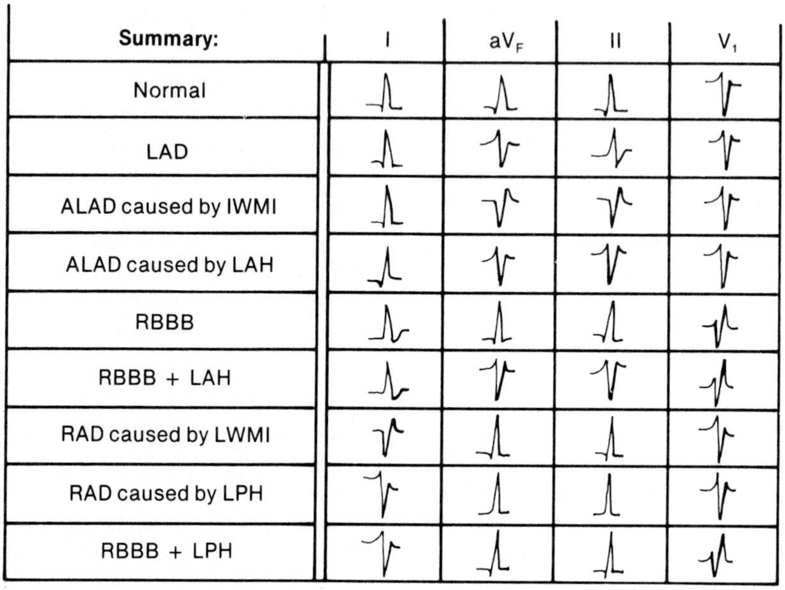

Summary:	I	aV$_F$	II	V$_1$
Normal				
LAD				
ALAD caused by IWMI				
ALAD caused by LAH				
RBBB				
RBBB + LAH				
RAD caused by LWMI				
RAD caused by LPH				
RBBB + LPH				

Fig. 7-14 Comparison of hemiblock, right and left bundle branch block, and bifascicular block patterns.

—Monitor for the development of Mobitz II, 2-1 or advanced AV block, and complete heart block with an idioventricular response. Choose whatever lead shows both clear P waves and QRS complexes so that AV block may be more easily detected.

5. Explain the purpose of all procedures and equipment to the patient and family.

ABERRANT CONDUCTION

If a premature atrial impulse finds one of the bundle branches refractory, the impulse will be blocked in that branch and will be conducted in a different direction using the other bundle branch (see Unit 6). This form of abnormal intraventricular conduction is called *aberrant conduction*. Aberrant conduction is associated with variations in the bundle branch refractory periods and is a form of temporary, functional, bundle branch block.[2,23,26,28]

Aberrantly conducted beats, although supraventricular in origin, produce wide, changing QRS complexes mimicking ventricular ectopy. The most common aberrantly conducted impulses are atrial ectopic beats. Junctional ectopic beats or rhythms may also be aberrantly conducted but are more difficult to differentiate from ventricular ectopy. Rate-dependent bundle branch block occurring during sinus bradycardia or sinus tachycardia is also considered a form of aberrant conduction.[2,9,23,28]

An aberrantly conducted premature atrial complex (PAC) is most easily differentiated from a ventricular ectopic beat (premature ventricular complex, or PVC) by the presence of a preceding premature P wave (Fig. 7-15).[9,23] Although PVCs may be preceded by P waves, these P waves are usually sinus

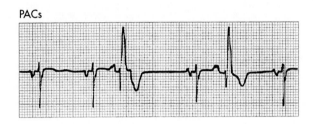

PACs

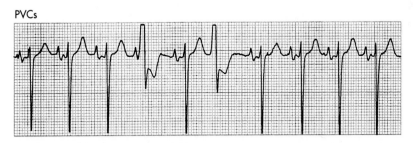

PVCs

Fig. 7-15 Differentiation of PACs with aberrant conduction from PVCs by preceding P waves. In the PACs the preceding P waves are premature, whereas in the PVCs preceding P waves, when present, are not premature.

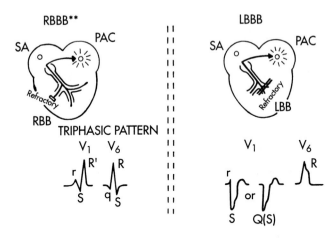

Fig. 7-16 RBBB versus LBBB aberrant conduction: mechanism and typical ECG patterns.

in origin and therefore are not premature. Other ECG criteria typical of aberrant conduction are the QRS complex morphology and Ashman's phenomenon.

Premature atrial beats may find either the right or the left bundle branch refractory.

Therefore, the characteristic QRS complex patterns associated with aberrant conduction assume either RBBB or LBBB morphology (Fig. 7-16). RBBB aberration is more common since the right bundle branch usually has a longer refractory period, especially at

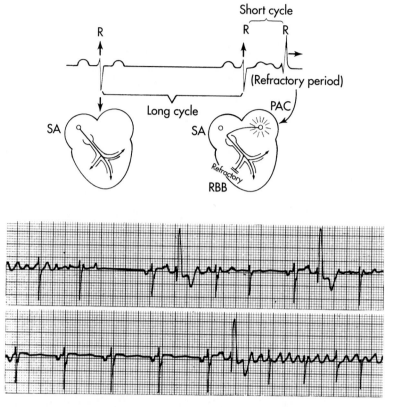

Fig. 7-17 Ashman's phenomenon. Aberrantly conducted atrial ectopic beats end short R–R cycles preceded by long cycles.

slow heart rates.[9,26,28,31] At faster heart rates, the left bundle branch may have a longer refractory period.[2,26] A triphasic pattern in both V1 and V6 favors aberrant conduction since this pattern is compatible with RBBB.[37] A small narrow r wave in V1 (0.03 second or less) with a rapid downstroke (0.06 second or less to the nadir or peak of the S wave) together with a wide monophasic R wave in V6, with or without notches or peaks, also favors aberrant conduction since this pattern is compatible with LBBB.[11,23,28] Although the QRS complexes of aberrantly conducted beats are wide, the width usually does not exceed 0.16 second.[1,28]

Bundle branch refractory periods vary according to the length of the preceding R–R interval or cycle.[8] A long R–R interval or cycle prolongs the refractory period of the impulse ending the cycle. When preceded by long R–R cycles, premature beats are more likely to find the bundle branches of the previous beat still refractory. Thus aberrant conduction is more likely to occur. The aberrantly conducted beat ends or forms a short R–R cycle preceded by a long R–R cycle (Fig. 7-17). This long-short cycle sequence favoring aberration is known as *Ashman's phenomenon.*[2,8,23,26,28,31]

The varying R–R cycles of atrial fibrillation predispose to Ashman's phenomenon. In atrial fibrillation, the impulse ending a short R–R cycle, preceded by a long R–R cycle, is likely to be aberrantly conducted

Lead V₁

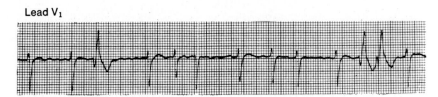

Fig. 7-18 Cycling (Ashman's phenomenon) in atrial fibrillation. Note the triphasic complex in V1, also supporting aberrant conduction.

(Fig. 7-18). Since the best indicator of aberrantly conducted atrial beats—the premature P wave—is lost in atrial fibrillation, this alternate characteristic is potentially useful. However, the occurrence of ventricular ectopic impulses may also be facilitated by long cycles.[23,31] Therefore, cycling or Ashman's phenomenon offers only weak support for aberrant conduction.[23] QRS morphology characteristics, if present in both V1 and V6, are more reliable. Aberrant conduction in atrial fibrillation typically disappears with slowing of the ventricular rate or conversion to sinus rhythm.[8]

Sinus rhythm with intermittent rate-dependent bundle branch block is differentiated from ventricular ectopy by the presence of a fixed P–R interval in consecutive beats. This form of aberrant conduction occurs less commonly than supraventricular ectopy and is usually associated with at least a slight increase or decrease in rate and R–R interval.

Aberrant conduction may also produce atypical QRS patterns. For example, in anteroseptal MI, RBBB assumes a qR configuration in lead V1, which usually favors ventricular ectopy (see Wide QRS Tachycardia). These and other similar variations may make it even more difficult to differentiate between aberrantly conducted supraventricular beats and ventricular ectopy. Therefore, QRS complexes different from the patient's normal complexes should be considered ventricular in origin unless there is *clear* evidence to the contrary, such as a preceding premature P wave or consecutive related P waves with fixed P–R intervals. Distinctly characteristic QRS patterns compatible with aberrant conduction also suggest a supraventricular origin.

VENTRICULAR ECTOPY PATTERNS

Criteria favoring the presence of ventricular ectopy in single or consecutive beats with changing QRS complexes include nonpremature P waves, fusion beats, QRS width, taller left "rabbit ear," AV dissociation, absence of cycling, and characteristic QRS patterns. Nonpremature P waves preceding different or changing QRS complexes rules out atrial ectopy—the most common form of aberrant conduction. The remaining criteria also help differentiate ventricular tachycardia (VT) from supraventricular tachycardia (SVT) in wide QRS tachycardia. Refer to the Wide QRS Tachycardia section for a more complete discussion of these criteria.

The most characteristic sign favoring ventricular ectopy is the presence of *fusion beats*. Ventricular fusion beats represent simultaneous depolarization of the ventricles by both supraventricular and ventricular impulses (Fig. 7-19). Fusion beats are thus evidence that a ventricular focus is firing if Wolff-Parkinson-White syndrome can be ruled out[26] (see Units 6 and 11).

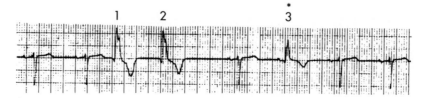

Fig. 7-19 Ventricular fusion confirming ventricular ectopy. The third ectopic beat from the left is the fusion beat. Note that the preceding P wave in this beat is not premature.

Right versus left ventricular ectopy

Leads V1 and V6 offer the best diagnosis of right versus left ventricular ectopy. These leads are useful in diagnosing conditions in which right to left or left to right ventricular activation changes. The specific morphology of ventricular ectopy in these leads varies from that of aberrant conduction and may also be helpful for problem solving in catheter-induced ventricular arrhythmias.

When a ventricular ectopic beat originates in the left ventricular His-Purkinje tissue, the predominant forces often travel from left to right toward the positive electrode of lead V1, producing a positive complex (Fig. 7-20).[12] These same forces travel away from the positive electrode of lead V6, producing a negative complex. Conduction occurs across ventricular muscle, usually resulting in a wide QRS complex. The wide, upright QRS complex in V1 produced by LV ectopy initially mimics the also upright and wide complex of RBBB aberration. However, the specific configuration or morphology in V1 and V6 differs (see Right Bundle Branch Block).

When a ventricular ectopic beat originates in the right ventricular His-Purkinje tissue, the predominant forces travel from right to left, away from the positive electrode of lead V1, producing a negative complex (Fig. 7-21).[12] These same forces travel toward the positive electrodes of V6, producing a positive complex. The wide, negative QRS complex in V1 initially mimics the also negative and wide complex occurring in LBBB aberration. The specific configuration or morphology in V1 and V6 differs, however (see Left Bundle Branch Block). In patients with

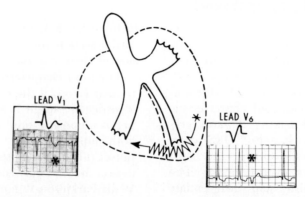

Fig. 7-20 The upright complex in V1: LV ectopy. Note the monophasic pattern in V1 and pattern in V6 inconsistent with either RBBB or LBBB.

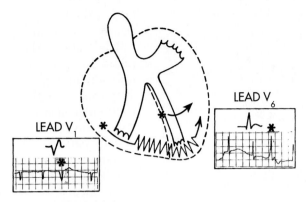

Fig. 7-21 The negative complex in V1: RV or LV (septal) ectopy. Note the slurred rather than rapid downstroke in V1.

coronary artery disease, ventricular ectopy in the LV septum can also produce negative complexes in V1.[9,12,24] Therefore, negative complexes in V1 may indicate *either* RV or LV ectopy. In the absence of coronary artery disease, the pattern is more likely to indicate RV ectopy.

Ventricular ectopic beats that originate in the right ventricle are more likely to result from mechanisms such as catheter irritation of the ventricular wall. We suggest monitor-ing patients on V1 (MCL1) during insertion of PA or pacing catheters and while the catheters remain in place unless there are indications to the contrary, such as inability to diagnose pacing spikes or sinus rhythm on these leads. Periodic inspection of V1 patterns during repetitive ventricular arrhythmias can also suffice. In catheter irritation, traditional treatments for ventricular ectopy, such as lidocaine, may not be indicated.

Fascicular ectopy

Ventricular ectopic beats may result in QRS complexes with only minimal widening, even when examined on multiple leads. These narrow PVCs may originate in one of the fascicles or divisions of the left bundle branch. The QRS configuration of fascicular ectopy resembles the patterns associated with bifascicular block due to delayed conduction through the other two fascicles (Fig. 7-22).[9]

WIDE QRS TACHYCARDIA

The defining characteristics of a wide QRS tachycardia are QRS complexes greater than or equal to 0.12 second in width and a ventricular rate greater than 100. The term is used most often to refer to sustained tachycardias. This frequently misdiagnosed and subsequently mistreated rhythm focuses on the differentiation of VT from SVT. The presence or absence of symptoms does not help differentiate between VT and SVT.[1,7,23,29,33] A particularly challenging diagnostic dilemma occurs when the underlying rhythm and onset of the arrhythmia are unavailable for comparison.

The four major mechanisms of a wide QRS tachycardia are (1) VT, (2) preexisting bundle branch block, (3) SVT with aberrant conduction, and 4) Wolff-Parkinson-White

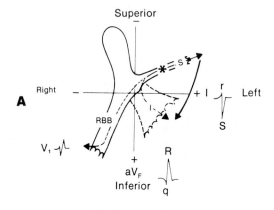

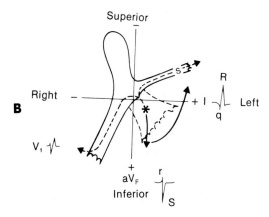

Fig. 7-22 Fascicular ectopy. The sequence of activation and corresponding ECG patterns in anterior fascicular beats *(A)* are contrasted with those of posterior fascicular beats *(B)*.

syndrome.[3,11,28,33] Ventricular tachycardia is the mechanism in 81% to 85% of the cases.[1,8,28,29] In patients with a history of acute MI, the probability of VT may be as high as 98%.[1,8,23,28–30] SVT with aberrant conduction or preexisting bundle branch block is the mechanism in approximately 14% of the cases. Wolff-Parkinson-White syndrome is the mechanism in the remaining 5%.[1,28] The differential diagnosis of preexisting bundle branch block is simplified when the QRS complex morphology in sinus rhythm is available for comparison. If the

QRS complex is the same, the rhythm is clearly supraventricular.[1,9,11]

The patient should be immediately assessed for presence or absence of *pulse* before attempting extensive ECG differential diagnosis. The absence of a pulse confirms ventricular tachycardia and allows for rapid critical intervention (see Unit 6). In a symptomatic patient with a pulse and a ventricular rate over 150, cardioversion may be initiated without the need for an accurate diagnosis since it is effective in both VT and SVT.[4,15,23,28] In the hemodynamically stable patient a trace of MCL1 (V1) and MCL6 (V6) can be quickly obtained for rapid ECG assessment. Leads I, aVF, and II may also be helpful. A standard 12-lead ECG can follow. A quick history should also be obtained, if previously not available, to rule out prior MI.[30]

Since the origin of the rhythm is most likely ventricular, an initial trial dose of lidocaine is currently recommended by the American Heart Association in the hemodynamically stable patient and may be administered prior to cardioversion.[15] Lidocaine administration may have diagnostic as well as therapeutic advantages. Intravenous procainamide (Pronestyl) is also acceptable initially and may be more effective in patients with chronic VT or Wolff-Parkinson-White syndrome.[9,15,23,28,33] If acceleration of the ventricular rate, though infrequent, occurs after either lidocaine or procainamide administration,[31] the patient should not receive further dosages (see Unit 9).[4,12,31] Supraventricular tachycardia may be diagnosed at this time, with subsequent treatment.

If lidocaine is ineffective, the American Heart Association recommends a trial dose of adenosine (Adenocard).[15] Adenosine is effective in SVT, and at least does no harm if the rhythm is VT (see Unit 9). Vagal maneuvers and carotid sinus pressure have similar effects.[15,31] Administration of verapamil (Calan, Isoptin, Verelan) in wide QRS tachycardias is contraindicated.[4,9,15,28,33] If the origin is ventricular or atrial fibrillation in Wolff-Parkinson-White syndrome, shock, ventricular fibrillation, or other forms of cardiac arrest can occur.[1,4,15,23] Diltiazem (Cardizem) is also best avoided because of its similarities in action to verapamil (see Unit 9). Compare the trace obtained after effective pharmacologic or electrical cardioversion with a trace of the tachycardia to retrospectively assist in confirming the diagnosis.

The four most common ECG characteristics used to differentiate between the major forms of wide QRS tachycardia are QRS width, AV dissociation, axis deviation, and QRS morphology or configuration. Wellens initially popularized these four differentiating characteristics. Although QRS morphology is a popular differentiating characteristic, it is the least accurate of these.[1,33] QRS morphology is more useful in supporting the diagnosis of VT than SVT, especially in the patient with MI. QRS width greater than 0.16 second favors ventricular ectopy.[1,11,28,33] QRS complexes less than 0.16 second do not confirm SVT, however, since these also occur in VT in a small percentage of patients.[1,16,28] QRS width should be determined from more than one lead.[4,11]

Since ventricular arrhythmias do not typically disturb the sinus rhythm, AV dissociation usually is present; studies have documented it in 50% to 60% of VT cases.[4,9,28] AV dissociation is one of the most accurate indicators of ventricular ectopy.[3,11,26,31,33] The ECG diagnosis, however, requires identification of P waves (see Unit 6). These P waves may be difficult to detect on the surface ECG at fast ventricular rates. Investigators report evidence of AV dissociation on the surface ECG in only 25% to 29% of VT cases.[1,26,33] Esophageal electrodes or intraatrial recordings may help to more clearly document AV dissociation. The presence of related P waves does not totally rule out VT since retrograde conduction with related P

waves has been reported in up to one third (25% to 60%) of patients with VT.[9,28]

The clinical signs of AV dissociation may be more evident than the ECG characteristics. Clinical signs of AV dissociation such as intermittent cannon waves (large neck vein pulsations) strongly support a diagnosis of ventricular ectopy (see Unit 6).[4,9,23,31,33] The patient may perceive these neck vein pulsations. Beat to beat variations in arterial pressure may be visible on an arterial pressure tracing.[4,9,23] Varying intensity of the S1 is also typically present.[4,23,31]

The presence of indeterminate axis favors ventricular ectopy.[1,4,9,11,23,26,28,33] This pattern occurs in approximately one in four cases of ventricular tachycardia.[11] The significance of left axis deviation is more controversial since it occurs in LBBB and fascicular block. Right axis deviation with negative complexes in V1 favors VT.[1,17,26,28,33]

An upright QRS complex in V1 is more common in wide QRS tachycardia than a negative complex and suggests either VT originating in the LV or SVT with RBBB.[1,28] Unlike RBBB aberration, the complexes produced by ventricular ectopy are typically monophasic or biphasic in V1 (Fig. 7-23).[7,9,11,31] When the QRS complex is *upright* in V1, the pattern in V6 often more clearly differentiates between VT and SVT. A predominantly negative complex (rS or QS) in V6 strongly favors VT.[7,9,11,17,26,31] This pattern is not compatible with either typical RBBB or LBBB patterns in V6. An essentially normal V6 with terminal delay is indicative of RBBB aberration, especially if triphasic. QRS complex morphology in V1, although typically triphasic (rSR'), is less helpful since atypical RBBB patterns mimicking patterns of LV ectopy are common (see Right Bundle Branch Block). Investigators also have reported the triphasic pattern in V1 and V6 in some cases of VT (10%).[1,9,17]

A negative QRS complex in V1 suggests ei-

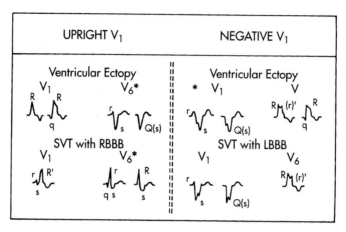

UPRIGHT V₁	NEGATIVE V₁

Ventricular Ectopy

V_1 V_6* * V_1 V

SVT with RBBB

V_1 V_6* V_1 V_6

Fig. 7-23 QRS morphology differences between ventricular ectopy (VT) and SVT with bundle branch block: leads V1 (MCL1) and V6 (MCL6). Note that when the QRS is upright in V_1, the pattern in V_6 is most diagnostic and when the QRS is negative in V_1, the pattern in V_1 is most diagnostic.

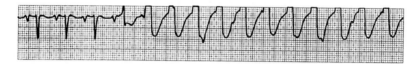

Fig. 7-24 Wide QRS tachycardia due to ventricular tachycardia (VT): confirmed by the onset of the tachycardia. Note the evidence of nonpremature P waves and a fusion beat (fourth complex from the left). AV dissociation is also clearly evidenced by the fusion beat.

ther VT (RV or LV) or SVT with LBBB. When the QRS complex is *negative* in V1, the pattern in V1 more clearly differentiates between VT and SVT, although the distinguishing characteristics are subtle. A wide initial R wave (>0.03 second) and/or slurred or delayed downslope (>0.06 second), especially with notching, favor VT,[7,9,16–18] whereas a narrow R wave, if present, and rapid downstroke favor LBBB.[1,9,11,16,23] The LBBB pattern should also be present in V2 to rule out VT.[7,9,11,17] The patterns of RV ectopy and LBBB aberration may be very similar in V6, so this lead is of limited value in differentiating between the two. A small q wave in VT is the somewhat subtle and infrequently seen major difference (Fig. 7-23).[7,9,18,23,28] The

primary value of lead V6 is with an upright QRS complex in V1.

A more recently discovered morphology characteristic is the presence or absence of an RS complex in the precordial leads.[3,9] The absence of an RS complex confirms the diagnosis of VT. The presence of an RS complex with a duration greater than 0.10 second from the beginning to the peak of the S wave also favors VT.

Other ECG criteria used by clinicians to differentiate between VT and SVT with wide QRS complexes include fusion or capture beats, concordance, taller left rabbit ear, the onset of tachycardia, and irregular R–R intervals.[4,23,28,31,33] Although fusion beats strongly favor the presence of ventricular ec-

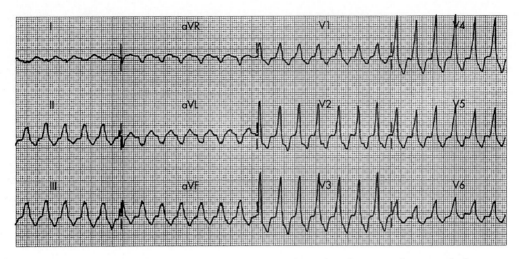

Fig. 7-25 Positive concordance in leads V1 through V6, suggesting ventricular tachycardia. The QRS width is non-specific (0.12 second) and the axis is normal. However, the complex in V1 is monophasic, and the complex in V6 looks obviously wide rather than essentially normal with only terminal delay (as in RBBB). In addition, there are no RS complexes in V1 through V6.

topy, these beats are not common in VT unless the ventricular rate of the underlying rhythm is approximately the same. Capture beats are occasional, normally conducted beats occurring during the tachycardia. Both fusion and capture beats indicate AV dissociation (Fig. 7-24).[31] Concordance is present when the QRS complexes are either all upright or all negative in V1 through V6. Positive concordance (all upright complexes) is more predictive, strongly favoring VT (Fig. 7-25).[1,28,33] Negative concordance occurs in LBBB.[1]

The dual peaks or notches appearing in some wide QRS complexes were described many years ago by Gozensky and Thorne as "rabbit ears." A taller left peak or rabbit ear in lead V1 favors ventricular ectopy (see Fig. 7-19).[7,9,16,23,31] A taller right peak is not helpful for diagnosis since it favors neither ventricular ectopy nor aberrant conduction.

A premature P wave at the onset of the tachycardia indicates an SVT, whereas a nonpremature P wave or fusion beat at the onset supports the diagnosis of VT (Fig. 7-24). We have found the presence of grossly irregular R–R intervals particularly helpful in identifying SVT (Fig. 7-26). Although slight irregularities are compatible with VT, if the R–R interval varies by more than 0.10 second the rhythm is more likely SVT (usually atrial fibrillation). Determination of irregular R–R intervals is more difficult at faster heart rates. Multiple criteria in single 12-lead ECG traces are common and further facilitate the diagnosis (Fig. 7-27).

The differential diagnosis of wide QRS tachycardia due to Wolff-Parkinson-White syndrome is the most difficult since the QRS patterns closely mimic ventricular ectopy. Clues include rapid, irregular QRS complexes (atrial fibrillation) with ventricular fusion and a history of palpitations or tachycardia without chest pain in a young patient.[4,9,11,28] A regular tachycardia at a ventricular rate of 300 that does not disintegrate rapidly into ventricular fibrillation is also likely to be Wolff-Parkinson-White syn-

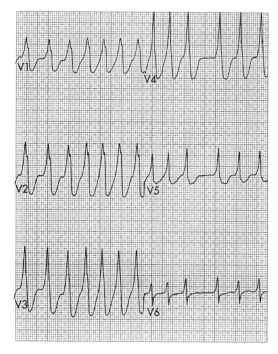

Fig. 7-26 Irregular wide QRS tachycardia (SVT). The rhythm is atrial fibrillation. The pattern in V6 is more suggestive of Wolff-Parkinson-White syndrome than RBBB since the QRS delay is initial rather than terminal.

drome. There is no qR pattern in the precordial leads.[17,28] Neither is there negative concordance.[9,26] Tracings of sinus rhythm recorded before the tachycardia or after its conversion may reveal a short P–R and delta wave[17,26] (see Unit 11).

A definitive diagnosis of VT or SVT in wide QRS tachycardia, and its specific mechanism, can be made only with His bundle electrophysiologic (EPS) studies.[4,28,33] EPS studies continue to be used as a research tool to validate proposed surface ECG criteria. These studies are not readily available in all institutions and are usually reserved for diagnosing or guiding therapy in individual patients with complex, recurrent tachycardia unresponsive to traditional therapy (see Unit

11). EPS studies may be particularly helpful when tachycardia episodes are infrequent.[26]

NURSING ORDERS: The patient with single ectopic beats with changing QRS complexes or sustained wide QRS tachycardia (Table 7-1).

RELATED NURSING DIAGNOSES: Alteration in cardiac output; impaired tissue perfusion; anxiety; knowledge deficit

1. When analyzing premature beats that have a different or wide QRS morphology:
   —Look for preceding premature P waves.
   —Also note the presence of preceding P waves with constant P–R intervals.
   —Look for the presence of fusion or taller left rabbit ear on V1.
   —Note whether the QRS width is greater than 0.16 seconds.
   —If no P waves are clearly visible, analyze the QRS configuration on lead V1 and V6 or their monitoring equivalents, MCL1 and MCL6.
   —Consider the clinical setting in which the ectopic beats occur. Has the patient been in heart failure? Does the patient have an acute MI? Is a catheter present in the right ventricle? Is the patient hypoxemic?
   —Consider the preceding and/or underlying rhythm. Is the patient in atrial fibrillation? If the patient was previously in sinus rhythm, were these beats present then? Has the patient been having PACs or PVCs?

2. In the presence of a sustained tachyarrhythmia with changing or wide QRS complexes:
   —Check the patient's pulse. If absent, treat as VF.
   —If the ventricular rate is over 150 and the patient is symptomatic, consider immediate cardioversion.
   —Check for history of MI. If yes, treat as ventricular.

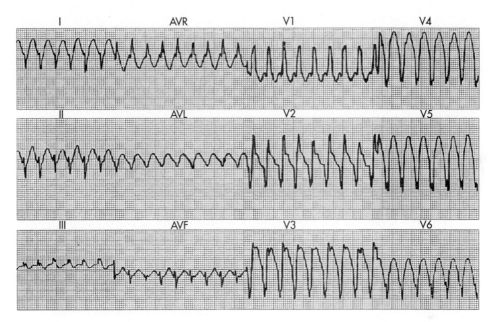

Fig. 7-27 Wide QRS tachycardia due to VT. Multiple confirming characteristics are present. The QRS complex is 0.16 second in width. The axis is indeterminate. The upright pattern in V1 is biphasic (qR) with a negative complex in V6, and there are no RS complexes in V1 through V6.

—Note whether the QRS width is over 0.16 seconds.

—Look for fusion beats or capture beats.

—Look for ECG or clinical signs of AV dissociation (cannon (e.g., waves, varying S1).

—Compare with previous tracing in sinus rhythm, if available.

—Look for preceding P waves at the onset, if available.

—In the asymptomatic patient, obtain a trace in V1 (MCL1) and V6 (MCL6), analyze the QRS configuration in these leads, and document changes on a standard 12-lead ECG. Note the presence of positive concordance or taller left rabbit ear in V1. Note the absence of RS complexes in leads V1 through V6.

—Note the presence of indeterminate axis deviation on leads I and aVF.

3. When in doubt, especially in a patient with an acute MI, consider the ectopic beat or tachycardia ventricular in origin and attempt an antiarrhythmic trial with lidocaine (Xylocaine) or procainamide (Pronestyl). In the presence of tachycardia, if this is ineffective, administer adenosine (Adenocard).

Table 7-1. Differential diagnosis of ventricular arrhythmias and supraventricular rhythms with bundle branch block or aberrant conduction

Single beats

Criteria favoring ventricular ectopy
1. If preceded by P wave, should *not* premature
2. QRS complex morphology
   —When *upright* in V1, monophasic (R) or biphasic (qR) with negative V6 (rS, QS); taller left rabbit ear in V1
   —When *negative* in V1, R wave >0.03 second with slurred downslope (0.06 second from the beginning of the complex to peak of S wave), small q wave in V6
3. QRS width >0.16 second
4. Fusion beats

5. Extreme axis deviation (IAD)—see sustained tachycardia

Criteria favoring aberrant conduction
1. Preceding premature P wave (indicates PAC)
2. QRS complex morphology
   —When *upright* in V1, triphasic in V1 (rSR) and V6 (qRS)
   —When *negative* in V1, R wave 0.03 second or less with rapid downslope (0.06 second or less from the beginning of the complex to peak of S wave)
3. QRS width not helpful
4. Long-short cycle sequence (weak criteria)
5. Preceding P wave with constant P–R

Sustained tachycardia

Criteria favoring VT

1. QRS width >0.16 second
2. AV dissociation (independent P waves, intermittent cannon "a" waves)
3. Fusion beats, capture beats, nonpremature P at onset
4. QRS complex morphology (see single beats); absence of RS complex in V1–V6
5. Axis deviation
   —Extreme axis deviation (IAD)— negative I/aVF
   —RAD with negative complex in V1, negative I, positive aVF
6. Positive concordance (V1–V6)
7. Conversion with lidocaine or procainamide

Criteria favoring SVT with bundle branch block
1. QRS width not helpful
2. Preceding P waves with constant P–R
3. Premature P wave at onset
4. QRS complex morphology (see single beats); QRS same a sin underlying rhythm
5. Grossly irregular R–R intervals

6. Slowing of ventricular rate or conversion with adenosine, vagal maneuvers, or carotid sinus pressure
7. Increase in ventricular rate with lidocaine or procainamide

SELF-ASSESSMENT

1 Mr. Bloch was admitted to the coronary care unit 2 days ago with the diagnosis of acute anterior wall MI.

In anterior wall MI, bundle branch blocks and hemiblocks (are/are not) common. The bundle branch block occurring most commonly in anterior wall MI is (RBBB/LBBB).

are

RBBB

2 The 12-lead ECG taken this morning showed the following:

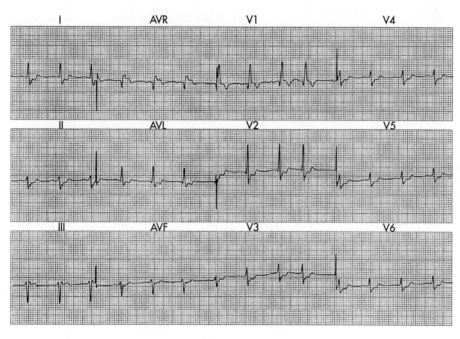

Fig. 7-28 Self-assessment trace 1.

The changes in leads V1 and V6 indicate (RBBB/LBBB). The axis in the frontal plane leads indicates (ALAD/RAD/IAD). The mechanism of this axis deviation is most likely (MI/hemiblock) or, more specifically, _____.

The combination of RBBB and LAH is called _____ block and (is/is not) an indication for a bifascicular temporary pacemaker in acute MI.

RBBB
ALAD
hemiblock
LAH
bifascicular
is

3 Mrs. Stevenson was admitted to the coronary care unit with inferior wall MI. Examination showed significant right ventricular infarction. On the morning of the third day she developed a wide QRS tachycardia. The 12-lead ECG showed the following:

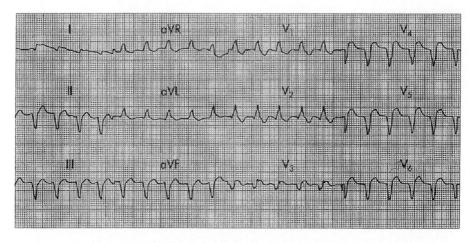

Fig. 7-29   Self-assessment trace 2.

The most common cause of wide QRS tachycardia is (VT/SVT with RBBB/Wolff-Parkinson-White syndrome). In coronary artery disease, VT is (more/less) common.

VT

more

The QRS complex morphology in V1 and V6 suggests (VT/SVT). RS complexes (are/are not) present in V1 through V6, confirming the diagnosis of (VT/SVT). The width of the QRS complex suggests (VT/SVT/neither). The axis is (RAD/ALAD/IAD). This axis (is/is not) the axis deviation most diagnostic for VT.

VT

are not

VT; neither (0.12)

ALAD; is not

4 Initial action when the rhythm in Fig. 7-29 appears on the monitor should be to (check the pulse/obtain 12-lead ECG). Since the ventricular rate is less than 150, cardioversion (is/is not) indicated. The initial drug recommended by the American Heart Association is

check the pulse

is not

_____.

Xylocaine

This VT most likely originates from the (RV/LV).

LV

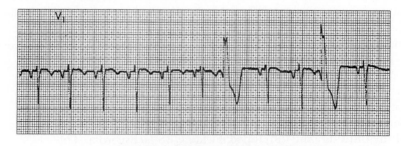

Fig. 7-30   Self-assessment trace 3.

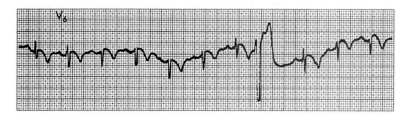

Fig. 7-30, cont'd.

5 INTERPRETATION: Sinus rhythm with PVCs

COMMENTS: A biphasic (qR) rather than triphasic complex is present in the ectopic beats in V1. Although this pattern is consistent with the RBBB in anteroseptal MI, it favors ventricular ectopy. Anteroseptal MI is unlikely since no Q waves are present in the underlying rhythm. A taller left rabbit ear is also present in the second of the ectopic beats. The negative QRS complex in V6 (RS configuration) in the presence of an upright complex in V1 helps confirm the diagnosis. The QRS width is nonspecific (0.14 second). Since they are upright in V1 and negative in V6, these PVCs most likely originate in the LV.

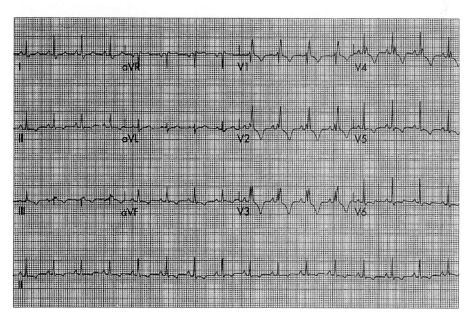

Fig. 7-31 Self-assessment trace 4.

6 INTERPRETATION: Sinus rhythm with complete RBBB

COMMENTS: The typical triphasic (rSR) pattern appears in V1. Repolarization is altered secondary to changes in depolarization. The pattern in V6 is essentially normal except for the terminal delay (S wave). A similar pattern with more distinct terminal delay is visible in lead I. The QRS width of 0.12 second is consistent with a complete bundle branch block. The axis is normal.

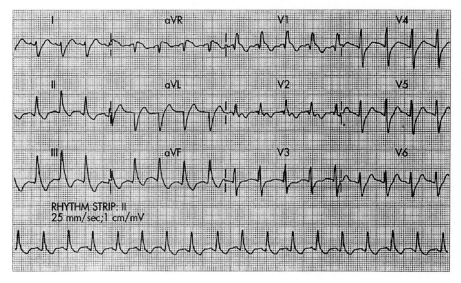

Fig. 7-32   Self-assessment trace 5.

7 INTERPRETATION: Sinus rhythm with bifascicular block (RBBB + LPH) COMMENTS: The pattern in leads I and aVF indicate RAD. The rS pattern in lead I rules out lateral wall MI as the mechanism and suggests LPH if other causes of RAD can be ruled out. No other evidence of pacing, Wolff-Parkinson-White syndrome, hyperkalemia, COPD, or RVH is present. The complex in lead V1 is upright and wide (0.12 second) with an atypical qR configuration consistent with RBBB in anteroseptal infarction. Although this qR pattern in V1 also favors ventricular ectopy, preceding P waves at a constant P–R interval confirm the diagnosis of RBBB. These related P waves are most clearly visible in lead I. The negative complex (RS) in V6 does not typically occur in RBBB but is most likely a reflection of the LPH and changes on lead I.

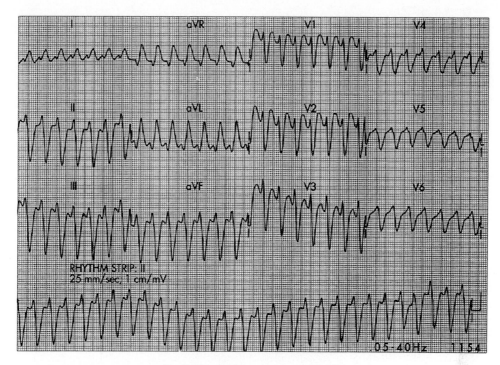

Fig. 7-33   Self-assessment trace 6.

8 INTERPRETATION: Wide QRS tachycardia due to VT

COMMENTS: The negative complex in V1 favors VT due to the wide R wave (0.04 second) in both V1 and V2 and a delayed downslope (0.10 second from the beginning of the complex to the peak negative deflection). The QRS width of more than 0.16 second also favors VT. Negative concordance is present in V1 through V6. This finding is nonspecific but rules out Wolff-Parkinson-White syndrome. The significance of the ALAD (leads I, II, aVF) is more controversial but not critical to the diagnosis since other confirming characteristics are present.

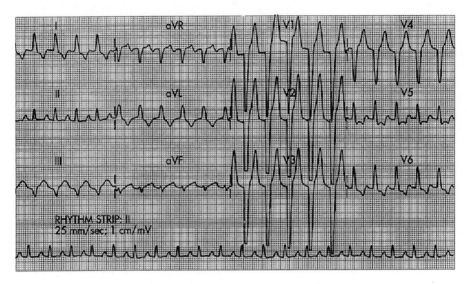

Fig. 7-34   Self-assessment trace 7.

9 INTERPRETATION: Wide QRS tachycardia due to SVT with LBBB
COMMENTS: The negative complex in V1 favors LBBB due to narrow R waves (<0.03 second) and a rapid downslope (0.04 to 0.06 seconds from the beginning of the complex to the peak negative deflection). The QRS width of 0.16 second is consistent with complete LBBB. The pattern in V6 is also consistent with LBBB. The axis is normal left. Without previous ECGs it is not possible to determine whether this LBBB is due to preexisting bundle branch block or aberrant conduction.

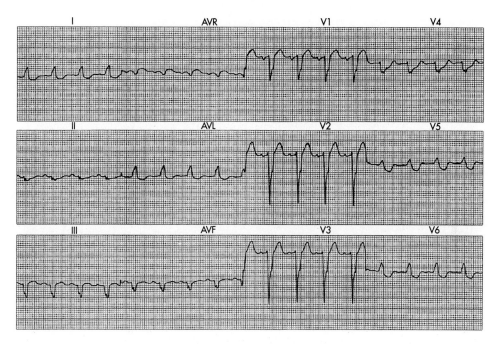

Fig. 7-35   Self-assessment trace 8.

10 INTERPRETATION: Sinus rhythm with complete LBBB

COMMENTS: The typical wide complex with medial delay appears in V6. Only slight notching occurs. The pattern in V1 is also typical with a narrow R wave (<0.03 second) and a rapid downslope (0.06 second from the beginning of the complex to the peak negative deflection). This same pattern is also present on V2. The QRS width of 0.14 second is consistent with complete LBBB. The ALAD (leads I, II, aVF) is also consistent with LBBB.

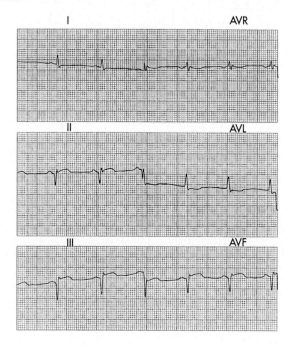

I   AVR

II   AVL

III   AVF

Fig. 7-36   Self-assessment trace 9.

11 INTERPRETATION: Sinus rhythm with inferior wall MI

COMMENTS: The axis indicates ALAD in leads I, II, and aVF. A Qr configuration occurs in the negative complexes in leads II and aVF. The abnormal Q waves indicate the mechanism of the axis deviation is MI. Since leads II and aVF reflect the inferior wall, the specific mechanism is inferior wall MI.

REFERENCES/SUGGESTED READINGS

1. Akhtar M et al: Wide QRS complex tachycardia: a reappraisal of a common clinical problem, Ann Intern Med 109:905, 1988.
2. Braunwald E, editor: Heart disease: a textbook of cardiovascular medicine, ed 3, Philadelphia, 1988, WB Saunders.
3. Brugada P et al: A new approach to the differential diagnosis of a regular tachycardia with a wide QRS complex, Circulation 83:1649, 1991.
4. Brzozowski LA: Wide QRS complex tachycardia, AACN Clin Issues 3(1):173, 1992.
5. Camm AJ, Garratt CJ: Adenosine and supraventricular tachycardia, N Engl J Med 325(23):1621, 1991.
6. Castellanos A, Myerburg A: The resting electrocardiogram. In Hurst WJ, Sclant RB, editors: The heart, arteries, and veins, ed 6, New York, McGraw-Hill, 1990.
7. Chapman EL, Strawn RM, Stewart BP: Differentiating between ventricular tachycardia and supraventricular tachycardia in the clinical setting, Focus on Crit Care 19(2):140, 1992.
8. Chenevert M et al: Ashman's phenomenon—a source of nonsustained wide-com-

plex tachycardia: case report and discussion, J Emerg Med 10(2):179, 1992.

9. Conover MB: Understanding electrocardiography, ed 6, St. Louis, 1992, Mosby–Year Book.

10. Cooper J, Marriott HJL: Why are so many critical care nurses unable to recognize VT on the 12-lead ECG? Heart and Lung 18(3):243, 1989.

11. Drew BJ: Bedside electrocardiographic monitoring: state of the art for the 1990s, Heart Lung 20(6):610, 1991.

12. Drew BJ: Differentiation of wide QRS complex tachycardias, Prog CV Nurs 2:130, 1987.

13. Geddes LE: Monitoring the patient with conduction disturbances and blocks, Nurs Clin North Am 22(1):33, 1987.

14. Grauer K: A practical guide to ECG interpretation, St. Louis, 1993, Mosby–Year Book.

15. Guidelines for cardiopulmonary resuscitation and emergency care—Part III: adult advance cardiac life support, JAMA 268(16):2199, 1992.

16. Hayes JJ et al: Narrow QRS ventricular tachycardia, Ann Intern Med 114(6):460, 1991.

17. Josephson ME, Wellens HJL: Differential diagnosis of supraventricular tachycardia, Cardiol Clin 8:411, 1990.

18. Kindwall KE, Brown J, Josephson ME: Electrocardiographic criteria for ventricular tachycardia in wide complex left bundle branch block morphology tachycardia, Am J Cardiol 61:1279, 1988.

19. Knapik ML: Determination of electrical axis deviation, Crit Care Nurs 10(6):57, 1990.

20. Kreger BE et al: Prevalence of intraventricular block in the general population: the Framingham study, Am Heart J 117(4):903, 1989.

21. Marcadet DM et al: Frequency of exercise-induced left hemiblock, Am J Cardiol 66(19):1390, 1990.

22. Marriott HJL: Practical electrocardiography, ed 8, Baltimore, 1988, Williams & Wilkins.

23. Marriott HJL, Conover MB: Advanced concepts in arrhythmias, ed 2, St. Louis, 1989, CV Mosby.

24. Miller JM et al: Relationship between the 12-lead electrocardiogram during ventricular tachycardia and endocardial site of origin in patients with coronary artery disease, Circulation 77:759, 1988.

25. Ricou F et al: Influence of right bundle branch block on short- and long-term survival after acute anterior myocardial infarction, J Am Coll Cardiol 17(4):858, 1991.

26. Rinkenberger RL, Naccarelli GV: Evaluation and acute treatment of wide complex tachycardias, Crit Care Clin 5(3):599, 1989.

27. Rosenfeld LE: Bradyarrhythmias, abnormalitites of conduction and indications for pacing in acute myocardial infarction, Cardiol Clin 6(1):49, 1988.

28. Sager PT et al: Wide complex tachycardias: differential diagnosis and management, Cardiol Clin 9(4):595, 1991.

29. Steinman RT et al: Wide QRS tachycardia in the conscious adult—ventricular tachycardia is the most frequent cause, JAMA 261(7):1013, 1989.

30. Tchou P et al: Useful clinical criteria for the diagnosis of VT, Am J Med 84:53, 1988.

31. Underhil SL et al: Cardiac nursing, ed 2, Philadelphia, 1989, JB Lippincott.

32. Wellens JJ, Brugada P: Diagnosis of ventricular tachycardia from the 12-lead electrocardiogram, Cardiol Clin 5(3):511, 1987.

33. Wrenn K: Management strategies in wide QRS complex tachycardia, Am J Emerg Med 9(6):592, 1991.

Mechanical Complications in Coronary Artery Disease: Heart Failure and Shock

Darie S. Gilliam, RN, MSN, CCRN

HEART FAILURE

The function of the heart is to provide an adequate supply of oxygenated blood to the body's tissues to meet their metabolic demands. In an attempt to meet these demands, the heart pumps out a certain amount of oxygenated blood per minute, known as the *cardiac output.* This pumping action of the heart muscle is considered the mechanical activity. When the cardiac output falls as a result of muscle or mechanical dysfunction and it no longer adequately meets tissue demands, the heart has failed to perform as an effective pump. This state is called *heart failure,* also known as "pump" failure.[17] Heart failure, then, may be defined as cardiac output that is inadequate to meet tissue demands and in which the pump is the direct cause of the imbalance.[13,24]

Congestive heart failure (CHF) currently affects more than 2 million Americans and is increasing in incidence. It is the most common diagnosis and cause of in-hospital mortality for patients with cardiac disease.[2,13,18,22,24,33] The most common cause of CHF is hypertension, followed by coronary artery disease (CAD). With the emphasis on early diagnosis and effective treatment of hypertension, CAD soon will be the

most common cause of CHF. Two factors that seem to increase the prevalence of CHF are the increasing age of the population and longer survival rates of people with CAD. As people survive longer, they are more likely to develop CHF and require hospitalization.[2,18]

The function of the heart as a pump depends on three main factors: (1) resistance to ejection of blood from the heart (systemic vascular resistance), (2) venous return to the heart, which is relative to venous tone and total intravascular blood volume, and (3) contractility of the heart muscle (Fig. 8-1). Disturbances in any of these factors may either cause or enhance mechanical dysfunction of the heart, resulting in heart failure.

The systemic vascular resistance (SVR) is also known as the heart's *afterload* (see Unit 1). The afterload is the sum of all the loads against which the myocardium must contract during systole or the resistance to ventricular ejection associated with aortic valve opening. Aortic valve opening and ventricular ejection are limited by the SVR, or the pressure in the aorta during diastole.[7]

Another way to view afterload is to think of the aortic valve as a door; one person is

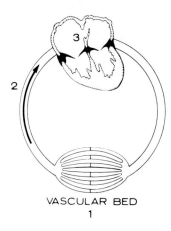

Fig. 8-1 Major determinants of pump function.

trying to push the door open (ventricular ejection) and on the other side someone is trying to hold it closed (SVR/diastolic pressure). If the person pushing the door open is not as strong as the person holding it closed, there is a greater pressure keeping it closed (i.e., increased afterload).

If the heart must pump against an increased SVR or afterload, heart failure may occur. Since SVR is a major determinant of the arterial blood pressure, systemic hypertension is an example of an increased pressure load or afterload.[13]

Venous return to the heart is also known as the *preload* to the heart (see Unit 1). Preload is the passive load of blood that establishes the stretch of the ventricular myocardium prior to contraction. It therefore corresponds to the volume of blood entering the ventricle during *diastole*. Starling's law of the heart states that an increase in preload will increase the muscle stretch and force of contraction and thus increase the cardiac output.[13] At some point, however, the increase in volume becomes an overload. The muscle becomes overstretched and contracts less effectively, actually decreasing cardiac output.

If the heart is presented with excessive volume or a preload that it is unable to pump, heart failure may occur. Administration of large amounts of intravenous fluids is one cause of increased volume load. Any fluid overload is a potential source of heart failure in patients with borderline cardiac reserve. Mitral insufficiency and ventricular septal defect (VSD) are examples of internal volume load problems that can occur in acute myocardial infarction (MI) and can further overload the heart.

Contractility, or *inotropy*, of the heart is reflected in the speed and force of each myocardial contraction.[7,14] If the heart muscle, or *myocardium*, is damaged, contractility is weakened and heart failure may occur. In acute MI, the myocardium is damaged and the practitioner can expect some manifestations of heart failure.

The right and left sides of the heart may fail together or separately. Therefore, heart failure may be left ventricular failure, right ventricular failure, or both. Heart failure in acute MI is usually left ventricular failure. Right ventricular failure usually occurs as a result of left ventricular failure. Right ventricular failure, however, may occur in the absence of left ventricular failure, in inferior wall MI with right ventricular infarction (see Unit 5). Right ventricular failure may also occur as a result of pulmonary hypertension in acute or chronic lung disease.

When the heart fails as a pump, the involved ventricle(s) cannot empty effectively. As a result, the blood becomes congested within the ventricle, causing an increased pressure in the heart and in the blood vessels that drain into the heart. The patient will exhibit symptoms caused by this congestion and increased pressure. Heart failure is thus frequently called *congestive* heart failure, or CHF.[2]

The initial sign of ventricular congestion is the appearance of the extra heart sound called an S_3 *gallop* (see Auscultation of the Heart).[2] However, the major symptoms of CHF are a consequence of either pulmonary

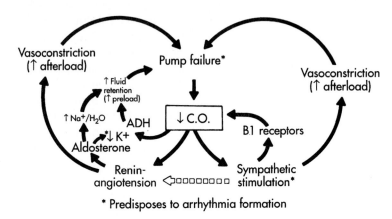

Fig. 8-2 Neurohormonal responses in congestive heart failure (CHF): potentiating effects.

or systemic pressure increases and congestion, depending on whether left or right ventricular failure is present. These symptoms occur secondary to the ineffective emptying of the heart, which in turn results in changes in ventricular filling or diastole, thus indirectly reflecting the changes in cardiac output.

The ineffective ventricular emptying associated with pump failure is also reflected by a decreased ejection fraction, which echocardiographic or nuclear diagnostic studies may detect (see Unit 5). *Ejection fraction* is the percentage of the ventricular diastolic volume ejected with each systolic event. Decreased left ventricular ejection fraction has functional and prognostic implications and may offer guidance for therapy such as exercise training and surgical intervention.

The major direct manifestations of an initial fall in cardiac output occurring in heart failure include tachycardia, fatigue, and serum and urine electrolyte changes, which reflect neurohormonal responses. The initial fall in cardiac output is sensed by systemic receptors and triggers activation of both the sympathetic and the renin-angiotension systems (see Unit 4). These neurohormonal changes often potentiate or aggravate the

problem and have implications for pharmacologic intervention (Fig. 8-2).[2,20]

Stimulation of the sympathetic nervous system results in vasoconstriction, increased heart rate, and increased contractility. Sustained activation of this compensatory mechanism is thought to eventually lead to exhaustion, with loss of these compensatory responses and deterioration of the heart failure. "Downregulation" of the sympathetic beta$_1$ (cardiac) receptors over time is at least partially responsible.[2,19] Researchers have reported a decrease in both numbers of the receptors and their sensitivity. Pharmacologic agents mediated by sympathetic channels may no longer be effective. Since the alpha (blood vessels) receptors are not downregulated, vasoconstrictive responses remain, producing an increased afterload for the failing heart.[2]

Stimulation of the renin-angiotension-aldosterone system results in vasoconstriction and aldosterone release, which triggers Na$^+$ and fluid retention and K+ excretion.[26] These changes promote fluid retention, increasing preload. Together with sympathetic signals, these changes can trigger arrhythmias, further compromising borderline cardiac reserve.[2,20] The renin-angiotension-al-

Table 8-1. The New York Heart Association Classification system for congestive heart failure based on functional limitations

Class	Limitations
I	No limitations (i.e., no symptoms of dyspnea, fatigue, or palpitation with ordinary physical activity)
II	Slight limitation (i.e., occurrence of the above symptoms with ordinary physical activity)
III	Marked limitation (i.e., occurrence of symptoms with less than ordinary activity)
IV	Symptoms present even at rest

Table 8-2. The Killip classification system for congestive heart failure (CHF) based on the presence and severity of symptomatology

Class	Symptomatology
I	Absence of crackles (rales) and S_3 (i.e., absence of CHF)
II	Crackles (rales) in the lower half of the lung fields and S_3 (i.e., mild to moderate CHF)
III	Acute pulmonary edema (i.e., severe CHF)
IV	Systolic blood pressure less than 90 mm Hg with oliguria and decreased level of consciousness (i.e., cardiogenic shock)

dosterone system is partially stimulated by sympathetic signals via beta$_1$ channels. Release of antidiuretic hormone (ADH) is also stimulated via the osmoreceptors, promoting further fluid retention and acting as an additional vasoconstrictor. Interruption of these neurohormonal cycles at any of various key points can prevent negative effects and restore positive compensatory efforts.[20]

The fall in cardiac output associated with CHF may produce functional limitations as a result of the associated decrease in oxygen supply and increase in energy demands. Pa-

tients can be classified into subsets describing the severity of these limitations or other symptoms of CHF. The popular New York Heart Association Classification system is based on functional limitations (Table 8-1).[13,21] The Killip classification system is based on the presence and severity of congestive symptomatology in patients with acute MI (Table 8-2).[1] As heart failure progresses to cardiogenic shock, signs of a significant fall in cardiac output appear. These symptoms include metabolic and cerebral signs of altered tissue perfusion (see Shock Syndrome).

Left ventricular failure

When the left ventricle is damaged, the heart cannot function efficiently as a pump. As a result, blood becomes backed up or congested within the left ventricle. This effect produces increased pressure within the left ventricle. The increase in ventricular contents and pressure interferes with effec-

tive filling. Thus the filling, or diastolic, pressure of the left ventricle rises. This pressure is transmitted retrogradely or backward to the communicating left atrium and to the pulmonary veins draining into the left side of the heart (Fig. 8-3). The atrial distention that occurs with the increased pressure

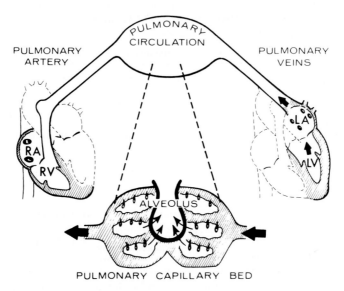

Fig. 8-3 Left ventricular failure: pressure changes and effects.

stretches the atrial muscle fibers, causing electrical instability and commonly producing atrial arrhythmias.[7]

In left ventricular failure the pressure may eventually back up into the pulmonary capillaries. The increase in pulmonary capillary pressure and congestion of blood in the pulmonary vascular bed cause fluid to escape from the alveolar capillaries into the interstitial spaces of the lungs (Fig. 8-3). This initial state is known as *interstitial pulmonary edema.*[15] Fluid may then transudate into the alveoli, interfering with gas exchange and leading to symptoms of hypoxemia.[8,13]

When the cause of pulmonary edema is cardiac disease, it is called *cardiogenic pulmonary edema* to differentiate it from other primary respiratory causes.[6,8,31]

Pulmonary congestion (edema) may be manifested by abnormal breath sounds, tachypnea, dyspnea, orthopnea, paroxysmal nocturnal dyspnea, and cough. Initially, these signs and symptoms occur with exertion but eventually they occur at rest. The abnormal breath sounds known as crackles can occur secondary to interstitial fluid changes and

may be present before tachypnea or other subjective symptoms appear. *Crackles,* previously called *rales,* are currently thought to be caused by pressure variations during the opening of small or medium airways. However, normal airway opening with inspiration does not produce these sounds. These pressure variations occur primarily with the opening of atelectatic airways or in the presence of interstitial fluid (see Unit 3). In early CHF, these extra or adventitious sounds are fine crackling sounds, most audible at the end of inspiration, and do not disappear with coughing.[13,16,21]

Crackles in CHF may be audible in the bases bilaterally or unilaterally on the right side.[2] The examiner may detect early left ventricular failure on chest x-ray films as pulmonary venous engorgement before hearing crackles at the bedside. With congestion in the pulmonary vasculature, enough irritation may exist to precipitate bronchoconstriction, producing *wheezes.*[7] The examiner will hear wheezing as musical sounds either at the mouth or through the stethoscope, usually on expiration.[8,21]

Dyspnea is a subjective sensation of difficulty in breathing, often described as shortness of breath and accompanied by tachypnea. In CHF this symptom is directly related to an increase in pulmonary pressure secondary to left ventricular failure. Pulmonary congestion causes the lungs to become stiff and less compliant. The result is an increase in the work of breathing, manifested symptomatically as dyspnea. The symptoms of dyspnea are related to position. *Orthopnea* implies that a patient with stiff, congested lungs has greater dyspnea when in the recumbent position and less dyspnea when in the upright position. In the upright position, venous return is decreased, hydrostatic pressure is decreased, and lung capacity is increased, thus decreasing the work of breathing. A severe form of orthopnea is *paroxysmal nocturnal dyspnea*. With this the patient awakens from sleep gasping for breath and sits up in an erect position.[13,21]

With acute or severe pulmonary edema these signs and symptoms of congestion are more dramatic. The patient is extremely breathless, anxious, and restless. The use of accessory muscles of the chest and neck is evident and the respiratory rate increases. Expectoration of pink, frothy sputum gives the patient a feeling of suffocation or drowning, further increasing anxiety. The increased work of breathing increases the work load on the heart, further compromising cardiac function.[7,13] In acute pulmonary edema tissue symptoms of hypoxia are evident and are reflected in the arterial blood gases as metabolic acidosis. In the early stage of pulmonary edema, respiratory alkalosis may occur as a result of hyperventilation. As the edema progresses, this changes to respiratory acidosis due to impairment in CO_2 excretion (see Unit 3).[7,13]

Right ventricular failure

The most common cause of right ventricular failure is left ventricular failure. Left ventricular failure increases the pressure in the pulmonary circulation. This pressure can eventually back up to the right ventricle, causing overload and congestion.[13,14] In acute and chronic pulmonary disease or right ventricular infarction, primary right ventricular failure is often present.

The earliest sign of right ventricular failure is an increased right atrial pressure, which is also called central venous pressure (CVP). CVP can be measured by placing a catheter into the right atrium, usually via the internal jugular or subclavian vein. This catheter can be used to infuse fluids and monitor the CVP. An increase in CVP *directly* indicates an increase in pressure of the right side of the heart.[13,14] An increased CVP may *indirectly* reflect left ventricular failure if left heart failure is the cause of the right heart failure. Patients with chronic left ventricular failure may develop right ventricular failure over time. However, in acute MI, the symptoms of right ventricular failure are uncommon unless the infarction is extensive or right ventricular infarction is present.

An increase in the right atrial pressure (CVP) can be evident clinically as distention of the neck veins, or jugular venous distention (JVD). These neck veins feed into the superior vena cava and the right atrium. As the right atrial pressure increases, the pressure and congestion back up into the venous side of the systemic circulation.[7] Just as pulmonary edema is a symptom of left ventricular failure, systemic edema is a symptom of right ventricular failure (Fig. 8-4).

The problem of systemic congestion may be manifested by liver enlargement (hepatomegaly) and peripheral edema. The liver becomes enlarged as a result of chronic, passive venous engorgement caused by the backup of blood from the increased pressure in the right heart. As the failure continues, the increased venous pressure results in in-

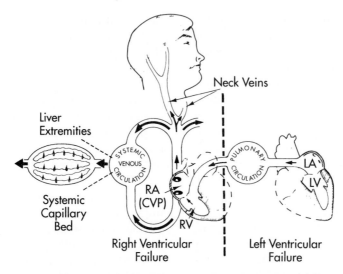

Fig. 8-4   Right ventricular failure: pressure changes and effects.

creased capillary permeability and leaking of fluid into the abdominal cavity, causing *ascites*. The increase in intraabdominal pressure may precipitate gastrointestinal complaints such as nausea, anorexia, or a feeling of fullness.[2,14]

Peripheral edema, a late sign of heart failure, is most obvious in the dependent parts of the body, usually in the feet and ankles in ambulatory patients. If the patient is bedridden, the edema will be most evident over the sacral area.[2,13,14] The patient may experience a weight gain of 10 to 15 pounds of fluid (4 to 7 liters) before the occurrence of pitting edema.[2,14] This peripheral edema be-

Therapy

Routine therapy in the management of heart failure focuses on decreasing the cardiac work load and supporting myocardial contractility. First-line pharmacologic therapy in the general management of heart failure is somewhat controversial. The choice of both pharmacologic and nonpharmacologic therapy depends on whether the patient presents with a normal or decreased cardiac output, hypotension or hypertension, myo-

gins in the lower extremities and ascends to the thighs, genitals, or abdomen. This state may eventually progress to an extensive generalized edema of the entire body referred to as *anasarca*.

In right ventricular failure secondary to right ventricular infarction, additional symptoms include Kussmaul's sign and a characteristic hemodynamic pattern mimicking cardiac tamponade. Kussmaul's sign refers to neck vein distention with inspiration and is associated with decreased compliance and increased right ventricular diastolic pressure. Signs of left ventricular failure, such as crackles, are absent.[3,10]

cardial ischemia, signs of significant pulmonary congestion, or arrhythmias.

Cardiac work load may be decreased by reducing preload, afterload, or both. Pharmacologic reduction of preload is routinely accomplished with venodilating agents and agents that limit or decrease circulating blood volume. Drugs that dilate veins such as the nitrates help to decrease preload.[1,13,24] Preload reduction is also accomplished by measures that decrease or limit circulating volume, such as the administration of diuretic agents or restriction of sodium and fluid intake.[2,15,24] Diuretics are commonly administered with vasodilating drugs, causing an additive effect.[2,23] Nitrates are especially helpful in the patient also presenting with chest pain secondary to myocardial ischemia.

Combined preload and afterload reduction is preferred to preload reduction alone in the patient with significant heart failure. A single drug or a combination of drugs may accomplish this goal. Vasodilators such as nitroprusside and the ACE inhibitors affect both veins and arteries, thus decreasing both preload and afterload. Nitroprusside is usually used in combination with inotropic therapy to achieve compensation in the acute setting. Nitroprusside is especially indicated in patients with severe hypertension suggestive of a significantly increased afterload. Hemodynamic monitoring is generally necessary to titrate nitroprusside, particularly in the normotensive patient with CHF. The ACE inhibitors reduce mortality in heart failure and are used in both acute and chronic management. Several clinical trials with enalapril (Vasotec) and captopril (Capoten) in combination with maintenance regimens of digoxin and diuretics have shown a significant reduction in mortality in heart failure.[2] ACE inhibitors also exert a diuretic effect by inhibiting aldosterone release.[15,17,34] Adding an ACE inhibitor may require a reduction or discontinuation of diuretic therapy.

Promoting physical and psychological comfort and rest can assist the patient in conserving energy and further decrease the work load on the heart.[15,24] Measures such as adequate pain management and positioning for comfort are helpful.[7,8] Positioning with legs dependent can also decrease venous return and pulmonary congestion, although it may aggravate peripheral vascular disease. Exercise training in cardiac rehabilitation centers can be helpful in maximizing energy conservation if initial ejection fractions are not severely decreased. Reassurance and explanations of therapies can allay many unwarranted fears.[24] Patients can be psychologically immobilized by the unknown. In addition, fear can stimulate the stress response, activating the sympathetic nervous system and increasing blood pressure, respirations, and heart rate, thus increasing O_2 demands.[13]

Therapy in heart failure may focus on increasing oxygen supply as well as decreasing oxygen demands. The use of supplemental oxygen via nasal cannula at 2 to 4 liters per minute is common in the first 24 to 48 hours. The goal of O_2 therapy is to maintain arterial oxygen saturation levels above 90%–92%.[1,2,13]

Therapy may also be directed toward supporting myocardial contractility. The questions of which positive inotropic agent to use, when drugs should be used, or whether they should be used at all are controversial. Inotropic agents such as dopamine (Intropin) and dobutamine (Dobutrex) are indicated with symptomatic hypotension.[2] Digitalis, once the classic treatment for CHF, is now the center of this controversy. Digitalis increases myocardial contractility but also increases O_2 demands.[23,25] Digitalis is still advocated in the treatment of CHF accompanied by atrial fibrillation with a fast ventricular response.[15,23] Newer inotropic agents reportedly are more effective in the short-term treatment of CHF. Inotropes such as amrinone (Inocor), a phosphodiesterase inhibitor,[2,23] and the sympathetic stimulators dopamine and dobutamine appear to have less harmful effects on O_2 demands.[2,15]

More controversial forms of therapy include the use of beta blockers in mild CHF to block sympathetic overactivity and prevent downgrading of the beta receptors. The use of atrial natriuretic stimulation is also under investigation (see Unit 4).[20]

The treatment of right ventricular failure secondary to right ventricular infarction varies significantly from the treatment of other forms of heart failure. Left ventricular filling pressures are reduced as a result of the decreased right ventricular output. Pulmonary congestion is not present; therefore, measures to decrease venous return are not indicated and may further compromise left ventricular filling. These patients should not receive morphine, nitroglycerin, and diuretics. Instead they require fluid administration to increase right ventricular stretch and output. Dobutamine is the inotrope of choice since it also dilates the pulmonary artery, reducing pulmonary vascular resistance or right ventricular afterload.[3,10] Dual chamber pacing may be necessary if blocks occur, since atrioventricular synchrony is more critical in maintaining cardiac output.

When severe pulmonary edema complicates left ventricular failure, initial therapy focuses on maintaining oxygenation and decreasing pulmonary congestion. The patient should receive supplemental oxygen to compensate for the interference in pulmonary oxygen transport.[1,2,8,9,13] To rapidly correct pulmonary congestion, the practitioner may initiate therapies to decrease the venous return to the heart and lungs, decrease the circulating blood volume, or both. Rapid reduction of venous return involves such measures as positioning, diuretics, morphine sulfate, nitroglycerin, continuous positive airway pressure (CPAP), and positive end-expiratory pressure (PEEP). These measures are currently considered first-line actions by the American Heart Association.[9] The use of rotating tourniquets is no longer routinely indicated.

The patient is positioned with the head of the bed elevated as high as the patient can tolerate (high Fowler's) and the legs dependent to facilitate pooling of venous blood in the lower extremities.[1,2,9,15] Intravenous furosemide (Lasix) is the diuretic of choice because of its immediate vasodilating effect as well as its effects in decreasing circulating blood volume. Improvement in pulmonary congestion can be expected within 20 minutes, often before the diuretic effect is visible.[9] Bumetanide (Bumex) acts similarly but is not advocated by the American Heart Association at this time as the initial diuretic of choice.

Morphine decreases venous return by dilating the peripheral veins and decreasing the respiratory rate. The negative inspiratory pressure associated with breathing increases venous return and pulmonary congestion. The sedative effect of morphine decreases the patient's anxiety, which also assists in stabilizing the patient's respiratory status, promotes patient comfort, and lowers O_2 demands.[1,7,8,13]

Nitroglycerin decreases pulmonary congestion by dilating the veins and decreasing venous return.[1,2,9,11,15] Sublingual nitroglycerin is the recommended initial treatment because of its availability, ease of administration, and rapid onset of action.[9] Isorbide dinitrate spray is another treatment option.

Second-line actions for the patient with acute pulmonary edema include the use of intravenous nitroglycerin (Tridil), nitroprusside (Nipride), dopamine (Intropin), and dobutamine (Dobutrex). The inotropic agents amrinone (Inocor) and digitalis are currently third-line agents. The use of digitalis is recommended primarily in supraventricular tachyarrhythmias. Aminophylline is reserved for patients with severe bronchospasm but without supraventricular tachyarrhythmias.

The use of complete positive-pressure ventilation measures, such as CPAP or PEEP, in the intubated patient decreases venous return to the heart due to the increase in intrathoracic pressure associated with these modalities. CPAP and PEEP also maintain a constant positive-airway pressure, which keeps the alveoli open and allows for improved gas exchange.[8,13,31]

Phlebotomy, which is called *plasmapheresis* when the red blood cells are returned, is a rapid way of decreasing circulating blood volume and venous return by manually withdrawing it from the circulation. In phlebotomy the blood is discarded, a practice now rarely followed.[6,21] More modern techniques such as hemodialysis, continuous arterial-venous hemofiltration (CAVH), ultrafiltration, and peritoneal dialysis may be useful if standard therapy is ineffective in reducing volume.[15,17,34]

NURSING ORDERS: For the patient with heart failure.

RELATED NURSING DIAGNOSIS: Impaired gas exchange related to pulmonary vascular congestion; decreased cardiac output related to alterations in preload, afterload, and/or contractility; activity intolerance; anxiety related to physical and psychological stress

1. Provide cardiac rest.
   —Place patient in semi-Fowler's or Fowler's position.
   —Encourage chair rest.
   —Allow use of commode chair.
   —To relieve psychological stress:
      Explain all procedures in simple terms.
      Allow patient contact with familiar objects.
      Encourage independence and self-care.
      Allow visitors, with limitations as needed.
   —Administer sedatives and analgesics as required.
2. Observe patient for the following overt signs of dyspnea:
   —Shortness of breath
   —Cough
   —Increased respiratory rate.
3. Auscultate the heart and lungs when checking vital signs. Check for:
   —Gallops
   —Murmurs
   —Variations in normal heart sounds
   —Crackles
   —Wheezes
   —Alterations in the quality of normal breath sounds
4. Check CVP and pulmonary artery (PA) readings with vital signs.
   —If there is no CVP or PA catheter, check for the development of neck vein distention or crackles.
5. Watch for the development of tissue symptoms indicating the heart failure is evolving to cardiogenic shock (see Shock Syndrome).
6. In the presence of severe pulmonary edema:
   —Support patient in high Fowler's position with legs dependent.
   —Start O_2 therapy.
   —Ensure patent IV route.
   —Maintain fluid restriction.
   —Obtain vital signs.
   —Have available:
      Resuscitation equipment
      PEEP or CPAP equipment
      Morphine
      Furosemide
      Vasodilators (nitrates, nitroprusside, ACE inhibitors, hydralazine)
      Positive inotropic agents (digitalis, amrinone, dopamine, dobutamine)

HEMODYNAMIC MONITORING

In acute CAD (angina or acute MI), the myocardial changes and resulting mechanical dysfunction alter the movement of blood through the heart and blood vessels. The study of the movement of blood is known as *hemodynamics*. The monitoring of hemodynamic changes is logically referred to as hemodynamic monitoring.

Assessment of cardiovascular function (i.e., hemodynamics) can be both invasive and noninvasive. Noninvasive assessment includes monitoring of heart sounds and detection of clinical signs of pulmonary congestion and decreased cardiac output mentioned earlier in this chapter. Two other currently used noninvasive methods of assessing left ventricular function (both systolic and diastolic) are echocardiography and radionuclide angiography (see Unit 5).

Noninvasive techniques of hemodynamic monitoring have not provided as practical, accurate, or early information about left ventricular function as the invasive modes to date. The advent of the flow-directed, balloon-tipped *pulmonary artery catheter* (first known as the Swan-Ganz catheter) popularized the use of invasive techniques at the bedside. The term *hemodynamics* is currently used more clinically to describe the invasive monitoring of cardiovascular function.

The focus of hemodynamic monitoring is assessment of actual or potential dysfunction of the cardiovascular *mechanical* structures. These mechanical structures include the cardiac muscle, blood vessels, and valves. Mechanical dysfunction within the cardiovascular system presents as either failure or shock.

The indications for invasive hemodynamic monitoring are varied; however, the necessity should exceed the potential risks. Hemodynamic monitoring is not usually indicated in an uncomplicated MI. Indications include hemodynamic instability (i.e., shock, heart failure); potential hemodynamic instability following major cardiovascular surgery; multiple vasoactive or inotropic pharmacologic support; or diagnostic purposes (i.e., to rule out VSD, right ventricular MI, tamponade).[5,13,14,56]

Flow, pressure, and resistance relationships

The three major physiologic parameters reflecting the mechanical function of the cardiovascular system are flow, pressure, and resistance. The heart as a pump creates the driving force that initiates blood *flow*. This flow of blood put out by the heart is more commonly called the cardiac output.[5] *Pressure* is generated within the blood vessels as the force of the blood flow from the heart (the cardiac output) meets resistance or "interference" in the vessel tubes. *Resistance* is determined primarily by the vasoconstriction and/or vasodilation of the smooth muscle lining of the vessels.[13] Systemic blood pressure is the measurement of this pressure within the blood vessels. More specifically, blood pressure reflects the force of the blood against the walls of the arteries during cardiac systole and diastole.

Pressure is also generated within the heart itself as the blood is forced against the chamber walls during systole and diastole. The *compliance* of the chamber wall determines the amount of "interference" to flow during ventricular filling or diastole. Compliance may be defined as the opposition to ventricular filling due to the natural distensibility or stiffness of the muscle wall. It is more accurately reflected by changes in pressure for a given change in volume ($\Delta P/\Delta V$).[7]

The movement of blood within the cardiovascular system is affected by the amount and force of the flow within the blood vessels or within the cardiac chambers and the corresponding resistance and compliance changes. The pressure generated within the blood vessels or heart itself is a reflection of these parameters. Complete hemodynamic monitoring involves the monitoring of all these parameters by information obtained from within both the blood vessels and the heart. Systemic blood pressure, which can be measured by cuff or invasive arterial catheters, reflects only the changes occurring within the blood vessels (i.e., the peripheral arteries). The cardiac pressures and output are monitored by invasive, pulmonary arteries (PA) catheters. Together these parameters provide a basis to assess cardiovascular function and circulating blood volume and guide in the planning and evaluation of therapy.[6,13]

Hemodynamic changes in acute myocardial infarction

The first clinically perceptible hemodynamic change in acute MI occurs within the left ventricle during diastole because of a decrease in compliance. This decrease in compliance is the result of an immediate inflammatory response to decreased coronary blood supply. Decreased compliance secondary to an inflammatory response can occur during episodes of angina as well as during MI (see Units 4 and 5). The muscle wall stiffens and does not stretch well in the presence of a decreased blood supply. As the left ventricle becomes stiffer or less compliant, it has difficulty accepting the entering blood volume and the diastolic pressure rises. Therefore, the first sign of left ventricular dysfunction in acute MI is a rise in left ventricular filling or diastolic pressure, secondary to a decrease in compliance.[7] The major exception is inferior wall MI complicated by right ventricular infarction.

The left ventricular pressure rises first at the *end* of diastole, when most of the blood has entered the ventricle, and is more commonly referred to as a rise in left ventricular end-diastolic pressure (LVEDP).[5] Changes in compliance result in only slight increases in LVEDP, which the patient usually tolerates asymptomatically. These changes are detected clinically either by invasive monitoring or by the presence of an S_4 gallop (see Auscultation of the Heart).[12]

The LVEDP reflects the stretch or load on the left ventricle prior to systole. This filling load is also known as the left ventricular preload.[52] Left ventricular filling pressure is affected not only by compliance changes but also by LV volume and pulmonary venous return, which in turn are affected by the systemic venous return or circulating blood volume.

The second clinically perceptible change in mechanical function affects ventricular systole, resulting in a fall in cardiac output. In the initial stages of myocardial damage, the unaffected fibers may increase their contractility and overcompensate for the loss of effective contractile structures. There is no initial net loss in contractility, and the heart's compensatory mechanisms maintain cardiac output.[7] Subsequent loss of myocardial function results in the inability of intact fibers to compensate for this loss. The cardiac output therefore falls, producing the clinical state of heart failure.

The fall in cardiac output associated with heart failure may be detected clinically by direct invasive techniques or may be inferred by its secondary effects on ventricular diastole. As the cardiac output falls, as a result of mechanical dysfunction, the fraction of the left ventricular diastolic volume ejected during systole (left ventricular ejection fraction) decreases. As a result, the residual volume remaining in the left ventricle at the end of systole rises. Thus at the onset of diastole the left ventricle is already partially full and has difficulty accepting even the initial amounts of entering blood. The left ventricular diastolic pressure rises significantly, initially generating an S_3 gallop (see Auscultation of the Heart).[7,52]

During ventricular diastole, the valve separating the left atrium from the left ventricle is open, forming one chamber with equal pressures. When ventricular diastolic pressure increases, atrial pressure also increases. This increase in pressure is further transmitted retrogradely to the communicating pulmonary veins and capillaries, resulting in the signs and symptoms of pulmonary congestion. The pulmonary congestion corresponds with the decrease in the left ventricular ejection fraction and further increase in LVEDP. In this hemodynamic phase, the diastolic changes are more clinically significant than those associated with simple compliance changes.

A compensatory rise in systemic vascular resistance occurs in response to the fall in cardiac output. This rise in SVR is the body's attempt to maintain the mean arterial pressure.[7] The rise in SVR is not accompanied initially by any significant change in cuff (arterial) pressure and thus may not be detected noninvasively. However, this reflexive rise in SVR (afterload) may further impede and actually decrease cardiac output. The decrease in cardiac output is due to the increased work load on the heart and increased O_2 consumption.[5]

With more extensive damage, a third major hemodynamic change occurs. The cardiac output continues to fall to the point that tissue perfusion becomes compromised in spite of compensatory efforts. When tissue symptoms of hypoxia result from this significant fall in cardiac output, the state is known as shock. When this state occurs as a consequence of severe heart failure, it is known as cardiogenic shock and is associated with a high left ventricular diastolic pressure.

O_2 needs of compromised tissue can be estimated by first determining the body surface area (BSA). The BSA is determined by obtaining the patient's height and weight and plotting them on a Dubois Body Surface Area Chart. The comparison of cardiac output to this BSA is referred to as the *cardiac index* (CI) and is a reflection of potentially compromised tissue O_2 needs.[5] Cardiac index is a more accurate reflection of the critical level of cardiac output in an individual patient and is a preferred hemodynamic measurement upon which to base clinical judgment. Cardiac index is also a key hemodynamic parameter in confirming the presence of shock. The determination of cardiac index requires an exact and, therefore, invasive measurement of cardiac output (see Monitoring Cardiac Output).

When considering the disturbances in myocardial function that occur in MI, the practitioner must also evaluate the factors affecting myocardial O_2 consumption (MVO_2). The determinants of MVO_2 are heart rate, preload, afterload, and contractility. These are also the major determinants of an adequate cardiac output. While a significant increase in any of these parameters can increase the MVO_2, a significant decrease in any of these may compromise the cardiac output. Thus both extremes are to be avoided.

Monitoring cardiac pressures

The goal of monitoring cardiac pressure changes in acute MI is to detect, as accurately as possible, early hemodynamic changes. The initial hemodynamic changes occurring in acute MI affect left ventricular diastolic pressure. Since maximum diastolic pressures are reached at the end of diastole, minor increases in filling pressures are first detectable at the end of diastole (i.e., LVEDP).

The most accurate measurement of LVEDP is obtained directly by a left atrial catheter, measuring the left atrial pressure (LAP). The LAP in diastole is equal to the LVEDP, because the mitral valve is open and they are like one chamber with the same pressure. The left atrial (LA) catheter must be placed, during cardiac surgery, directly into the left atrium, exiting through the chest wall to be attached to monitoring equipment. The use of this catheter poses a risk of air emboli to the brain from accidental introduction through the line. Another high risk is cardiac tamponade after removal of the line. Therefore, this catheter is not often used.[8,13]

Since the right side of the heart is more

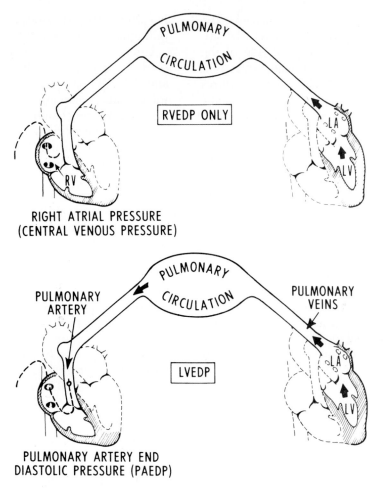

Fig. 8-5 Right atrial (central venous) pressure versus pulmonary artery diastolic pressure. Detection of critical right ventricular versus left ventricular changes with catheters in each location.

easily accessible via the venous system, indirect monitoring of left ventricular pressures is now accomplished with catheters introduced into the right side of the heart. Early attempts to monitor left ventricular function were made through catheters introduced into the right atrium to record right atrial (RA) pressures, also known as central venous pressure (CVP).

The RA pressure is the same as the right ventricular end-diastolic pressure (RVEDP) since the tricuspid valve is open during dias-

tole, allowing the right atrium and right ventricle to communicate with each other and act as one chamber (Fig. 8-5).[56] In the absence of tricuspid valve disease, RVEDP and RA pressure (CVP) are equal and range from 0 to 6 mm Hg.[12] In low cardiac output states, higher pressures may be necessary to maintain the cardiac output. Significant venous congestion typically occurs when these pressures exceed 12 mm Hg. The RA pressure and RVEDP are not considered *critically* elevated until they exceed this upper therapeutic limit of 12 mm Hg.

The RA pressure (CVP) and RVEDP reflect venous return to the right side of the heart (right ventricular preload) and right ventricular function.[12] However, pressures from the right side of the heart are usually poor indicators of left ventricular function.[12] During diastole, the closed pulmonic valve limits communication with the pulmonary circulation and left side of the heart. In acute MI, the CVP and RVEDP may be normal in the presence of an elevated LVEDP. The CVP is used to detect the presence of right ventricular failure especially in pulmonary disease or right ventricular infarction. In right ventricular failure secondary to right ventricular infarction, the CVP and RVEDP are elevated as a result of both decreased compliance and congestion of blood within the right ventricle. The LV pressures are usually normal or low because of decreased left ventricular filling from poor right ventricular contraction.[4,60]

Pressures recorded from the pulmonary artery correlate more closely with left ventricular function than RA pressures. The PA catheter is situated beyond the pulmonic valve. Closure of this valve during ventricular diastole interrupts communication with the right side of the heart. However, direct communication is maintained with the pulmonary circulation (which has no valves) and the left atrium (see Fig. 8-5).[5]

Since the left atrium and left ventricle are like one chamber in diastole, communication is then established between the pulmonary artery and left ventricle. Thus pulmonary artery end-diastolic pressure (PAEDP) closely approximates the pressure in the pulmonary circulation and, in the absence of pulmonary or mitral valve disease, LA pressure and LVEDP.[4,5] Normal PAEDP ranges from 6 to 12 mm Hg and is usually only slightly higher than the LVEDP (2 to 4 mm Hg). The PAEDP is not considered *critically* elevated until it exceeds the upper therapeutic limits of 18 mm

Hg which may be associated with significant pulmonary congestion.[5,12]

Unlike the CVP, PA pressures are recorded separately as PA systolic pressure and PAEDP. During systole the pulmonic valve is open, making the PA and the right ventricle as one chamber. Therefore the PA and right ventricular systolic pressures are the same. The normal PA and right ventricular systolic pressures range from 15 to 30 mm Hg.[12]

In pulmonary disease, the pulmonary vascular resistance and systolic and diastolic pressures are typically elevated. These pressures may also be elevated in severe CHF. Thus PA systolic and diastolic pressures alone are not helpful in differentiating pulmonary disease from CHF.[4,5]

Although the monitoring of PA diastolic pressure in acute MI is a useful index of left ventricular function, there is a more accurate measurement. The balloon of the PA catheter can be intermittently reinflated, allowing the catheter to float or advance farther into a smaller PA branch. When the catheter is in this position, it is said to be wedged in the vessel. The pressure obtained after the catheter is wedged is known as the *pulmonary artery wedge pressure* (PAWP or PAW).[4,8] Because the catheter, when wedged in this position, is closer to the pulmonary capillary bed than it is to the main PA, the pressure is more accurately called the *pulmonary capillary wedge pressure* (PCWP).[6,52] Since a PA branch is temporarily occluded while obtaining this reading, it is also known as the *pulmonary artery occlusion pressure* (PAOP).

The wedging of the catheter in a small PA branch interrupts communication with the right side of the heart and part of the pulmonary circulation. When the balloon is inflated, the distal tip can no longer "see" the main PA or the right side of the heart behind the balloon.[6] Instead, the tip "sees" directly through the capillary bed, which has no valves, into the left atrium, which com-

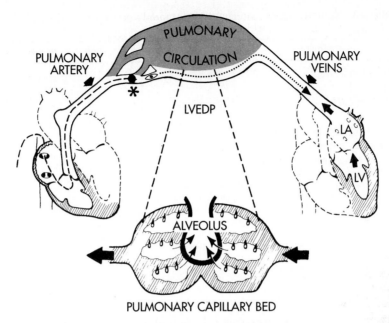

Fig. 8-6 Pulmonary capillary wedge pressure (PCWP) or pulmonary artery occlusion pressure (PAOP). Monitoring of left ventricular diastolic pressure.

municates with the left ventricle in diastole (Fig. 8-6). Since there is no forward flow in the small vessel while the balloon is inflated, the tip does not read the pressure in the rest of the pulmonary circulation nor is it affected by pulmonary vascular resistance. Therefore, as compared with the PA pressure, the PCWP is a more accurate index of left atrial and left ventricular end-diastolic function. The PCWP is considered equal to LVEDP in the absence of pulmonary and mitral valve disease.[4,5]

Normally, LVEDP is approximately 6 to 12 mm Hg. Some sources quote lower normal limits of 4 to 12 mm Hg.[4,5,54] Elevations in LVEDP of up to 15 mm Hg can be expected in acute MI and may be caused by altered compliance, even in the absence of CHF.[12] However, the LVEDP is not considered critically elevated until it exceeds 18 mm Hg.[5,12] Since the PCWP usually reflects LVEDP, PCWP readings should not exceed 18 mmHg in acute MI. Increases in pressure

beyond this level may indicate greater left ventricular dysfunction and predict impending pulmonary congestion. Interstitial pulmonary edema usually occurs when the PCWP ranges between 18 mm Hg and 25 mm Hg, as manifested by symptoms such as dyspnea and crackles. As the PCWP exceeds 25 mm Hg, the fluid transudates into the alveoli, causing severe pulmonary edema, with expectoration of pink, frothy sputum.[14]

Although still within the normal limits, a PCWP of 5 mm Hg indicates a low LVEDP if the cardiac output is compromised. The most likely explanation for this would be decreased left ventricular filling caused by blood volume depletion (hypovolemia). Even a damaged myocardium requires a certain amount of stretch during diastole to promote effective contraction and cardiac output during systole. Stretching of the myocardium during diastole actually promotes contraction (Starling's law).[7] The detection of a low PCWP in the presence of a low cardiac

Table 8-3. Hemodynamic patterns that commonly occur in certain clinical conditions

Condition	CVP	PAS	PAD	PCWP	CI
Hypovolemia	↓	↓	↓	—↓	—↓
AMI c̄ LVF	*—↑	↑	↑	↑	—↓ †
RVF 2° RVMI	↑	↑	—↑	—	↓
Tamponade	↑	↑	↑	↑	↓
Acute lung disease (pulmonary embolus, ARDS)	—↑	↑	↑	—↓	—↓ ‡
Chronic lung disease (COPD, cor pulmonale)	↑	↑	↑	—	—

CVP = central venous pressure; PAS = pulmonary artery systolic pressure; PAD = pulmonary artery diastolic pressure; PCWP = pulmonary capillary wedge pressure; CI = cardiac index; AMI c̄ LVF = acute myocardial infarction with left ventricular failure; RVF 2° RVMI = right ventricular failure secondary to right ventricular myocardial infarction; ARDS = adult respiratory distress syndrome; COPD = chronic obstructive pulmonary disease; ↓ = decreased; ↑ = elevated; — = normal.
*CVP may be elevated if RVF occurs from LVF.
†Progressed to cardiogenic shock if CI is low.
‡CI may decrease with the use of PEEP.

output indicates inadequate left ventricular filling pressures (left ventricular preload).[4] Optimization of preload consists of IV fluid administration until the cardiac output is adequate. During this time the PAEDP and PCWP should be carefully maintained below 18 mm Hg to prevent pulmonary edema.[12,57]

The PAEDP is usually 2 to 4 mm Hg higher than the PCWP and LVEDP. When the PAEDP is essentially equal to the PCWP (+2 to 4 mm Hg) in a given patient, this parameter can be used in lieu of wedge pressure readings.[4,5] Complications associated with prolonged balloon inflation or rupture are thus avoided.

PAEDP more than 4 to 5 mm Hg higher than the PCWP indicates increased pulmonary vascular resistance (PVR). The elevated PVR may be caused by such pulmonary problems as chronic obstructive pulmonary disease (COPD), pulmonary embolus, or adult respiratory distress syndrome (ARDS). In this situation the PAEDP no longer reflects the LVEDP and requires separate measurement of the PCWP.[4,5]

Under certain circumstances neither the PAEDP nor the PCWP accurately reflects the LVEDP. With mitral valve dysfunction or heart rates greater than 130 to 140, ventricular filling may be inadequate. With mitral valve regurgitation blood flows back into the right atrium during systole, causing higher pressures in the left atrium. Thus both the PAEDP and PCWP are increased over the LVEDP. In mitral valve stenosis less blood gets through the stenotic valve, and with fast heart rates the ventricular filling time decreases. In both of these conditions left atrial pressure increases, raising the PAEDP and PCWP but not the LVEDP.[4,12]

The nurse should remember to observe for trends occurring in hemodynamic patterns rather than reacting to single values. Awareness of commonly occurring hemodynamic patterns is important (Table 8-3).[5,12] Understanding the implications of an increase or decrease in these pressures assists the nurse in planning and implementing care.

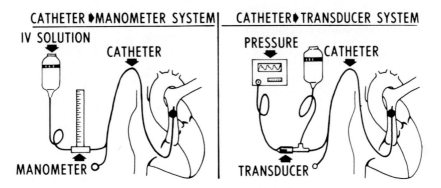

Fig. 8-7 Methods of recording pressures.

Atrial patterns (or pulmonary capillary wedge pattern)

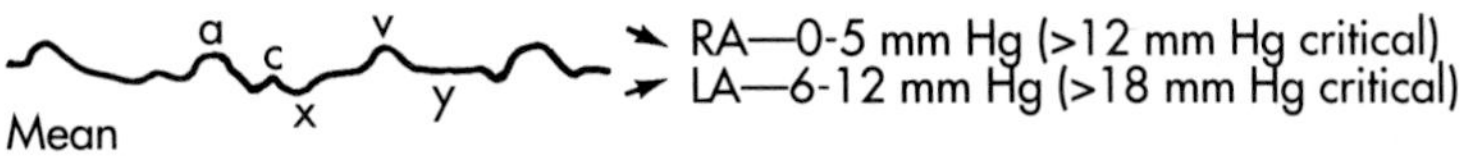

Mean

RA—0-5 mm Hg (>12 mm Hg critical)
LA—6-12 mm Hg (>18 mm Hg critical)

a = Atrial contraction
c = Bulging of AV valve into atria with early ventricular contraction
        (usually not seen with PCWP)
v = Ventricular contraction
x and y = Drop in pressure with atrial relaxation and filling

Fig. 8-8 Atrial pressure waveform pattern—right atrial (RA/CVP) or left atrial (PCWP).

Normal pressure waveforms

Continuous monitoring of the pressure waveforms is necessary to effectively monitor catheter position, assess for acute changes in hemodynamic status, record pressures accurately, and avoid some of the complications of invasive monitoring. Although pressure values can be recorded with a catheter-manometer system, a record of the pressure waveform can be obtained only with the use of a catheter-transducer system (Fig. 8-7). A transducer is a device that changes one form of energy into another.[56] In this case a transducer changes pressure into an electrical signal that can provide an oscilloscope pattern and record. The water manometer was the original technique for measuring CVP.[5] The advent of the catheter-transducer systems allowed characteristic patterns to be recorded from either atria, ventricles, or arteries. Recognition of these characteristic patterns is now fundamental in the nursing management of critical care patients.

The waveforms most often monitored are those corresponding to the PA, CVP (RA), and arterial pressures. PCWP (LA) patterns are obtained intermittently. Each waveform is discussed separately here.

Pressures within the right and left *atria* rise quickly with onset of atrial contraction, producing an atrial systolic pulse wave recorded as the *a wave* (Fig. 8-8). The *c wave* represents the bulging of the AV valve into the atria with AV valve closure and early ventricular contraction and coincides with the carotid pulse. The *v wave* is caused by an increase in pressure from atrial filling that occurs during ventricular contraction. The x and y descents reflect the drop in pressure with atrial relaxation and ventricular filling, respectively.[5,14,56]

Because the force of atrial contraction is not as great as the force of ventricular contraction, the atrial systolic pulse (a wave) is not as distinctly recorded on the oscilloscope or recording paper. The atria are also influenced by ventricular contraction, which produces extra pulsation (c,v waves) in the pressure pattern. As a result, atrial waveforms do not exhibit the distinct systolic and diastolic fluctuations noted in ventricular and arterial patterns. Instead, atrial waveforms usually assume a wavy configuration, especially at low pressures. The separate atrial waves are more clearly differentiated at higher pressures or in the presence of pathology. The RA (CVP) and LA (PCWP) waveforms have the same configuration, but the LA pressures are normally higher (see Fig. 8-8). The c wave in the PCWP waveform is not always visible because of the distance of the mitral valve from where the PA catheter is wedged. An average, or mean, pressure level is calculated, displayed, and recorded using the formula:

1/3 (systolic-diastolic) + diastolic = mean (systole = 1/3 and diastole = 2/3 of the cardiac cycle).[5]

Pressure within the right and left *ventricles* rises quickly with the onset of ventricular contraction, or systole. It rapidly reaches a point referred to as the peak systolic pressure. As systolic ejection is completed, the semilunar valves close, separating the ventricles from the great vessels (pulmonary artery and aorta) leaving them. The pressure in the ventricles drops abruptly as ventricular filling, or diastole, begins. The ventricular end-diastole pressure is recorded just before the

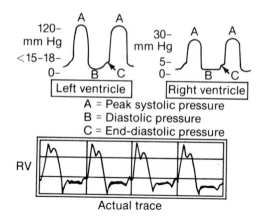

Fig. 8-9 Ventricular pressure waveform pattern—right ventricular (RV) or left ventricular (LV).

onset of the next systole (Fig. 8-9). Right and left ventricular patterns are not monitored routinely but are important for understanding hemodynamics and the relationship with other pressures and waveforms. A right ventricular pattern may signify inadvertent displacement of a PA catheter back into the right ventricle, where ventricular ectopy may be induced.

The pressure within the major *arteries* (pulmonary artery and aorta) rises quickly as blood is ejected into them with the onset of ventricular systole and it rapidly reaches a peak systolic pressure. As previously discussed, the PA and the right ventricular pressures are equal in systole. The aortic and left ventricular pressures also are equal in systole. Arterial systolic pressures reflect the changes occurring in the arteries (PA, aorta, and periphery) during systole.

With the onset of ventricular diastole, the semilunar valves close, separating the great vessels from the ventricles. As the valves snap shut, a small notch is produced in the waveform, which is called the *dicrotic notch*. The dicrotic notch in the PA waveform represents closure of the pulmonic valve and, in

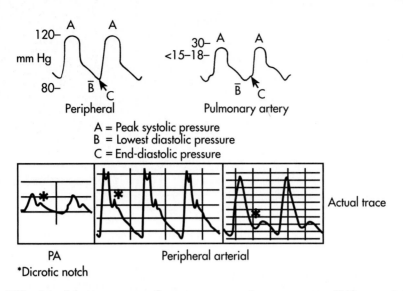

A = Peak systolic pressure
B = Lowest diastolic pressure
C = End-diastolic pressure

*Dicrotic notch

Fig. 8-10 Arterial pressure waveform pattern—pulmonary artery (PA) or peripheral artery (radial/femoral). The dicrotic notch in the PA waveform represents pulmonic valve closure and in the peripheral waveform represents aortic valve closure.

an aortic or peripheral arterial waveform, closure of the aortic valve (Fig. 8-10).[4,5]

With the onset of diastole the pressure in the vessels drops gradually as the blood still within them is dispersed throughout the vascular bed (PA → pulmonary capillary bed; aorta → systemic vascular bed). Ventricular diastolic pressure drops abruptly; therefore, the ventricular and arterial systolic patterns are similar but their diastolic patterns are distinctly different.

The PA waveform should be continuously monitored while the PCWP is taken intermittently. To minimize complications of balloon inflation, inflating the balloon can be limited to once an hour, or to every 4 hours if the PCWP correlates with the PAEDP. The PCWP waveform should make a distinct change from the PA waveform on inflation of the balloon with air. The oscilloscope should be observed for this change as the balloon is slowly inflated. After the change in waveform is observed, the balloon should not be further inflated (Fig. 8-11). The catheter should wedge with approximately 1.25 to 1.5 ml of air but never fluid.[54,56] Inflation with fluid or more than 1.5 ml of air could cause the balloon to rupture, resulting in air embolism or PA rupture. If less than 1.25 ml of air results in a wedge waveform, the catheter has migrated to a small branch and should be repositioned to prevent spontaneous inadvertent wedging.[5,54,56,65] The catheter should be wedged the minimal time required to take a reading and recording but no longer than 15 seconds.[4,5] Deflation of the balloon should be confirmed by the return of the PA pattern.

The peripheral arterial pressure waveform (radial/femoral) is similar to the PA waveform but usually has a sharper upstroke and higher pressures (see Fig. 8-10). It also requires continuous monitoring and the alarms should be appropriately set for high and low levels for both the systolic and diastolic pressures. These levels must be individual for each patient depending on the patient's baseline pressure. The average mean arterial pressure (MAP) is calculated, dis-

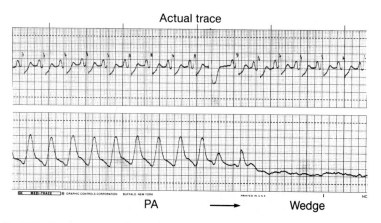

Actual trace

PA ⟶ Wedge

Fig. 8-11   Pressure waveform changes with PA catheter balloon inflation.

played, and recorded using the same formula as with atrial pressures. Normal MAP is 70 to 90 mm Hg.

Simultaneous monitoring of the ECG and arterial pressure allows concurrent assessment of beat to beat perfusion. As discussed, the ECG is first (electrical), followed by the arterial pressure (mechanical). The arterial pressure is also affected by the timing of the ECG. Any arrhythmia may alter the arterial pressure. Both tachycardias and bradycardias as well as irregular rhythms can significantly alter pressures.

Single ectopic beats may alter arterial pressure due to their timing, origin, or both. When a PAC occurs, the ventricular filling time is shortened and the stroke volume may be decreased (Fig. 8-12). In atrial fibrillation atrial contribution is lost to ventricular filling and stroke volume. The ventricular filling pressure and arterial pressure also vary according to irregular R–R cycle lengths. When PVCs occur, the filling time is also decreased, there is no contribution from atrial contraction, and the strength of the ventric-

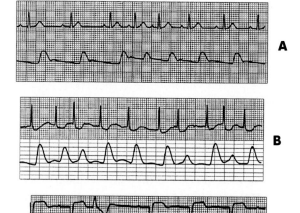

Fig. 8-12   Effects of arrhythmias on peripheral arterial pressure waveforms. PACs *(A)*, atrial fibrillation *(B)*, and PVC *(C)*.

ular contraction may be altered, all decreasing the arterial pressure.[5]

Distorted pressure waveforms

The changes in intrathoracic pressure occurring with inspiration and expiration are transmitted to the RA, PA, and wedge pressure tracings as cyclic increases and decreases in pressure. The intrathoracic pressure is more negative on spontaneous inspiration,

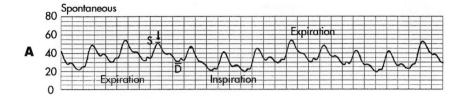

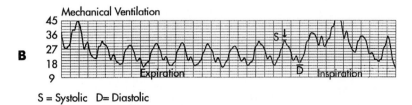

S = Systolic   D= Diastolic

Fig. 8-13 Effects of spontaneous *(A)* and mechanical ventilation *(B)* on PA waveforms. Note inspiratory distortion with return to baseline on expiration. The arrow indicates end expiration.

commonly resulting in a decrease in pressure. Labored breathing, as with severe pulmonary congestion, magnifies these effects. With mechanical ventilation, in contrast to spontaneous breathing, the intrathoracic pressure and corresponding pressure readings are increased on inspiration. With intermittent mandatory ventilation (IMV), inspiratory pressures vary in response to either spontaneous or mechanical ventilation. The heart pressures at end expiration are the least affected by respiration. Therefore, the most accurate readings are obtained at end expiration for all waveforms, with either spontaneous or mechanical ventilation or a mixture of the two (Fig. 8-13).[4,5,47,48] End expiration occurs at a higher (more positive) pressure during spontaneous breaths and at a lower (more negative) pressure during mechanical ventilation.[5,56] The addition of PEEP increases expiration pressure and causes compression of the pulmonary vascular bed, thus elevating the PCWP. However, distortions are minimal in normovolemic patients unless PEEP levels exceed 10 cm H_2O.[47] Placement of the catheter tip below the left atrium minimizes distortions at PEEP levels above 10 cm H_2O. To correct for levels of PEEP in excess of 10 cm H_2O, subtract 1.8 mm Hg for every 5 cm H_2O from the measured wedge pressure.[47]

Normal breathing has a less significant effect on peripheral arterial pressure or waveforms. The increase in right ventricular filling during normal inspiration limits left ventricular filling, producing a paradoxical decrease in left ventricular output and a slight drop in systolic pressure of less than 10 mm Hg. A drop in systolic arterial pressure of more than 10 mm Hg with inspiration is considered abnormal and is called *pulsus paradoxus* (Fig. 8-14). Pulsus paradoxus is a classic sign in cardiac tamponade, which further limits left ventricular filling. Pulsus paradoxus may also occur in patients with constrictive pericarditis or obstructive airway disease. During mechanical ventilation an increase in systolic pressure occurs during inspiration. The positive inspiratory pressure occurring with mechanical ventilation squeezes the blood out of the lungs, increasing LV filling

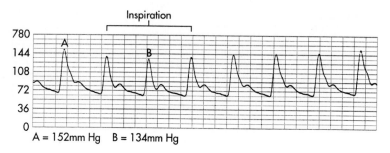

Fig. 8-14   Pulsus paradoxus.

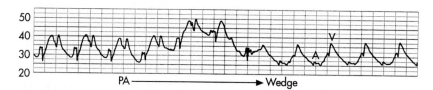

Fig. 8-15   Effects of mitral regurgitation on PA pressure waveforms. A = a wave,
V = v wave.

and output. Hypovolemia magnifies this inspiratory increase in systolic pressure because of a lower baseline cardiac output during expiration. A systolic increase of greater than 10 mm Hg is referred to as reversed or "positive" pulsus paradoxus, and is usually effectively treated with an increase in fluid therapy.[4,63]

To ensure that pressures are an accurate reflection of hemodynamic status, take readings with the patient in the same position. Have the patient supine, with the head of the bed at 60 degrees or less. Initially compare readings obtained in these positions with those obtained with the patient flat to detect occasional discrepancies in individual patients.[47] Do not alter the position of the backrest in the 20 minutes before taking readings. The patient should not be in a side-lying position.[47,50,53] Follow the proper procedure for leveling the transducer to the phlebostatic axis and zeroing the transducer, routinely and after any position change.[49,51,58]

Mitral regurgitation produces a giant V wave distorting both the PA and wedge trac-

ings, making it more difficult to distinguish between them. The V wave immediately follows the systolic peak in the PA tracing, resulting in a notched appearance. As the balloon is inflated, this notch disappears, leaving only the V waves (Fig. 8-15).[5] Mitral regurgitation or insufficiency occurs in angina and/or MI owing to papillary muscle ischemia or infarction. In this case the a wave pressure of the PCWP (instead of the mean) correlates the most closely with LVEDP and should be recorded. Diseases of the aorta or aortic valve can cause alterations in the arterial pressure waveform. With aortic insufficiency there is usually a wide pulse pressure due to an elevated systolic and very low diastolic pressure. The low diastolic pressure reflects the incompetent mitral valve and regurgitation. Since the aortic valve does not close completely, the dicrotic notch is usually not present.[4]

When aortic stenosis is present, the waveform is similar to a damped waveform, which is discussed later in this section. The systolic pressure is lower because ejection is

Table 8-4. Equipment-related distortions of heart and arterial pressure patterns causing inaccurate measurements.*

Problem	Cause	Intervention
Damped tracing	Blood or clot in catheter or transducer system	Aspirate clot with syringe, then flush with heparinized saline and check for loss of pressure of infusion bag or loose connections. If problem persists, change catheter or transducer system as appropriate.
	Air in transducer or tubing or tubing too long	Close stopcock to patient and flush out of system, maintain < 3–4 feet of tubing between patient and transducer.[56,61]
	Catheter tip against vessel wall or kink in catheter	Reposition extremity (arterial line) while observing waveform, and tape securely or notify physician to reposition catheter.
Catheter whip	High-frequency interference	Keep lines free from other equipment and patient. Add high-frequency filter to system. If unresolved, consider using mean pressures.[56]
	PA catheter looped in right ventricle or tip near turbulent flow (pulmonic valve)[56]	Confirm looping on chest radiograph, notify physician to reposition catheter, or add high-frequency filter to system.
	Hemodynamically unstable patient[65]	Consider using mean pressures.
Abnormal high or low meaure-ments	Transducer not level with right atrium	Rezero, with air-fluid interface of stopcock (open to air) level with midanteroposterior position of chest at 4th intercostal space.[47,56,61] Read pressures with patient in same position each time and record position.
Flatline waveform	System disconnect or stopcock open	Check system for breaks, or disconnect, reconnect, or change system if contaminated. Close all stopcocks and cover with sterile caps.

*Any of these problems may represent true patient changes. Always assess the patient first.

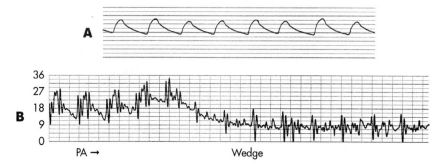

Fig. 8-16 Equipment-related distortions in arterial tracings. Trace A illustrates a dampened PA or A line. Trace B illustrates catheter whip.

inhibited by the stenosis and the upstroke of the arterial waveform is slowed. The dicrotic notch is also distorted or absent as a result of the stiffened closure of the aortic valve.[4,5]

Equipment-related distortions in the pressure patterns, which may result in inaccurate measurements, include damped tracing, catheter whip (Fig. 8-16), abnormally high or low readings, and flat line. These distortions may be caused by catheter kinks or clots, air bubbles in the system, incorrect leveling (referencing) or zeroing of the transducer, loss of pressure in the infusion bag, line disconnect or improper positioning of a stopcock,

or a true change in patient status.[5] Troubleshooting and interventions for these distortions are similar for PA and arterial waveforms (Table 8-4).[4] Always assess the patient first, to determine if the problem is related to deterioration in condition, before looking at the equipment. Note that a damped tracing from technical distortions mimics the arterial waveform seen in hypotension. A flat line may be the result of a disconnection was well as cardiac or circulatory arrest. Always begin differentiation of patient-related as opposed to equipment-related problems with a rapid assessment of the patient.

PA catheter: insertion, lumens, and complications

Continuous monitoring of PA pressures was made possible with the *balloon-tipped, flow-directed pulmonary artery catheter,* originally known as the Swan-Ganz catheter. The catheter is inserted percutaneously or by a surgical cutdown approach, using the subclavian, jugular, brachial, or femoral veins. The optimal site depends on the clinician's experience and individual patient's needs. Each site has advantages and disadvantages, such as restriction of mobility and difficulty keeping dressings intact with the use of neck and extremity sites. Although there is risk of bleeding from any site, the risk with the sub-

clavian site is greater because it is more difficult to compress the vessel and stop the bleeding.[4,5]

Before insertion of the PA catheter, the procedure is explained in terms the patient and/or family can understand and informed consent obtained. Insertion requires aseptic conditions and administration of local anesthesia. Necessary equipment, including the transducer, heparinized saline, catheter, and insertion kit, is assembled. The components of the monitoring system are zeroed according to the manufacturer's recommendation. The balloon integrity is checked and each lu-

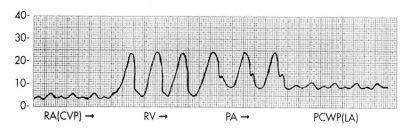

Fig. 8-17 Pressure waveform changes during PA insertion.

men of the catheter flushed before insertion.[56] The patient is positioned for comfort and ease of venous access according to the clinician's preference.

Once venous access is achieved, the catheter is manually advanced under fluoroscopy, or by recognition of right heart pressure waveforms on the oscilloscope. The balloon is kept deflated while in the venous system and is inflated once the catheter enters the right atrium. The force of blood flow behind the balloon carries the catheter (like wind pushing a sailboat) through the tricuspid valve into the right ventricle, up through the pulmonic valve, and into the pulmonary artery. The inflated balloon also cushions the catheter tip, minimizing ventricular arrhythmias.[56] As the clinician continues to advance the catheter the balloon remains inflated until the catheter floats through the PA tree and wedges in a small branch, occluding the pulmonary artery.[6] The PA wedge or pulmonary occlusion pressure is obtained in this position. The syringe is then removed from the balloon port and the balloon is allowed to passively deflate, with the tip remaining in the pulmonary artery.[56] Accurate wedge position may be confirmed by obtaining a venous blood gas sample from the distal port with the balloon inflated and comparing it with an arterial blood gas. The PaO_2 will be up to 19 mm Hg higher, and the $PaCO_2$ will be at least 11 mm Hg lower on the arterial blood gas (ABG).[61]

As the catheter advances through each chamber and into the pulmonary artery there is usually a distinct change in waveform and pressure (Fig. 8-17). A postinsertion radiograph is obtained to rule out the development of a pneumothorax and to confirm the location of the catheter tip in the preferred position below the left atrium. To prevent spontaneous wedging, the nurse also confirms that no less than 1.25 to 1.5 ml is required to wedge the catheter from the resting PA position.[56,65]

The original double-lumen catheter has undergone many modifications, including the addition of both standard and optional features (Fig. 8-18). All catheters have a PA distal port that runs the length of the catheter and ends at the distal tip, positioned in the pulmonary artery. Through this distal port the PA systolic and diastolic patterns are monitored and wedge readings are taken. True mixed venous blood samples are also aspirated from this port with the balloon deflated for use in estimating cardiac output (see Unit 3). A heparinized IV saline solution enclosed in a pressurized device is attached to the distal port by a continuous low flush device to keep the lumen open. No hyperosmotic solutions or medications are administered through this port. The caustic effect of such solutions on the small pulmonary artery may cause local damage to the vessel wall.[5] In addition, the PA waveform cannot be continuously monitored if IVs are infused through

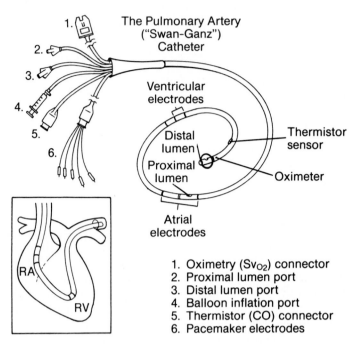

1. Oximetry (Sv_{O2}) connector
2. Proximal lumen port
3. Distal lumen port
4. Balloon inflation port
5. Thermistor (CO) connector
6. Pacemaker electrodes

Fig. 8-18   Possible PA catheter lumens.

the distal port since the stopcock would be turned off to the transducer.

PA catheters also have a lumen that opens into the RA when the distal tip is in the PA. Through this lumen, usually referred to as the proximal (injectate) port, mean RA (CVP) pressures can be monitored and IV infusions or medications delivered. This port is also used to draw RA or routine blood samples. The thermistor connector of the PA catheter is used in conjunction with the proximal (injectate) port for the measurement of cardiac output. If the O_2 saturation abruptly increases when comparing samples obtained from the proximal and distal ports, the diagnosis of ventricular septal defect may be confirmed. A second proximal (infusion) port that opens a few centimeters below the first, in the RA, may be available for all the previous uses (except to obtain car-

diac outputs). This port serves as another venous access when the patient has multiple IVs infusing.

The balloon inflation port extends through the catheter and terminates in the balloon just before the distal tip. The balloon is inflated by using the syringe provided by the manufacturer. This syringe is designed with two safety features. One special feature prevents aspiration of more than 1.5 ml of air, and the other, a Luer-Lock tip, prevents inadvertent disconnection of the syringe.

Optional features currently available include an outlet for concurrent monitoring of venous O_2 saturation (SVO_2) and electrodes for atrial, ventricular, or dual-chamber pacing (see Units 3 and 10).

The most common complications occurring during insertion and maintenance of PA catheters are right ventricular PVCs and nonsustained ventricular tachycardia (VT). These ventricular arrhythmias result from mechanical stimulation of the ventricular wall during insertion or if the catheter slips back into the right ventricle. Although these rhythms are usually transient, there is a risk of deterioration to sustained VT or ventricular fibrillation (VF). Therefore, lidocaine and a defibrillator should be readily available.[4,5,62]

A right bundle branch block (RBBB) may occur during insertion if the catheter scrapes the right bundle located in the anterior wall of the right ventricle. RBBB is usually transient and clinically insignificant, unless there is a preexisting left bundle branch block (LBBB), which would result in complete heart block. Therefore, in patients with LBBB a pacing PA catheter should be inserted and connected to a temporary pacer or a trancutaneous pacer should be readily available.[4,5,56]

Other patient complications associated with PA catheters include infection, pulmonary infarction, and pulmonary rupture. Both insertion and daily maintenance carry a potential for local and systemic infection. The incidence of infection rises significantly after the catheter has been in place for more than 4 days. The general recommendation is to replace the catheter after 4 days and change the IV solutions, tubings, and dressing every 24 to 48 hours.[4,5] Meticulous use of sterile techniques during insertion and daily maintenance are important in decreasing the risk of infection.[4]

Pulmonary infarction can occur as a result of prolonged balloon inflation when obtaining wedge pressures or spontaneous migration of the catheter into the wedge position. The PA waveform should be continuously monitored to detect changes indicative of spontaneous wedging.[4,5] Refer to the nursing orders at the end of this section for the recommended nursing actions.

Pulmonary artery rupture occurs rarely as a result of migration of the catheter tip into a small branch, overinflation of the balloon, eccentric inflation of the balloon, and forced flushing of the PA distal lumen. The extent of damage determines how symptomatic the patient will be. With minor damage the patient may be asymptomatic or have minimal hemoptysis. If the rupture is large, massive hemoptysis will occur, resulting in shock and possibly death. If PA rupture is suspected, the patient should be placed in the lateral position, with the affected side down, to prevent spillage of blood into the unaffected lung.[4,5] Since the PA catheter is usually inserted into the right pulmonary artery, the affected side is usually the right side. Emergency surgery or intubation with a double-lumen endotracheal tube may be necessary to prevent bleeding into the unaffected lung and to allow mechanical ventilation.[4,5]

Equipment-related complications include catheter knotting and balloon rupture. Knotting of the catheter usually occurs during insertion, but the danger is during removal when the valves may be damaged or torn. Before a PA catheter is removed a chest radiograph should confirm that the catheter is not knotted.[62] Balloon rupture occurs as a result of overinflating the balloon, inflating the balloon with any fluid, or actively withdrawing air from the balloon. Balloon rupture results in loss of the ability to obtain the wedge pressure and possibly air embolus. The initial introduction of 1.5 ml of air into the PA will probably not be problematic, but additional injections of air may be. When the catheter is in the proper position, there is a slight resistance to inflation and the air should passively fill the syringe when the plunger is released. If neither of these conditions is present, the valve of the balloon port should be closed and a piece of tape labeled "Do not inflate, balloon broken" applied to the port.[4,56]

Monitoring cardiac output

The current, most accurate method of determining cardiac output at the bedside is by *thermal dilution* technique using a PA catheter (Fig 8-19).[59,65] The thermistor lumen communicates with the distal tip of the PA catheter located in the pulmonary artery. The external thermistor lumen is attached to a computer, which calculates the cardiac output. The patient's backrest is elevated no more than 20 to 30 degrees during cardiac output measurements.[51,65] A 5- to 10-ml bolus of room temperature or iced saline or D5W is rapidly injected through the CVP injectate port and mixes with the patient's warm blood. As the fluid, still cooler than the patient's blood, passes the thermistor sensor at the catheter tip, the temperature change is recorded. The computer calculates the cardiac output using the time from the beginning of the bolus until the temperature change is sensed. This calculation is expressed as the cardiac output in liters per minute.[4,5,65]

Inaccurate cardiac output readings may occur because of catheter-, technique-, or patient-related factors. If the PA catheter tip is positioned too far within the pulmonary artery, the thermistor may rest against a small vessel wall. Before taking cardiac output measurements, the nurse should verify that the PA tracing is not damped and that at least 1.25 to 1.5 ml is required to obtain a wedge tracing.[65] Cardiac output measurements should never be made while the catheter is in the wedge position. The injectate should be administered in a smooth, rapid fashion with minimal handling. Accuracy is verified by a smooth thermodilution curve with a rapid upstroke and a more gradual downslope.[65]

Patient-related factors that may interfere with accurate readings include patient movement, arrhythmias, catheter whip due to hemodynamic instability or varying flow rates, valvular disorders, and the effects of respiration, especially in the mechanically ventilated patient. Measurements may be inaccurate in the presence of frequent premature beats or sustained arrhythmias such as atrial fibrillation. Alternate methods of determining cardiac output may be necessary in these patients as well as in patients with valvular disorders. Obtaining an average of three readings can also help minimize discrepancies. Patient movement should be limited during measurement, and the injectate should be delivered at end expiration.[65] In the presence of catheter whip, 10 ml of iced injectates is preferred to minimize signal noise.[65]

The purpose of maintaining effective cardiac output is to meet tissue O_2 demands. Tissue O_2 demands can be estimated by determining the BSA from the patient's height and weight using a Dubois Body Surface Area Chart.[4] The effectiveness of cardiac output relative to these tissue O_2 demands is then determined by dividing the measured cardiac output by the BSA to obtain the cardiac index. The normal cardiac index is 2.5 to 4.2 $L/min/m^2$. A cardiac index is considered critically low when it drops below 1.8 $L/min/m^2$.[1,2,14,80] At that point shock is imminent.

Cardiac output may also be determined by

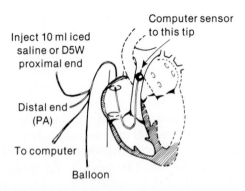

Inject 10 ml iced saline or D5W proximal end

Computer sensor to this tip

Distal end (PA)

To computer

Balloon

Fig. 8-19 Determination of cardiac output by thermodilution technique.

estimating or calculating the A-VO$_2$ difference and relating this to the Fick principle.[5,65] The introduction of continuous Svo$_2$ monitoring allows for the continuous evaluation of cardiac output changes relative to tissue oxygenation needs (see Unit 3).

Other methods of determining cardiac output currently under investigation include noninvasive measurement using Doppler echocardiography, thoracic electrical bio-impedance, and thoracocardiography.[65] Thoracic electrical impedance uses electrodes placed on the patient's chest and neck to record volume and velocity changes with each heartbeat. Thoracocardiography uses specialized transducers to record cardiac oscillations from the outer thoracic surface and translate these to volume changes. Continuous thermodilution cardiac output using a PA catheter is also in the experimental phase.[56]

Systemic and pulmonary vascular resistance

Systemic vascular resistance (SVR) and pulmonary vascular resistance (PVR) cannot be directly measured invasively or noninvasively. Therefore, calculation of these parameters is mathematically determined from established relationships between the pressures in the arterial and venous vascular beds and the cardiac output (see below). The SVR reflects the afterload of the left ventricle. The PVR reflects the afterload of the right ventricle.[4]

NURSING ORDERS: Hemodynamic monitoring.

RELATED NURSING DIAGNOSIS: Decreased cardiac output related to hypovolemia, CHF, or shock; fluid volume deficit or excess; potential for injury related to PA catheter complications

1. While monitoring the PA pressures, note the characteristic PA waveform on oscilloscope:

—Watch for changes in the waveform that might indicate the catheter has slipped back into the right ventricle (Fig. 8-20). If this occurs, inflate the balloon to cushion the catheter tip, monitor closely for inadvertent wedging, and notify physician to reposition. If hemodynamically significant arrhythmias occur, the balloon may be deflated and the catheter withdrawn into the right atrium.[56]

—Monitor in lead V$_1$ for right ventricular PVCs during catheter insertion and throughout monitoring period.

—Keep lidocaine (Xylocaine) at bedside; may be given prophylactically during insertion or as per routine criteria.

—Obtain all PA pressures at end expiration.

—Note the presence or development of pulmonary complications that might invalidate correlations between PAEDP and

Formulas for calculating SVR and PVR

$$SVR = \frac{MAP - MVP\ (CVP)}{CO} \times constant\ 80*$$

$$PVR = \frac{MPAP - MLAP\ (wedge)}{CO} \times constant\ 80*$$

MAP = mean arterial pressure; MVP = mean venous pressure; CO = cardiac output; CVP = central venous pressure; MPAP = mean pulmonary arterial pressure; MLAP = mean left atrial pressure.
*Converts the result to resistance units or dynes/sec/cm^{-5}.

LVEDP. Increased PA systolic pressure may be an indication of these complications.

2. When obtaining PCWP:

— Inflate balloon with 1.25 to 1.5 ml until a change in waveform from PA to PCWP occurs, and record volume required. If tracing gradually moves up and off the screen with loss of waveform (overwedging), remove syringe and notify physician to reposition.[56]

— Inflate the balloon slowly to allow time for it to float into the wedge position. Notify physician if it requires less than 1.25 ml.

— Do not introduce more air than is designated on balloon catheter (i.e., 1.5 ml).

— Record the mean wedge pressure quickly (within 15 seconds), allowing passive deflation of the balloon thereafter[4,56]; verify that the catheter is no longer wedged by return of PA waveform on scope.

— If the wedge waveform cannot be obtained with maximum inflation, allow balloon to passively deflate. Notify physician, and record the PAEDP in the interim.

— If there is no air return, and balloon rupture is suspected, label port "Do not inflate"[4,56] and notify physician. Do not insert additional air.

3. While monitoring pressures invasively, watch concurrently for:

— Noninvasive signs of increased LVEDP, such as S_4 or S_3 gallop.

— Atrial and ventricular arrhythmias.

— Signs of pulmonary congestion, such as increased respiratory rate, Valsalva (forced) respiration, and end-inspiratory rales not clearing with cough.

4. Watch for spontaneous wedging detected by change in waveform from PA to wedge. Have the patient turn on side opposite to distal tip location (usually left), deep breathe, and cough.[56] If not successful immediately, notify physician.

5. Monitor for equipment-related distortions, including damped tracings and catheter whip. Refer to Table 8-4 for specific causes and interventions. Always assess the patient first.

6. Take initial readings and rezero with offgoing shift to confirm accuracy.

7. Institute nursing measures to minimize O_2 demands by preventing and/or quickly correcting factors that might increase myocardial O_2 consumption.

8. Provide increased O_2 supply with supplementary oxygen.

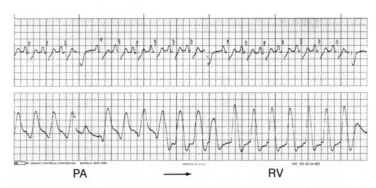

PA ⟶ RV

Fig. 8-20 PA catheter slipped into the right ventricle. Characteristic pressure pulse pattern changes.

9. Watch for intermittent changes in the waveform that might indicate alterations in contractility or CO.

   —Every other pressure waveform may be smaller in a patient with CHF because the heart cannot sustain strong pulses (pulsus alternans).

   —With arrhythmias, the waveform may become irregular and/or diminished because the output with these is less.

   —The voltage of the pattern may also vary with respiration because of respiratory influences on cardiac output (pulsus paradoxus).

10. In the event of suspected PA rupture, turn patient to affected side (usually right) and notify physician immediately.

11. To prevent sepsis, give special care to catheter site in the form of routine preparation, dressing changes, and use of carefully sealed dressings; monitor temperature.

12. Record serial changes in cardiac output; when evaluating the cardiac output results, relate them to the patient's BSA (cardiac index) and SVR.

13. As cardiac index begins to drop, monitor clinical signs of decreased tissue perfusion (noting a symptomatic fall in cardiac output) that might indicate heart failure is evolving to the shock state.

AUSCULTATION OF THE HEART

Heart sounds serve as parameters outlining the mechanical events of the heart. Alterations in the heart's mechanical activity are reflected by extra heart sounds and variations in the normal heart sounds. The earliest mechanical alterations occurring in acute MI effect ventricular diastole. Minor changes in filling pressures are best detected at the end of diastole. Variations in heart sounds are produced that correlate with these changes in LVEDP. The heart sounds thus provide a means for clinically evaluating the mechanical and hemodynamic changes in acute MI.[4]

Normal heart sounds are produced by the mechanical events that accompany valve closure. Although older theories claim that valve closure is the major factor responsible for production of the sound, more recent theories are less definite. Heart sounds may be produced by any of three factors or a combination of them. These factors include valve closure, vibrations of the ventricular wall associated with ventricular contraction, and vibrations associated with acceleration and deceleration of blood by the force of ventricular contraction.[5,6,13]

S_1 marks the onset of ventricular systole. During ventricular systole the AV valves close, the ventricular muscle wall contracts, and the blood is ejected into the blood vessels. S_2 marks the onset of ventricular diastole. During ventricular diastole, the semilunar valves close, the ventricular wall relaxes, and blood enters the ventricles from the atria.[32] The heart sounds allow noninvasive correlation of electrical and mechanical activity at the bedside (Fig. 8-21).

Both S_1 and S_2 are most audible with the diaphragm of the stethoscope. These heart sounds form the characteristic "lub-dub" (S_1 = lub, S_2 = dub) in the normal heart. S_1 is most audible at the apex and S_2 at the base of the heart where the corresponding valves are located (Fig. 8-22).

Normal variations of heart sounds

The intensity of S_1 may be either loud or soft, as a result of the dual component of AV valve closure. The AV valves begin closing passively because of increases in ventricular pressure occurring with ventricular filling. If the AV valves have had enough time

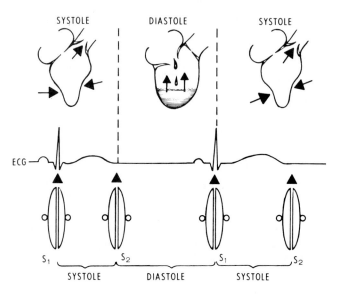

SYSTOLE   DIASTOLE   SYSTOLE

ECG

S_1 S_2 S_1 S_2

SYSTOLE   DIASTOLE   SYSTOLE

Fig. 8-21   Correlation of normal heart sounds with mechanical and electrical events.

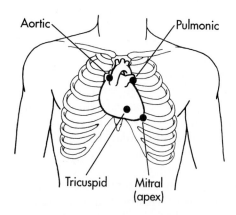

Aortic   Pulmonic

Tricuspid   Mitral (apex)

Fig. 8-22   Areas for auscultation.

to start closing passively before active closure with ventricular systole, the S_1 sound will be soft. If the AV valves are still wide open when ventricular systole begins, the valves will slam shut, producing a loud S_1 sound (Fig. 8-23).[5,6] Conditions producing a loud S_1 by decreasing passive closure time are a short P–R interval, tachycardias, and early beats.

Conditions producing a soft S_1 are a long P–R interval, bradycardia, and CHF. The first two conditions increase passive closure time. In CHF there is incomplete emptying of the ventricles during systole. As a result, during diastole there is an increase in ventricular contents. This increase in contents creates an increased pressure against the AV valves, forcing closure to begin earlier and producing a softer sound.[6,32]

Varying intensity of S_1 may indicate rhythms with varying P–R intervals. This varying intensity is a bedside clue to the diagnosis of complete heart block and other forms of AV dissociation.[32] The presence or absence of varying intensity may also aid in differential diagnosis of VT versus SVT with aberration (see Unit 7).

The characteristics of S_2 can be affected by normal respiration. Inspiration creates a negative pressure within the chest, drawing blood into the right side of the heart. As a result of this increased right ventricular filling, right ventricular systole is longer in duration. This creates a splitting of the S_2 sound. The S_2 has both a pulmonic and an

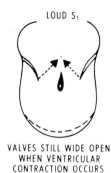
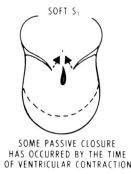

LOUD S₁ ... SOFT S₁

VALVES STILL WIDE OPEN WHEN VENTRICULAR CONTRACTION OCCURS

SOME PASSIVE CLOSURE HAS OCCURRED BY THE TIME OF VENTRICULAR CONTRACTION

Fig. 8-23 Intensity of the first heart sound: production of loud or soft S_1.

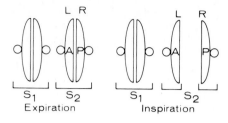

S_1 S_2
Expiration

S_1 S_2
Inspiration

Fig. 8-24 Normal splitting of the second heart sound (S_2) with inspiration.

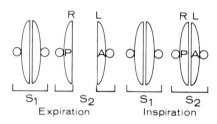

S_1 S_2
Expiration

S_1 S_2
Inspiration

Fig. 8-25 Abnormal paradoxical splitting of the second heart sound (S_2) on expiration.

aortic component. The pulmonic component denotes the end of right ventricular systole, which is delayed during inspiration and separated from the aortic component, creating a split S_2 (Fig. 8-24).[32] Conditions that further delay right ventricular systole, such as RBBB or left ventricular pacing, may augment this normal splitting.[32]

Anything that delays left ventricular systole causes delayed closure of the aortic valve. This delay produces an abnormal paradoxical splitting of S_2 on expiration (Fig. 8-25).[32] Examples of conditions causing par-

Gallops

The most clinically significant abnormal heart sounds in acute MI are *gallops* and *murmurs*. The abnormal heart sounds that reflect left ventricular diastolic changes are gallops.

Gallops are extra sounds created by gushes of blood entering resistant, or stiffened, ventricles. Gushes of blood enter the ventricles twice during ventricular diastole—during the initial filling phase (early to mid-diastole) and at the time of atrial systole (at the end of ventricular diastole). Therefore, gallops occur during early and late ventricular diastole.[6]

Ventricular diastole begins after the closure of the semilunar valves denoted by S_2.

adoxical splitting of S_2 on expiration are LBBB, right ventricular pacing, left ventricular failure, ventricular aneurysm, and angina pectoris.

The abnormal extra sound created within the ventricles at the beginning of ventricular diastole, immediately following the S_2, is known as an *S_3 gallop* (Fig. 8-26). This sound is usually pathologic in adults over 30 years of age. It is produced as the gush of blood during the rapid ventricular filling phase enters a congested ventricle, as in CHF. An S_3 heard in children and adults less than 30 years of age with normal hearts is referred to as a physiologic S_3.[5,6] Other terms used to describe this extra sound are *ventricular gallop* and *protodiastolic gallop*.[6,32]

Another abnormal sound can occur as the blood enters the ventricles at the end of ventricular diastole. This sound is known as an

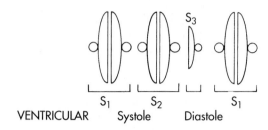

Fig. 8-26 Timing of S₃ gallop.

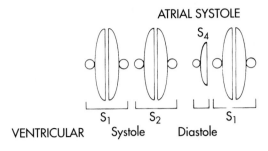

Fig. 8-27 Timing of S₄ gallop.

S_4 *gallop* and is associated with atrial contraction. (atrial systole). Although all gallop sounds are created in the ventricles, the S_4 gallop, because it is associated with atrial systole, is called an *atrial gallop*.[32] The S_4 sound occurs with active atrial contribution to ventricular filling and will not occur in the absence of atrial contraction such as with atrial fibrillation.[29] The S_4 is audible at the end of ventricular diastole, or just before S_1, and may also be called a presystolic gallop (Fig. 8-27).[6]

A physiologic S_4, may be heard in the healthy hearts of small children and adults over 50 years of age. It is otherwise considered pathologic and referred to as a gallop. The S_4 gallop is associated with diseases such as acute MI that cause a decrease in ventricular compliance.[5,6,32] The S_4 reflects the corresponding slight increase in LVEDP. Other myocardial pathologic conditions that produce alterations in ventricular compliance resulting in an S_4 gallop include left ventricular hypertrophy secondary to hypertension and the cardiomyopathies. Myocardial ischemia occurring during episodes of angina produces transient changes in compliance, resulting in an S_4 that disappears after the pain subsides.[5,6]

A slightly damaged, noncompliant left ventricle can accommodate the blood that enters through the initial filling phase. However, it cannot accommodate the added volume that enters with atrial contraction. Therefore, the S_4 is an early expected find-

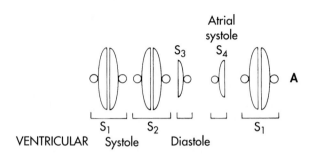

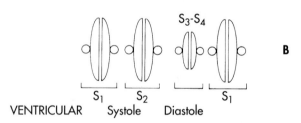

Fig. 8-28 Quadruple rhythm *(A)* leading to summation gallop *(B)* in faster heart rates.

ing in patients with acute MI and may occur without an S_3. When heart failure complicates acute MI, the cardiac output falls, and the injured left ventricle may not completely eject its contents. As a result, residual volume remains in the left ventricle at the end of systole and at the beginning of diastole. When this condition occurs, the left ventricle cannot fully accommodate blood that enters, even during initial stages. Thus, in left ventricular failure an abnormal sound may also be audible at the beginning of diastole.[6,29] This abnormal sound produced at the beginning of diastole is an S_3 gallop and is associated with significant increases in LVEDP.

Finding both an S_3 and S_4 gallop is not unusual in a patient with left ventricular failure resulting from an acute MI. The resulting sound is a quadruple rhythm (Fig. 8-28,*A*).

Murmurs

The other major abnormal heart sound is a *murmur*. Murmurs occur because of alterations in the movement of blood. These alterations occur as a result of abnormal or diseased valves or vessels. The movement of blood is significantly altered when there is leakage through insufficient valves or when turbulence occurs across a narrowed outlet as with stenotic valves.[4]

Murmurs are described according to when they occur in the cardiac cycle (systolic or diastolic), intensity (loudness), pitch (high or low), quality (i.e., blowing, musical, harsh), shape (i.e., crescendo, decrescendo), and duration (i.e., holosystolic). They may radiate to characteristic locations on the chest wall, such as the pulmonic or aortic region and sternal borders. The intensity is graded on a scale of 1 to 6, with 6 being the loudest.[32] A systolic murmur graded 3/6 would be of average intensity.[5,29,32]

A systolic murmur occurs between the heart sounds S_1 and S_2 (Fig. 8-29). In systole the AV valves should be closed and semilunar valves should be open. Insufficient AV valves or stenotic semilunar valves may cause

systolic murmurs.[4,29,32] Mitral insufficiency is the most likely cause of a systolic murmur heard during angina or after an acute MI. This insufficiency is usually caused by papillary muscle ischemia or infarction. Another possible cause is ventricular dilation resulting from CHF. If a sudden, very loud systolic murmur occurs, possible causes are ruptured interventricular septum resulting in a ventricular septal defect (VSD), or papillary muscle rupture.[5]

A diastolic murmur is audible between the heart sounds S_2 and S_1 (see Fig. 8-29). In diastole the AV valves should be open and the semilunar valves should be closed. Insufficient semilunar valves or stenotic AV valves, then, may cause diastolic murmurs.[6,29] The turbulent blood flow through either stenotic AV valve produces a low-pitched, rumbling murmur. Regurgitant blood flow through insufficient semilunar valves produces a soft, high-pitched murmur.[4]

NURSING ORDERS: Auscultation

RELATED NURSING DIAGNOSIS: Alteration in cardiac output related to decreased compliance, CHF, mitral insufficiency, or VSD

1. In the patient with MI, auscultate the heart with each set of vital signs and listen for:
   —Gallop sounds
   —Murmurs, especially systolic
   —Changes in the intensity of S_1
   —Paradoxical splitting of S_2 on expiration.
2. Identify the normal heart sounds first.
3. When auscultating the heart, listen at the apex to hear the most significant changes.
4. When listening for paradoxical splitting

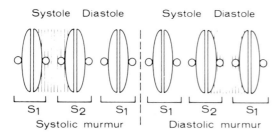

Systole Diastole   Systole Diastole

S_1 S_2 S_1 S_1 S_2 S_1
Systolic murmur   Diastolic murmur

Fig. 8-29 Relationship of systolic and diastolic murmurs to normal heart sounds.

of S_2, listen only at the second intercostal space. Do not report normal splitting heard on inspiration.

5. When auscultating gallops:
—Listen for both S_3 and S_4 during diastole.
—Listen for S_3 together with S_2.
—Listen for S_4 at the end of diastole together with S_1.
—Listen with light pressure, using the bell of the stethoscope; these are low-frequency sounds and are easily obliterated.
—Do not except to hear two distinct sounds; gallops often sound like mere distortions of the normal heart sound.
—Note that left ventricular sounds may be augmented on expiration; with patient supine (increased venous return) or on the left side (left ventricle closer to chest wall); or with mild strain, such as coughing or squeezing the examiner's hand.

6. Report any new murmurs immediately.
—Listen for murmurs, especially between S_1 and S_2, because these are the most significant in acute MI.

—If the murmur is loud and the onset is sudden, watch the patient closely, checking the vital signs until the physician has checked the patient.
—For complete auscultation of a murmur, note whether it is systolic or diastolic; if it occurs early, late, or throughout the cycle; where it is heard most loudly on the chest; where it radiates; its quality (blowing, musical, harsh); and exactly how loud it is on a scale of 1 to 6.

7. When you hear varying intensity of S_1, look at the monitor for an arrhythmia indicating a form of AV dissociation.

8. If you hear paradoxical splitting, rule out aneurysm, LBBB, right ventricular pacing, and angina when considering it is a sign of heart failure.

9. Abnormal heart sounds are frequently of very low intensity and therefore very difficult to hear. When you first are starting to listen, ask another nurse or physician to verify your findings. Ability to hear these changes develops only with practice.

SHOCK SYNDROME

Shock is a clinical syndrome that occurs as a result of acute circulatory failure. The shock syndrome can be defined as a state in which there is a significant reduction in cardiac output, effective tissue perfusion, and tissue oxygenation, resulting in multiorgan tissue symptoms.[41,44]

In heart failure resulting from acute MI, a fall in cardiac output occurs. Therefore, CHF caused by acute MI has the potential, if the patient's condition deteriorates, to lead to a more severe fall in cardiac output and shock. Other factors discussed later in this section may also lead to the shock state in acute MI. The practitioner should also recognize these and take them into consideration.

The common denominator in all forms of shock is the critical reduction in the supply of oxygenated blood to the tissues.[45] The demands of the tissues for oxygen are met by an adequate O_2 supply and an adequate blood supply (see Unit 3). Maintenance of an adequate blood supply in dependent on the integrity of the cardiovascular system (see Fig. 8-1). This integrity is affected by any of four variables influencing cardiac output: (1) heart rate and rhythm, (2) blood volume or venous return (preload), (3) systemic vascular resistance or tone (afterload), and (4) myocardial contractility.[6,40] Significant alterations in any of these four variables may cause a marked decrease in the supply of oxygenated blood to the tissues. This decrease is eventually reflected by a significant fall in cardiac output and blood pressure, changes

Table 8-5. Clinical and hemodynamic responses in different types of shock

Response	Cardiogenic	Hypovolemic	Septic (Distributive)	
			Warm	Cold
Heart rate	↑	↑	↑	↑
Blood pressure	↓	↓	↓	↓
Respiratory rate	↑	↑	↑	↑
Urine output	↓	↓	↑	↓
Skin	Cool	Cool	Warm	Cool
Color	Pale	Pale	Flushed	Pale
PCWP	↑	↓	↓	↑
CVP (neck veins)	↑	↓	↓	↑
CO/CI	↓	↓	↑	↓
SVR	↑	↑	↓	↑
SVO$_2$	↓	↓	↑	↓

↑ = elevated; ↓ = decreased; CO = cardiac output; CI = cardiac index.

in cellular metabolism, and a group of characteristic symptoms.[41,45] Cardiac index measurements less than 1.8 L/min/m^2 are consistent with the shock syndrome.[1]

Shock may occur simply as a result of a tachyarrhythmia or bradyarrhythmia (see Unit 6).[9] The three major traditional classifications of shock, however, are hypovolemic, distributive, and cardiogenic.[6,41,44] There are some similarities as well as distinct differences in the clinical and hemodynamic presentation of these major classifications of shock (Table 8-5).[6,45] Obstructive shock is a fourth frequently added and clinically helpful classification with its own distinct characteristics.[2,4,7,9]

Hypovolemic and distributive shock are loosely related. *Hypovolemic shock* results from a severe reduction in intravascular blood volume. Causes include hemorrhage, excessive diuresis, gastrointestinal losses, severe dehydration, or internal fluid shifts.[6,41,45] *Distributive shock,* also known as *vasogenic* shock, results from a maldistribution of blood flow and volume, primarily as a result of decreased vascular tone. This classification of shock includes septic, anaphylactic, and neurogenic shock.[6,41,44] Drugs that produce vasodilation, such as morphine, nitroglycerin, and nitroprusside, may also contribute to va-

sogenic or distributive shock in the patient with an acute MI. Although massive vasodilation is the major contributing factor, other factors characterize these forms of shock.

Septic shock is the most common type of distributive shock. Chemical mediators are released as a result of the infection, causing vasodilation and increased capillary permeability.[44,45] These reactions occur during the first phase of septic shock, referred to as *warm shock* or the hyperdynamic phase. Massive vasodilation decreases both preload and afterload, triggering compensatory mechanisms that increase cardiac output. The patient's skin during this phase is warm and pink as a result of peripheral vasodilation and increased CO. In the second phase of septic shock, chemical mediators cause depression of the myocardium, leading to decreased contractility and intense vasoconstriction. This stage is referred to as *cold shock* or *the hypodynamic phase,* characterized by cold, clammy skin. All factors combined eventually cause a severe decrease in cardiac output and blood pressure, resulting in critically low tissue perfusion. Cold shock is usually irreversible, leading to multisystem organ failure.[41,44-46]

Anaphylactic shock follows a severe allergic

reaction, resulting in an antigen-antibody reaction that stimulates the release of chemical mediators. These mediators produce massive vasodilation, increased capillary permeability, and intense bronchoconstriction. As fluid leaks out of the vascular compartment, a relative hypovolemia occurs as well. Shock secondary to these changes coupled with respiratory distress secondary to bronchial edema and spasm creates an acutely life-threatening situation.[40,44,45]

Cardiogenic shock

Cardiogenic shock usually results from severe impairment of cardiac muscle contractility, presenting initially as heart failure. Specific causes include MI, valvular disease, cardiomyopathy, and myocardial dysfunction after cardiac surgery. Although some authorities consider shock secondary to arrhythmias a form of cardiogenic shock, this is misleading since the treatment and prognosis differ significantly.[2,9] Causes of obstructive shock are also sometimes included under the heading of cardiogenic shock.[14,38] These causes include cardiac tamponade, massive pulmonary emboli, and tension pneumothorax. The clinical presentation and treatment of these also differ significantly from cardiogenic shock due to heart failure.

In cardiogenic shock secondary to coronary artery disease (CAD), 40% or more of the myocardium is necrotic or injured and as such does not contribute to contractility.[41,45] By definition, therefore, cardiogenic shock in CAD usually implies the presence of extensive muscle damage. The prognosis for this shock state is extremely poor, and the mortality is high. Early, aggressive clinical intervention may contain the area of infarction. Without appropriate clinical management, however, areas of critically ischemic tissue may subsequently become necrotic, thus extending the area of infarction and increasing the potential for developing cardio-

Neurogenic shock occurs as a result of a sudden loss of vasomotor or sympathetic tone. This leads to massive dilation of the veins, increasing vascular capacity and therefore significantly decreasing venous return. Some causes of neurogenic shock are deep general anesthesia, spinal anesthesia, spinal cord damage, severe emotional stress or pain, and barbiturate overdose.[40,41,44]

genic shock.[39] Papillary muscle rupture and ventricular septal defects complicating MI may also result in cardiogenic shock but are surgically correctable if detected early. Cardiogenic shock following cardiac surgery or other reperfusion measures is more likely to be due to stunning rather than permanent muscle damage. Therefore this form of shock is often short term and reversible (see Unit 5).[2]

A more simplistic, practical approach to the classification of shock has been recently proposed to facilitate emergency intervention.[9] This approach incorporates most of the traditional categories and focuses on *rate, volume,* or *pump* problems. Distributive shock is included under the heading of a volume problem since relative hypovolemia is present and initial volume replacement is indicated. Obstructive causes of shock and their treatment are not fully addressed when using this approach and may need to be simultaneously considered.

The precise clinical picture or symptoms of the patient in shock may vary. It is dependent on the cause of the disorder and the stage of the shock. In general, there are three stages of shock: early or compensated, intermediate or progressive, and irreversible.[7,14,40]

With a decrease in systemic blood pressure, the body initiates a series of compensatory mechanisms to maintain an adequate

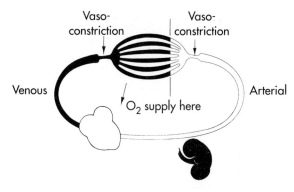

Fig. 8-30 Constriction of arterial and venous capillary beds in response to sympathetic stimulation.

blood supply to the brain and heart. Epinephrine and norepinephrine are released, resulting in sympathetic stimulation.[39,40,45] In acute MI, the most important compensatory mechanisms occurring as a result of sympathetic stimulation are increased heart rate and vasoconstriction. The heart rate increases to assist in improving cardiac output and blood pressure. The blood vessels to the skin, abdominal viscera, voluntary muscle, and finally the kidneys constrict in an attempt to maintain the blood pressure and redirect blood flow to the more critical areas of the brain and heart. Both the arterial and venous ends of the capillary bed constrict (Fig. 8-30).[7,40] The SVR increases in response to this vasoconstriction. Initially, blood pressure is maintained and symptoms may be limited to tachycardia, which can occur from a variety of causes.[7] In the absence of invasive hemodynamic monitoring, this phase of shock is easy to miss.

As shock progresses, the systolic blood pressure falls and the diastolic blood pressure remains elevated secondary to the increased SVR. The pulse pressure, or difference between the systolic and diastolic pressure, is reduced. As shock progresses to this more typical intermediate phase, tissue compromise becomes evident, producing the classic symptoms of shock.[7] The skin assumes a dusky, cool, moist appearance (i.e., cold and clammy). Secondary to intense vasoconstriction, the earlobes, tip of the nose, and distal portions of the extremities become cyanotic.[2] The fall in cardiac output and vasoconstriction of the vessels to the kidneys cause decreased renal perfusion, which results in oliguria and eventually anuria. In spite of the compensatory mechanisms, the supply of oxygenated blood to the brain decreases resulting in decreased cerebral perfusion. Decreased cerebral perfusion is manifested by sensorium changes, such as dizziness, confusion, agitation, and lethargy. These changes may further progress to a state of significant decrease in level of consciousness and coma.[6,41,45]

The inadequate cellular perfusion causes cell anoxia and changes in cellular metabolism. During cellular anoxia, the cells are forced to metabolize glucose without O_2 (glycolysis). This abnormal process is described as *anaerobic metabolism*. As a result, lactic acid accumulates within the cell, leading to lactic acidosis or metabolic acidosis and a decrease in serum pH levels.[2,40,44]

In the end stages of shock, no matter what the initiating factor, shock causes more shock.[40] Severe lactic acidosis occurs secondary to hypoxia. Because of decreased blood flow, carbon dioxide removal decreases, potentiating the acidosis. Since the arterial ends of the capillary bed are not accustomed to an acidic environment, vasodilation occurs. The venous link from the capillary bed, however, remains constricted (Fig. 8-31). Blood flows into the capillary bed but cannot return to the heart.[2,7] Stasis and pooling of large volumes of blood occur in the capillary beds. Cellular, tissue, and organ death are imminent. Hypoxia, decreased serum pH, and cellular acidosis also contribute directly to cell membrane destruction.[40,44]

As shock progresses to the irreversible phase, cellular destruction occurs, leading to multisystem organ failure.[2,7,14] The major

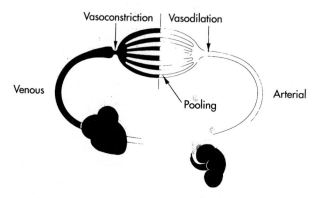

Fig. 8-31 Response of the capillary bed to severe lactic acidosis in end stages of shock. Note the arterial vasodilation in the presence of sustained venoconstriction.

complications involve the heart, lungs, kidneys, and blood clotting factors.

Chemical mediators, thought to be released as a result of cellular destruction and inadequate myocardial nutrition, cause myocardial depression. An increase in pulmonary capillary permeability and inadequate oxygenation of the alveolar cells can cause leaking of fluid into the interstitial spaces and/or alveoli, producing adult respiratory distress syndrome (ARDS).[2,40,41] The kidneys require 25% of the cardiac output each minute. Therefore, prolonged hypotension leads to acute tubular necrosis (ATN) and renal failure.[40,43] Disseminated intravascular coagulation (DIC) also occurs as a complication of shock. This condition results from decreased perfusion of the microvasculature and acidosis, causing increased stickiness of blood cells, sludging, then activation of the clotting cascade, which eventually depletes clotting stores. Depletion of the clotting stores leads to bleeding.[36,41]

As the recently proposed American Heart Association ACLS algorithm suggests, the development of shock in any patient, including a cardiac patient, requires assessment from at least three major parameters: rate, volume, and pump problems.[9] Initial therapy focuses on correcting these disturbances. Treatment of significant tachycardias or bradycardias is considered first since they may be the easiest to correct (see Unit 6). Because the common denominator of all shock states is a critically low tissue perfusion, the goal of all therapy is to increase delivery of O_2 to meet the tissue demands. Some clinicians calculate the O_2 delivery (Do_2), O_2 consumption (Vo_2), and O_2 extraction ratio in order to manipulate and assess therapy.[5,35,45]

A PA catheter is indicated for monitoring hemodynamics in the patient with potential cardiogenic shock. The patient with right ventricular infarction or with a normal or low wedge pressure may require volume administration. For optimal cardiac output in cardiogenic shock the PCWP should be between 15 and 18 mm Hg.[1,5,39] Fluid balance in these patients is an important challenge for the critical care nurse. Fluid resuscitation may be necessary for a PCWP of less than 18 mmHg, to maintain an acceptable cardiac index of greater than 2.2 L/min/m^2.[7,14,38] This cardiac index is preferred, athough slightly higher than the critical level of 1.8 L/min/m^2 (see Monitoring cardiac output). More commonly, the PCWP is greater than 18 mm Hg, and the use of diuretics and vasodilators (e.g., nitroglycerin) is indicated to decrease circulating fluid volume.[37,39,41]

The practitioner should consider the presence of obstructive shock in the form of cardiac tamponade. Although the hemodynamic pattern may mimic right ventricular infarction, heart sounds may be absent and pulseless electrical activity (PEA),[9] formerly called EMD, may be present. Therefore, volume administration will not be effective and pericardiocentesis is indicated.

In patients with PCWP greater than 18 mm Hg, the pump disorder or cardiogenic component is then addressed. Administration of norepinephrine (Levophed) at 0.5 to 30 mcg/min or dopamine (Intropin) at 5 to 20 mcg/kg/min is recommended if the systolic blood pressure is less than 70 mm Hg.[9] Dopamine is recommended initially in the patient with a systolic blood pressure between 70 and 100 mm Hg.[9] Diuretics or nitroglycerin may also be administered in conjunction with an inotropic agent.[37,39,41] Emergency surgery is considered in the presence of papillary muscle rupture, severe valvular insufficiency, or ventricular septal rupture. Toxic effects of myocardial depressants such as beta blockers or calcium channel blockers require correction.

Circulatory assist measures such as the intraaortic balloon pump and ventricular assist devices are indicated in coronary cardiogenic shock since they increase coronary blood and O_2 supply, lower myocardial demands, and improve cardiac output (see Circulatory Assist Devices). These temporary measures can stabilize the patient by relieving the strain on the heart until angioplasty or surgical coronary revascularization can be attempted.[5,9,39]

Other important therapies include adequate analgesia and respiratory support.[7] Morphine sulfate can be given intravenously for pain and anxiety. The vasodilatory effects of morphine may also help decrease preload. To promote tissue oxygenation, administration of higher oxygen concentrations may be necessary. Some patients may require mechanical ventilation and PEEP to increase tissue oxygenation.[39,40] Other metabolic imbalances such as acidosis or hypoglycemia also need correction.

NURSING ORDERS: For the patient with coronary artery disease in shock

RELATED NURSING DIAGNOSES: Alteration in tissue perfusion related to decreased cardiac output; impaired gas exchange related to pulmonary vascular congestion; alteration in comfort related to myocardial ischemia; alteration in urine output related to decreased cardiac output

1. Evaluate underlying cause.
   —Place patient in flat position.
   —Treat dysrhythmias or other abnormalities evident on ECG.
   —Check for hypovolemia by elevating the patient's legs to increase venous return, then checking blood pressure; checking CVP, PAP, and PCWP.
   —Monitor vital signs closely.
   —Have resuscitation equipment at the bedside.
   —Rule out any vasoactive mechanism such as morphine, meperidine, nitroglycerin, or sepsis, and elevate patient's legs to increase venous return. Have narcotic antagonists available.
   —Monitor cardiac output via PA catheter by thermodilution technique.
   —If mechanism is determined to be cardiogenic and is associated with CAD, institute measures to limit discrepancy between myocardial O_2 supply and demand.
   —Take the following actions to limit MVO_2:
   Rate: Watch for and correct any significant dysrhythmias quickly.
   Preload: Monitor fluid intake and output carefully; administer diuretics as ordered; check PCWP for effectiveness.
   Afterload: Correct any hypertensive state; relieve stress factors, such as pain and anxiety.
   Contractility: Correct any acid-base or electrolyte imbalances quickly; limit peripheral demands by investigating and

managing any other systemic diseases such as diabetes, COPD, or sepsis; if inotropic agents are ordered, monitor vital signs and other hemodynamic parameters carefully for signs of deterioration.
— To increase O_2 supply, administer supplementary oxygen.
— Document all nursing actions and effectiveness.
2. Evaluate vascular response:
— Monitor vasoactive drugs carefully (see Unit 9).
— Determine endpoint of therapy with physician.
3. Evaluate and assist tissue metabolism:
— Monitor blood gases for metabolic acidosis.

— Watch for Kussmaul-type respirations as signs of respiratory compensatory efforts.
— Evaluate patient symptoms of tissue perfusion; watch for deterioration, such as deepening of sensorium changes.
— Administer and monitor effects of drugs that may aid in stabilizing tissue metabolism, such as steroids or osmotic diuretics.
4. Assess the patient for signs of cardiac tamponade.
5. Assess the patient for acute mitral insufficiency or ventricular septal defects.
6. Consider circulatory assist devices and revascularization to support the remaining myocardium.

CIRCULATORY ASSIST DEVICES

Circulatory assist devices help maintain coronary and systemic circulation in the failing heart while decreasing the heart's work load.[2,4,66,72,75] These devices are indicated in the treatment of cardiogenic shock when medical therapy has been ineffective or during weaning from cardiopulmonary bypass.

Intraaortic balloon pump (IABP)

The *intraaortic balloon pump* (IABP) is currently the most common mode of circulatory assist in the critical care unit. It is effective in improving coronary and systemic circulation, may be inserted at the bedside even in acute situations, and has a lower incidence of complications than other assist devices.[4,66,72,77]

The intraaortic balloon catheter is usually inserted percutaneously under fluoroscopy through the femoral artery and positioned in the descending aorta just below the origin of the left subclavian artery.[4,5] The balloon is connected to a console that controls the balloon inflation and deflation, or pump action (Fig. 8-32). Although the balloon is synchronized to the cardiac cycle, inflation occurs during ventricular diastole while deflation occurs during ventricular systole.[39,73] Since the balloon pulsations occur opposite the natural cardiac pulsations, this system is also called *counterpulsation.*

The usual volume of gas required to inflate the balloon is 40 ml. During inflation the gas-filled portion of the balloon catheter lies just below the left subclavian artery and just above the renal arteries. The gas most commonly used is helium because it is lighter than air and can be mobilized more rapidly during inflation and deflation.[73]

Inflation of the balloon occurs at the beginning of diastole, with closure of the aortic valve. The inflated balloon raises the aortic diastolic pressure and displaces the blood in the aorta proximally into the coronary artery openings within the aortic root and toward the cerebral arteries. Balloon inflation also displaces the blood in the aorta distally toward the renal arteries and other peripheral arteries. Since the openings to the coronary arteries are in the aortic root and fill during diastole, balloon inflation causes an increase in coronary blood flow and myocardial oxygen supply.[4,73,77]

When the IABP is effective in the patient with CAD, episodes of angina and ventricular ectopy decrease and ischemic ECG changes resolve.[14] Deflation of the balloon just before systole decreases the aortic root pressure, thus facilitating systolic emptying by decreasing the afterload of the left ventricle. The deflation action of the balloon exerts a sucking effect as the left ventricle ejects its contents.[4,39,73] Thus the cardiac output increases while the workload and oxygen demands of the heart decrease. However, only small increases in cardiac output can be expected.[14,80] When effective, PCWP and heart rate decrease, urine output in-

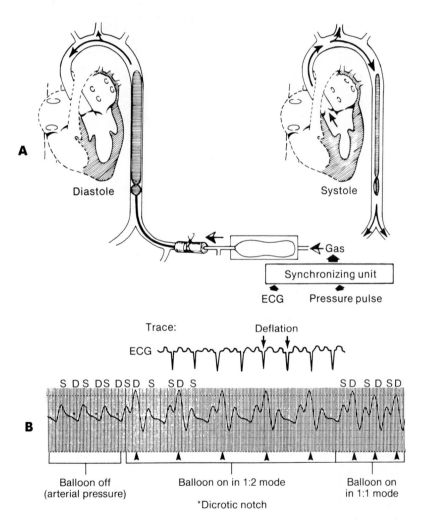

Fig. 8-32 The intraaortic balloon pump. The effects of balloon inflation and deflation on (A) the patient, (B) the ECG and pressure waveforms, and (C) the IABP console. *Continued.*

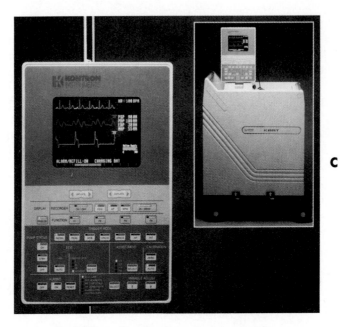

C

Fig. 8-32, cont'd.   For legend see page 351.

creases, and skin color, temperature, breath sounds, and consciousness improve.[14]

Use of the intraaortic balloon may reverse the shock state or stabilize the patient to allow time for cardiac catheterization, angioplasty, cardiac surgery, or cardiac transplantation. Other indications include unstable angina, refractory life-threatening arrhythmias, and inability to wean from cardiopulmonary bypass.[4,39,73,75,77,79] The IABP also may be useful in acute MI after thrombolytic therapy or angioplasty to assist with reperfusion.[69,70,72,74]

IABP therapy is contraindicated in patients with aortic valvular insufficiency and aortic aneurysm dissection. Relative contraindications include aortic aneurysms, severe peripheral vascular disease, blood dyscrasias, end-stage diseases, and terminal illnesses.[4,73,74]

Either the ECG or arterial waveform can be used as the initial signal or "trigger" for balloon inflation and deflation. Although the ECG pattern is the automatic initial signal or trigger, optimal timing requires subsequent manual adjustment using the arterial line waveform from the IABP catheter. Thus the examiner should see both a clear ECG and arterial line waveform on the console before beginning counterpulsation.[4,77] When the arterial waveform is significantly damped, the ECG becomes the trigger. Conversely, the arterial waveform may be used when the ECG signal is poor. If the ECG signal is altered by an irregular rhythm, wide QRS complex, or a paced rhythm, alternate trigger modes are preferred. These modes include A-Fib (for any grossly irregular rhythm), ECG peak (for rhythms with wide QRS complexes), or A or V paced (for single- or dual-chamber pacing). If there is no ECG signal or arterial waveform as in cardiopulmonary bypass, the internal trigger mode is preferred. During cardiopulmonary resuscitation (CPR) the arterial trigger mode is preferred, using the arterial waveform generated by compression as the signal.

The aortic arterial pressure obtained from

the IABP catheter provides a more accurate basis for timing than a peripheral arterial line. The time it takes the blood to travel from the aortic valve to the tip of the balloon is about 25 milliseconds. If a peripheral line is used, an adjustment should be made for a time delay of up to 60 milliseconds.[4,73]

The dominant QRS deflection of the ECG (generically called the R wave) triggers balloon deflation. To determine balloon inflation time, the IABP console senses the average R-R cycle length to determine the exact onset of diastole. The onset of diastole usually corresponds with the end of the T wave on the ECG complex.[4]

Manual adjustment of timing

Although the automatic trigger for inflation and deflation of the balloon is usually the ECG, the pump operator fine tunes the timing using the patient's aortic arterial waveform.[4] Timing is adjusted by the use of slide controls located on the front of the IABP console. Accurate timing of inflation and deflation is critical for optimal augmentation (Fig. 8-33). Manual timing of deflation may not be permitted in some alternate trigger modes (i.e., A-Fib). In rapid heart rates (greater than 120), changing augmentation from 1:1 to 1:2 can facilitate timing.

Balloon pump manufacturers provide options for balloon assist that range from augmentation of every beat to augmentation of every eighth beat (i.e., 1:1 to 1:8). This allows the nurse to make adjustments in the assist rate for different clinical conditions and allows for a gradual decrease in augmentation as the patient is weaned from the balloon pump. Some patients may benefit more from a 1:2 to 1:4 assist mode than from a 1:1 mode. This judgment is based on clinical parameters, such as the patient's blood pressure, heart rate, and rhythm, and requirements for pharmacologic support.[4,73]

The practitioner should adjust balloon inflation and deflation timing only when the balloon pump is in the 1:2 mode or less.

1. Patient arotic end diastolic pressure (PA$_o$EDP)
2. Unassisted systole–Peak systolic pressure (PSP)
3. Augmentation pressure (balloon inflation)–Peak diastolic pressure (PDP)
4. Balloon aortic end diastolic pressure (BA$_o$EDP)
5. Assisted systole–Balloon assisted peak systolic pressure (BAPSP)
6. Dicrotic notch

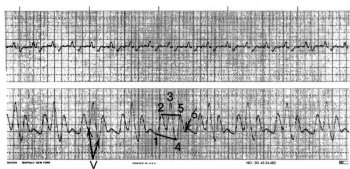

Fig. 8-33 Assessment of normal IABP timing on 1:2. Key waveform components routinely recorded. Note the V configuration before and after the balloon inflation waveform (arrows).

This allows for comparison between the patient's normal arterial pressure waveform and the *assisted* arterial waveform and for visualization of the dicrotic notch.[4,14,73] The dicrotic notch signifies closure of the aortic valve and beginning of diastole.

The goal of timing is to augment coronary blood flow and maximize afterload reduction for the left ventricle. Augmentation of coronary blood flow is a function of balloon *inflation*. Afterload reduction is a function of balloon *deflation*.

Inflation is typically adjusted first. Inflation of the balloon should start at the onset of diastole or the dicrotic notch on the IABP arterial waveform (Fig. 8-33). The inflation upstroke should form a V when aligned with the unassisted arterial waveform (Fig. 8-33). Balloon inflation pressure or *peak diastolic augmented pressure* is usually higher than *peak systolic pressure* (PSP). The PSP is the pressure reached at the height of the patient's systole and is also called unassisted systole.[4,73]

Late inflation occurs when the dicrotic notch is visible before inflation begins, losing the V configuration (Fig. 8-34, *A*). Late inflation poses no danger to the patient, but optimal augmentation is not achieved. Since some of the aortic volume has already been dispersed before inflation begins, less blood remains in the aortic root to perfuse the coronary arteries during balloon inflation.[77] Late inflation can be corrected by moving the inflation slide control to the left.

With early inflation the balloon waveform is superimposed on the patient's arterial waveform (Fig. 8-34, *A*). Early inflation is detrimental to the patient because it increases the afterload of the LV. If the balloon inflates early, the LV has to pump against it to open the aortic valve, actually increasing resistance to left ventricular emptying. Early inflation of the balloon may

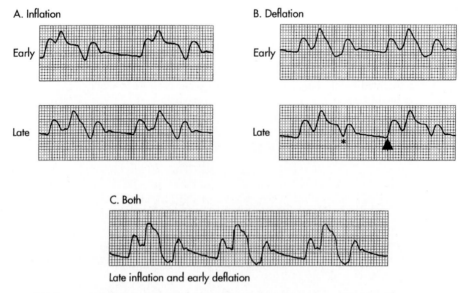

A. Inflation

Early

Late

B. Deflation

Early

Late

C. Both

Late inflation and early deflation

Fig. 8-34 Improper balloon timing. The major distinguishing characteristic in late deflation is that the BAoEDP(*) is not lower than the PAoEDP (▲). Note the normal plateau seen in the early inflation and late deflation patterns.

force the aortic valve to close prematurely, decreasing stroke volume and cardiac output and increasing LV end-diastolic volume.[73,77] Early inflation can be corrected by moving the inflation slide control to the right.

Deflation of the balloon is adjusted to occur exactly at the end of diastole or just before systole to maximize the assist to the left ventricle. As the balloon deflates, aortic root pressure is decreased, thereby reducing systemic vascular resistance or the afterload of the left ventricle.[77] The deflation downstroke should also form a V when aligned with the assisted arterial waveform on the IABP console (Fig. 8-33). The normal balloon waveform pattern may have either a sharp peak (Fig. 8-33) or a plateau (Fig. 8-34) between inflation and deflation.

The reduction of left ventricular afterload assists the LV in ejecting blood during systole, which follows balloon deflation. The arterial waveform following balloon deflation is thus known as the *balloon-assisted peak systolic pressure* or *assisted systole*. This pressure should be equal to or lower than the unassisted systole, reflecting the afterload reduction (Fig. 8-33).[73,77]

With proper deflation, the *balloon aortic end-diastolic pressure* (BAoEDP) should be lower than the *patient's aortic end-diastolic pressure* (PAoEDP) (Fig. 8-33).[77] The PAoEDP

and the BAoEDP are the lowest pressures before the upstroke of systole. The PAoEDP is the naturally occurring diastolic pressure after the assisted systole on 1:2. BAoEDP is determined by the timing of the balloon deflation after the peak diastolic augmented pressure, just before the assisted systole.

Late deflation of the balloon results in an increased afterload for the left ventricle as it is trying to eject its contents against a higher than normal pressure (i.e., from inflated balloon in aorta).[73,77] Late deflation is evident on the balloon tracing by the absence of a drop or an actual rise in the BAoEDP (on 1:2) (Fig. 8-34,B). This problem can be corrected by moving the deflation slide control to the left until a proper waveform is achieved (i.e., BAoEDP < AoEDP).

Early deflation is recognized by a U-shaped effect in the deflation curve rather than the V shape (Fig. 8-34,B).[77] Early deflation minimizes the assist to the left ventricle and may allow for retrograde flow from the coronary arteries into the aortic root, thereby jeopardizing coronary blood flow.[73] With early deflation the balloon-assisted peak systolic pressure is not lowered. This problem can be corrected by moving the deflation slide control to the right and observing the waveform.

Patient assessment and problem solving

The three major patient complications associated with the use of the IABP are (1) impaired peripheral circulation, (2) infection, and (3) bleeding.[4,14,73,77] The most common complication is impaired peripheral circulation distal to the balloon insertion site.[4] Loss of peripheral circulation may occur as a result of occlusion of the vessels by the balloon catheter, thrombus, or embolus. Close monitoring of sensation, temperature, and pulses in the limb distal to insertion of the balloon catheter is a high priority in the nursing assessment. Peripheral pulses, especially of the

lower extremities, require hourly assessment and careful documentation.[77] It is not unusual to have some decrease in pulse amplitude in the limb of insertion and some slight difference in temperature. However, the nurse should report any perceived significant loss, such as total loss of pulses or acute pain or other sensory abnormalities, to the physician immediately.

Anticoagulant therapy may be used during IABP therapy to prevent clot formation on the balloon catheter. Both heparin or low-molecular-weight dextran can be used.

For this reason, as well as a high occurrence of stress ulcers, closely monitoring coagulation studies, testing N/G and stool for occult blood, and instituting measures to reduce physiologic and psychological stress are also important. Anticoagulation should be used cautiously, if at all, in patients following open heart surgery due to the evidence of coagulopathy. All patients who require IABP support should receive histamine$_2$ inhibitors and antacids prophylactically. Increased bleeding times also lead to oozing at the balloon catheter insertion site or any puncture site and require bleeding precautions.[4,73]

Scrupulous use of sterile technique when dressing the insertion site and care to prevent cross-contamination with other patients in the unit are imperative.[14,73] These steps are especially important when managing patients awaiting cardiac transplant who may already be in a seriously debilitated state; infection would mean they are no longer candidates for transplant. Special instructions and precautions to visitors are also indicated.

Other problems that may occur with patients requiring IABP support are (1) compromise of renal, cerebral, and left arm circulation as a result of malposition of the balloon catheter, (2) alteration in sleep patterns due to the critically ill state and sounds of the balloon pump, and (3) alteration in nutritional status.[4,14,77]

Problems related to the balloon catheter or the balloon console include kinking of the catheter, slow gas leaks, improper timing, balloon rupture, and console failure.[4,77] Newer balloon pumps have sophisticated alarm systems that alert the operator to all of these problems except improper timing. Most manufacturers provide troubleshooting guidelines for dealing with these problems. Only nurses trained in the operation of the balloon pump should assume responsibility for this device. A backup plan in the event of console failure should always be delineated.

Other assist devices

In a small percentage of patients, aggressive medical therapy and IABP support are not effective in controlling or reversing the shock syndrome. More aggressive therapies such as *cardiopulmonary support* (CPS) or ventricular assist devices are indicated. CPS, sometimes called *extracorporeal membrane oxygenation* (ECMO), may be used during cardiac arrest as well as shock for short-term therapy (8 to 48 hours).[2,67,68,72,76,79] CPS systems can be instituted at the bedside within 30 minutes to provide adequate perfusion of vital organs and time for further evaluation.[2]

CPS provides full cardiac, circulatory and pulmonary support. Venous blood is aspirated from a femoral percutaneous catheter, oxygenated and warmed in the CPS system, and returned to the femoral artery. The membrane oxygenator also removes excess carbon dioxide from the blood before reinfusing it into the patient. In most institutions trained perfusionists are required to operate the CPS equipment. However, the critical care nurse is responsible for assessment and plan of care for the patient. This assessment is similar to the care of the patient with an IABP.[67,68,76,79]

Ventricular assist devices (VADs) provide temporary support for the right ventricle (RVAD), left ventricle (LVAD), or both ventricles (BiVAD). Most of the blood flow bypasses the natural pump (the heart) and travels through an artificial pump, reducing the work load of the heart to a significantly greater extent than with the IABP.[75] The heart receives the opportunity to rest and recover. The artificial pump usually maintains flow rates of up to 2 to 4 L/min, although rates up to 10 L/min are possible.[2,80] These flow rates supplement the natural cardiac output or provide total support, enhanc-

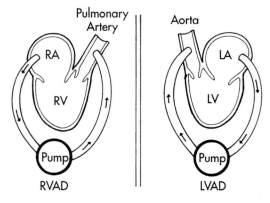

Fig. 8-35 Typical LVAD and RVAD circuits. The combination of an LVAD and RVAD is known as a BiVAD.

ing tissue perfusion. These devices also facilitate weaning from cardiopulmonary bypass.[66,79,80]

The LVAD circuit usually begins with a large cannula in the left atrium or ventricle that pulls blood into a pump device and returns it to the ascending aorta. The RVAD circuit connects a cannula from the right atrium to a pump and then back to the main pulmonary artery. The BiVAD incorporates both of these circuits running concurrently (Fig. 8-35).[66,79]

Current pumps provide either continuous or pulsatile flow.[14] Continuous-flow devices such as the Bio-Medicus centrifugal force pump are useful in patients requiring more intensive support than the IABP can provide but in whom short-term support (usually under 1 week) is anticipated.[2,14,71] Candidates include patients who have had acute MI or cardiac surgery. Heparin administration is usually necessary after 48 hours.[14]

Pumps providing pulsatile flow are the most physiologic and may be pneumatically or electrically powered. Examples include the Pierce-Donachy Thoratec, Novacor, and Jarvik pumps. The artificial chamber fills passively during contraction of the natural atrium or ventricle and periodically compresses to provide pulsatile flow. The pulsatile flow maximizes coronary, cerebral, and renal perfusion. Inflow and outflow valves prevent backflow, similar to a natural heart. Pulsatile pumps can be used longer than other assist devices, including the continuous-flow VAD systems. This characteristic makes them ideal for use in patients awaiting cardiac transplantation.[66,79,80] Systems requiring cannulation or removal of parts of the left ventricle are usually reserved for this population. Circulatory support has been maintained successfully for up to 1 year with these devices.[2] Heparinization is not usually required, minimizing complications. Implantable forms of electrically powered pulsatile systems are currently under investigation. At this time the power source although smaller and portable, is still external but has the potential to be fully implantable.

Hemodynamic indications for a VAD are consistent with signs of cardiogenic shock. These indications include cardiac index less than 1.8 L/min/m^2, RA or LA pressures (PCWP) greater than 20 to 25 mm Hg, and urine output less than 20 ml/hr together with low systolic blood pressure and high systemic vascular resistance.[2,80] If these parameters do not improve after pharmacologic therapy, pacing, and 1 to 2 hours of IABP, the decision may be made to use a VAD. In rapidly deteriorating patients, a VAD may be the initial mode of circulatory assist. Even with hemodynamic improvement, VAD insertion may be considered if the patient requires high doses of inotropic agents or IABP for longer than 48 hours and especially for longer than 1 week.[2] Contraindications include end-stage renal or hepatic failure, peripheral vascular disease, cancer, CVA, coagulopathy, severe infection, or psychosocial history incompatible with eventual cardiac transplantation (see Unit 11).[2,71] Most of these conditions are also contraindications to IABP and transplantation.

As with CPS, a trained perfusionist is required to operate short-term VADs. Patients requiring these short-term VADs are usually hemodynamically unstable and need complex care from specially trained critical care nurses. Hourly hemodynamic measurements are obtained and VAD flow rates are correlated with the patient's clinical status. Inotropic and vasoactive agents are often infusing. Chest tubes are usually in place. Arrhythmias, although not desirable, do not physiologically affect the patient since pumping occurs independent of the natural heart's electrical activity.

With later-generation, long-term pulsatile pumps, after the patient is stabilized and optimal pumping parameters are established, regular hemodynamic monitoring is no longer required. All invasive lines and intravenous pharmacologic support are discontinued. The patient may be transferred to a routine cardiac nursing unit. In the more recently developed models the artificial chamber is implanted, although the power source is external, facilitating progressive ambulation and rehabilitation. Treadmill protocols should be followed by patients to guide activity (see Unit 5). Nurses caring for these patients should monitor the patient's response to the set parameters. They should be aware of interventions in the event of VAD failure and should be familiar with the alarm features of the particular model being used.

With both continuous-flow (short-term) and pulsatile VADs, the nurse should monitor the patient for potential complications. Thrombocytopenia occurs secondary to platelet activation and depletion.[2] Right ventricular failure commonly occurs with LVADs and may be due in part to an increase in venous return secondary to the improved flow.[2,80] If pharmacologic support and pacing are ineffective, additional insertion of an RVAD may be required. Other complications include thromboembolism, renal failure, and infection.[2,66,79,81]

Weaning the patient from the VAD usually involves gradually decreasing the VAD flow rates over a period of about 12 to 14 hours.[80] Heparin is administered at this time to prevent clotting associated with the lower flow rates. Arterial blood gases, cardiac index, and atrial and arterial pressures are measured. Echocardiograms or nuclear studies may also be used to evaluate the return of effective ventricular function.[80]

A multidisciplinary approach is important in planning the care of these unstable and complex patients. Open communication among the health care team members is essential in delivering optimal care.[66,78-80]

NURSING ORDERS: For patients requiring circulatory assist with the IABP and other devices

RELATED NURSING DIAGNOSES: Alteration in tissue perfusion related to decreased cardiac output, device malfunction, right ventricular failure, or hypovolemia; potential for injury related to bleeding from anticoagulation, infection, or thromboembolism; impaired mobility related to invasive lines and assist devices; anxiety or fear related to prognosis, sensory overload, lack of understanding of equipment and procedures, separation from family and friends; impaired gas exchange related to atelectasis and immobility

1. Explain to the patient and family the purpose of balloon insertion (or other assist devices) and what to expect with insertion and operation; obtain signed informed consent.
   —Equipment (console, balloon catheter, A-line, or other devices as ordered)
   —Premedication for discomfort
   —Sensations associated with balloon or device function
   —Activity limitations
2. Record baseline vital signs and clinical observations regarding temperature and skin color of legs before catheter or cannula is inserted.
3. Guard against sepsis; following balloon/

device insertion, apply occlusive sterile dressing to site and inspect frequently for bleeding; change dressing every 24 hours or as ordered.
—Maintain nutritional support.
—Use scrupulous aseptic technique with invasive lines.
—Request blood cultures for patients with a temperature greater than 38° C (101° F).
—Monitor white blood cell and differential blood count.

4. With IABP evaluate timing and effectiveness of counterpulsation.
—Compare pressure waveform with ECG to determine if augmentation is timed appropriately. Does inflation begin at the dicrotic notch? Is BAoEDP less than PAoEDP? Is presystolic dip present? Observe for effects of arrhythmias
—Correlate wedge pressure, cardiac output, arterial pressure, and SVR with clinical parameters such as neurologic status, respiratory status, and renal function. Are these parameters improving with augmentation? If so, can augmentation be decreased to every second or third beat (1:2 or 1:3 as opposed to 1:1)?
—Titrate vasoactive drugs as indicated.

5. With VADs, monitor flow rates and patient response
—Collaborate with perfusionist to monitor specific alarm settings on model.
—Correlate flow rates with hemodynamic parameters.
—Monitor volume status.
—Monitor respiratory status and arterial blood gases (ABG).

6. Check blood flow to areas potentially involved with balloon insertion or other large-bore catheters.
—Verify balloon position by chest radiograph.
—Check pulses, temperature, and color of leg and foot distal to insertion; compare to uninvolved leg (Q1H). Report any pain, numbness, temperature, or color change; loss of motor function in the involved leg is usually a medical emergency requiring immediate removal of the catheter.
—Check pulses, temperature, and color of arms, especially left arm, to rule out balloon occlusion of left subclavian artery, particularly if there is a loss of radial artery tracing.
—Monitor neurologic status to rule out embolic phenomena or occlusion of left carotid artery by the balloon.
—Monitor renal status; if urine output diminishes rather than improves with assist devices, check for possible occlusion of renal artery by IABP or development of renal failure.
—Avoid raising head of bed greater than 45 degrees to prevent displacement of balloon or kinking of catheter.

7. Avoid unnecessarily flexing the patient's leg at the groin to prevent kinking of balloon or other large-bore catheters. Periodically inspect catheters for kinking, cracking, disconnections, or leaks.

8. In patients with a recently inserted LVAD, watch for signs of right ventricular failure; anticipate possible RVAD insertion.

9. Assess the following laboratory values relating to balloon/device complications or prophylactic anticoagulation:
—Red blood cell count; with IABP or pulsatile pumps, anemia may result from hemolysis.
—Platelet count; thrombocytopenia may result from mechanical destruction.
—BUN/creatinine.
—Liver function studies.
—Other coagulation studies (PT, PTT, ACT).

10. In the patient with IABP and/or assist devices anticipate high stress levels caused

by critical physiologic state, sensory overload, activity restriction, discomfort, or fear of prognosis.

—Provide consistent personnel and optimum emotional support.

—Maintain family contact as much as possible.

—Administer antacids or agents that decrease acid levels rising in response to stress.

11. If IABP shutoff is required, notify patient to allay anxiety; if balloon console breaks and backup unit is not available, patient support is imperative. Psychological dependence on the balloon may predispose the patient to physiologic crisis if balloon is abruptly withdrawn.

NOTE: The balloon should be manually inflated at least every 10 minutes to prevent clot formation on the balloon.

12. Wean the patient from IABP or assist device according to planned protocol, with frequent observation of cardiac hemodynamic profile.

SELF ASSESSMENT

Mr. Jackson, a 54-year-old construction worker, was admitted to the coronary care unit yesterday with the diagnosis of extensive anterior wall MI. Although TPA was administered in the emergency room, a large akinetic area was visible on echocardiogram, together with an ejection fraction of 40%. Over the past few hours Mr. Jackson has become progressively short of breath, with respirations increasing to 26 per minute. Inspiratory crackles, not clearing with coughing, were auscultated over the lower third of the lower lobes posteriorly. Both an S3 and S4 were present. The ECG trace also showed frequent PACs.

1 The clinical signs are compatible with (right/left) ventricular failure. Heart failure is defined as inadequate _____ _____ secondary to mechanical or _____ dysfunction.

The most common cause of heart failure is _____, which is a manifestation of the effects of an increased (preload/afterload) on a weakened pump.

> left
> cardiac output
> pump
> hypertension
> afterload

2 In heart failure, blood becomes congested within the involved ventricle secondary to ineffective (filling/emptying). The major symptoms of CHF are a consequence of either _____ or _____ pressure increases.

Serum and urine electrolyte (Na^+/K^+) changes occur secondary to neurohormonal responses to a fall in cardiac output (increasing/decreasing) fluid retention.

> emptying
> pulmonary; systemic
> increasing

3 Both S_3 and S_4 are extra (systolic/diastolic) heart sounds called _____. An S_4 reflects increases in left ventricular pressure related to changes in _____ and (is/is not) a common finding in acute MI. An S_3 reflects increases in left ventricular pressure related to _____.

Crackles occur secondary to opening of _____ airways or in the presence of _____ _____. In

> diastolic
> gallops
> compliance; is
> CHF
> atelectatic
> interstitial fluid

360

early CHF, these sounds are audible at the (beginning/end) of inspiration. Arterial blood gases drawn at this time can be expected to show respiratory (alkalosis/acidosis).

end

alkalosis

4 Mr. Jackson received oxygen, diuretics, and topical nitrates. Nitrates act primarily to decrease (preload/afterload). The initial diuretic of choice for severe pulmonary congestion is _____ _____ because of an immediate effect in dilating (veins/arteries).

Mr. Jackson should be positioned with the head of the bed in high Fowler's and legs _____. Morphine may be administered to decrease anxiety, _____ rate, and _____ return.

Digitalis is currently considered a (second-/third-) line agent in the management of severe CHF (acute PE). Preferred inotropic agents are _____ and _____.

preload
furosemide (Lasix)
veins

dependent
respiratory; venous
third-

dopamine; dobutamine

5 As Mr. Jackson's condition deteriorates, a PA line is inserted. After insertion, the following trace is recorded from the distal port.

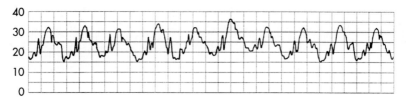

Fig. 8-36   Self-assessment trace 1.

This tracing is a (normal/abnormal) PA trace. In the spontaneously breathing patient, the PAEDP should be obtained at the end of (inspiration/expiration). In the preceding trace, it is _____ mm Hg and should be 2 to 4 mm Hg (higher/lower) than the PCWP (LVEDP).

The remaining hemodynamic values are RA, 12 mm Hg; PCWP 20 mm Hg, cardiac index 2.5 L/min/m^2, SVR 2000 dynes/sec/cm^5. This pattern indicates hypovolemia/CHF/shock).

normal
expiration
20–22
higher

CHF

6 A few hours later the following trace is recorded from the distal port.

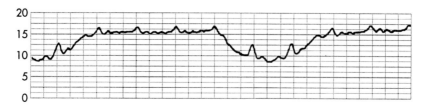

Fig. 8-37   Self-assessment trace 2.

This tracing suggests (catheter whip/RV pattern/spontaneous wedge). Nursing action includes (inflation/deflation) of the balloon, having the patient (cough/deep breathe), and _____ the patient on one side.

spontaneous wedge
deflation
cough; turning

7 Mr. Jackson becomes confused. His urine output decreases to less than 20 ml/hr. The cardiac index drops to 1.8 L/m^2. These signs and symptoms indicate the presence of (CHF/shock), which results in ABGs that typically show metabolic (acidosis/alkalosis).

shock
acidosis

An IABP is inserted. The IABP inflates during (systole/diastole) to (increase/decrease) coronary and cerebral perfusion. As the balloon deflates, (preload/afterload) is decreased, facilitating _____ _____.

diastole
increase
afterload; cardiac output

8 The following trace is recorded from the arterial line.

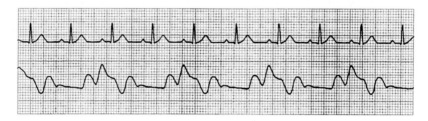

Fig. 8-38   Self-assessment trace 3.

This tracing suggests (early inflation/late inflation/normal IABP effects). Early inflation and late deflation can compromise the patient's status by causing an increased (preload/afterload).

normal IABP effects

afterload

The three major patient complications associated with IABP pumps are (1) impaired peripheral _____, (2) infection, and (3) _____.

circulation
bleeding

9 Although the hemodynamic parameters improve with IABP therapy, after 1 week Mr. Jackson still cannot be weaned off the pump. Since long-term support is anticipated, the decision is made to insert a pulsatile LVAD. The LVAD (is/is not) another mode of circulatory assist that differs from the IABP in that (some/most) of the blood flow bypasses the natural pump, primarily (increasing coronary supply/decreasing cardiac work).

is
most
decreasing cardiac work

The LVAD circuit connects the left _____ or ventricle to the artificial pump, then returns the blood to the _____. The pump and/or power source at this time is usually (internal/external).

atrium
aorta
external

Potential complications associated with LVAD systems include low _____ count, _____ ventricle failure, and _____.

platelet; right (bi)
infection

Table 8-6. Intervention in patients with hemodynamic imbalance: congestive heart failure or shock

Management goal	Intervention
1. Preload	
To decrease preload (with pulmonary or systemic congestion)	Decrease venous return
	High Fowler's position with legs dangling
	Morphine sulfate
	Diuretics (Lasix/Bumex)
	Nitroglycerin, isosorbide (Isordil) (decreases afterload also)
	PEEP
	Fluid restriction, decrease IV fluids
To increase preload (with decreased cardiac output and wedge)	Increase volume
	Crystalloids
	Dextran
2. To decrease afterload	Nitroprusside (Nipride)
	Hydralazine (Apresoline)
	Captopril (Capoten)
	IABP
3. To increase contractility	Dopamine
	Dobutamine
	Amrinone
	Digitalis
	Correction of arrhythmias
	Repair of mechanical defects
4. To increase O_2 supply and decrease O_2 demands	Oxygen
	Psychological support
	Rest
	Morphine sulfate
	IABP
	Ventricular assist devices
	Coronary bypass
	Decrease of preload/afterload
5. To support tissue metabolism	Hyperalimentation
	Steroids

10 Mrs. Miller is admitted to the coronary care unit with the diagnosis of inferior wall MI. Her neck veins are distended, but her lungs remain clear.

The nurse should suspect the presence of (right/left) ventricular failure secondary to _____ ventricular infarction. A PA line was inserted in anticipation of hemodynamic instability.

The RA and PA systolic pressures are usually (high/low), and the PA diastolic and PCWP pressures are usually (high/normal). Equalization of right and left heart pressures may occur. These findings are also seen in cardiac _____.

right

right

high

tamponade

363

Treatment of right ventricular failure secondary to right ventricular infarction includes (fluids/diuretics). The patient should not receive M.S. and _____. The inotropic agent of choice is _____.

fluids

nitrates

dobutamine

REFERENCES/SUGGESTED READINGS

General

1. Albarran-Sotelo R et al: Textbook of advanced cardiac life support, ed 2, Dallas, 1990, American Heart Association.
2. Braunwald E, editor: Heart disease: a textbook of cardiovascular medicine, ed 4, vol 1, Philadelphia, 1992, WB Saunders.
3. Clausen P: Right ventricular infarction: how to recognize hidden cardiac damage, Nursing 20:(3):34, 1990.
4. Daily EK, Schroeder JS: Techniques in bedside hemodynamic monitoring, ed 4, St. Louis, 1989, CV Mosby.
5. Darovic GO: Hemodynamic monitoring: invasive and noninvasive clinical applications, Philadelphia, 1987, WB Saunders.
6. Holloway NM: Nursing the critically ill adult, ed 3, Menlo Park, 1988, Addison-Wesley Publishing Company.
7. Hurst JW, Schlant RC, editors: The heart arteries and veins, ed 7, vol 1, New York, 1990, McGraw-Hill Information Services Company.
8. Kinney MR, Packa DR, Dunbar SB: AACN's clinical reference for critical care nursing, ed 2, New York, 1988, McGraw-Hill Book Company.
9. Lundberg, GD, editor: Guidelines for cardiopulmonary resuscitation and emergency cardiac care: recommendations of the 1992 national conference, JAMA 268(16):2171, 1992.
10. McMillan JY, Little-Longeway CD: Right ventricular infarction, Focus on Critical Care 18(2):157, 1991.
11. Rippe JM, editor: Manual of intensive care medicine, ed 2, Boston, 1989, Little, Brown and Company.
12. Rippe JM, et al, editors: Intensive care medicine, ed 2, Boston, 1991, Little, Brown.
13. Thelan LA: Textbook of critical care nursing: Diagnosis and management, St. Louis, 1990, CV Mosby.
14. Underhill SL et al: Cardiac nursing, ed 2, Philadelphia, 1992, JB Lippincott.

Congestive heart failure and auscultation of the heart

15. Alpert JS, Rippe JM: Manual of cardiovascular diagnosis and therapy, ed 3, Boston, 1988, Little, Brown.
16. Bates B: A guide to physical examination and history taking, ed 4, Philadelphia, 1987, JB Lippincott.
17. Chent TO: Cardiac failure in coronary heart disease, Am Heart J 120(2):396, 1990.
18. Chent TO: Congestive heart failure in coronary artery disease, Am J Med 91:409, Oct 1991.
19. Francis GS: Interaction of the sympathetic nervous system and electrolytes in congestive heart failure, Am J Cardiol 65:24E, 1990.
20. Francis GS: Neuroendocrine manifestations of congestive heart failure, Am J Cardiol 62:9A, 1988.
21. Harvey AM et al, editors: The principles and practice of medicine, ed 22, Norwalk, CT, 1988, Appleton & Lange.
22. Kannel WB, Belanger, AJ: Epidemiology of heart failure, Am Heart J 121(3):951, 1991.
23. Keller KB, Lemberg L: Changing concepts in the management of congestive heart failure, Heart Lung 9(4):425, 1990.
24. Letterer RA et al: Learning to live with congestive heart failure, Nursing 92 22(5):34, 1992.
25. Luce JM, Pierson DJ: Critical care medicine, Philadelphia, 1988, WB Saunders.
26. Marino PL: The ICU book, Philadelphia, 1991, Lea & Febiger.
27. Packer M. Pathophysiology of heart failure, Lancet 340(8811):88, 1992.
28. Packer M: Treatment of chronic heart failure, Lancet 340(8811):92,1992.

29. Perloff JK: Heart sounds and murmurs: physiological mechanisms. In Braunwald E, editor: Heart disease: a textbook of cardiovascular medicine, ed 4, vol 1, Philadelphia, 1992, WB Saunders.

30. Perret C: Heart failure myocardial infarction: principles of treatment, Crit Care Med 19(1):6, 1990.

31. Shoemaker WC et al, editors: Textbook of critical care, ed 2, Philadelphia, 1989, WB Saunders.

32. Stein E, Abner JD: Rapid interpretation of heart sounds and murmurs, ed 3, Philadelphia, 1990, Lea & Febiger.

33. Williams JF: Evolving concepts in congestive heart failure, part 1, Modern Concepts of Cardiovascular Disease 59(8):43, 1990.

34. Williams JF: Evolving concepts in congestive heart failure, part 2, Modern Concepts of Cardiovascular Disease 59:(9):49, 1990.

Shock

35. Barone JE, Snyder AB: Treatment strategies in shock: use of oxygen transport measurements, Heart Lung 20(1):81, 1991.

36. Bell TN: Disseminated intravascular coagulation and shock, Crit Care Nurs Clin North Am 2(2):255, 1990.

37. Burns KM: Vasoactive drug therapy in shock, Crit Care Clin North Am 2(2):167, 1990.

38. Daily EK: Use of hemodynamics to differentiate pathophysiologic causes of cardiogenic shock, Crit Care Nurs Clin North Am 1(3):589, 1989.

39. Gawlinski A: Saving the cardiogenic shock patient, Nursing, 12:34, Dec 1989.

40. Guyton AC: Textbook of medical physiology, ed 8, Philadelphia, 1991, WB Saunders.

41. Houston MC: Pathophysiology of shock, Crit Care Nurs Clin North Am 2(2):143, 1990.

42. Killip T: Cardiogenic shock complicating myocardial infarction, J Am Coll Cardiol 14:47, 1989.

43. Lancaster LE: Renal response to shock, Crit Care Nurs Clin North Am 2(2):221, 1990.

44. Rice V: Shock, a clinical syndrome: an update, part 1, Crit Care Nurse 11(4):20, 1991.

45. Summers G: The clinical and hemodynamic presentation of the shock patient, Crit Care Nurs Clin North Am 2(2), 1990.

46. Wahl SC: Septic shock: how to detect it early, Nursing 1:52, Jan 1989.

Hemodynamic monitoring

47. Bridges EJ, Woods SL: Pulmonary artery measurement: state of the art, Heart Lung 22(2):99, 1993.

48. Campbell ML, Greenberg CA: Reading pulmonary artery wedge pressure at end-expiration, Focus on Critical Care 15(2):60, 1988.

49. Cason CL et al: Effects of backrest elevation and position on pulmonary artery pressures, Cardiovasc Nurs 26(1):1, 1990.

50. Ciaccio JM: Measurements of hemodynamics in side-lying positions: a review of the literature, Focus on Critical Care 17(3):250, 1990.

51. Cline JK, Gurka AM: Effect of backrest position on pulmonary artery pressure and cardiac output measurements in critically ill patients, Focus on Critical Care 18(5):383, 1991.

52. Dennison RD: Understanding the four determinants of cardiac output, Nursing 20(7):35, 1990.

53. Doering LV: The effect of positioning on hemodynamics and gas exchange in the critically ill: a review, Am J Crit Care 2(3):208, 1993.

54. Enger EL: Pulmonary artery wedge pressure: when it's valid, when it's not, Crit Care Nurs Clin North Am 1(3):603, 1989.

55. Feigenbaum H: Echocardiography. In Braunwald E, editor: Heart disease: a textbook of cardiovascular medicine, ed 4, vol 1, Philadelphia, 1992, WB Saunders.

56. Gardner PE: Pulmonary artery pressure monitoring, AACN Clinical Issues 4(1):98, 1993.

57. Harvey AM et al, editors: The principles and practice of medicine, ed 22, Norwalk, CT, 1988, Appleton & Lange.

58. Lambert CW, Cason CL: Backrest elevation and pulmonary artery pressures: research analysis, Dimensions of Critical Care Nursing 9(6):327, 1990.

59. Pesola GR, Rosata HP, Carlon GC: Room temperature thermodilution cardiac output: central venous vs right ventricular port, Am J Crit Care 1(1):76, 1992.

60. Proulx R et al: Detection of right ventricular myocardial infarction in patients with inferior wall myocardial infarction, Crit Care Nurse 12(5):50, 1992.

61. Qaal SJ: Quality assurance in hemodynamic monitoring, AACN Clinical Issues 4(1):197, 1993.
62. Rountree WD: Removal of pulmonary artery catheters by registered nurses: a study in safety and complications, Focus on Critical Care 18(4):313, 1991.
63. Stock MC, Perel A: Handbook of mechanical ventilatory support, Baltimore, 1992, Williams & Wilkins.
64. Urban N: Integrating the hemodynamic profile with clinical assessment, AACN Clinical Issues 4(1):161, 1993.
65. Woods SJ, Osguthorpe S: Cardiac output determination, AACN Clinical Issues 4(1):81, 1993.

Circulatory assist devices

66. Barden C, Lee R: Update on ventricular assist devices, AACN Clinical Issues in Critical Care Nursing 1(1):13, 1990.
67. Bavin TK: Cardiac considerations for patients requiring cardiopulmonary support, AACN Clinical Issues in Critical Care Nursing 2(3):500, 1991.
68. Cone M et al: Cardiopulmonary support in the intensive care unit, Am J Crit Care 1(1):98, 1992.
69. Goodwin M, et al: Safety of intraaortic balloon counterpulsation in patients with acute myocardial infarction receiving streptokinase intravenously, Am J Cardiol 60:937, 1989.
70. Ishihara M et al: Intraaortic balloon pumping as the postangioplasty strategy in acute myocardial infarction, Am Heart J 122(2):385, 1991.
71. Ley SJ: Myocardial depression after cardiac surgery: pharmacologic and mechanical support, AACN Clinical Issues 4(2):293, 1993.
72. Nawa S et al: Evaluation of conventional circulatory assist devices, Chest 95(2):261, 1989.
73. Odom BS: Managing the challenge of IABP therapy, Crit Care Nurse 11(2):60, 1991.
74. Ohman EM et al: The use of intraaortic balloon pumping as an adjunct to reperfusion therapy in acute myocardial infarction, Am Heart J 121(3):895, 1991.
75. Quaal SJ: Cardiac assist devices, AACN Clinical Issues in Critical Care Nursing 2(3):475, 1991.
76. Reedy, JE et al: Mechanical cardiopulmonary support for refractory cardiogenic shock, Heart Lung 19(5):514, 1990.
77. Schott KE: Intra-aortic balloon counterpulsation as a therapy for shock, Crit Care Nurs Clin North Am 2(27):187, 1990.
78. Simpson M, Luguire r, Dewitt L: TCI left ventricular assist device: nursing implications, Dimensions of Critical Care Nursing 9(6):318, 1990.
79. Smith RG, Cleavinger M: Current perspectives on the use of circulatory assist devices, AACN Clinical Issues in Critical Care Nursing 2(3):488, 1991.
80. Teplitz L: An algorithm for ventricular assist devices, Dimensions of Critical Care Nursing 9(5):256, 1990.
81. Vaska PL: Biventricular assist devices, Critical Care Nurse 11(8):52, 1991.

Pharmacologic Intervention in Coronary Artery Disease

Colleen Counsell, RN, MSN
Marielle Vinsant Crawford, RNC, MS

OVERVIEW

Pharmacologic intervention is frequently indicated for the complications of coronary artery disease. The three major life-threatening problems complicating coronary heart disease are arrhythmias, heart failure, and cardiogenic shock. Arrhythmias reflect alterations in electrical activity, and heart failure and cardiogenic shock reflect alterations in mechanical activity (Fig. 9-1). Arrhythmias may occur during angina or acute myocardial infarction (MI). Heart failure and cardiogenic shock, however, are typically related to the permanent structural changes in the muscle wall associated with acute MI. When electrical or mechanical disorders occur in other forms of heart disease, treatment in a coronary care unit includes the same pharmacologic agents as those used in patients with coronary artery disease.

Pharmacologic management of arrhythmias varies according to the three major clinically significant forms: (1) ventricular tachyarrhythmias, (2) supraventricular tachyarrhythmias, and (3) bradyarrhythmias. The primary pharmacologic agents in the management of ventricular tachyarrhythmias are the antiarrhythmic agents. The major mechanism of action of these drugs, as a group, is to depress ectopic impulse formation in the ventricles. The initial goal of therapy in supraventricular tachyarrhythmias is to decrease the ventricular rate. A variety of pharmacologic agents from different classification systems can accomplish this goal, including the inotropic agent digitalis, the beta blockers, the calcium channel blocking agents, and adenosine (Adenocard)—the only currently available cardiac nucleoside. The initial goal of therapy in bradyarrhythmias is to increase the ventricular rate. The primary drugs used for this purpose are autonomic agents such as atropine, epinephrine (Adrenalin), and isoproterenol (Isuprel).[3]

Pharmacologic intervention in the management of heart failure includes the use of diuretics, vasodilating agents, and inotropic agents. Cardiogenic shock, as well as other forms of shock, may require a variety of autonomic agents.

Pharmacologic intervention is also indicated in the management of hypertension, which represents altered mechanical activity in both the heart and the vascular bed. Hypertension occurs in coronary artery disease as a predisposing risk factor and as an aggravating factor. Although not directly life-threatening, hypertension can aggravate heart failure and precipitate coronary chest pain. Control of hypertension may require administration of diuretics, vasodilators including calcium channel blocking agents and angiotensin-converting enzyme (ACE) inhibitors, and a variety of autonomic agents.

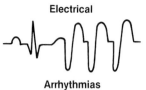

Electrical

Arrhythmias
• Angina or
  acute MI

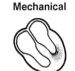

Mechanical

Heart failure
Shock (cardiogenic)
• Acute MI

Fig. 9-1 General functional disorders: electrical versus mechanical.

Another complication occurring in the patient with coronary artery disease is chest pain. Chest pain is usually the initial symptom in both angina and acute MI. It is most significant in the context of structural coronary artery disease because of the potential life-threatening complications. Narcotic analgesics may be required to suppress the pain associated with myocardial ischemia.

Cardiac arrest is usually a manifestation of extreme electrical or mechanical dysfunction associated with hypoxia or metabolic complications. Therefore, the drugs used in cardiac arrest include agents to manage arrhythmias, chest pain, heart failure, and shock, as well as additional agents to manage related complications.

ROLE OF THE AUTONOMIC NERVOUS SYSTEM

The autonomic nervous system plays a significant role in the pharmacologic management of problems associated with acute coronary artery disease. Drugs that mimic, support, or block the effects of the sympathetic and parasympathetic (autonomic) nervous systems on the heart and blood vessels are commonly used in the pharmacologic management of supraventricular tachyarrhythmias, bradyarrhythmias, heart failure, shock, chest pain, and hypertension.

The cardiovascular system is richly innervated by the autonomic nervous system. Sympathetic and parasympathetic receiving or receptor sites line the surface of cardiac electrical and muscle cells. Certain chemicals in the body act as mediators, or *messengers,* carrying sympathetic and parasympathetic information from the nerves and central nervous system (CNS) to receptor sites. The receptors act as doors, allowing the chemical messengers to enter the cell (Fig. 9-2).

The sympathetic nervous system exerts its major influence on the blood vessels, heart, and lungs. The chemical mediators of the sympathetic nervous system are epinephrine (Adrenalin) and norepinephrine (Levophed). Both are produced within the adrenal medulla and are released into the bloodstream after sympathetic stimulation. Norepinephrine is also produced and stored in granules at sympathetic nerve endings and within the CNS. Because of their common production site within the adrenal medulla, these sympathetic chemicals are routinely referred to as *adrenergic.* Another term used to refer to norepinephrine and epinephrine is *catecholamines,* because of their catechol ring—a key chemical structure contained in both.

The sympathetic nervous system has two major types of receptors: alpha and beta. Alpha receptors are predominantly located in the peripheral and coronary blood vessels. Beta receptors are located in the heart and lungs but also in the blood vessels. Norepinephrine is primarily attracted to alpha-receptor sites, although it can also stimulate beta receptors to some extent. It is therefore called an *alpha-adrenergic agent.* The major effect of norepinephrine is on the blood vessels. Epinephrine is primarily attracted to beta sites, although it can also stimulate the alpha receptors. It is therefore referred to as a *beta-adrenergic agent.* Epinephrine has a primary dose-related effect on the heart and

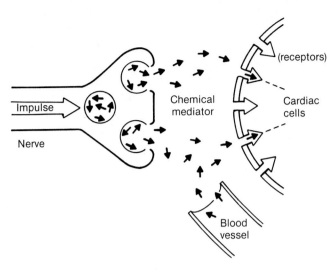

Fig. 9-2 Autonomic nervous system: role of receptors and chemical mediators.

lungs. Dopamine (Intropin), which ultimately converts into norepinephrine, is attracted to a third type of receptor (dopaminergic) that is selectively located in the renal and mesenteric blood vessels (Fig. 9-3).[6,146]

Stimulation of *alpha* receptors results in peripheral vasoconstriction and coronary spasm. Systemic vascular resistance is increased, producing increases in both systolic and diastolic blood pressure. Clinical manifestations include cold or clammy skin and decreased urine output. Coronary and cerebral perfusion increase secondary to increases in diastolic pressure. However, the accompanying increase in afterload may compromise the cardiac output. Vasoconstriction secondary to alpha stimulation can limit bleeding and decrease edema. Related nursing diagnoses include impaired tissue perfusion, alteration in elimination, and alteration in cardiac output.

Beta receptor sites can be further differentiated into B_1 sites on cardiac muscle and conduction structures and B_2 sites on bronchial smooth muscle. Stimulation of the B_1 receptors affects the heart. The effects of autonomic stimulation of the heart can be classified as (1) *chronotropic,* affecting heart rate, (2) *dromotropic,* affecting conduction through the atrioventricular (AV) junctional tissue, or (3) *inotropic,* affecting contractility. To describe these responses of the heart to a drug, the terms *positive* and *negative* can be used. For instance, a drug that increases contractility has a positive inotropic effect. Responses to B_1 receptor stimulation include (1) increase in heart rate (positive chronotropic effect), (2) increase in AV conduction (positive dromotropic effect), (3) increase in contractility (positive inotropic effect), and (4) increase in automaticity. B_1 stimulation also causes the release of renin from the juxtaglomerular apparatus of the kidney, ultimately resulting in the release of the vasoconstrictor angiotensin and aldosterone (see Units 4 and 8).[6] Related nursing diagnoses include alteration in cardiac output and potential fluid overload.

Stimulation of the B_2 receptors in the lungs results in bronchodilation (smooth muscle relaxation). The peripheral and coronary vascular smooth muscles also contain

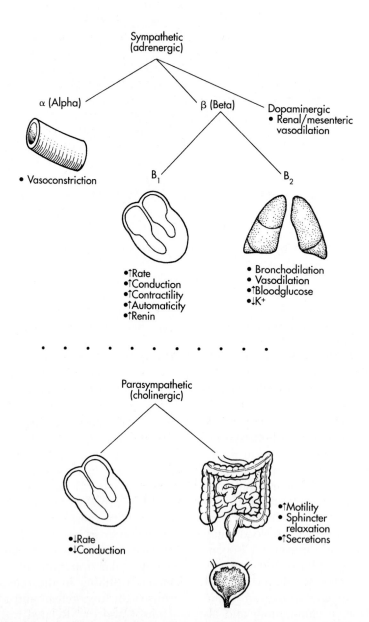

Sympathetic
(adrenergic)

α (Alpha)

• Vasoconstriction

β (Beta)

Dopaminergic
• Renal/mesenteric
  vasodilation

B$_1$

•↑Rate
•↑Conduction
•↑Contractility
•↑Automaticity
•↑Renin

B$_2$

• Bronchodilation
• Vasodilation
•↑Bloodglucose
•↓K+

Parasympathetic
(cholinergic)

•↓Rate
•↓Conduction

•↑Motility
• Sphincter
  relaxation
•↑Secretions

Fig. 9-3 Sites of action and effects of sympathetic and parasympathetic stimulation. Major sympathetic and parasympathetic blockade can be expected to produce the exact opposite effects.

B_2 receptor sites. Stimulation of these receptor sites results in relaxation as well, offsetting the effects of alpha-receptor stimulation. These effects are mediated by the opening and/or closing of the vascular calcium channels. B_2 stimulation also causes an increase in blood glucose secondary to the breakdown of glycogen stores and can promote the movement of potassium into the cells, potentiating hypokalemia.[5,6] Dopaminergic stimulation results in the selective relaxation of the renal and mesenteric vascular beds.[3,136] The urine output increases secondary to increased renal perfusion. Related nursing diagnoses include ineffective airway clearance, impaired gas exchange, impaired tissue perfusion, nutritional or metabolic imbalance, and electrolyte imbalance.

Drugs affecting the sympathetic nervous system are classified into alpha-adrenergic stimulators or blockers and beta-adrenergic stimulators or blockers. Drugs that stimulate beta receptors affect the heart and lungs. Selective B_2 (lung) agents are commonly available for use in patients with pulmonary disorders. These agents have only weak B_1 (heart) effects. However, many sympathetic drugs that significantly affect the heart have significant lung effects as well. These agents possess both B_1 and B_2 effects.

Drugs that block the beta receptors produce effects opposite to those of beta simulation. In the heart, beta blockers produce (1) a negative chronotropic effect (decreased heart rate), (2) a negative dromotropic effect (depressed AV conduction), (3) a negative inotropic effect (decreased myocardial contractility), and (4) decreased ventricular automaticity (decreased ventricular ectopic beats). Because of their effects on heart rate and contractility, beta blockers decrease myocardial O_2 consumption. In the lungs, beta blockers cause bronchoconstriction.

Drugs that block the alpha receptors produce an effect opposite to that of alpha simulation. Therefore, alpha blockers produce dilation of the peripheral blood vessels, lowering blood pressure and relaxing or reversing coronary spasm. Systemic vascular resistance and cardiac afterload are reduced. However, alpha blockers compromise coronary perfusion and may facilitate postoperative bleeding.

The parasympathetic nervous system exerts a major influence on the heart, smooth muscle of the gastrointestinal (GI) and genitourinary (GU) tracts, and respiratory system as well as on GI secretions. The chemical mediator of the parasympathetic nervous system is acetylcholine. For this reason, this parasympathetic chemical and other synthetic parasympathetic drugs that mimic or enhance its action are commonly referred to as *cholinergic*. The major nerve of the parasympathetic nervous system is the vagus nerve. Therefore, parasympathetic agents are also referred to as *vagomimetic*. In the heart, parasympathetic stimulation produces (1) a negative chronotropic effect (decreased heart rate), (2) a negative dromotropic effect (depressed AV conduction), and (3) no effects on inotropy or ventricular automaticity.

Drugs that block or inhibit the effects of the parasympathetic nervous system are called anticholinergic, or vagolytic. In the heart, parasympathetic blockers produce (1) a positive chronotropic effect (increased heart rate) and (2) a positive dromotropic effect (accelerated AV conduction). In the GI and GU tracts, parasympathetic blockade decreases motility and contracts the sphincter muscle, thus inhibiting emptying. In the GI and respiratory tracts, parasympathetic blockade decreases secretions. Related nursing diagnoses include alteration in cardiac output, alteration in elimination, and ineffective airway clearance.

Atropine

Atropine is an example of a drug that blocks the parasympathetic nervous system. Because the parasympathetic nerve that innervates the heart is the vagus nerve, atropine is also known as a vagolytic drug. Parasympathetic blockers such as atropine increase sinus rate and accelerate AV conduction, thus increasing the ventricular rate.

Atropine sulfate is indicated in the management of asystole and bradyarrhythmias with or without a pulse. Atropine is the initial drug of choice in the management of symptomatic bra... arrhythmias, although its use requires caution in type II AV blocks (see Unit 6).[1,3,6] The indicated IV dosage is 0.5 to 1 mg every 3 to 5 minutes, with a maximum of 3 mg.[3,4] Atropine administration via the endotracheal tube is 2 to 2.5 times the dosage.[3,4]

Accelerating the heart rate in a recently injured ischemic myocardium requires caution. The practitioner should accelerate the ventricular rate gradually, using small increments of atropine until the patient's symptoms disappear. Even moderate acceleration of ventricular rate can increase myocardial O_2 consumption, causing ischemia, infarct extension, or rarely ventricular tachycardia (VT) and ventricular fibrillation (VF).

Epinephrine

Epinephrine (Adrenalin) is a commonly used drug during cardiac arrest because of its adrenergic stimulating properties. The actions of epinephrine include B_1 effects (increased heart rate and contractility) and alpha effects (increased systemic vascular resistance). The increase in arterial diastolic pressure, occurring secondary to changes in systemic vascular resistance, results in increased coronary and cerebral perfusion and may provide the greatest benefit during cardiopulmonary resuscitation.[3,6] Epinephrine also has bronchodilating effects in asthma

Another undesirable effect of atropine is its ability to produce urinary retention. The bladder is innervated by parasympathetic fibers; thus blockage of these nerves may lead to difficulty in voiding for some patients. Prolonged atropine therapy may cause mental confusion, which has been labeled "atropine madness" or "atropine psychosis." Additional side effects associated with atropine therapy include dryness of the mouth, flushing of the face, and dilation of the pupils. Atropine is generally contraindicated in patients with glaucoma; however, in emergency settings it may be used if mitotic eye drops are concomitantly administered.

NURSING ORDERS: For patients receiving atropine for bradyarrhythmias

1. Monitor the heart rate for the therapeutic response when administering atropine.
2. Assess for the development of urinary retention.
3. With prolonged atropine therapy, watch for changes in sensorium.
4. Do not administer atropine in patients with glaucoma.
5. Do not administer doses less than 0.5 mg since this may produce a paradoxical slowing effect.[1,3,6]

and anaphylactic reactions (B_2 effects).

Epinephrine is currently indicated in the management of bradyarrhythmias, asystole, ventricular fibrillation, and electrical mechanical dissociation (EMD), also known as pulseless electrical activity (PEA).[3] It is the first drug indicated after cardiopulmonary resuscitation (CPR) and intubation to treat asystole, EMD, and ventricular fibrillation that has not responded to defibrillation.[3,6] Ventricular fibrillation may become more responsive to defibrillation as a result of epinephrine administration. In all three of these disorders, the initial IV dosage is 1 mg every 3 to 5 minutes. If this is ineffective, administration options include the following: 2 to 3 mg every 3 to 5 minutes; 1 mg, 3 mg, and 5 mg 3 minutes apart; 0.1 mg/kg (5 to 10 mg) every 3 to 5 minutes; or a continuous infusion at 200 mcg/min (equivalent to 1 mg every 3 to 5 minutes).[3,149]

Investigators have recently recommended an IV infusion of epinephrine in the treatment of symptomatic bradyarrhythmias unresponsive to atropine, transcutaneous pacing (if immediately available), and dopamine.[3,149] In this situation the infusion rate is 2 to 10 mcg/minute. Epinephrine is also effective when administered via the endotracheal tube at 2 to 2.5 times the peripheral IV dose.[3,149]

NURSING ORDERS: For patients receiving epinephrine

1. Monitor for coarsening of VF pattern after administration, return of pulse in EMD, and return of or increase in heart rate in asystole and bradyarrhythmias.
2. Assess for tachycardia, ventricular arrhythmias, and increased blood pressure.
3. Follow each IV push dose with a 20 cc flush.[3]
4. To prepare an infusion for treatment of bradyarrhythmias, add 2 mg to 500 ml of D_5W or normal saline for a concentration of 4 mcg/cc. To provide 2 mcg/min, set the infusion pump at 30 gtt/min (cc/hr).
5. To prepare an infusion for treatment of asystole, EMD, or VF, add 30 cc of 1:1000 multidose vial (30 mg) to 250 ml D_5W or normal saline for a concentration of 120 mcg/cc. Set the infusion pump at 100 gtt/min (cc/hr), providing approximately 200 mcg/min.[3]
6. Administer IV infusion via a central line. If infiltration occurs in a peripheral line, administer phentolamine (Regitine) subcutaneously to prevent necrosis and sloughing of tissue (secondary to alpha effect).
7. Do not administer together with alkaline solutions such as bicarbonate or aminophylline.

Isoproterenol

Isoproterenol hydrochloride (Isuprel) is an example of a pure beta stimulator. Drugs that stimulate the beta receptors of the sympathetic nervous system produce effects on the heart and lungs identical to epinephrine (Adrenalin). However, the effects on the blood vessels differ. Unlike epinephrine, isoproterenol causes vasodilation, lowering the diastolic blood pressure. As a result, coronary and cerebral perfusion decreases while O_2 consumption increases through its other beta actions, and ischemia is potentiated. The systolic pressure remains elevated secondary to increased cardiac output.

The major benefit of isoproterenol is an increase in the ventricular rate secondary to effects on the sinoatrial (SA) node, AV conduction, and ventricular automaticity. For this reason, isoproterenol may be helpful in the management of bradyarrhythmias. However, the use of isoproterenol is limited to those bradyarrhythmias refractory to atropine, dopamine, and epinephrine only when a transcutaneous pacemaker is not available.[3] Isoproterenol is more effective than atropine in patients with denervated hearts after cardiac transplantation (see Unit 11).[3]

Administration of isoproterenol is by a continuous low-dose intravenous infusion of 2 to 10 mcg/min. The drug requires careful titration to prevent tachyarrhythmias and ventricular arrhythmias[3,6]; these side effects may also occur when isoproterenol is used in respiratory therapy as a bronchial dilator.

NURSING ORDERS: For patients receiving isoproterenol for bradyarrhythmia

1. Monitor cardiac status closely.
2. Watch for the development of tachyarrhythmias and ventricular arrhythmias. If ventricular tachyarrhythmias occur, discontinue drip and institute alternate mode of rate control.
3. Prepare infusion by adding 2 mg to 500 cc of D_5W or normal saline for a concentration of 4 mcg/cc. To provide 2 mcg/min, set the infusion pump at 30 gtt/min (or cc/hr).
4. Use as a temporary measure only. Prepare for immediate pacemaker insertion.

ADENOSINE

A relatively new drug, Adenosine (Adenocard), is an extremely short-acting, highly effective agent for the management of supraventricular tachyarrhythmias.[19,20] Adenosine is a biologic compound found in human cells. It is an endogenous nucleoside produced from the breakdown of adenosine triphosphate (ATP).[9,10,17,19]

The chief indication for adenosine is in the treatment of paroxysmal supraventricular tachycardia (PSVT), which usually presents as a regular, narrow complex tachycardia. In PSVT, adenosine acts primarily to slow AV conduction and interrupt the tachycardia circuit, thus restoring sinus rhythm. It is the preferred drug for treating patients with this supraventricular arrhythmia.[3,9,19,20] Administration of adenosine is usually preceded by treatment with vagotonic physical maneuvers or by electrical cardioversion if the patient demonstrates signs of hemodynamic compromise.[3,9,20] Adenosine is as effective as verapamil (Isoptin, Calan) in terminating PSVT and is considered superior to verapamil in this situation because of its slightly faster onset of action, absence of significant hemodynamic effects, and short half-life, which allows side effects, although common, to be transient.[3,11,17,18] Adenosine is considered safer in patients with significant left ventricular failure.[10] Administration of verapamil is reserved for patients with recurrent PSVT in whom more sustained effects are needed and the blood pressure remains stable.[3,19,20]

In the irregular, narrow complex tachycardias associated with atrial flutter or fibrillation, treatment with verapamil is usually preferred unless hypotension is present.[3,9,20] In atrial flutter and fibrillation the effects of adenosine are primarily diagnostic since they are short term. The rhythm is not terminated. However, the ventricular response is decreased, allowing for detection of characteristic P wave changes.[10,11,20] Atrial flutter with a regular response may also be differentiated from PSVT after adenosine administration.

The second major indication for adenosine is in the diagnosis of regular, wide complex tachycardias. These tachycardias, although usually ventricular in origin, may also represent supraventricular tachycardias with preexisting bundle branch block or aberrant conduction (see Unit 7). These rhythms are initially treated as VT. In the hemodynamically stable patient, anticipate administration of adenosine after trial doses of lidocaine.[3,19,20] Supraventricular rhythms convert to sinus rhythms (if PSVT) or manifest a transient slowing of the ventricular rate, facilitating the diagnosis. Ventricular rhythms are usually unaffected and the hemodynamic deterioration associated with accidental verapamil in VT does not occur.[3,10,17,19,20]

Because of its extremely short half-life of 10 to 30 seconds, administer adenosine initially as a rapid IV bolus of 6 mg followed by a 10 ml flush. If this dose is not effective within 1 to 2 minutes, give a 12-mg bolus, which may be repeated once.[3] Side effects are transient, lasting no more than 1 to 2 minutes, and most commonly include dyspnea, flushing, and chest pain.[3,9,11,14] Transient arrhythmias also commonly occurring after conversion of PSVT with adenosine include AV block, bradycardia, sinus arrest, and ventricular ectopic beats.[3,10,17,19,20] The AV block is unresponsive to atropine but rarely sustained.[9,10] Researchers have reported bronchospasm, primarily with inhaled adenosine in asthmatic patients. Sufficient data are not available as yet in asthmatic patients to rule out this possibility with IV administration.[9,17] Related nursing diagnoses include alteration in comfort, alteration in cardiac output, and anxiety or knowledge deficit.

Adenosine is also a potent coronary vasodilator and is used in conjunction with echocardiography or nuclear imaging in the diagnosis of coronary artery disease as an alternative to exercise stress testing (see Unit 5).[9,13,17] Although similar doses are used, they are administered more slowly so that the effects on AV conduction are minimized.[9,17]

NURSING ORDERS: For patients receiving adenosine for supraventricular tachyarrhythmias

1. Instruct patient to report all unusual sensations. Assess patient for dyspnea, flushing, and chest pain. Reassure patient that these are transient and expected.
2. Administer adenosine as a rapid IV bolus at the most proximal port. Follow boluses with a 10- to 20-cc flush of normal saline.[3,10,18] Store adenosine at room temperature since it may crystallize with refrigeration.[5,10]
3. Do not exceed 30-mg total dose in a 10-minute period.[9,12]
4. Anticipate therapeutic response within 10 to 30 seconds depending on whether administered centrally or peripherally.[10,17,18,19]
5. Use with caution, if at all, in patients with a history of asthma.[9,17] Monitor breath sounds in these patients.
6. Monitor ECG for significant AV block exceeding 60 seconds.
7. Although usually not necessary, reverse toxic effects with theophylline (aminophylline).[9,10,17]
8. Patients on theophylline (aminophylline) may require a higher dose of adenosine.[10]
9. Patients on dipyridamole (Persantin) require approximately one quarter the dose to avoid cumulative effects, or should not receive adenosine at all.[3,17] Cardiac transplant patients are also more sensitive to adenosine because of accompanying denervation.[17]
10. Like verapamil, adenosine is contraindicated in patients with sick sinus syndrome.[10,18]
11. If supraventricular tachycardia recurs, consider alternate agents such as verapamil with more sustained effects.

ANTIARRHYTHMIC AGENTS

The antiarrhythmic agents as a group act to depress ventricular ectopic impulse formation and are usually indicated in the management of ventricular arrhythmias. Some also depress impulse formation in the atria and/or AV junction. Ventricular ectopic activity is suppressed by (1) directly depressing automaticity, (2) altering conduction and repolarization so that reentry circuits are broken, or (3) both. All antiarrhythmic drugs are depressants, and the practitioner should administer them with caution when the patient shows signs of either electrical or mechanical depression.

The antiarrhythmic drugs are most commonly grouped into four classes according to the system proposed by Singh and Vaughn-Williams.[4,5] These classes and examples of currently available agents are as follows:

- *Class I agents:* Suppress Na^+ channels
- Quinidine sulfate (quinidine)
- Procainamide HCl (Pronestyl)
- Disopyramide phosphate (Norpace)
- Lidocaine HCl (Xylocaine)
- Phenytoin sodium (Dilantin)
- Tocainide HCl (Tonocard)
- Mexiletine HCl (Mexitil)
- Flecainide acetate (Tambocor)
- Encainide (Enkaid)
- Propafenone HCl (Rythmol)
- Moricizine HCl (Ethmozine)

Class II agents: Inhibit sympathetic responses (see Beta Blockers)

Class III agents: Act selectively on repolarization and reentry circuits and are most effective in abolishing ventricular tachycardia and fibrillation
- Bretylium tosylate (Bretylol)
- Amiodarone HCl (Cordarone)

Class IV agents: Suppress Ca^{++} channels
- Verapamil (Isoptin, Calan)
- Diltiazem (Cardizem)

Class I antiarrhythmic drugs

Ventricular arrhythmias are usually most effectively managed by agents that suppress Na^+ channels (class I agents). The most commonly used antiarrhythmic agents belong to this category. The specific effects of class I agents differ with regard to depolarization and repolarization. Class I agents may be further divided into classes IA, IB, and IC according to these differences (Table 9-1).

Moricizine is a more recently introduced class I agent that is indicated in the treat-

Class IA agents

Class IA agents prolong both depolarization and repolarization. Prolongation of de-

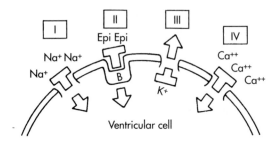

Fig. 9-4 Major differences between the four main antiarrhythmic classes.

Figure 9-4 illustrates differences between these four classes.

Sotatol (Betapace) is a recently released drug that has characteristics of both class II and class III agents. It is a unique drug with antiarrhythmic and beta blocking activities and is effective and well tolerated in treating a variety of supraventricular and ventricular arrhythmias. It has potential to become a first-line agent. Another advantage of sotatol is twice daily dosing. Side effects include dyspnea, bradycardia, chest pain, and torsades de pointes.[4,21]

ment of life-threatening ventricular arrhythmias.[4,29,30] This drug has characteristics of IA, IB and IC agents. Moricizine produced proarrhythmic effects in the CAST study in patients with structural heart disease, ischemia, and congestive heart failure (CHF). Lack of demonstration of improved survival with this agent led to termination of the study. To obtain the desired antiarrhythmic effect, a dose between 600 and 900 mg is administered in three equally divided doses.[4,29,30]

polarization results in widening of the QRS complex at toxic levels. Prolongation of re-

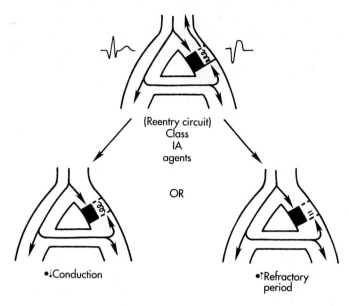

Fig. 9-5 Effects of Class IA antiarrhythmic agents on reentry circuits.

Table 9-1. Class I antiarrhythmics: major differences

	Class IA	Class IB	Class IC
Depolarization (QRS)	Prolonged	Minimal effect	Prolonged
Repolarization (QT/U)*	Prolonged	Shortened	No effect
Spectrum of activity	A/V/WPW	V	A/V/WPW

*Torsades de pointes is most typically produced by agents that prolong the QT(U) interval.

polarization results in prolongation of the Q–T interval with an accompanying risk of torsades de pointes.

The class IA antiarrhythmic agents include quinidine sulfate (quinidine), procainamide HCl (Pronestyl), and disopyramide phosphate (Norpace). These agents, although pharmacologically different, have certain common actions. They depress impulse formation in both the atria and the ventricles. Therefore, these drugs can be used in the management of both atrial and ventricular arrhythmias. These agents are also effective in the management of the atrial arrhythmias of Wolff-Parkinson-White syndrome (see Unit 11). In addition to suppressing automaticity, the class IA drugs have specific effects on repolarization and conduction that may affect reentry circuits. Class IA drugs abolish intraventricular reentry circuits by slowing conduction in ischemic tissue so the impulse is extinguished, or prolonging the refractory period of the ischemic cells within the circuit so that the impulse is blocked from reentering the ischemic area (Fig. 9-5).

By prolonging the refractory period of cardiac cells, quinidine, procainamide, and disopyramide prolong repolarization. Prolonged or delayed repolarization may be manifested on the ECG by the appearance of a U wave, TU fusion, and "pseudo" QT prolongation. This ECG manifestation of the group IA antiarrhythmic drugs mimics the ECG pattern of hypokalemia. It is often referred to as the quinidine effect and usually does not represent a toxic effect of these drugs. Toxic effects of group I agents may be manifested by severe prolongation of the refractory period, with extreme prolongation of the Q-T interval and enhancement—rather than suppression—of ectopic activity. Q-T intervals greater than 0.5 second or one half the preceding R-R interval are considered significant. Repolarization is so prolonged that recovery in adjacent cells becomes less uniform. Ventricular tachycardia or ventricular fibrillation can occur, producing the pattern known as torsades de pointes since it gives the appearance of twisting around a central baseline (see Unit 11).

The toxic effect of class IA drugs on intraventricular conduction appears on analysis of the QRS complexes of the normal beats. Widening of the normal QRS complexes by 50% of the original width is a toxic manifestation of these drugs and an indication to discontinue therapy.[3] Administration of class IA drugs requires caution in patients who normally have wide QRS complexes, indicating preexisting intraventricular conduction abnormalities. These agents are also contraindicated in the presence of hyperkalemia. The antidote for the QRS widening associated with toxicity from class IA drugs is sodium bicarbonate or sodium lactate. The sodium ion acts as a stimulus to the heart and overcomes some of the Na^+ channel blocking. Alkalinization promotes binding of the drug to serum proteins, thus lowering toxic levels.

Class IA drugs at therapeutic blood levels slow AV conduction. With initial administration, however, they may accelerate AV conduction. This transient vagolytic effect of class IA agents necessitates administering digitalis or verapamil before using these agents in the initial therapy for supraventricular arrhythmias, such as atrial fibrillation.

Class IA drugs also have hemodynamic side effects. They depress myocardial mechanical function. They may cause a rise in left ventricular end-diastolic pressure (LVEDP) (filling pressure) and a fall in cardiac output and therefore require caution in the patient with heart failure. The effects of disopyramide are the most pronounced. The practitioner should use caution when administering this agent in conjunction with other myocardial depressants, particularly beta blockers, and calcium blockers.

Procainamide is the only group IA agent commonly administered by the IV route. It is therefore used more often in the acute management of ventricular arrhythmias than are disopyramide or quinidine. Procainamide is indicated for premature ventricular contractions (PVCs) and VT unresponsive to lidocaine (Xylocaine).[3,6] The drug is also indicated in VF unresponsive to lidocaine, bretylium, and magnesium.[3,4] IV administration potentially causes more pronounced toxic effects. Procainamide is a peripheral vasodilator and therefore may cause hypotension when received intravenously. The usual initial dose of procainamide is 100 mg with a maximum of 17 mg/kg (850 to 1700 mg).[3,4,6] IV procainamide should be administered slowly (no more than 20 to 30 mg/min) to minimize QRS widening and prevent marked vascular effects (hypotension). Maintain therapeutic effects by continuous procainamide infusion at a rate of 1 to 4 mg/min.[3,6]

Other reported side effects of class IA agents vary with the specific agents. They may cause GI disturbances such as nausea and vomiting, which can be minimized by concurrent administration with milk or meals. Quinidine and procainamide, to a lesser extent, cause diarrhea.[5] A side effect specifically associated with disopyramide therapy is urinary retention. Dryness of the mouth has also been reported. Other specific side effects include thrombocytopenia and hemolytic anemia, which are associated with quinidine therapy. Quinidine administration has also been linked with the occurrence of a cinchonism, a syndrome associated with administration of cinchona bark derivatives such as quinine and quinidine. Symptoms include tinnitus, blurring of vision or diplopia, loss of hearing, headache, and confusion. Concurrent administration of quinidine and digitalis has been known to raise serum digitalis levels by various mechanisms such as displacing the digitalis bound to serum proteins. The potential for digitalis toxicity is thus enhanced.

NURSING ORDERS: For patients receiving quinidine, procainamide, or disopyramide for ventricular or atrial arrhythmias

RELATED NURSING DIAGNOSES: Alteration in cardiac output related to uncontrolled arrhythmias, torsades de pointes, heart failure, or hypotension; alteration in elimination; volume deficit; potential impaired skin integrity; anxiety or knowledge deficit

1. When administering procainamide intravenously, watch for the development of hypotension and widening of the QRS complex to 50% of baseline (the antidote is sodium bicarbonate).

—Administer IV boluses slowly, at a rate of no more than 20 mg/min.

—Following procainamide boluses, anticipate continuous IV infusion in dosages similar to those for lidocaine.

2. Procainamide infusion may be prepared by adding 2 g to 500 ml of D5W or normal saline for a concentration of 4 mg/cc. To provide 2 mg/min, set the infusion pump at 30 gtt/min (cc/hr).

3. Monitor for QT prolongation greater than 0.5 second 00 > one half the preceding R–R cycle, especially within the first 2 hours. Watch for torsades de pointes until this QT prolongation is corrected.

4. Administer oral class 1A agents with milk or food to minimize GI disturbances such as nausea and vomiting. Watch for the development of diarrhea with quinidine or procainamide therapy.

5. Watch for the development of urinary retention with disopyramide therapy and for aggravation of CHF, especially with disopyramide.

6. Watch for signs and symptoms of lupus with oral procainamide administration.

Class IB agents

The current class IB agents include lidocaine HCl (Xylocaine), phenytoin sodium (Dilantin), tocainide HCl (Tonocard), and mexiletine (Mexitil). These agents share certain common mechanisms of action that allow them to be grouped together. The clinical effectiveness differs significantly, however.

The antiarrhythmic drug most commonly used in the management of acute ventricular arrhythmias is lidocaine. Lidocaine is ideal for use in acute MI because of its rapid onset of action and its relative lack of toxic effects on the heart. Traditional specific indications for lidocaine include six or more PVCs per minute, PVCs on the T wave ("close coupled"), multiformed (multifocal) PVCs, two or more consecutive PVCs with a ventricular rate greater than 100 (includes VT), and VF after defibrillation and epinephrine.[1,6,62,64]

The route of administration in the acute setting is intravenous. Lidocaine can be given in a single bolus of 1 to 1.5 mg/kg (usually 50 to 150 mg) and by a continuous infusion of 2 to 4 mg/min. Bolus doses can be repeated every 5 to 10 minutes at half the initial dose, up to a maximum of 3 mg/kg.[3,6] The American Heart Association recently increased the initial bolus dose recommendation.[3] The higher limit is suggested as an initial and repeated dose in VF. The second bolus in VF is given within 3 to 5 minutes. When an infusion is started, a bolus should be given simultaneously to ensure that adequate blood levels are achieved rapidly.[1] Researchers currently are disputing the use of prophylactic lidocaine in the first 24 to 48 hours after acute MI.[3,62,64]

If bursts of ectopic beats decrease in frequency or stop after the administration of lidocaine, the beats are likely to be ventricular. If the ectopic beats seem to increase after the administration of lidocaine, they are less likely to be ventricular, and aberrant conduction is a possibility. Lidocaine does not appear to have a significant direct effect on either AV node refractoriness or conduction. However, lidocaine may decrease ectopic rates of atrial flutter and atrial fibrillation, indirectly facilitating AV conduction. This potential effect does not minimize the value of a lidocaine trial in differentiating ventricular ectopy from aberrant conduction (see Unit 7).

Lidocaine also does not significantly affect automaticity and conduction in the SA node. Therefore, lidocaine is relatively safe to use in sinus bradycardia; atropine should be readily available as a precaution. Lidocaine should never be administered in a patient with a sustained idioventricular rhythm. Asystole may occur, caused by elimination of this compensatory ventricular ectopic rhythm.

Class IB agents depress ventricular automaticity by decreasing Na^+ influx during phase 4 of unstable cells. Reentry circuits are interrupted by production of a bidirectional block. Lidocaine acts preferentially on ischemic myocardium. Depressed conduction within the circuit may also extinguish the impulse. The effects of class IB agents on normal cardiac cells are to only minimally prolong depolarization and shorten repolarization. Therefore, these agents do not widen the QRS complex or prolong the Q–T interval. Class IB agents may actually shorten the

Q–T interval slightly, and clinicians therefore have suggested them as therapy for torsades de pointes or as alternate antiarrhythmics in patients with borderline or prolonged Q–T intervals.

Class IB agents rarely cause adverse cardiac effects. They have the least negative inotropic effects of all the antiarrhythmic agents and minimal proarrhythmic effects. The most significant cardiovascular side effect is hypotension, which is uncommon except with IV lidocaine.

Mexiletine and tocainamide are administered orally, and therefore these drugs do not have the rapid onset of action characteristic of lidocaine. Their mechanisms of action and spectrum of activity are very similar to those of lidocaine. Unlike lidocaine, however, they may be used in the management of both acute and chronic ventricular arrhythmias. Mexiletine and tocainide are less effective than lidocaine or other antiarrhythmics, especially in VT or VF, unless combined with a class IA agent.[4] Class IB agents are ideal for combination therapy because of their minimal cardiotoxicity. Lower doses of both class IB and class IA agents may be sufficient.

Lidocaine, mexiletine, and tocainide share similar neurologic side effects. These include tremors, hot and cold flashes, dysarthria, diplopia or blurred vision, confusion, ataxia, dizziness, paresthesias, and numbness. Both mexiletine and lidocaine may cause seizures. Nausea and vomiting can also occur, but taking the drug with food may minimize these effects. Cases of agranulocytosis, lupus, severe neutropenia, and pulmonary fibrosis have been reported with tocainide. These three agents are predominantly metabolized in the liver, with some renal excretion with tocainide. Patients with renal or hepatic failure or hepatic congestion secondary to CHF require lower dosages for mexiletine and tocainide.

Unlike the other class IB agents, phenytoin sodium (Dilantin) depresses ectopic impulse formation in the atria, ventricles, and AV junctional tissue. It accelerates AV conduction and shortens the refractory period. Phenytoin sodium is effective primarily in the management of digitalis-induced arrhythmias, both ventricular and supraventricular. It is especially effective in digitalis-induced junctional tachycardia. The arrhythmias of digitalis toxicity represent increased automaticity in the presence of decreased conduction. Phenytoin sodium decreases automaticity and increases conduction, thus reversing the toxic effects of digitalis.

Phenytoin sodium does not produce significant hemodynamic alterations, although it may cause hypotension and bradycardia, which is rate dependent. In toxic dosages it can produce hypotension, bradyarrhythmias, and cardiac standstill. The degree of cardiac depression produced appears related to the dose and speed of administration. Other side effects that may be associated with phenytoin sodium therapy are visual disturbances (nystagmus, blurred vision), CNS changes (confusion, ataxia, slurred speech), gingivitis, and an autoimmune blood dyscrasia known as Stevens-Johnson syndrome, manifested dermatologically by the sloughing of tissues.[8] The usual IV dose is 10 to 15 mg/kg (500 to 1500 mg).[5,8]

NURSING ORDERS: For patients receiving class IB drugs (lidocaine, mexiletine, phenytoin) for ventricular arrhythmias

RELATED NURSING DIAGNOSES: Alteration in cardiac output related to uncontrolled arrhythmias or hypotension, alteration in comfort, potential for infection, impaired skin integrity, and knowledge deficit

1. Analyze the need for the drug within the clinical context of the arrhythmias, especially before administering IV lidocaine. Note whether the underlying rhythm is fast or slow. Clarify traditional indications for treatment with physician (e.g., Will PVCs >6/min on T wave multifocal etc. be treated?).

2. Evaluate possible causes of ventricular arrhythmia.

3. Lidocaine infusion may be premixed or may be prepared by adding 2 g to 500 cc of D_5W for a concentration of 4 mg/cc. To provide 2 mg/min, set the infusion pump at 30 gtt/min (cc/hr).

4. During IV infusion of lidocaine, monitor cardiac status, blood pressure, and sensorium.
   —Evaluate the response of the rhythm to the drug. Has the lidocaine therapy suppressed the arrhythmia?
   —Observe the patient for signs of lidocaine toxicity, such as hypotension, changes in sensorium, and seizures. If these occur, stop the infusion. With hypotension, also have the patient lie flat and raise the patient's legs.

5. Monitor for neurologic and GI side effects with tocainide, mexiletine, and phenytoin. Administer with food.[8]

6. If the patient has liver failure or congestion secondary to CHF, consider small amounts of the drug for initial administration.

7. When administering phenytoin:
   —Note that IV rate should not exceed 50 mg/min. Administer 25 mg/min if patient has a significant cardiac history.[8]
   —Inject as close to the catheter as possible.
   —Mix only in normal saline. Flush IV line slowly with normal saline before and after administration.

Class IC agents

The three currently available class IC agents are flecainide acetate (Tambocor), encainide (Enkaid), and propafenone (Rythmol). Rythmol has beta blocking and calcium blocking effects, actually combining three classes in one drug.[4,22] At this time, encainide has been voluntarily withdrawn from the market but remains available on a limited basis.[4]

Class IC agents have a broad spectrum of activity affecting most areas of the heart. Therefore, these drugs are effective in the control of both atrial and ventricular arrhythmias. They are also the only class I agents effective in both the paroxysmal atrial tachycardia (PAT) and atrial fibrillation of Wolff-Parkinson-White syndrome as a result of effects on both the AV node and accessory pathway.

These agents are highly effective in the control of ventricular arrhythmias since they are the most potent class I agents. They may be considered when class IA and/or class IB agents have been ineffective or toxic effects have limited their use. However, class IC agents possess significant proarrhythmic effects, ironically more when used with malignant, complex ventricular arrhythmias, such as VT or VF, where they are also most effective. The use of these agents has been significantly curtailed following the results of the CAST study, which reported serious proarrhythmic complications.[4,42]

In addition to suppressing automaticity, class IC agents abolish intraventricular reentry circuits by depressing conduction so that the impulse is extinguished. This action results from prolongation of depolarization, similar to the action of class IA agents. Unlike class IA agents, however, class IC agents have no effect on repolarization and the refractory periods of reentry circuits. Since these agents do not prolong the Q–T(U) interval (beyond the QRS complex), they can be used in patients at risk for torsades de pointes. These agents do not have selective effects on ischemic tissues like the class IB agents.

Because of the profound effect on conduction of class IC agents, widening of the QRS complex may occur therapeutically with these drugs and is not necessarily an indication for discontinuing therapy. Other cardiac side effects include negative inotropic effects, which are most pronounced with flecainide. Avoid flecainide in patients with significant preexisting heart failure. Monitor patients for signs of CHF. The newest agent, propafenone, possesses slight negative inotropic effects. Additive effects can occur when class IC agents are combined with beta blockers, calcium channel blockers, or disopyramide. These agents may also significantly suppress SA and AV node function when combined with agents such as digitalis, calcium channel blockers, or beta blockers.

Class II antiarrhythmic drugs

Sympathetic (beta) blocking drugs, such as propranolol (Inderal), can also act as antiarrhythmic agents by depressing ectopic formation in the ventricles. They are currently used in the management of *chronic* ventricular arrhythmias as a backup or alternative to class I agents, with the exception of the intravenous beta blocker esmolol (Brevibloc). Esmolol is used exclusively in the management of acute supraventricular arrhythmias (see Beta Blocking Agents).

Beta blockers are most effective in suppressing automaticity (whether mediated by Na^+ or Ca^{++}) and reentry circuits that are catecholamine induced. These disorders include arrhythmias that are either stress-related or triggered-sustained by stimulation of sympathetic nervous system activity. Because of their effect on AV junctional node automaticity and conduction, beta blockers are also useful in the management of supraventricular arrhythmias.

Class III antiarrhythmic drugs

The two currently available class III anti-arrhythmic agents are bretylium tosylate (Bretylol) and amiodarone (Cordarone). Class III agents act on repolarization and re-entry circuits and are most effective as a group in abolishing VF.

Prolongation of repolarization and refractory periods prevents or interrupts reentry circuits by producing bidirectional block. Bretylium also promotes homogeneity between normal and ischemic cells as a result of a differential effect on ischemic tissues similar to that of lidocaine (see Class IB Agents). Class III agents also raise the VF threshold.

The indications for, spectrum of activity of, and side effects of these two agents vary significantly. Amiodarone has a diffuse effect on the heart, affecting all conduction structures, and is associated with many significant cardiac and extracardiac side effects. In contrast, bretylium acts selectively on ventricular fibers and is associated with fewer side effects.

Bretylium is a sympathetic blocking drug that causes an initial displacement of norepinephrine from nerve terminals with subsequent depletion of this chemical mediator. Since bretylium initially displaces norepinephrine (a sympathetic chemical transmitter) from nerve terminals, it may cause a transient increase in automaticity with tachycardia, hypertension, increased ventricular ectopic activity, or all of these.[3,6] For this reason it is not appropriate for initial therapy for single, malignant PVCs. Thus bretylium is not a first-line agent in the management of all malignant ventricular arrhythmias. Because of this transient increase in norepinephrine release, bretylium may also potentiate the effects of digitalis toxicity.[6,8] Thus it should be administered to a patient receiving digitalis only when the ventricular arrhythmias do not appear to be related to digitalis toxicity.

Bretylium is used primarily in the management of recurrent VF, when defibrillation, epinephrine, and lidocaine are ineffective.[3,6] In therapy for VF, bretylium is given as an undiluted rapid bolus of 5 mg/kg (250 to 500 mg) followed by boluses of 10 mg/kg (500 to 1000 mg) every 5 minutes up to 30 to 35 mg/kg.[3] The effect of bretylium in raising the VF threshold is usually visible rapidly. Unlike lidocaine and procainamide, bretylium has a long half-life (6 to 8 hours). Therefore, initiation of continuous IV infusion therapy can often be postponed for several hours without a significant drop in blood levels. The usual dose is 1 to 2 mg/min.

Bretylium is also used to manage VT associated with a pulse that is unresponsive to lidocaine or procainamide. When used to manage VT, a 5 to 10 mg/kg dose of bretylium is diluted in 50 cc and administered as an infusion over a minimum of 8 to 10 minutes. The effect occurs less rapidly in this situation, usually within 20 minutes to 2 hours after administration.[4,6]

Although it may produce hypotension, bretylium does not appear to affect LVEDP or cardiac output adversely. In fact, it is thought to stimulate cardiac contractility (positive inotropic effect). Other side effects reported with the use of bretylium include vertigo, light-headedness, and dizziness.

Amiodarone has a diffuse effect on the cardiac conduction structures; it is not limited to the ventricular myocardium. It prolongs the refractory period of the SA node, AV node, atria, and accessory bypass tract tissues, as well as the ventricular Purkinje fibers and myocardium. It is most useful in Wolff-Parkinson-White syndrome, in recurring VT and VF, and where a variety of arrhythmias unresponsive to standard antiarrhythmic therapy are present.[27,32] Amiodarone has a slow onset of action (averaging 4 to 10 days) and therefore is *not* currently indicated in the acute management of ventricular arrhythmias. However, clinical trials with IV Amiodarone are in progress.

Significant therapeutic effects may be delayed for weeks. The use of loading doses can provide antiarrhythmic effects within a few days. Because of this delayed onset of action and significant side effects, patients may require 2 to 3 weeks of in-hospital monitoring. Although amiodarone may be administered intravenously, it is currently approved only in oral form in the United States.

Amiodarone produces significant cardiotoxicity. Its significant negative inotropic effects are associated with aggravation of CHF. Its proarrhythmic effects are related to significant prolongation of the refractory periods and Q–T(U) interval, resulting in torsades de pointes.[34,40] Maintaining normal serum K^+ and Mg^{++} levels may minimize this toxic effect. Ironically, bretylium does not share this toxic effect and may actually be beneficial in therapy for torsades. An explanation may be bretylium's differential, more selective effect on abnormal conduction tissue.

Investigators also have reported AV block and bradycardia as complications of amiodarone therapy owing to its effects on the SA and AV nodes. Extracardiac side effects include corneal microdeposits, neurologic toxicity, GI symptoms, and skin photosensitivity with gray or blue discoloration (pseudocyanosis). The corneal deposits may cause blurring of vision or orange and yellow halos at night or in dim light. Administration of artificial tears can help decrease these side effects. Neurologic toxic effects include tremors, insomnia, ataxia, peripheral polyneuropathy, and thigh muscle weakness. GI symptoms include nausea, vomiting, and constipation.[32]

Both hypothyroidism and hyperthyroidism can occur from a release of high levels of iodine from amiodarone metabolism. Pulmonary toxicity, including pulmonary fibrosis, is the most common serious toxic effect.

Researchers also have reported hepatic and renal toxicity. Asymptomatic abnormalities in liver function tests occur more commonly.

Most of the extracardiac side effects of amiodarone are reversible, but because of the long duration of action, these, like the electrophysiologic effects, may continue for 3 to 12 months after cessation of therapy. The pulmonary fibrotic changes are the least likely to revert.

NURSING ORDERS: For patients receiving bretylium tosylate or amiodarone for arrhythmias

RELATED NURSING DIAGNOSES: Alteration in cardiac output, alteration in comfort, alteration in metabolism, impaired gas exchange, anxiety or knowledge deficit

With bretylium tosylate:
1. Monitor for hypotension, nausea, and vomiting when administering bretylium. Evaluate response to therapy.
2. To prepare bretylium infusion, add 2 g to 500 cc of D_5W for a concentration of 4 mg/cc. To provide 2 mg/min, set the infusion pump at 30 gtt/min (cc/hr).

With amiodarone:
1. Assess for neurologic side effects including both motor and sensory deficits.
2. Administer artificial tear solution to minimize corneal microdeposits.
3. Instruct the patient to avoid sun exposure: cover exposed areas with clothing and use sunscreen.
4. Instruct the patient to report new onset of cough, fever, or shortness of breath immediately.
5. Assess for and report any signs of possible hyperthyroidism or hypothyroidism, including tremors, weight loss or gain, lethargy, palpitations, mental dullness, or hyperexcitability.
6. Monitor for increased sensitivity to digitalis, calcium blockers, beta blockers, class IA agents, and warfarin.

7. Assess the Q–T(U) interval for risk of torsades de pointes.
8. Auscultate the heart and lungs for signs of increased CHF, i.e., rales, new S_3 gallop.

9. Obtain baseline liver and pulmonary function tests and thyroid profile before initiating therapy and monitor regularly thereafter.

Class IV antiarrhythmic drugs

Class IV agents act by blocking the entry of extracellular calcium into the cardiovascular cells. They are therefore called calcium channel blockers and do not alter total serum calcium. The currently available Ca^{++} channel blockers with significant electrophysiologic effects include verapamil (Isoptin, Calan) and diltiazem (Cardizem).

Ventricular arrhythmias that are unresponsive to usual antiarrhythmic therapy (class I and/or II agents) may be produced by Ca^{++}-dependent (slow) cells rather than Na^+-dependent (fast) cells. Ca^{++} channel antagonists such as verapamil may be more effective. Verapamil also is effective in the control of ventricular arrhythmias related to coronary spasm. However, the significant depressant effect of verapamil on the AV node limits its application in ventricular arrhythmia unless the patient receives a temporary or permanent pacemaker. Verapamil and diltiazem are used primarily in the management of supraventricular tachyarrhythmias. A thorough discussion of the use of verapamil in supraventricular arrhythmias is presented in the section on calcium channel blocking agents (see Calcium Channel Blocking Agents).

ANTILIPEMIC AGENTS

Hyperlipidemia can have a significant effect on the development of coronary artery disease. A diet low in saturated fats and cholesterol is the first treatment for the patient with elevated lipids (see Unit 5). When hyperlipidemia persists after a usual 6-month trial with diet and exercise, the physician may institute drug therapy.[67,75,78] The goal of drug therapy is to attain optimal control of hyperlipidemia as evidenced by low-density lipoprotein (LDL) levels of less than 130 to 160 mg/dl, depending on the presence of coronary risk factors or actual coronary artery disease.[75,78] A combination of drugs may be necessary to minimize the side effects and increase their potential.

Bile acid sequestrants

Cholestyramine (Questran) and colestipol (Colestid) act to irreversibly bind with bile acids, which are derivatives of cholesterol. After binding, bile acids are unable to reabsorb into the system. This action causes the liver to convert an increased amount of cholesterol into bile acids. When this occurs, the liver demand for cholesterol rises. The end result is a decrease in the total cholesterol and LDL.[67]

Major disadvantages are the patient effort and education required, an increase in plasma triglycerides, and other side effects.[67,75,78] These agents are dispensed in powder form, which must be diluted in a palatable fluid or alternative. A candy bar alternative, although more expensive, is now available. The strength and frequency are gradually increased up to 4 doses per day.[8,75,78]

The primary side effects associated with these agents include constipation, heartburn, abdominal cramps, and flatulence.[67] A lower dose or a period of adaptation lessens side effects. The bile acid sequestrants interfere with the absorption of digoxin, anticoagulants, thyroxine, thiazides, beta blockers, phenytoin (Dilantin), and fat-soluble vita-

mins.[5,75,78] Therefore, these drugs should be given 1 hour before the administration of the sequestrant or 4 hours after.

Nicotinic acid

The basic effect of nicotinic acid (niacin) is to inhibit the lipolysis of adipose tissue.[8] Nicotinic acid lowers the plasma LDLs including the triglyceride component, very low-density lipoprotein (VLDL). It consistently elevates the high-density lipoproteins (HDLs). In addition, nicotinic acid is the least costly of all the antilipemic agents.[75,78]

Nicotinic acid has numerous side effects, including flushing, dizziness, pruritus, and GI irritation. The flushing decreases over

time with continued administration of the drug.[67] Administering aspirin 30 minutes before each dose may lessen the flushing. Switching to a timed-release form may also be helpful. Abnormal liver function, hyperuricemia, and hyperglycemia may occur.[75,78] Obtain baseline levels and check levels regularly. Avoid this agent in patients with liver disease, gout, arthritis, peptic ulcer, and diabetes.

Gemfibrozil

Gemfibrozil (Lopid) is an effective agent in decreasing lipid levels. As the recent Helsinki Heart Study showed, it is useful primarily in patients with high triglycerides and low HDL levels; LDL levels are also lowered but to a lesser extent than with bile acid sequestrants and nicotinic acid.[5,67,75,78] Heart attack risk may be reduced as much as 50% in these individuals. Gemfibrozil is a fibric

acid derivative. Clofibrate (Atromid S), another fibric acid derivative, is used minimally due to more significant toxic effects.[75,78]

The side effects of gemfibrozil are minimal and include primarily GI side effects. Administer it with caution in patients receiving warfarin as it potentiates its effect, causing bleeding. There may also be a slight increase in blood glucose.[8]

Probucol

Probucol (Lorelco) lowers both the serum HDL and LDL cholesterol. It appears to interfere with cholesterol synthesis and increases LDL catabolism and cholesterol excretion in bile.[8,67] Its use is limited, however, by the effect on HDL, so the drug is reserved for combination therapy or when

other antilipemic agents cannot be used.

Avoid probucol in patients with a preexisting prolonged QT or with drugs that might produce an abnormal Q–T interval. GI side effects include nausea, vomiting, flatulence, and diarrhea.

HMG-CoA reductase inhibitor

The three agents currently available in this category include lovastatin (Mevacor), pravastatin (Pravachol), and simvastatin (Zocor). These newer agents lower LDL levels by inhibiting the enzyme HMG-CoA reductase, which is necessary for cholesterol synthesis.[8,78] Major advantages include patient con-

venience and lower frequency of side effects. All three agents are available in pill form with once-a-day dosing.

The most common side effects are headache, fatigue, nausea, constipation, and myalgia. These side effects may lessen after the patient develops a tolerance. Creatine kinase

(CK) and transaminase levels may become elevated. Liver function tests require periodic monitoring.

When these drugs are administered with warfarin, the anticoagulant effect may increase, requiring monitoring of the prothrombin time. Rhabdomyolysis or severe myopathy may occur with a combination of lovastatin and cyclosporine, erythromycin, gemfibrozil, and niacin.[5]

The ideal lipid-lowering drug does not exist. Combination therapy may help to achieve optimal control of hyperlipidemia. It maximizes the effect on cholesterol while minimizing side effects. An example of combination therapy might include a bile acid sequestrant and an HMG-CoA reductase inhibitor. Several combinations have been used to enhance effectiveness. Lower doses of both medications may be possible.[78] Improvement should occur within 3 months of a change in medication.[5]

NURSING ORDERS: For patients receiving an antilipemic agent

RELATED NURSING DIAGNOSES: Impaired tissue perfusion, alteration in comfort, alteration in elimination, and knowledge deficit

1. Instruct patient to take bile sequestrants in fruit juice, puddings, yogurt, or oatmeal.
2. Administer antilipemic agents 30 minutes after meals to minimize GI side effects. Remind patient vitamins and certain medications should be taken 1 hour before bile sequestrants.
3. Encourage adequate fluid intake and high fiber diet. Use stool softeners if necessary.
4. Instruct patient on measures to reduce flushing with nicotinic acid.
5. Reinforce the importance of taking follow-up cholesterol levels initially, usually after 1 month, then 3 months.[74,78] With nicotinic acid and the HMG-CoA reductase inhibitors, also monitor liver function tests.
6. Instruct patient on self-monitoring techniques and provide feedback regarding cholesterol levels.

ANTITHROMBOTIC AGENTS

Drugs that alter the clotting process may be referred to collectively as antithrombotic agents. These drugs have a potential role in reversing acute coronary stenosis and preventing or minimizing myocardial infarction and its thrombotic complications. The process of sealing potential vascular leaks with a clot is called *hemostasis*. It is a major body defense mechanism designed to prevent the escape of blood and involves a process of clot formation *balanced* by a process of clot lysis (Fig. 9-6).

Disruption of this balance leads to an abnormal response, resulting in either thrombosis or hemorrhage. The focus of this discussion is thrombosis, since this is the major disorder affecting the patient with coronary artery disease.

The process of clot formation is activated in response to either extravascular or intravascular injury. It involves three interrelated steps: a vascular response, platelet activation, and formation of a fibrin clot. The primary purpose of this clotting, hemostatic mechanism is to provide a simple seal (plug) in the presence of vessel breaks or disruption. *Thrombosis* is defined as inappropriate or exaggerated hemostasis. It is triggered by endothelium vascular injury and is no longer limited to the simple sealing off of a vascular break. The normal process of repair is extended or exaggerated until an abnormal mass develops. This mass obstructs the lumen of the artery or vein, limiting or arresting blood flow. An interplay between five major factors determines whether a signifi-

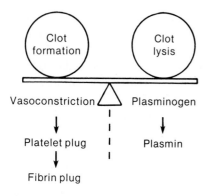

Fig. 9-6   Clotting process: overview.

cant thrombus will form within the vascular system: (1) state of the vessel wall, (2) activity of the blood platelets, (3) activity of the clotting factors, (4) rate of blood flow, and (5) activity of the fibrinolytic or clot lysis system.

Like the normal hemostatic mechanism, thrombus formation involves the initial deposition of a primary platelet plug. This primary plug may or may not be followed by the formation of a fibrin clot (the secondary plug). Three types of thrombi may occur in coronary artery disease: arterial, venous, and mural. Arterial thrombi are triggered by *vessel wall* changes such as those occurring in the process of atherosclerosis. Venous and mural thrombi are primarily triggered by *stasis* and may or may not be associated with vascular wall change or injury.

The site of origin of an arterial thrombus is usually a roughened intimal lining such as occurs in atherosclerosis. This vessel wall abnormality predisposes to platelet activation, and a thrombus slowly forms. Usually a minimal deposition of fibrin occurs in an initial arterial thrombus because rapid flow rates in arteries allow for washout of the required clotting factors. The amount of fibrin deposited in an arterial thrombus thus relates to the degree to which the atherosclerotic process has slowed blood flow. Atherosclerosis narrows the lumen of the coronary artery.

Fibrin thrombus formation is often the final event, resulting in complete or significant occlusion. The antithrombotic agents most effective in preventing coronary artery disease are thus those that inhibit platelet activation. Drugs that inhibit platelet aggregation include aspirin, dipyridamole (Persantine), sulfinpyrazone (Anturane), and dextran 40 (Rheomacrodex).

Thrombus formation in the venous system is usually slower and involves extensive fibrin deposition. The slow-flow venous system promotes stasis, allowing time for the clotting factors to accumulate and react. Restricting activity in the patient with acute MI promotes venous stasis. This activity restriction predisposes to thrombus formation with potential embolization. Emboli from a venous thrombus can travel rapidly to the pulmonary circulation, resulting in pulmonary embolus and infarction.

When MI occurs, contractility diminishes, resulting in areas of relative stasis within the left ventricular wall. Thrombi formed on these areas of ventricular wall stasis are called *mural thrombi*. Emboli from a left ventricular mural thrombus can travel rapidly to the cerebral circulation, resulting in a cerebral embolus and infarction.

Stasis predisposes to more complete thrombus formation with the deposition of fibrin. Antithrombotic agents used to prevent the formation of venous and mural thrombi are those that inhibit fibrin formation. The two drugs most commonly used in coronary care for this purpose are warfarin (Coumadin) and heparin. They are considered true anticoagulants.[5,8,164] These drugs have no effect on an established thrombus. Once a thrombus has occurred, however, anticoagulant treatment prevents further clot formation and minimizes embolization.

Let us now review in more detail the normal processes of platelet activation and fibrin formation to understand the exact mechanism of action for drugs that alter the clotting

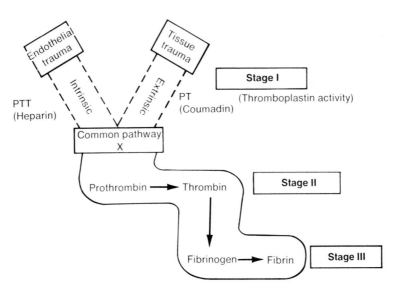

Fig. 9-7 Pathways of fibrin formation.

process. As mentioned earlier, hemostasis is a function of three interrelated processes: a vascular response, platelet activation, and fibrin formation. The vascular response to vessel disruption primarily involves contraction of the smooth muscle within the vessel wall and probably does not play a significant role in coronary artery disease.

Platelet activation is triggered when the smooth inner lining of the blood vessel (endothelium) is disrupted or roughened. The first response to the disruption of the endothelial tissue is platelet *adhesion,* which refers to the process by which platelets are attracted to and stick to something other than platelets. Following adhesion, platelets undergo a change in shape and are activated. With activation, a complex series of reactions occurs, resulting in the release of compounds that promote platelet aggregation. *Aggregation* refers to the process by which platelets are attracted to and stick to other platelets, forming larger clumps. Platelet release factors have also been implicated as contributing factors for coronary artery spasm and the development of atherosclero-

sis. Platelets may contribute to the development of atherosclerosis by altering permeability and thus allowing for lipid deposition and/or aggravating smooth muscle proliferation (medial layer changes).

Platelet aggregation follows platelet adhesion and results in the formation of larger clumps. Many substances, such as epinephrine, collagen fibers, immune complexes, serotonin, adenosine phosphate, thrombin, and microorganisms, can induce platelet aggregation.[5] Risk factors associated with coronary artery disease have also been implicated in platelet aggregation. These include high serum cholesterol values, type II hyperlipidemia, cigarette smoking, stress, birth control pills, diabetes, and a high-fat diet.

Fibrin formation occurs in three major stages: thromboplastin activity, conversion of prothrombin to thrombin, and conversion of fibrinogen to fibrin (Fig. 9-7). Thromboplastin activity may be generated by either the intrinsic or the extrinsic clotting factor pathways. The intrinsic pathway is stimulated by intravascular trauma. Disruption or roughening of the endothelial layer of the blood vessels results. Platelet activation is also triggered by intravascular damage. Platelets therefore exert a major influence on the intrinsic pathway. The extrinsic pathway for the generation of thromboplastin activity is stimulated by extravascular tissue trauma. With tissue trauma a clotting factor referred to as *tissue juice* is released, which activates the extrinsic pathway. Fibrin deposition is probably a result of simultaneous activation of both pathways.

Certain clotting factors are unique to each pathway. However, there is a common point or junction at which the two pathways become one. This common pathway begins with factor X. Immediately after the activation of factor X, stage II of the fibrin formation process begins, with the conversion of prothrombin to thrombin. Thrombin subsequently converts fibrinogen to fibrin, completing stage III.

Fibrin formation is accompanied by activation of a fibrin breakdown or fibrinolytic (clot lysis) system. A delicate balance normally exists between the fibrin formation and fibrinolysis. A thrombus in the vascular system indicates that the rate of fibrin formation has exceeded the body's fibrinolytic capacity.

The proteolytic enzyme plasmin is the active component of the fibrinolytic system. The action of plasmin is to digest fibrin clots. Plasmin is a nonspecific proteolytic enzyme and depletes many circulating proteins. Plasminogen is the inactive precursor of plasmin. Conversion of plasminogen to plasmin depends on contact with specific activator substances. Plasminogen activators have an affinity for fibrin threads, thus allowing for plasmin to be generated at the site of thrombus formation. The end products of this fibrinolytic or clot breakdown process are called *fibrin split products* (FSP) or *fibrin degradation products* (FDP). These end products exert anticoagulant effects themselves.

Antithrombotic therapy in coronary artery disease focuses on one or more of the following: (1) prevention of thrombus formation, (2) prevention of embolic complications, and (3) disruption of existing thrombi. Three major categories of drugs may be effective. They include the antiplatelet, antifibrin, and fibrinolytic agents.

Antiplatelet agents

The antiplatelet agents are most effective in the prevention of coronary artery thrombosis, since thrombus formation in arteries consists primarily of platelets. Agents that prevent arterial thrombi have a potential role in the prevention of acute MI. Although researchers have not conclusively established the exact pathogenesis of acute coronary artery occlusion, they have implicated the triad of atherosclerosis, spasm, and thrombus in the syndromes of angina and MI. Investigators also have shown that antiplatelet agents prevent closure of vein grafts after bypass surgery. Many agents inhibit platelet activity and thus have potential as antithrombotic agents. The three major antiplatelet agents currently in use are aspirin, dipyridamole (Persatine), and sulfinpyrazone (Anturan, Anturane).

Aspirin

Aspirin inhibits the formation of arterial thrombi by preventing the release of platelet-activator substances. When platelets adhere to a roughened endothelium, they release *platelet-activator substances,* which cause platelets to clump, or aggregate.[5,175] Arterial thrombi are primarily composed of platelet aggregates.

The use of low-dose aspirin (160 to 325 mg daily) in the prevention of initial MI and reinfarction has been supported by recent data, including the ISSI-2 MI trial.[1,5,175,179]

Aspirin administration is recommended primarily in patients with confirmed coronary artery disease, such as those with unstable angina, with previous infarction, or who have received thrombolytic therapy.[1,5] Aspirin is also prescribed before coronary angioplasty to prevent thrombus formation, after coronary bypass surgery to prevent graft clo-sure, in patients with peripheral vascular disease, and in men with transient ischemic attacks (TIAs) to prevent strokes. The antithrombotic effects of aspirin do not usually cause bleeding except in patients with a history of ulcers or bleeding disorders. Avoid the use of aspirin in these patients.

Dipyridamole and sulfinpyrazone

Although pharmacologically different, both dipyridamole (Persantine) and sulfinpyrazone (Anturan, Anturane) act as antiplatelet agents. Both are currently under clinical investigation in the prophylaxis of acute MI as well as in the prevention of vein graft closure after bypass surgery. Aspirin is generally preferred and considered more effective in the patient with coronary and cerebrovascular disease at this time.[5,179] Dipyridamole, a coronary vasodilator, was initially used in the treatment of angina pectoris. Side effects associated with its use are primarily related to its peripheral vasodilating actions; they include headache, dizziness, weakness, hypotension, flushing, and fainting. Sulfinpyrazone is classified as a uricosuric agent because it promotes the excretion of uric acid. Associated side effects primarily relate to its antithrombotic effects and include epigastric pain, blood loss, and reactivation of peptic ulcers.

Ticlopidine HCl (Ticlid) was recently approved as a platelet aggregation inhibitor.[4] This dose-dependent agent produces an irreversible effect on the platelet membrane. Ticlopidine HCl is indicated in thrombotic stroke and may be beneficial in unstable angina and acute infarction.[5] Neutropenia and thrombocytopenia may occur with the administration of ticlopidine.

Antifibrin agents

The antifibrin agents warfarin (Coumadin) and heparin are effective in the prevention of venous and mural thrombi. These agents potentially decrease thrombus formation, thrombus growth, and pulmonary or cerebral thrombus formation. Heparin and warfarin are generally thought to be ineffective in preventing arterial thrombi or resolving a thromboembolic event unless flow is compromised. Compromised flow occurs with stenosis or in the presence of mechanical devices, such as the intraaortic balloon pump (IABP) or arterial line catheters.

Heparin is currently used, preferably with aspirin, after thrombolytic therapy to prevent reocclusion.[1] Heparin is also used in conjunction with coronary angioplasty to prevent thrombosis. Administering heparin to the patient with unstable angina may prevent MI.[5] A new antithrombin agent, hirudin, with antiplatelet and thrombolytic effects, is currently under investigation as an alternative to Heparin in these settings.[204a] Side effects are minimal.

Heparin

Heparin sodium is a naturally occurring substance found in many tissues, including the liver, lung, and intestine. Heparin inhibits the formation of fibrin clots primarily by inactivating thrombin. The main role of the enzyme thrombin is to convert fibrinogen to fibrin. Heparin also exerts a significant inhibitory effect on the clotting factors within the intrinsic pathway.

Heparin may be administered intravenously as a bolus or as a continuous infusion. It may also be given subcutaneously. It is generally not given intramuscularly because of the risk of intramuscular or retroperitoneal hematomas. Administering small doses of heparin (5000 units) subcutaneously at 12-hour intervals, known as *low-dose heparin,* is considered effective in the prevention of venous thrombosis and pulmonary embolism in patients with acute MI.[1] Most deep venous thrombi in patients with acute MI form within the first 3 days. Therefore, in patients not receiving thrombolytic therapy, administer low-dose heparin for the first 24 to 48 hours.[1] In patients over 70 years old, with CHF, with shock, or otherwise immobilized for longer than 3 days, continue heparin until the patient is ambulatory.

Effective prevention of left ventricular thrombi and arterial embolization requires higher doses of heparin (12,000 units subcutaneously every 12 hours).[1,175] These subcutaneous or similar IV doses are indicated in patients with extensive anterior wall MIs, where the incidence of mural thrombi formation is reported to be as high as 60%.[1,175] Therapy should be continued until discharge or up to 10 days. The risk of mural thrombus formation is higher in patients with dilated ventricles secondary to CHF. Patients with heart failure may receive calcium heparin rather than sodium heparin to avoid further Na^+ retention.[2]

Still higher therapeutic dosages of heparin are required once a coagulation disorder, such as thrombophlebitis or pulmonary emboli, is established in a patient with acute MI. Heparin should be administered in the form of a continuous infusion at a rate of approximately 1000 units per hour.[2] Heparin may neutralize the effects of many other agents because of its acid pH. Therefore, it should generally not be administered in conjunction with other drugs by the intravenous route.

The anticoagulation study most commonly used to control heparin therapy is the partial thromboplastin time (PTT). This study tests for the clotting factors unique to the intrinsic pathways as well as those involved in the common pathway. Heparin exerts a significant effect on the intrinsic pathway. Maintaining the PTT between 1.5 and 2.0 times the control values ensures anticoagulation in most patients.[1,5,175]

The plasma recalcification time (PRT) and activated clotting time (ACT) may also be used to monitor heparin therapy. These studies test the overall fibrin formation process or clotting time. This normally slow process may be accelerated by adding the clotting factor Ca^{++} to the patient's blood sample.

The most common complication of heparin therapy is bleeding. Monitoring coagulation studies as well as observing for signs and symptoms of bleeding are primary nursing responsibilities. If bleeding requires rapid reversal of the effects of heparin, protamine sulfate is the specific antidote; the usual method of administration is a slow IV bolus of 50 mg over 10 minutes.[5] Protamine sulfate in excessive amounts may itself act as an anticoagulant.

Warfarin

The most commonly used anticoagulant of the coumarin group is warfarin sodium (Coumadin). Warfarin competes with vitamin K and thus depresses the synthesis of vitamin K–dependent clotting factors in the liver. There are four vitamin K–dependent clotting factors, the most well known of which is prothrombin (factor II).

Warfarin is usually given orally. It may take several days to achieve the full anticoagulant effect. Therefore, when switching from heparin to warfarin, the patient must receive the two drugs concomitantly for 3 to 5 days. Warfarin can be administered up to 3 months after acute MI in documented mural thrombi or aneurysm.[1] Warfarin is also prescribed before cardioversion of atrial flutter or fibrillation and in chronic atrial fibrillation. The coagulation study most commonly used to control warfarin therapy is the prothrombin time (PT). The PT tests for the factors unique to the extrinsic pathway as well as for those of the common pathway. Warfarin thus exerts its main influence on the extrinsic pathway of fibrin formation. Maintaining the PT at approximately 1.3 to 1.5 times the control value ensures anticoagulation in most patients.[1,5]

Many commonly used drugs interact with the coumarin anticoagulants. Some drugs antagonize the action, producing warfarin resistance, and may lead to overdosage when they are withdrawn. Commonly used drugs that antagonize coumarins are the barbiturates and oral contraceptives. Other drugs may potentiate the action of the coumarins, including aspirin, quinidine, neomycin, chlo-ral hydrate, clofibrate, indomethacin, amiodarone, sulfamethoxazole (Septra), ciprofloxacin (Cipro), and allopurinol. A complete list of drugs with which warfarin can interact should be available to the prescribing physician. The physician will need to readjust the warfarin dosage when withdrawing or prescribing interacting drugs.

The most common complication of warfarin therapy is bleeding. Patient education regarding covert signs of bleeding as well as the importance of follow-up coagulation studies is crucial for patients receiving warfarin at home. Warfarin exerts its anticoagulant effect by competing with vitamin K. Thus the antidote for bleeding resulting from warfarin therapy is vitamin K, or phytonadione (Aquamephyton).The patient should be made aware of dietary sources of vitamin K^+ which could alter the effectiveness of warfarin.

Thrombolytic agents

The common denominator of all thrombolytic drugs is that they in some way activate the body's own clot lysis or *fibrinolytic* system. For this reason these agents may also be called fibrinolytic agents. Four agents—streptokinase, recombinant tissue-type plasminogen activator or rt-PA, anisoylated plasminogen streptokinase activator complex, and urokinase—currently are approved for use as thrombolytic agents in acute myocardial infarction. These agents are most commonly administered today by the intravenous rather than the intracoronary route.

Streptokinase (Kabikinase, Streptase) is an extract of nonpathogenic hemolytic streptococci that exerts its action systemically, converting plasminogen to plasmin in the circulating blood pool. This action results in high levels of plasmin, which ultimately deplete the blood pool of fibrinogen and other clotting factors for as long as 24 to 36 hours. High levels of fibrin split and degradation products are also present, which together with depletion of clotting factors potentially expose the patient to serious bleeding complications. The usual dose of streptokinase is 1.5 million units administered as an IV infusion over 60 minutes.[8,182] Streptokinase is recognized as a foreign protein by the body and is thus antigenic. Therefore, resistance, sensitivity, and allergic reactions may develop with the use of the drug. Streptokinase may produce serious hypotension with initial administration in some patients and may require vasopressor support. Rash and fever are the most common reactions; treatment is with IV steroids and antihistamines. This agent should not be used in patients with a recent streptococcal infection.[5,178,182]

Tissue plasminogen activator (rt-PA, Alteplase, Activase) is a substance that naturally occurs in the endothelium, circulating blood, and other human tissue. It normally plays a role in the fibrinolytic system. Although it was first isolated in the 1940s, it was not until the 1980s through recombinant

DNA genetic engineering techniques that it could be produced in quantities sufficient for commercial use. Tissue plasminogen activator is nonantigenic and, unlike streptokinase, reportedly causes no allergic reactions. Unlike both streptokinase and urokinase, the action of rt-PA is clot specific. It activates only the plasminogen that is incorporated into the thrombotic fibrin clot and does not alter circulating plasminogen. Because of its short half-life, the usual 100 mg dose is staggered over 3 hours: 10 mg over 1 to 2 minutes, then 50 mg the first hour, and 20 mg over each of the next 2 hours.[8,173,178,182]

The recently published GUSTO study suggests benefits with "accelerated" administration of this same 100 mg dose over 1½ hours (15 mg over 1-2 min, then 50 mg over 30 min, and the remaining 35 mg over the next hour).[176a]

Anisoylated plasminogen streptokinase activator complex (APSAC, Anistreplace, Eminase), a more recently introduced clot-specific agent, is a streptokinase plasminogen complex that is chemically modified to be inactive until it binds with fibrin. However, the antigenic reactions triggered by streptokinase still occur. The usual dose is 30 units given intravenously over 2 to 5 minutes.[5,182]

Urokinase (Abbokinase, Breokinase, Win-Kinase) is a naturally occurring human enzyme derived from kidney cells and is a direct activator of plasminogen. Like streptokinase but unlike rt-PA and APSAC, urokinase is not clot specific and exerts its action systematically on circulating plasminogen. Urokinase is nonantigenic and is generally well tolerated when administered intravenously, with no reports of allergic reactions. The usual dose is 2 to 3 million units, administered intravenously over 30 minutes. A clot-specific derivative, single-chain urokinase-type plasminogen activator (SCUPA, prourokinase) is currently under investigation.[173,182]

The goal of thrombolytic therapy in acute MI is to achieve sustained reperfusion of the infarct-related vessel, thereby maintaining left ventricular function, limiting infarct size, and improving immediate and long-term survival. Reperfusion is accomplished by reversing the thrombotic component of coronary thrombosis or occlusion. Perfusion is maintained by the administration of heparin (5000 units IV, followed by continuous infusion of 800 to 1000 units per hour) either during or after thrombolysis with rt-PA. Administration with APSAC or streptokinase is more controversial because of reports of increased bleeding.[3,174a]

The triad of lipidemia, vasospasm, and thrombosis contributes to coronary stenosis or occlusion associated with acute MI. Thrombolytic therapy in acute MI was first attempted in the 1950s using streptokinase. Without the benefit of coronary arteriography to confirm the pathology and results of therapy, however, the findings were inconclusive and this mode of intervention was abandoned.

Enthusiasm for the use of thrombolytic drugs was rekindled in the 1970s by the work of Chazov and later Rentrop, who dramatically showed the opening of a coronary artery in acute MI with intracoronary streptokinase. De Wood and associates in 1980 even more clearly established the rationale for the use of thrombolytic therapy in acute MI. Performing coronary arteriograms within 6 hours of the onset of symptoms of acute MI, they demonstrated that a thrombus was present in 87% of those patients evaluated. Their work also confirmed the safety of catheterization in acute MI, which had been controversial until this time.

Since 1980, researchers have conducted many large-scale trials using thrombolytic drugs in acute MI. Results repeatedly have demonstrated that the time from onset of symptoms until reperfusion of the involved muscle is the critical factor in achieving success. One large study involving over 12,000 patients in Italy (GISSI) demonstrated little benefit in patients treated beyond 6 hours. The greatest benefit was in those treated within 1 hour.[1] Despite reperfusion in a large percentage of patients receiving thrombolytic drugs, reocclusion occurs in 20% to 40% of patients. The most important determinant for acute reocclusion appears to be the degree of residual stenosis.

Ideal candidates for thrombolytic therapy are patients with an MI in progress, as evidenced by ST segment elevation of 1 to 2 mm on at least two leads, less than 6 hours' duration of symptoms, no response to nitroglycerin, and age less than 70 to 75 years.[1] Age over 75 years is associated with an increase in hemorrhagic complications. ST segment elevation suggests probable Q wave infarction. ASA and heparin are preferred in non−Q wave infarction.[184] Relative and absolute contraindications for thrombolytic therapy include history of actual bleeding disorders such as hemorrhagic CVA, hypertension, hematocrit less than 33%, major surgery within 2 months, chest trauma, intracranial tumors, or aneurysms.[1,5,8] Routine laboratory tests include complete blood count, CK isoenzymes, PT, PTT, fibrinogen, and thrombin.

Indications of effective reperfusion include abrupt cessation of chest pain, a rapid fall in ST segments, and rapid peaking of the CK enzymes 3 to 4 hours after treatment ("CK washout").[5,166,173] The major complications associated with any form of reperfusion are arrhythmias. These include accelerated idioventricular rhythm, ventricular tachycardia, ventricular fibrillation, and bradycardia primarily with inferior wall MI. Prophylactic lidocaine can be administered but most of the arrhythmias are minor or transient.[5] Hypotension may also occur.

The major complication associated with thrombolytic drugs is bleeding. Periaccess bleeding or bleeding at puncture sites may be serious and can occur with all of the thrombolytic drugs in use, including rt-PA. This bleeding occurs most often at femoral access sites used for catheterization or arterial or venous sheaths; thus limiting venous and arterial punctures is recommended. Anticoagulants administered to maintain patency, such as heparin, may also contribute to bleeding episodes. Intracranial hemorrhages have been reported with all the thrombolytic drugs in high-risk patients. Other reported bleeding sites include gastrointestinal and retroperitoneal.[182] Risk factors for bleeding include female gender, advanced age (more than 70 to 75 years), and long-standing or acute hypertension. The incidence of bleeding is approximately 1 in every 200 patients.

The practitioner will want to compare currently available thrombolytic agents according to cost, ease of administration, side effects, and effectiveness. Streptokinase is the least expensive. APSAC is the easiest to administer but is more expensive than both streptokinase and rt-PA. Both streptokinase and APSAC are associated with the development of sensitivity and allergic reactions.[3,173,178] The incidence of hemorrhagic side effects is similar with all four agents regardless of clot-specific characteristics, probably due in part to the concurrent heparin administration.[173,178,182] Studies have shown tissue plasminogen activator (rt-PA) to be more effective than streptokinase in opening occluded coronary vessels (TIMI, ECSG studies).[1,5,8,166,182] Differences in other indices of success such as ventricular function and mortality are not as significant, however.[1,184,194] One study comparing APSAC and rt-PA reported no difference. The addition of aspirin seems to increase the effectiveness of at least streptokinase (ISI-II study). The recently completed GISSI-II and ISIS-III studies found no difference in mortality when comparing aspirin combined with APSAC, streptokinase, or rt-PA.[176a,184] The more recently published GUSTO study found a significant decrease in mortality with rt-PA plus IV herparin when compared to streptokinase regimens.[176a] However, this study is currently under scrutiny due to cost-benefit issues.[174a] Research has not yet clearly determined the overall preferred agent (Table 9-2).

NURSING ORDERS: For patients receiving antithrombotic therapy for coronary artery disease

RELATED NURSING DIAGNOSES: Alteration in comfort, volume deficit, potential for injury, knowledge deficit

1. Before initiating therapy, check for a history of bleeding disorders, GI ulcers, gastritis, and liver disease. Anticipate use of antiplatelet and antifibrin agents within a specified time after surgery in selected cases (e.g., after bypass surgery or valve replacement).
2. Check other medications for possible interactions with anticoagulants, especially with warfarin and heparin. Do not infuse IV heparin with other drugs.
3. Regularly inspect the patient for signs of bleeding. Assess urine, stools, and emesis for occult blood; check gums and nose for bruising and ecchymotic areas.
4. Report any new pericardial friction rub to the physician; anticoagulant therapy may need to be withdrawn.
5. Follow coagulation studies closely; PTT with heparin therapy should be 1.5 to 2.0 times normal; PT with warfarin therapy should be 1.3 to 1.5 times normal. Thrombin time (TT) with thrombolytic therapy should be 2 to 5 times normal.[8]
6. During thrombolytic therapy:
   —Support the patient and family and provide them with information as required regarding the therapy.
   —Monitor patient for signs of reper-

fusion during IV administration of thrombolytic drugs, i.e. arrhythmia, sudden end to chest pain, hypotension and bradycardia with inferior wall MI, early peaking of the creatine phosphokinase (CPK) enzyme. Note CPK higher than normal and falls faster than normal.
   —Monitor ECG on a lead where you can watch ST elevation carefully. Note any increases or decreases with therapy.
   —Be alert for the development of life-threatening reperfusion arrhythmias, i.e. VT, VF, accelerated idioventricular rhythm (AIVR).
   —Monitor clinical signs of ischemia closely, i.e. chest discomfort, ST segment shift, arrhythmias.
   —Report continued chest discomfort following thrombolytic therapy or any ECG changes suggestive of further ischemia that could signal reocclusion. Alert the physician immediately if these occur.
   —Monitor carefully at catheter insertion sites for signs of bleeding, hematoma formation, unusual bruising. Monitor laboratory values that may indicate covert bleeding.
   —Limit IV puncture to use of large-gauge intracaths for blood sampling and IV therapy. Avoid IM injections.[8]
   —Maintain heparin infusion and follow PTTs carefully.
   —Monitor neurologic status carefully for subtle signs of possible intracranial bleeding.
7. After thrombolytic therapy:
   —Maintain pressure at the catheter-introducer site as prescribed to avoid excessive bleeding.
   —Handle the patient gently to avoid bruising.
   —Administer no IM medications until the effects of therapy are resolved.

Table 9-2. Antithrombotic drugs

	Antiplatelet	Antifibrin	Thrombolytic
Drug	Acetylacetic acid (aspirin) Dipyridamole (Persantine) Sulfinpyrazone (Anturane)	Warfarin sodium (Coumadin) Heparin	Streptokinase (Streptase, Kabikinase) Urokinase APSAC (Eminase) rt-PA (Activase)
Major use in coronary artery disease	Prevent arterial thrombus/vein graft closure before and after MI bypass surgery	Prevent venous/mural thrombus after MI; prevent left atrial thrombus in chronic atrial fibrillation	Disrupt coronary arterial thrombus with acute obstruction
Severity of associated side effects	Mild	Moderate	Potentially severe
Treatment of complications	Withdraw medication; no specific therapy usually required	Administer medication: for warfarin, vitamin K; for heparin, protamine sulfate; for extreme cases , fresh frozen plasma (FFP)	Discontinue drug; administer blood products
Related coagulation test(s)	Platelet count	PT: warfarin PTT: heparin	PTT: concomitant heparin administration

—Note that no exact antidote exists for thrombolytic drugs.

8. Administer subcutaneous heparin between the iliac crests in the lower abdomen. Rotate the injection sites and do not massage. Use of a standardized card is desirable for this purpose. Obtain PTT approximately 30 minutes before the next dose of heparin. The antidote for bleeding from heparin therapy is protamine sulfate.

9. Give warfarin at the same time daily. Elderly patients and those with renal and liver disease are particularly susceptible to bleeding if given warfarin, and they should wear a Medic Alert bracelet. The antidote for bleeding from warfarin therapy is vitamin K.

10. Include the following in patient teaching:
    —Have patients receiving anticoagulants at home wear a Medic Alert bracelet.
    —Instruct patients to keep a "vial of life" with medical information and a list of all cardiac medications in the refrigerator.
    —Teach patients the subtle signs and symptoms of bleeding.
    —Avoid over-the-counter medications that may potentiate anticoagulant effects.
    —Instruct patients to take warfarin at the same time daily.
    —Instruct patients to use an electric razor and a soft toothbrush.
    —Instruct patients to report any changes in menses.
    —Stress to patients the importance of a pressure dressing or bag.
    —Instruct patients regarding dietary sources of vitamin K^+ (e.g., green, leafy vegetables)

BETA BLOCKING AGENTS

Beta-adrenergic blocking agents are indicated in the management of arrhythmias, angina, MI, and hypertension. They are also currently used in the management of other cardiovascular disorders such as aortic dissection, migraine, hypertrophic cardiomyopathy, and mitral valve prolapse (see Unit 11). Noncardiovascular indications include thyrotoxicosis, glaucoma, and anxiety.

Twelve beta blockers are currently available in the United States. These specific agents are propranolol (Inderal), metoprolol (Lopressor), nadolol (Corgard), atenolol (Tenormin), timolol (Blocadren), pindolol (Visken), labetalol (Normodyne, Trandate), acebutolol (Sectral), penbutolol (Levatol), betaxolol (Kerlone), bisoprolol (Zebeta), carteolol (Cartrol), and esmolol (Brevibloc).[4] The available beta blockers differ primarily according to their selectivity for B_1 receptors, partial agonist or intrinsic sympathetic activity, vasodilating properties, and fat solubility.

B_1 receptor blockade is essential for most therapeutic effects of the beta blocking agents. Drugs that block the B_1 receptors of the sympathetic nervous system have the following effects: (1) decreased heart rate, (2) decreased AV conduction, (3) decreased contractility, and (4) decreased automaticity.[5] Related side effects include bradycardia, hypotension, and CHF. Ironically, patients with mild CHF may benefit from beta blockade because of the effect on heart rate and neurohormonal responses (see Unit 8). Beta blockade prevents exhaustion of the compensatory sympathetic responses occurring in CHF, which ultimately results in decreased numbers and sensitivity ("down regulation") of the beta receptors.[82] However, heart failure can deteriorate as a result of the direct effect on contractility. For this reason, beta blockers should be administered with caution in the patient with CHF and should not be administered at all to patients with severe CHF. Beta blockers with vasodilating effects may be more beneficial as a result of offsetting effects on afterload.

B_2 blockade is not critical for the therapeutic effects of beta blockade and is often associated with side effects. Cardioselective beta blockers block B_1 receptors with minimal or decreased effects on B_2 receptors. This selectivity is dose dependent, however, and is lost at higher doses. Selective B_1 blockers have fewer bronchospastic, vasospastic, and metabolic side effects. B_2 receptor sites are located on the bronchial smooth muscle. B_2 blockade produces bronchospasm; thus all beta blockers should be avoided in patients with severe chronic obstructive pulmonary disease (COPD) or asthma. In less severe lung disease, the cardioselective beta blockers provide the least risk. B_2 receptors also control glucose release from glycogen stores in response to hypoglycemia. Nonselective beta blockers may precipitate insulin-induced hypoglycemia in diabetic patients. Therefore, cardioselective beta-blocking agents may be preferable in diabetic patients. The cardioselective beta blockers are atenolol (Tenormin), acebutolol (Sectral), betaxolol (Kerlone), and metoprolol (Lopressor).

Coronary and peripheral vascular tone is maintained by a balance of alpha-adrenergic and beta-adrenergic (sympathetic) activity. Alpha-adrenergic activity causes vasoconstriction while beta$_2$-adrenergic activity causes vasodilation. B_2 blockade allows alpha-adrenergic activity to predominate, which may result in coronary or peripheral vascular spasm. Therefore, nonselective beta blockers should be avoided or used with caution in patients with vasospastic coronary or peripheral vascular disease. Nonselective beta blockers are also associated with negative effects on the blood lipids. HDL levels are decreased, and VLDL levels are increased.[4,5]

The beta blockers pindolol (Visken) and acebutolol (Sectral) differ from the others by possessing some intrinsic sympathetic activity (ISA), also called partial agonist activity (PAA).[5] Acebutolol is cardioselective, whereas pindolol is nonselective. The ISA of acebutolol is also milder. This activity is evident primarily when overall sympathetic tone is low, such as at rest, rather than during exercise. Reduction in resting heart rate induced by the beta blockade is balanced by this slight beta stimulation. Therefore, administration of pindolol or acebutolol produces less resting bradycardia. Vasodilation occurs as a result of B_2 stimulation, thereby decreasing the risk of coronary and peripheral spasm and more effectively lowering the peripheral vascular resistance in hypertensive disease. This mild inherent sympathetic stimulation may also minimize the typically aggravating effect of beta blockade in CHF but has not yet been proved clinically significant. Intrinsic B_2 activity may produce tremors.

Although vasoconstriction is typical in nonselective beta blockade, vasodilation may occur either secondary to ISA activity or alpha-blocking activity. Labetalol (Normodyne, Trandate) has the unique property of alpha blockade in addition to beta blockade. Alpha receptors are located in the peripheral and coronary blood vessels. Stimulation of the alpha receptors causes vasoconstriction. Blockade of the alpha receptors, therefore, causes vasodilation. Labetalol thus lowers peripheral vascular resistance. Labetalol is available in IV form and acts more rapidly on severe hypertension than any other beta blocker administered intravenously. These properties make labetalol a useful alternative to nitroprusside (Nipride) for the management of hypertensive crisis. Labetalol also can be continued in oral form. Although labetalol is not cardioselective, it combines the effects of beta blockade with vasodilation.

The fat-soluble beta blockers are metabolized in the liver and are associated with CNS side effects including insomnia, nightmares, hallucinations, and depression. These effects may be prevented or minimized by the use of water-soluble beta blockers that do not penetrate the blood-brain barrier, such as nadolol (Corgard), atenolol (Tenormin), or carteolol (Cartrol).[5,8] Water-soluble beta blockers are excreted by the kidneys. Patients with liver failure are sensitive to the fat-soluble beta blockers, and patients with renal failure are sensitive to the water-soluble beta blockers.

All beta blockers are associated with fatigue and rebound effects if abruptly withheld. Although the exact mechanism of the fatigue is unknown, it may occur because of bradycardia, hypotension, CHF, or altered skeletal muscle metabolism. Beta blockers such as propranolol lower free fatty acids, which act as a skeletal muscle energy source. Beta blockers also inhibit the catecholamine-induced breakdown of muscle glycogen stores in response to hypoglycemia or increased energy demands. Switching to another beta blocker may decrease fatigue. The use of beta blockers with cardioselective or vasodilating effects may be associated with less fatigue.[5] Abrupt withdrawal may be associated with a rebound increase in angina, arrhythmias, or hypertension.

Beta blockers are particularly effective in controlling arrhythmias that are stress related. Propranolol (Inderal) and the other beta-blocking agents are used primarily in the chronic management of both ventricular and supraventricular arrhythmias and are also classified as class II antiarrhythmics (see Antiarrhythmics). However, the sympathetic beta-blocking drug esmolol (Brevibloc) was introduced exclusively for the acute management of supraventricular tachyarrhythmias. It is shorter acting than the prototype beta-blocking agent propranolol. Esmolol is cardioselective, producing less toxic effects on the lungs and vascular bed than propranolol and mimicking most closely the action of the more selective beta blocking agent metopro-

lol (Lopressor). Unlike metoprolol, esmolol is available for IV use only. Titration can be complex. A loading dose of 0.5 mg/kg (25 to 50 mg) is administered over 1 minute followed by an infusion of one tenth the amount (2.5 to 5 mg/min). The sequence is repeated every 5 minutes, increasing the infusion by 2.5 to 5 mg, up to a maximum of 10 to 20 mg/min.

Esmolol has been shown to be as effective as IV propranolol in controlling supraventricular tachyarrhythmias. The major adverse reaction reported is hypotension, which is usually asymptomatic and resolves within 30 minutes of discontinuing the drug. This side effect occurs more often than with IV propranolol. Merely lowering the dose range may also be effective. The infusion is gradually decreased as oral agents are initiated.

The American Heart Association currently recommends three beta blockers for the acute management of supraventricular arrhythmias: propranolol (Inderal), esmolol (Brevibloc), and metoprolol (Lopressor).[3] The action of beta blockers in supraventricular arrhythmias is to slow AV conduction. Therefore, they slow the ventricular rate of these arrhythmias, convert them, or prevent them from occurring.

Beta blockers are indicated in therapy for effort angina. They relieve chest pain by lowering O_2 balance. Beta blockers such as propranolol reduce myocardial O_2 consumption (MVO_2) or demands by *decreasing heart rate* and *depressing contractility*. Myocardial O_2 consumption is a function of rate, preload, afterload, and contractility. Beta blockers may also indirectly increase the O_2 supply secondary to a decrease in rate and prolonged diastolic filling time.

Although beta blockade is effective in relieving the chest pain of effort angina, it may aggravate chest pain caused by coronary spasm or rest angina. The administration of beta blockers in Prinzmetal (variant) angina has potential risks and is best avoided. The use of beta blockers in unstable angina probably represents a mixture of fixed disease and spasm. Concurrent administration of nitrates of calcium antagonists may offset any negative vasospastic effects.

Most beta-blocking agents are equally effective in the control of angina and hypertension. Control of hypertension may provide further benefits in angina control because of the reduction in afterload. The primary mechanism of action in chronic hypertension is thought to be a lowering of cardiac output. Peripheral vascular resistance may actually increase in response to the fall in cardiac output or B_2 blockade. Inhibition of renin secretion from B_1 cells in the kidney is likely to be a contributing factor. The full antihypertensive effect may take as long as 1 to 4 weeks. Labetalol is the only beta blocker indicated in the acute management of severe end-stage hypertension where systemic vascular resistance is typically high.

Beta blockers may also be used during or after MI to limit infarction size, prevent extension of the infarction, and prevent complications such as ventricular fibrillation or cardiac rupture. [1,5,8,97,101] When administered intravenously in the initial hours of acute infarction, beta blockers lower myocardial O_2 demands by decreasing heart rate, blood pressure, and contractility. Coronary perfusion may also increase secondary to the effects on heart rate and diastole. Early administration of beta blockers is primarily recommended at this time for patients with tachycardia, hypertension, and no contraindications to beta blockade.[1,97,101] Contraindications include bradycardia, systolic blood pressure lower than 100 mm Hg, severe COPD, and moderate to severe CHF. Only metoprolol (Lopressor) and atenolol (Tenormin) are approved in the United States at this time for IV administration in acute MI.[4,5] However, propranolol (Inderal) is also frequently used. The recommended dosage for metoprolol in this setting is 5 mg every 5 minutes to a total of 15 mg, then 100 mg PO bid for 3 months. The recommended dosage of atenolol is 5 to 10 mg the first day, followed by oral therapy. Propranolol is administered in 0.5 mg doses up to a total of 0.1 mg/kg.[4,5]

Beta blockers are recommended for most patients after acute MI, except those with uncomplicated MIs (low risk) and those with non−Q wave infarction, and unless contraindications to beta blockade exist.[1,5,97,101] Beta blockers currently considered effective include atenolol, metoprolol, timolol, and propranolol. Therapy is initiated within the first few weeks and is continued for at least 2 years, or indefinitely.[1,5,97,101]

NURSING ORDERS: For patients receiving a beta blocker

RELATED NURSING DIAGNOSES: Alteration in cardiac output, alteration in comfort, activity intolerance, ineffective airway clearance, alteration in metabolism, impaired tissue perfusion, anxiety or knowledge deficit

1. Check pulse and blood pressure before administering each dose. Watch for bradycardia and/or hypotension. Establish a target pulse rate and blood pressure with the physician. Hold for a heart rate of less than 40 beats per minute. Notify physician of heart rate less than 60 beats per minute.
2. Auscultate for wheezes or increased crackles (rales) with each set of vital signs. Do not administer to patient with a history of asthma.
3. Administer with caution to patient with:
   —CHF
   —Diabetes, who is receiving insulin therapy or oral hypoglycemics
   —Peripheral vascular disease
4. To avoid potential withdrawal syndrome, do not discontinue beta blockers abruptly.

5. Instruct patient not to stop taking these medicines abruptly, and explain why.
6. Observe patient for (or instruct patient to report):
   —Increased peripheral vascular spasm (e.g., claudication, paresthesias)
   —Increased angina (especially rest angina)
   —Excessive fatigue
   —Nightmares
7. Watch for interaction with disopyramide.
8. When administering esmolol:
   —Use a 10 mg/ml vial to administer the loading dose of 0.5 mg/kg (25 to 50 mg).
   —Prepare the same infusion concentration (10 mg/cc) by adding two 2.5-g vials to 500 cc of D5W or normal saline. To deliver 5 mg/min, set the infusion pump at 30 gtt/min (cc/hr).
   —Monitor for hypotension and effective response. Monitor breath sounds (wheezes or crackles) at higher dose ranges.
   —Administer before but not after verapamil (because of the longer half-life of verapamil).
   —Thirty minutes after the administration of an oral agent, reduce the esmolol infusion rate by half. Discontinue the infusion 1 hour after the second dose.

CALCIUM CHANNEL BLOCKING AGENTS

Calcium channel blocking agents are indicated in the management of supraventricular arrhythmias, angina, and hypertension. The calcium channel blockers are also effective in many other cardiovascular disorders, including migraine headaches, cerebrovascular spasm, peripheral vascular spasm (Raynaud's disease), pulmonary hypertension, and hypertrophic cardiomyopathy. Effects in inhibiting platelet function may also be beneficial in coronary artery disease.[8,122,132,134]

Calcium channel blocking agents act by blocking the entry of calcium into cardiac or vascular cells. Although these agents are also frequently called calcium antagonists, the label can be misleading since they do not significantly alter serum calcium levels.

Calcium has major cardiac and vascular actions. Therefore, calcium channel blockers can be *cardioactive* and/or *vasoactive*. There are three major categories of currently available calcium channel blockers: (1) the cardioactive agents; (2) the dihyropyridine vasoactive agents, and (3) the mixed Na^+ and Ca^{++} channel blockers. The two currently available cardioactive agents are verapamil (Isoptin, Calan, Verelan) and diltiazem (Cardizem). The six dihydropyridine vasoactive agents currently available in the United States are nifedipine (Procardia), nicardipine (Cardene, Syntex), nimodipine (Nimotop), isradipine (DynaCirc), felodipine (Plendil), and amlodipine besylate (Norvasc).[4] Nimodipine has selective effects on the cerebrovascular bed and is indicated primarily for the spasm associated with subarachnoid hemorrhage. Bepridil (Vascor) is the only mixed Na^+ and Ca^{++} channel blocker currently available. This drug also has class I antiarrhythmic effects related to its effects on Na^+ channels. Its use is limited by significant Q–T prolongation, which can lead to torsades de pointes.[8]

Calcium plays a significant role in the contraction of the peripheral and coronary arterial bed as well as other types of smooth muscle. Vasoactive calcium channel blocking agents block these actions, resulting in vasodilatation (Fig. 9-8). Systemic vascular resistance, blood pressure, and afterload are decreased. Relaxation of both coronary and peripheral vascular spasm also occurs.

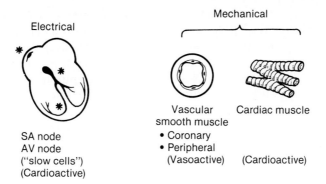

Fig. 9-8 Calcium channel blockade: electrical and mechanical, cardioactive and vasoactive effects.

The cardioactive consequences of calcium channel blockade can be classified as either electrical or mechanical. The electrical effects result in suppression of Ca^{++}-dependent, slow cell depolarization in the SA and AV nodes. These actions may also be referred to as *negative chronotropic* and *dromotropic*. The mechanical effects result in suppression of contractility. This action may also be referred to as *negative inotropic*.[120]

The cardioactive calcium channel blocking agents such as verapamil and diltiazem actually have both cardioactive and vasoactive effects. Therefore, they have a wide spectrum of potential clinical usage.

Specific cardioactive actions on the electrical structures of the heart include (1) SA block, (2) AV block, and (3) suppression of slow cell ectopy (supraventricular or ventricular). These actions are related to depression of SA and AV node automaticity and prolongation of SA and AV node refractory periods and conduction time. The calcium channel blockers may also influence the abnormally slow conduction within the ischemic zone of selected reentry circuits (see Units 4 and 6).

Both verapamil and diltiazem are currently indicated in the acute management of supraventricular arrhythmias.[1,3,102] The clinical effects of calcium channel blockers in supraventricular tachyarrhythmias are (1) decreased ventricular rate and/or (2) conversion or prevention of supraventricular arrhythmias with an AV node reentry circuit. Supraventricular arrhythmias such as PSVT typically use an AV node reentry circuit. Therefore, the effects of verapamil in PSVT are conversion and prevention. Verapamil is preferred to diltiazem at this time in recurrent PSVT. Verapamil is indicated after the administration of adenosine if the blood pressure remains stable.[3,12,17,18] Supraventricular arrhythmias such as atrial flutter or fibrillation do not use AV node reentry cicuits. However, AV node refractory period and conduction time determine the ventricular rate of these arrhythmias. Therefore, the effect of verapamil and diltiazem in atrial flutter and/or fibrillation is primarily to decrease the ventricular rate.[1,3,6,109,130] The supraventricular arrhythmias occurring in Wolff-Parkinson-White syndrome constitute a special category that requires extra precautions to ensure safe administration of verapamil or diltiazem (see Unit 11). Unlike verapamil or adenosine, diltiazem can be administered as a maintenance infusion.[3,109.130]

Sustained control of the ventricular rate may be accomplished by the concurrent administration of IV diltiazem (5 to 15 mg/hr) or digitalis, usually followed by oral digitalis. Oral verapamil may later be added if digitalis is not effective. However, the digitalis dosage should then be reduced, since chronic verapamil therapy increases serum digoxin levels from 50% to 70% and may increase the risk of digitalis toxicity. Subsequent digitalis levels should be monitored carefully.

The major toxic effects of the cardioactive calcium channel blockers are hypotension caused by peripheral vasodilation and bradycardia. Bradycardia occurs primarily with preexisting SA or AV node disease. Therefore, verapamil and diltiazem are contraindicated in patients with sick sinus syndrome, second-degree or third-degree AV block, and severe hypotension. Use atropine or dopamine as indicated to manage these adverse reactions. Avoid calcium since it may unnecessarily increase the total serum calcium. Administer IV verapamil slowly to minimize these side effects. Administer an initial dose of 2.5 to 5 mg over 2 to 3 minutes. A 3-minute period is recommended for patients over 55 years of age. After 15 to 30 minutes, this dose may be repeated up to 10 mg for a total of 15 mg. A continuous IV drip is not required and may be difficult to monitor. Administer diltiazem in an IV dose of 20 mg (0.25 mg/kg for the average person) over 2 minutes, followed after 15 minutes with a 25-mg bolus, also administered over 2 minutes.[3,5,109,115]

Both verapamil and diltiazem are contraindicated in severe CHF, although diltiazem reportedly has fewer negative effects on contractility.[3,106,124] Myocardial depression may also be magnified when these agents are used in combination with either disopyramide or IV propranolol. Disopyramide should not be administered within 48 hours before or 24 hours after verapamil. Concurrent administration of IV verapamil and IV propranolol produces significant electrical and mechanical depression and is contraindicated.[3] Combined oral administration of these agents does not usually produce these effects, but this method probably should be used with caution in situations in which electrical and/or mechanical function is already significantly depressed.

The use of either verapamil or diltiazem in wide QRS tachycardias to differentiate between ventricular tachycardia and supraventricular tachycardia is contraindicated.[3,5,7,8] Inadvertent administration of verapamil in ventricular tachycardia is associated with severe hypotension and ventricular fibrillation. Verapamil and diltiazem can also cause harmful effects in patients with the wide QRS tachycardias of Wolff-Parkinson-White syndrome.[3,6]

Calcium channel blockers are indicated as therapy for both rest and effort angina.[103,105,111] All currently available calcium channel blockers are equally effective in the management of rest angina or angina caused by coronary spasm. Their effectiveness in effort angina varies, however, according to the mechanism and ability of the specific agent to lower demands in individual patients. Effort angina is triggered by increased O_2 demands. The most effective treatment is rest or drugs that lower these demands. Decreasing afterload, heart rate, or contractility may lower O_2 demands. Rest angina is triggered by coronary spasm or decreased O_2 supply. Its most effective treatment is drugs that relieve the coronary spasm, thus increasing O_2 supply. Calcium channel blockers can both increase coronary (O_2) supply and lower O_2 demands. They are therefore potentially effective in both effort and rest angina or a mixture of the two. Calcium channel blockers are effective in postinfarction angina as well as chronic or unstable angina since the mechanisms are similar. These agents may also be useful during and after coronary angioplasty to prevent vasospasm.[1,112,113,119,127]

The major mechanism of action of the dihydropyridine vasoactive agents in effort angina is to decrease afterload by peripheral arterial dilation. In selected cases these agents, particularly nifedipine, may increase heart rate as a reflex response to the vasodilation, thus limiting its antianginal action.[103,133] However, treatment of angina with vasoactive agents may be safer than with cardioactive agents in patients with SA or AV node disease, patients with severe heart failure, or those receiving other cardiac depressant medications.

The cardioactive agents act on effort angina by a combination of actions, including decreasing heart rate and contractility as well as afterload. For this reason, verapamil may prove effective in cases in which nifedipine has not proved beneficial. It is ideal for patients requiring a combination of arrhythmia and angina control. Diltiazem also has a potential combined mode of action in effort angina but is weaker than verapamil. Its use is ideal for cases in which side effects from nifedipine or verapamil prevent their use.

Therapy with calcium antagonists offers certain distinct advantages over therapy with beta blockers alone, especially in regard to side effects. None of the calcium antagonists possesses any bronchoconstricting activity. They are thus safer in the patient with asthma. Even the cardioactive agents produce fewer myocardial depressant effects than do the beta blockers in dosages used for either arrhythmia or angina control, despite some blockade of myocardial calcium channels. They are thus safer in the patient with CHF. The afterload reducing effects are also beneficial to the patient with CHF.[8,106,124]

Calcium channel blockade relaxes coronary and peripheral vascular spasm, whereas beta blockade may aggravate it. Thus calcium channel blockade is safer than beta blockade in the patient with rest angina or peripheral vascular disease. Coronary spasm probably complicates unstable angina even in patients with fixed disease or a history of effort angina. The addition of calcium channel blockade to beta blockade can minimize detrimental effects on coronary supply while maximizing lowered demands.

Calcium channel blockade does not offer advantages over nitrate therapy in the first-line management of effort or mixed angina syndromes. Nitrates act primarily to decrease preload but can also relax coronary spasm, thus decreasing O_2 demands and increasing O_2 supply, similar to calcium channel blockade. However, fewer significant side effects have been reported with nitrates, despite extensive use of these drugs over many years. The lower incidence of side effects may result from the absence of myocardial depressant activity and the lessening of peripheral arterial activity. The effect of calcium channel blockade on afterload may complement the action of the nitrates in angina. Calcium channel blockers may be added to the therapeutic regimen in patients unresponsive to nitrate therapy or in those receiving combined nitrate and beta-blocker therapy.

Diltiazem is the only calcium channel blocking agent to date that has been shown to be beneficial in the management of acute MI.[115,127,133] In patients with non−Q wave infarction oral diltiazem may be more effective than beta blockade in preventing reinfarction, postinfarction angina, and mortality.[1,115,127] Administration usually begins within the first 48 hours after infarction.

All calcium channel blockers are effective antihypertensive agents, especially for the patient with coronary artery disease.[5,135] The vasoactive dihydropyridines are the most popular. Current uses are as (1) a third-line agent after diuretics and beta blockers, (2) a second-line agent in conjunction with an ACE inhibitor or beta blocker, or (3) an initial single agent.[5,7,8] There is some evidence that the calcium channel blockers may be more effective in black patients, elderly patients, and patients with low renin levels, and beta blockers and ACE inhibitors may be more effective in patients with high serum renin levels.[5,7] Calcium channel blockers may also be an effective alternative to beta blockade in the patient at risk for pulmonary, vascular, or metabolic side effects, or in whom these or other side effects have already occurred. The major mechanism of action of the calcium channel blockers is to lower peripheral vascular resistance, which is a characteristic of end-stage hypertensive disease. For this reason, they are often more effective than beta blockers in severe hypertension. Most beta blockers act on the heart to lower cardiac output and, at least initially, increase peripheral vascular resistance. Labetalol (Normodyne, Trandate) is the major exception. The dihydropyridine calcium channel blockers also produce diuresis with sodium loss secondary to increases in glomerular filtration rate.[5,8]

Sublingual nifedipine (10 mg) is commonly used in the acute management of severe diastolic hypertension. The dose may be repeated once after 30 to 60 minutes.[2,116] Sustained effects require the use of other oral agents. The mode of delivery varies considerably between practitioners, and studies do not consistently support a more rapid onset or peak effect.[116,123] Methods vary from puncturing the capsule with a needle and squeezing out the contents to aspirating the contents into a syringe. Biting the capsule, then swallowing it with water is recommended for patients who can do this.[116] In others, the best method is unclear and requires further investigation.

Side effects of calcium antagonists are related to cardiovascular, CNS, and GI actions. The cardiovascular effects include hypotension, headache, facial flushing, and dizziness.[5] Bradycardia occurs with cardioactive agents, especially when used in combination with other cardiac depressants or in the presence of conduction system disease.

CNS effects include tremors, nervousness, and mood changes. They are less commonly reported than the CNS effects occurring with beta blockers. Peripheral edema occurs often, especially with nifedipine. However, this edema is not thought to be related to cardiovascular deterioration. The exact mechanism is unclear but may be related to local protein shifts. Significant peripheral and facial edema has also been reported with amlodipine and diltiazem.[5]

NURSING ORDERS: For patients receiving a calcium channel blocker

RELATED NURSING DIAGNOSES: Alteration in cardiac output, alteration in comfort, alteration in elimination, knowledge deficit

1. Check blood pressure before administering each dose. Watch for hypotension and establish target blood pressure with the physician.
2. Check the pulse rate before administering verapamil or diltiazem. Establish a target pulse rate with the physician. Hold for a heart rate of less than 40 beats per minute. Notify physician of heart rate less than 60 beats per minute.
3. Instruct the patient to report dizziness, headache, or constipation.
4. Evaluate the effectiveness in anginal relief and document it.
5. Do not administer a calcium channel blocker in patients with severe hypotension, CHF, sick sinus syndrome, or severe AV block. (Always check pulse before administering.)
6. Administer verapamil slowly when giving intravenously (2.5-5 mg over 2 to 3 minutes). Have patient on a cardiac monitor; use only amount of verapamil necessary to control rate. This dose may be repeated up to 10 mg after 15 to 30 minutes for a total of 15 mg. An IV infusion is not typically used. Request follow-up orders for digitalis, oral verapamil, or beta blockers.

7. Do not administer verapamil or diltiazem in wide QRS tachycardia.
8. Never administer IV verapamil and IV propranolol together.

9. When administering sublingual nifedipine, instruct patient to bite the capsule, then swallow it with water if possible.

INOTROPIC AGENTS

Inotropic agents may be administered to patients with CHF to stimulate myocardial contractility and thus to improve cardiac output. However, positive inotropic agents increase myocardial O_2 consumption and may prove harmful to ischemic myocardium, resulting in further myocardial necrosis. These agents require caution in acute MI and are usually administered in conjunction with unloading agents. Their use is limited to cases of severe left ventricular failure. The inotropic agents used most commonly in the management of CHF include the cardiac glycoside digitalis, the beta-stimulating agents dopamine (Intropin), and dobutamine (Dobutrex), and the phosphodiesterase inhibitor amrinone (Inocor). The inotropic agents dopamine, dobutamine, and amrinone are more potent and less arrhythmogenic and are associated with fewer deleterious effects on ischemic myocardium than digitalis. Therefore, these agents are currently preferred over digitalis in the acute, short-term management of severe CHF caused by MI.[3,6,150]

Digitalis

Digoxin (Lanoxin) is by far the most commonly prescribed digitalis glycoside because of its onset and duration of action, stability, and ease of administration. Digitalis is currently used in the chronic management of supraventricular tachyarrhythmias and as an inotropic agent. The mechanism of action of digitalis on cardiovascular cells is probably twofold; it includes (1) parasympathetic stimulation and (2) local cellular metabolic action.[8,141,147,150] Drugs that stimulate the parasympathetic nervous system decrease heart rate and depress AV conduction.

Digitalis may be indicated in the management of heart failure because it has a positive inotropic effect and thus stimulates myocardial contractility. However, inotropic agents also increase myocardial O_2 consumption. Therefore, when O_2 supply to the heart is already critically reduced, digitalis must be used with caution. In acute MI, digitalis may cause extension of the infarcted area. The ischemic myocardium is also more sensitive to the effects of digitalis toxicity.

Therefore, digitalis has been associated with increased mortality and is not the drug of choice in the initial management of heart failure caused by MI.[3,5,8,150] It may be indicated in the management of CHF that persists or is caused by other mechanisms.

The effect of digitalis on myocardial contractility is caused by a direct effect on the myocardial cells and is independent of its parasympathetic action. Digitalis enhances contractility by partial inhibition of the Na^+-K^+ pump.[5,6,8] The accumulation of intracellular Na^+ triggers the uptake of Ca^{++}, which activates contractile proteins. Improved contractility may result in further reductions in rate or prevent atrial arrhythmias caused by CHF. Inhibition of the Na^+-K^+ pump also results in a deficit of intracellular K^+. The deficit in intracellular K^+ produces electrical instability by enhancing automaticity. Arrhythmias associated with digitalis toxicity are magnified by hypokalemia. The arrhythmias of digitalis toxicity are also enhanced by a low serum Mg^{++} level, since

Mg^{++} is necessary to activate the Na^+-K^+ pump. In therapeutic dosages, digitalis decreases heart rate, depresses AV conduction, and increases myocardial contractility.

Toxic effects of digitalis therapy include anorexia, nausea, vomiting, fatigue, restlessness, nightmares, yellow-green halos around visual images, other visual changes, and digitalis toxicity arrhythmias. Hyperkalemia also may occur with severe digitalis toxicity. Serum levels of digitalis alone do not accurately confirm or rule out digitalis toxicity since they may not be a true reflection of myocardial levels or related electrolyte imbalances.[5,6,147] Digitalis toxicity should be suspected primarily when elevated serum levels are corroborated by typical clinical findings. Verapamil, quinidine, and amiodarone interact with digitalis to further raise digitalis levels and potentiate digitalis toxicity.[5,138,147]

The arrhythmias of digitalis toxicity are a manifestation of either enhanced automaticity, depressed conduction, or both. Recent evidence also implicates delayed afterdepolarizations (triggered activity) secondary to severe inhibition of the NA^+-K^+ pump and calcium overload (see Unit 6).[5,138,147] Digitalis has the ability to increase automaticity in the atria, AV junctional tissue, and ventricles. In digitalis toxicity, this property together with the development of afterdepolarizations may lead to the development of the following arrhythmias: (1) PAT with block, (2) accelerated junctional rhythms including junctional tachycardia, and (3) ventricular arrhythmias, especially ventricular bigeminy and bidirectional VT. Atrial arrhythmias with very slow ventricular rates may also represent digitalis toxicity. The arrhythmias of digitalis toxicity typically occur in combinations of two of these arrhythmias (Fig. 9-9).[138,147]

In PAT with block, the atrial rate is within the range characteristic of atrial tachycardia. Unlike typical atrial tachycardia, however, not all P waves are followed by QRS complexes, indicating AV block. The conduction block is most commonly second degree 2:1 or Wenkebach. The P–P intervals may be "ventriculophasic" or shorter when a QRS complex occurs between P waves.[138] The bidirectional VT is a form of fascicular VT, alternating every other beat between the two fascicles. On leads I, aVF, and II, the beats alternate between the patterns of right and left axis deviation with an incomplete right bundle branch pattern on lead V_1 (see Unit 7).[138] When junctional tachycardia secondary to digitalis toxicity develops in a patient with atrial fibrillation, the ventricular rhythm either becomes regular or assumes a repeating pattern of grouped beating (groups of two or three beats).[138]

The ventricular arrhythmias of digitalis toxicity may be treated with lidocaine (Xylocaine) but may also respond to diphenylhydantoin (Dilantin). Symptomatic junctional tachycardia may be treated with either diphenylhydantoin or propranolol (Inderal). The ventricular rates of PAT with block are usually not rapid, and therefore aggressive therapy is rarely indicated. Cessation of the digitalis and/or electrolyte replacement as needed may suffice. Although triggered activity should logically respond to calcium channel blockers, these agents are not used in the management of digitalis toxicity at this time. Symptomatic AV block caused by digitalis is usually responsive to atropine therapy. Epinephrine, isoproterenol, and/or temporary pacing can also be used if necessary.

Severe, potentially life-threatening digitalis toxicity, including severe AV block, can also be treated with digoxin immune Fab (Digibind).[5,6,141,147] Digibind consists of fragments of digoxin-specific antibodies obtained from sheep serum. The key antigen binding fragments, referred to as *Fab*, bind to the digoxin, inactivating it and facilitating its excretion through the kidney. Antibody fragments are less antigenic and allow for an earlier onset of

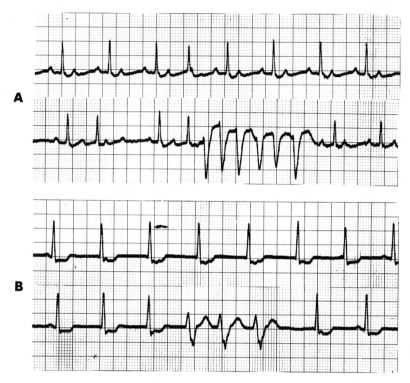

Fig. 9-9 Arrhythmias of digitalis toxicity. **A,** The p wave rate close to 150 (@ 180) without QRS complexes for every p is consistent with PAT with block. The presence of a second arrhythmia compatible with digitalis toxicity (VT) is also typical. **B,** VT is present in combination with an accelerated junctional rhythm.

action than a completed antibody. No allergic reactions have been reported. The dose is determined from the serum level or the amount of tablets ingested.

A therapeutic effect of arrhythmia control may be visible within minutes of administration. Resolution of all toxic effects usually occurs within 2 to 3 hours. Serum digitalis levels typically rise after administration of Digibind and remain distorted for up to 1 week. This increase in digitalis concentration includes the bound fragments that have been inactivated and should not be of concern. When toxicity is reversed too rapidly, hypokalemia may occur. For this reason, serum and ECG effects require monitoring during administration of Digibind.

Digitalis also has an effect on the ECG that is not necessarily associated with toxicity and may appear only during exercise. This fact makes it difficult at times to distinguish digitalis effects from ischemic changes. The electrolyte that affects contractility is calcium. Ca^{++} affects the ST segment on the ECG. The effect of digitalis on the ECG is to shorten the ST segment, typically causing it to "sag" (Fig. 9-10).

NURSING ORDERS: For patients receiving digitalis

RELATED NURSING DIAGNOSES: Alteration in cardiac output, alteration in nutrition, fluid volume deficit, knowledge deficit

1. Observe for the therapeutic effects of digitalis. Digitalis may slow the heart

Fig. 9-10 Digitalis effect on ECG.

rate simply by improving myocardial function.
—Is heart failure improving?
—Is heart rate slowing?
2. Observe for the development of anorexia. This development is often the first sign of digitalis intolerance.
3. Watch for the development of nausea and vomiting or visual changes.
4. Check pulse before administering. Establish target pulse rate with physician.

Hold for a heart rate less than 60 unless otherwise specified.
5. Monitor the patient carefully for development of the following arrhythmias:
—PAT with block
—Junctional tachycardia
—Ventricular arrhythmias, especially ventricular bigeminy and bidirectional VT
—Sinus bradycardia
—AV block
6. Monitor renal function, serum digitalis levels, K^+ and Mg^{++}.
7. When administering Digibind for severe digitalis toxicity, monitor for high temperature or low blood pressure due to allergic reactions. Monitor ECG for K^+ effects.

Beta-stimulating agents

Dopamine (Intropin) and dobutamine (Dobutrex) are examples of beta-adrenergic-stimulating agents that act as inotropic agents. Both agents have the unique ability, within carefully controlled dose ranges, to produce a selective increase in myocardial contractility, without significant increase in heart rate or arrhythmia formation.

Dopamine is a natural sympathetic chemical mediator with both alpha- and beta-stimulating properties within specific dose ranges. It is a catecholamine that acts as a precursor to norepinephrine and is used by the body predominantly for its alpha effects. Dopamine is the drug of choice for cardiogenic shock with moderate hypotension (70 to 100 mm Hg).[1,3,146] Also, the American Heart Association currently recommends it for hypotension associated with bradycardia unresponsive to atropine when a transcutaneous pacemaker is unavailable.[3]

In a moderate dosage range (2 to 10 mcg/kg/min), selective B_1 stimulation occurs.[3,8,146,147] B_1 receptors line the cardiac musculature. Stimulation of B_1 receptors routinely produce an increase in heart rate (chro-notropic effect), an increase in conduction (dromotropic effect), an increase in contractility (inotropic effect), and enhanced automaticity. However, the beta effects are initially selective, allowing only the inotropic effects to occur. For inotropic effects an initial dose range of 2.5 to 5 mcg/kg/min is recommended.[3,146,147] In dosages approaching and exceeding 10 mcg/kg/min, other B_1 properties begin to appear. These effects are visible in the form of tachycardia, ventricular arrhythmias, or both. Tachycardias increase myocardial O_2 consumption and may further compromise an ischemic myocardium.

In low dosage ranges (1 to 2 mcg/kg/min) dopamine has the unique ability to produce vasodilation selectively in certain vascular beds, such as the renal and mesenteric arteries.[3,5,8,146,147] Dopamine enters the renal vessels via special dopaminergic receptors and may be indicated to improve renal blood flow, prevent renal failure, and increase urine output in low-output states, such as CHF.[5,146,147] In CHF the fall in cardiac output produces a decrease in renal perfusion, with a corresponding fall in urine output.

Dopamine is a precursor of the alpha-adrenergic chemical norepinephrine (Levophed). Alpha-adrenergic receptors line the blood vessels. Stimulation of these receptors produces vasoconstriction and increases vascular resistance, blood pressure, and afterload. In dosages exceeding 10 mcg/kg/min, alpha-adrenergic properties appear.[3,5,146,147] These effects further increase myocardial O_2 consumption and may counterbalance any benefits obtained by dopamine administration. Necrosis and sloughing of tissues may also occur with IV infiltration, particularly in these dosage ranges. Phentolamine (Regitine), an alpha blocker, may be administered subcutaneously to treat the IV infiltration.[8] In high dosage ranges, dopaminergic effects are lost. Renal blood flow and urine output may actually decrease as the alpha-adrenergic effects on the renal vessels dominate. If dosages more than 20 mcg/kg/min are required to maintain the blood pressure, norepinephrine should be used instead.[3]

Careful calculation of the dosage range is critical in determining the beneficial effects and preventing the potential toxic effects of dopamine administration. Concurrent monitoring of cardiac output and wedge pressure can provide documentation of improvement or deterioration in left ventricular function. The wedge pressure typically remains unchanged or decreases slightly as the cardiac output increases and left ventricular emptying improves. Thus an increase in wedge pressure indicates a toxic response, possibly related to increased MVO_2, that can occur even in the usual therapeutic dose ranges. The afterload reducing agent nitroprusside (Nipride) or preload reducing agent NTG may be then commonly added to facilitate

improvement in cardiac output and to minimize increases in O_2 consumption. Dopamine may also be administered in conjunction with inotropic agents having arterial vasodilating effects, such as dobutamine or amrinone for similar reasons.

Dobutamine hydrochloride (Dobutrex) is a synthetic catecholamine with inotropic properties similar to those of dopamine, also mediated by B_1 receptors. Its inotropic action begins at the same dosage of dopamine but continues up to higher ranges before toxic effects appear (2 to 20 mcg/kg/min). At dosages greater than 20 mcg/kg/min, tachycardias occur.[3,5,8]

In contrast to dopamine, dobutamine does not have direct renal vasodilating effects and has mild peripheral vasodilating effects, resulting in a reduction of both preload and afterload; the exact mechanism is unclear.[5,8] Thus dobutamine has a more significant, consistent effect in lowering wedge pressure than dopamine. Pulmonary congestion decreases as the cardiac output increases. Dobutamine appears to possess the unique ability to combine the benefits of both inotropic and vasodilator therapy.

Dobutamine is the inotropic agent of choice in the normotensive patient with heart failure.[1,3,5,147] Dobutamine is preferred over dopamine as a vasopressor agent in the patient with right ventricular infarction since dopamine increases pulmonary vascular resistance whereas dobutamine lowers it.[1,3] Unlike dopamine, dobutamine may also be administered by intermittent infusion for the management of chronic CHF and is associated with an unexplained prolonged duration of action.

Phosphodiesterase inhibitors

Amrinone lactate (Inocor) is an intravenous inotropic agent with effects similar to those of dobutamine but with a totally different mechanism of action. It can be used

when dopamine or dobutamine is no longer effective or as an initial agent.[5,8,139,152] Amrinone is commonly referred to as a nonglycoside, noncatecholamine inotropic agent.

The initial dose is 0.75 mg/kg over 2 to 3 minutes followed by an infusion of 10 mcg/kg/min.[5,8,139] Amrinone acts as a phosphodiesterase inhibitor (similar to the bronchodilator aminophylline), resulting in an increased level of cAMP, an intracellular sympathetic messenger.[5,8,139,152] However, its action is more selective than that of aminophylline, acting primarily in cardiovascular tissues to produce an increase in contractility and vasodilation.

Tachyarrhythmias are uncommon but can occur at higher dose ranges. Thrombocytopenia has also been reported. The incidence of nausea and vomiting associated with administration has limited its long-term use.

Experimental agents within this classification system include fenoximone and sulmazole. Milrinone lactate (Primacor) has been recently released and is approved for IV use. It is significantly more potent than amrinone with a similar action. Milrinone has the benefit of an inotropic and vasodilating effect without a significant change in the heart rate or blood pressure.[4,144,152]

NURSING ORDERS: For patients receiving beta-stimulating or phosphodiesterase-inhibiting agents

RELATED NURSING DIAGNOSES: Alteration in cardiac output, impaired tissue perfusion, impaired gas exchange, knowledge deficit

1. Monitor the wedge pressure and cardiac output before and immediately after onset of therapy; continue to evaluate them at regular intervals thereafter.
2. Determine the patient's weight and calculate the dosage accordingly.
3. Monitor for the following toxic effects, depending on dosage:
   —Tachycardias/ventricular arrhythmias
   —Increased blood pressure
   —Decreased urine output
   —Increased wedge pressure
   —Sloughing of tissues primarily with Dopamine due to its alpha effects (Antidote is intradermal phentolamine if infiltration occurs.)
4. Document improvement in urine output with a low-dosage range (dopamine only).
5. Administer with an infusion pump.
6. Avoid peripheral IV line; watch for infiltration and necrotic areas.
7. Do not administer with sodium bicarbonate or other alkaline solutions. Mix amrinone only with saline solutions. Do not administer furosemide (Lasix) in the same line as amrinone.[139]
8. Monitor for thrombocytopenia when administering amrinone.[8,139,147] Assess for bleeding. Monitor liver function tests, blood urea nitrogen (BUN), and creatine also.[139]

DIURETIC AGENTS

The primary goals in the management of heart failure are to decrease pulmonary congestion and to improve cardiac output. Diuretic agents act principally to decrease pulmonary congestion. They also improve cardiac output by decreasing cardiac work load. Cardiac work load, or myocardial O_2 consumption, is a function of (1) heart rate, (2) preload (radius) or venous return, (3) afterload, and (4) contractility. Diuretics decrease pulmonary congestion and cardiac work load by decreasing volume and venous return. Diuretics thus decrease the radius of the heart during diastole and lower the preload. Diuretics are also useful in the treatment of hypertension, especially in blacks and older patients, as either the first or second drug of choice.[7] The major action in hypertension is the excretion of Na^+ and water.

Diuretics are classified according to their mechanism of action and site of action in the nephron of the kidney. The action common to most diuretic agents is inhibition of tubular reabsorption of Na^+. Diuretics may also act by increasing renal blood flow or altering hormonal effects on the kidney tubules. Water usually moves with Na^+. When sodium is excreted, so is water. Excretion of water acts to decrease circulating volume and thus decrease venous return, preload, and pulmonary congestion.

Loop diuretics

Furosemide (Lasix), bumetanide (Bumex), and ethacrynic acid (Edecrin) are classified as loop diuretics because they act primarily by inhibiting sodium resorption in the ascending loop of Henle.[156,157,159] Furosemide has other characteristics that add to its usefulness in acute care. It decreases pulmonary congestion and reduces cardiac work load by at least two mechanisms.

IV furosemide is usually the preferred diuretic for severe CHF because of its immediate venodilating effect and its effectiveness even in the presence of a low renal blood flow.[3,5,156,157] The venodilating effect decreases the venous return to the heart and lungs and reduces the preload. The left ventricular filling (wedge) pressure falls. Furosemide also reduces circulating blood volume by its diuretic effect. The immediate fall in LVEDP with IV furosemide may precede the diuretic effect and provide immediate symptomatic relief.[3,156,157] Bumetanide differs from furosemide primarily in its potency, allowing for small dosages to be effective, even in patients not responsive to furosemide.[5,157] Ototoxicity (deafness) is less with bumetanide, but renal toxicity is greater.

Therapy with potent diuretics, such as furosemide or ethacrynic acid, may result in hypovolemia and electrolyte depletion. Hypovolemia may result in hypotension from the reduction in circulating blood volume. Patients with right ventricular infarction should not receive diuretics.[1] The most common electrolyte disturbance associated with the use of furosemide is hypokalemia. Chloride (Cl^-), an anion, is frequently lost with the K^+. When an anion, in this case Cl^-, is lost, the body attempts to compensate by retaining another anion, HCO_3^-. This may eventually cause a metabolic alkalosis. Loss of H^+ also may contribute to the alkalosis. Potassium replacement solutions must contain chloride in order to prevent metabolic alkalosis.

Reports of ototoxicity and abnormal liver function tests after large doses of ethacrynic acid have discouraged routine use of this diuretic. An additional limitation is the preparation time. However, in an occasional patient refractory to furosemide therapy, ethacrynic acid may produce significant diuresis and thus be clinically useful. Ototoxicity may also occur with the use of furosemide but is more transient than that caused by ethacrynic acid.

The focus of this discussion is those diuretic agents commonly used in acute coronary settings. These drugs include the loop diuretics, the osmotic agents, and the selective renovascular dilator dopamine. Other commonly used diuretic agents, summarized in Table 9-3, include the thiazides, potassium-sparing agents, and carbonic anhydrase inhibitors.

Osmotic diuretics

The osmotic diuretic most commonly used in patients with coronary artery disease is mannitol. Albumin (25%), although not specifically classified as a diuretic, has osmotic diuretic effects similar to those of mannitol. Osmotic diuretics increase urine flow by (1) increasing plasma tonicity (osmolality) and thus mobilizing excess fluid from the cells

Table 9-3. Summary chart: diuretics

Classifications	Common agents	Chief site of action*	Primary complications
Loop diuretics	Furosemide (Lasix) bumetanide (Bumex) ethacrynic acid (Edecrin)	Ascending limp; loop of Henle	Hypokalemia; hypovolemia; metabolic alkalosis; ototoxicity
Thiazides and related agents	Chlorothiazide (Diuril); hydrochlorothiazide (HydroDIURIL, Esidrix, Oretic); chlorthalidone (Hygroton) indapamide (Lozol) metolazone (Zaroxolyn)	Distal tubule	Hypokalemia; metabolic alkalosis; hyperglycemia; uric acid; cholesterol
Renovascular dilator	Dopamine (Intropin) (in low dosage)	Increases cardiac output; selectively dilates renal arteries in low doses; proximal tubule	Tachyarrhythmias (higher doses only)
Osmotic agents	Mannitol; albumin (25%); glucose	Proximal tubule	Cellular dehydration; worsening of heart failure
Potassium-sparing agents	Spironolactone (Aldactone); triamterene (Dyrenium); amiloride (Midamor)	Distal tubule; collecting duct	Hyperkalemia
Carbonic anhydrase inhibitors	Acetazolamide (Diamox)	Proximal tubule	Hyperchloremia; metabolic acidosis

*The sites of action of most diuretic agents are multiple. The chief site listed is a general consensus derived from several texts.

and interstitial spaces and (2) increasing the osmolality of the glomerular filtrate.

Mannitol is a hypertonic solution and is given only by the IV route. A hypertonic solution has a greater concentration of dissolved particles. Administration of a hypertonic agent into the plasma causes fluid to move from the intracellular and interstitial spaces into the vascular space. Hypertonic agents produce an immediate increase in circulating blood volume.

Subsequent increased fluid flow to the kidneys promotes diuresis. The use of hypertonic solutions in fluid overload requires caution because of the ability of these solutions to expand circulating blood volume rapidly. If diuresis does not occur, the nurse should rapidly assess the patient for an increase in heart failure caused by fluid overload. Administration of mannitol is less hazardous in the treatment of local fluid accumulation, such as cerebral or myocardial edema caused by a hypoxic injury.

After IV administration, mannitol is freely filtered by the kidneys but cannot be resorbed. It thereby increases the osmolality (tonicity) of the glomerular filtrate and promotes Na^+ and water loss through the proximal tubules of the nephrons. The major diuretic effect of mannitol is probably by means of this mechanism.

Mannitol is most commonly used in coronary care to establish urine flow in oliguria with suspected impending acute tubular necrosis or in refractory pulmonary edema. It may also be helpful in confirming the presence of prerenal, as opposed to intrarenal, mechanisms in states of low urine output. Mannitol is generally not used in the acute management of heart failure because of its initial effect of increasing circulating volume. Potential complications of mannitol therapy include cellular dehydration and worsening of heart failure.

Albumin, a plasma protein, is not classified as a diuretic. However, it may be used to mobilize edema fluid because of its influence on colloid osmotic or oncotic pressure. The major force responsible for holding fluid within the vascular compartment is the serum colloid osmotic pressure (osmotic pressure). This force is exerted by the largely nondiffusible plasma proteins, the primary one being albumin (see Unit 4).

When hypoalbuminemia occurs because of stress, liver disease, or malnutrition, oncotic pressure decreases. As a result, fluid moves more easily from the vascular compartment into the interstitial spaces. Albumin restores plasma oncotic pressure and promotes fluid movement back from the interstitial spaces to the plasma.

Because of its ability to increase circulating blood volume, albumin (25%) should be administered slowly in patients with heart failure. Close monitoring of hemodynamic parameters, such as pulmonary artery pressures, PCWP, arterial pressure, and cardiac output profiles is desirable to prevent worsening of heart failure.

Selective renovascular dilator: dopamine

Dopamine (Intropin) is a sympathomimetic drug that has both alpha-stimulating and beta-stimulating properties and selective renal actions in specific dose ranges. It is used primarily for its B_1 stimulating effects or its action on the heart and is most commonly known as a positive inotropic agent. When administered at low dosages, dopamine selectively dilates the renal arteries, thereby promoting renal blood flow and inducing diuresis. When dopamine is administered in moderate to high dosages, the cardiotonic effects predominate. Improvement in cardiac output by these effects also enhances renal blood flow and thus induces diuresis. A more thorough discussion of dopamine and nursing orders relating to its administration are presented in the section on inotropic agents.

NURSING ORDERS: For patients receiving diuretic agents for management of heart failure

RELATED NURSING DIAGNOSIS: Alteration in cardiac output, impaired gas exchange, fluid deficit, electrolyte imbalance (Na^+, K^+, Mg^{++}), knowledge deficit

1. Observe for therapeutic effects following administration.
   — Is urine output increasing?
   — Is heart failure improving?
   — Is symptomatology diminishing?
   — Is wedge pressure decreasing?
   — Are rales diminishing?
2. Accurately record intake and output.
3. Watch for development of the following complications:
   — Hypovolemia and hypotension: Assess hydration status.
   — Hypokalemia: Check serum K^+ levels; note whether patient is receiving potassium chloride supplements.
   — Metabolic alkalosis: Check arterial pH and HCO_{-3} levels on arterial blood gas (ABG) samples; check total carbon dioxide on serum electrolytes.
   — Hypomagnesemia: Check serum Mg^{++} levels.
4. Monitor daily serum electrolytes, BUN, and creatinine.
5. With administration of furosemide and ethacrynic acid, watch for symptoms of ototoxicity (tinnitus, deafness).
6. With albumin (25%) and mannitol administration, watch for worsening of heart failure caused by an initial increase in circulating blood volume.

NARCOTIC ANALGESICS

The drugs most commonly used in the management of the chest pain of acute MI are the narcotic analgesics. Therapy focuses on relieving discomfort rapidly and effectively, with as few side effects as possible.[206-208] The two narcotics used most often in coronary care are morphine sulfate and meperidine hydrochloride (Demerol).[1,8,206-208] Narcotic analgesics act by blocking pain perception in the CNS. The concurrent use of beta blockers may decrease the need for narcotics.[206,207]

Morphine

Morphine sulfate is a CNS depressant that exerts a narcotic effect. Because of its ability to relieve pain rapidly and effectively when administered intravenously, morphine is the drug of choice for the management of chest pain associated with acute MI.[1,8,207] Another manifestation of the effect of morphine on the CNS may be vasodilation caused by depression of sympathetic pathways.[1,206,207] Thus morphine administration may result in hypotension. Significant hypotension may occur if the patient is volume depleted before the administration of morphine.

Morphine not only decreases arteriolar constriction but also produces venodilation. Venodilation results in peripheral pooling and thus reduces preload. This effect on preload is desirable in the relief of pulmonary edema. The hemodynamic actions associated with morphine administration are beneficial in reducing the myocardial oxygen demands (MVO_2). Another effect of morphine that is beneficial in the management of pulmonary edema and myocardia ischemic episodes is its ability to decrease the respiratory rate and anxiety.

Morphine slows the heart rate in some settings by creating autonomic imbalance. Therefore, the use of morphine requires caution in patients with bradycardias or enhanced vagal tone, such as occurs in inferior wall MIs.

Morphine decreases the sensitivity of the respiratory center to arterial CO_2 levels, thereby depressing respirations.[8,206–208] These effects occur within several minutes after IV administration. The administration of morphine to patients known to have limited respiratory reserves therefore requires a cautious approach. A narcotic antagonist such as naloxone hydrochloride (Narcan) can reverse respiratory depression.

The initial dose of morphine is 1 to 3 μg IV push at a rate of 1 mg/min. This dose may be repeated at intervals of 5 to 30 minutes until pain is relieved.[1,4] Adjust the dose if the patient shows signs of toxicity such as hypotension, decreased respiratory rate, or severe vomiting.

Meperidine

Meperidine hydrochloride (Demerol), another narcotic analgesic, is structurally different from morphine but has a similar mechanism of action. Because of its ability to relieve pain rapidly and effectively when administered intravenously, it is also commonly used in the management of chest pain associated with acute MI. Researchers have suggested it as an alternative to morphine in inferior wall MI because of its vagolytic effect.[1,8]

Meperidine depresses respirations by decreasing the tidal volume rather than by depressing the respiratory rate. Hypotension may occur after the IV administration of meperidine, with a compensatory increase in the heart rate. Meperidine is not recommended for use in patients with renal failure.

NURSING ORDERS: For patients receiving narcotic analgesics for management of chest pain

RELATED NURSING DIAGNOSIS: Alteration in comfort, alteration in cardiac output

1. Monitor for hypotension after IV administration; elevate the patient's legs as indicated.
2. Observe for respiratory depression after administration; administer with caution in patients known to have limited respiratory reserve, i.e., patients with emphysema, asthma, bronchitis, or pneumonia.
3. Administer morphine with caution to patients with increased vagal tone, i.e., patients with inferior wall MI or bradyarrythmia. Have atropine available.
4. The following side effects may occur with the administration of morphine or meperidine:
   —Dizziness
   —Sweating
   —Nausea and vomiting
   —Weakness
   —Syncope
   —Palpitations
5. Evaluate patient response.
6. Determine dosage and interval of administration by patient's response.

VASODILATOR AGENTS

The *vasodilators* are currently being used in the management of heart failure and hypertension. These agents are typically indicated in severe CHF when either diuretics or digitalis or both have proved ineffective. Vasodilators are also in use in acute settings to treat angina and preserve ischemic myocardium. The general effect of the vasodilators is to decrease the cardiac work load or unload the heart by acting on either preload, afterload, or both (Fig. 9-11). Pulmonary congestion and cardiac output may also improve. Certain va-

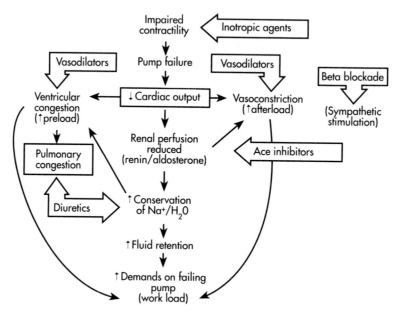

Fig. 9-11 Management of heart failure. The effects of vasodilators are contrasted with those of other agents used in the management of heart failure.

sodilators produce a greater improvement in cardiac output, whereas others primarily decrease pulmonary congestion. These selective actions are related to the dilating effects of the agents on either the arterial or venous systems or both (Table 9-4).

The major categories of vasodilators used in the management of CHF include (1) the direct vasodilators, such as nitroprusside, the nitrates, and hydralazine; (2) the alpha-adrenergic blocking agents, such as prazosin, and (3) ACE inhibitors, such as captropril and enalapril.

Dilation of the venous bed increases venous capacity and decreases venous return, thus reducing ventricular preload. Reduction of preload reduces LVEDP and decreases pulmonary congestion. Cardiac output may also improve, since the heart is able to function more efficiently with optimal filling pressures. Dilation of the arterial bed decreases arteriolar resistance and thus reduces

afterload. Reduction of afterload decreases resistance to left ventricular emptying, facilitating left ventricular ejection. As a result, the cardiac output increases.

In the normotensive patient with heart failure, the systemic vascular resistance (SVR) is typically high. In this case the cautious use of vasodilators affecting the arterial bed facilitates left ventricular ejection and improves cardiac output. The reduction of SVR with vasodilators may produce little or no change in the arterial pressure while improving the cardiac output, because the improvement in cardiac output usually offsets the reduction in SVR. As a precaution in this setting, however, initially administer these drugs slowly and in small doses. Also carefully monitor their effects on hemodynamic parameters.

The hypertensive patient with severe, chronically sustained elevations in SVR and heart failure usually requires larger doses.

Table 9-4. Summary of the vasodilators used in congestive heart failure

| Vasodilator drug | Predominant effect | | Effect on cardiac output |
	Afterload reduction (arterial bed)	Preload reduction (venous bed)	
Nitroprusside (Nipride)	X	X	Increase
Nitroglycerin		X	Slight increase or no change
Isosorbide dinitrate (Isordil)		X	Slight increase or no change
Hydralazine (Apresoline)	X		Increase
Prazosin (Minipress)	X	X	Initial increase
Captopril (Capoten)	X	X	Increase
Enalapril (Vasotec)	X	X	Increase

The increase in SVR compromises the cardiac output. However, administration of vasodilators in this patient is less hazardous and may not require such aggressive hemodynamic monitoring. Check the arterial blood pressure frequently, and preferably use invasive hemodynamic monitoring.

Because of their effect on preload, or the venous bed, the use of venous vasodilators in patients with normal or low filling pressures may result in hypotensive episodes and re-flexive tachyarrhythmias. The systemic pressoreceptors are activated, resulting in a compensatory tachycardia.

The vasodilators most commonly used in the acute management of coronary artery disease complicated by CHF, chest pain, or hypertension are the nitrates and nitroprusside since they may be administered intravenously. The general effect of these agents is to unload the heart by reducing preload, afterload, or both.

Nitrates

The nitrates are the only agents equally effective in the management of all forms of angina. They are also well established in clinical use with few reported side effects. For these reasons, they are currently indicated in the first-line management of effort or mixed angina syndromes and CHF.[3,147,150,209,216] The most commonly used nitrates are nitroglycerin (NTG) and isosorbide dinitrate (Isordil). Erythrityl tetranitrate (Cardilate) and pentaerythritol tetranitrate (Peritrate) are two other forms.[4,8,216]

Nitrates increase coronary supply as well as lower demands. They are therefore effective in the treatment of both effort and rest angina. In this way they differ from the beta blockers, which are effective in effort angina but may aggravate rest angina by facilitating spasm. They also differ from the calcium channel blockers (calcium antagonists), which are most effective in rest angina but whose effectiveness in effort angina varies with the specific agent.

The predominant effect of nitrates in chronic stable angina is to decrease O_2 demands. The nitrates act directly on the smooth muscle of the peripheral and coronary vascular beds. They act to lower O_2 demands by reducing both preload and afterload. The nitrates reduce preload by producing venous dilation and reduce afterload by producing arterial dilation. The predominant effect is on the venous bed.[8,147,209,216]

Reduction of both preload and afterload results in the lowering of myocardial O_2 demands and relief or prevention of anginal chest pain. Reduction of preload and left ventricular filling pressure can also decrease the pulmonary congestion associated with CHF. Cardiac output improves because of the changes in preload and afterload. For these reasons the nitrates are also in common use in the acute and chronic management of heart failure. The combination of IV nitrates and dobutamine (Dobutrex) is particularly beneficial to the patient in heart failure who also has ischemic heart disease.[3]

Nitrates also act to increase coronary supply by increasing blood flow in the normal collateral vessels or by relaxing spasm.[6,8,209,216] Diseased vessels lose their responsiveness to vasodilators unless spasm is involved. Reductions in LV filling pressure may also facilitate coronary flow by reducing impedance to coronary filling. Because of these effects on coronary blood flow, in an acute MI or unstable angina, nitroglycerin may be more beneficial than nitroprusside in the management of heart failure.[3,6,216]

The pain of angina is usually quickly relieved by a rapidly acting nitrate, such as sublingual nitroglycerin (Nitrostat) or isosorbide dinitrate (Isordil). Nitroglycerin spray is also available.[4,5] Use of these agents immediately before anticipated stressful events may also prevent anginal attacks. The chest pain of unstable angina usually requires the intravenous nitrates. Longer-acting nitrates, such as the topical ointment (Nitrol) or oral nitrates (Nitrospan, Nitro-Bid, Iso-Bid, Sorbitrate), are useful prophylactically on a continuous basis to prevent anginal attacks. Transdermal nitroglycerin patches (Nitro-Dur, Nitroderm) have become popular in the management of chronic stable angina, since they enhance patient compliance. However, their absorption rate may be less predictable and/or reliable, making these agents less ideal in the acute setting. In severe heart failure, sublingual nitroglycerin is recommended as a first-line agent, followed by IV nitroglycerin as a second-line agent as long as the blood pressure remains above 100 mm Hg systolic.[3,214] Short periods of withdrawal or alternating with other vasodilators can minimize the development of nitrate tolerance.[1,5,8]

Administration of IV nitrates, as in the chest pain of unstable angina, requires more careful monitoring. IV nitroglycerin (Tridil) is administered as a continuous drip. The usual dose is 50 to 200 mcg/min.[4,6] Nitrates may also be administered by the intravenous route within the first 2 to 4 hours of evolving MI, especially anterior wall, in an attempt to reverse coronary stenosis and limit infarct size.[1,215,217,218] IV nitrates may also reduce complications of reperfusion.[1,215,217,218]

Like other vasodilators, nitroglycerin may cause hypotension. Hypotension results primarily from venous dilation and is usually preceded by a drop in filling (wedge) pressure or preload. Thus patients with right ventricular infarction should not receive nitrates.[1] Significant hypotension is otherwise unusual with continuous IV drip nitroglycerin. A PA catheter can most closely monitor filling pressure; however, the use of a PA catheter is not critical. Frequent monitoring of arterial blood pressure via arterial line or cuff is usually adequate.

Hypotension more commonly occurs with sublingual, oral, or topical administration of nitrates for the management of chronic stable angina. The physician should establish the blood pressure end point and communicate it to the nurse. Nursing actions in the event of hypotensive episodes should focus on supporting preload or venous return. Measures such as lowering the head of the bed and raising the legs may provide rapid symptomatic relief.[6] Patients also require observation for reflexive tachycardias, especially with normal or low filling pressures. These effects are uncommon when using nitroglycerin in the management of heart failure. Orthostatic hypotension is often reported with sublingual nitroglycerin. Patients should sit or lie down before taking sublingual nitroglycerin and should remain in this position for at least 15 minutes.

Headaches are also common with nitrate administration; treatment is with acetaminophen (Tylenol) or by decreasing the nitrate dosage. These headaches may also disappear over time. A less common side effect of nitrate administration is methemoglobinemia, which can affect the O_2 saturation (see Unit 3).[5,6]

NURSING ORDERS: For patients receiving a nitrate (nitroglycerin or isosorbide) for the management of chest pain or CHF

RELATED NURSING DIAGNOSIS: Alteration in comfort, impaired gas exchange, alteration in cardiac output, knowledge deficit

1. Check blood pressure before administering a vasodilator for chest pain.
2. Watch for episodes of symptomatic hypotension and tachyarrhythmias after the administration of nitrates.
   —Lower the head of the bed.
   —Elevate the patient's legs.
3. Repeat nitroglycerin as ordered by the physician if chest pain is still not relieved; administer a narcotic as prescribed.
4. Report closely recurring episodes of chest pain to the physician; administration of nitrates on a continual basis may be necessary.
5. Instruct the patient regarding the administration of nitroglycerin:
   —Instruct the patient always to sit or lie down when taking sublingual nitroglycerin.[8,216] Sitting is preferred since venous return and cardiac work load are decreased.[5]
   —Caution the patient to report chest pain that is unrelieved by taking nitroglycerin three successive times at 5-minute intervals.[3]
   —Caution the patient that nitroglycerin tablets may deteriorate and lose effectiveness in as short a time as 3 months; thus the patient should replace the tablets every 6 months with a fresh supply. Instruct the patient to store tablets in the original container and to avoid hot, humid storage locations.
   —Inform the patient that potent tablets characteristically produce a transient headache because of meningeal vasodilation, a burning sensation under the tongue, or both.
   —Instruct the patient that sublingual nitroglycerin may be taken prophylactically before stressful activity.[8]
6. Instruct the patient in the proper application of the dermal patch to ensure adhesion and proper absorption. Make the patient aware that any site having access to blood flow is adequate. Have the patient avoid distal portions of the extremities. Encourage the rotation of patch sites.
7. Instruct patients to take oral nitrates on an empty stomach and not to chew sustained-release forms.[8]
8. When administering IV nitroglycerin infusion, initiate the infusion at 10 to 20 mcg/min and increase the dose by 5 mcg every 3 to 5 minutes as needed up to 500 mcg/min.[1,3,6,8] Mix nitroglycerin in glass containers. Use the special non-polyvinyl tubing provided.[8,216] One method of preparing the infusion is to add 25 mg to 250 cc of D5W or normal saline for a concentration of 100 mcg/

cc. At this concentration every 3 gtt/min (or cc/hr) provides 5 mcg. Monitor for relief of chest pain or reduction in wedge pressure or rales with relief of shortness of breath, depending on indication.

Nitroprusside

Sodium nitroprusside (Nipride) acts directly on the smooth muscle blood vessels, dilating both the venous and arterial beds. Nitroprusside reduces preload by producing venous dilation and afterload by producing arterial dilation. Nitroprusside may also help preserve ischemic myocardium by reducing afterload and preload. Its effects on preload and afterload reduction are balanced, so that neither effect predominates.[8,216]

The hemodynamic improvements with nitroprusside therapy are related to both preload and afterload reduction. Reduction in preload reduces LVEDP and thereby decreases pulmonary congestion. Reduction in arterial resistance, or afterload, reduces impedance to left ventricular emptying and increases cardiac output. Nitroprusside is indicated in the short-term management of acute hypertensive crisis and in normotensive or hypertensive patients in CHF.[8,216]

Nitroprusside is administered only by the IV route and therefore is used only in an acute setting. The therapeutic action of nitroprusside is evident within minutes after initiation. Dosages of 0.1 to 5 mcg/kg/min are titrated to achieve the desired effect.[3,4] Lower dosages, are indicated in the normotensive patient with heart failure, whereas higher dosages, up to 10 mcg/kg/min, are indicated in the patient with hypertensive crises whose SVR is usually much higher. An abrupt discontinuance of nitroprusside may cause rebound hypertension; therefore, the dose is gradually titrated until discontinued. The major goal of nitroprusside therapy in CHF is improvement in cardiac output. Invasive monitoring of cardiac output offers the best evaluation of this effect currently. The major toxic effects of nitroprusside administration are excessive reduction in preload and a fall in both arterial pressure and cardiac output in afterload.[8,216] In the normotensive patient with heart failure, excessive reduction of afterload (mean arterial pressure) may significantly compromise coronary filling and jeopardize the ischemic myocardium.

Excessive preload reduction can be detected by monitoring wedge pressures; excessive afterload reduction can be detected by monitoring arterial pressures. Thus before and immediately after initiating nitroprusside therapy, especially in the normotensive individual, obtain measurements of at least arterial pressure and wedge pressure.[8] Preferably, also measure cardiac output, SVR, and PVR. Measure these parameters at regular intervals throughout the course of therapy. Therefore, in normotensive patients, administer the agent only in intensive cardiac care units capable of hemodynamic monitoring.

Nitroprusside contains cyanide as part of its molecular structure. Metabolism of nitroprusside by the liver results in the release of cyanide, which is subsequently converted to thiocyanate. Long-term therapy with nitroprusside may result in cyanide or thiocyanate toxicity, which impairs tissue O_2 use. Renal dysfunction increases the risk of toxicity because these metabolic end products are excreted by the kidneys. If patients require therapy with nitroprusside for longer than 3 days, anticipate evaluation of blood levels of cyanide and thiocyanate. Levels greater than 12 mg/100 ml indicate toxicity.[8]

Signs of thiocyanate toxicity include tinnitus, blurred vision, and delirium. Signs of cyanide poisoning include coma, imperceptible pulse, tinnitus, dilated pupils, pink color, hypotension, shallow breathing, seizures, confusion, and metabolic acidosis.[3,8,216] When signs of cyanide toxicity are present, discontinue the infusion. Administer amyl nitrite inhalations for 15 to 30 seconds each minute until a 3% sodium nitrate solution can be prepared for IV administration.

NURSING ORDERS: For patients receiving IV nitroprusside in the management of hypertension or heart failure

RELATED NURSING DIAGNOSES: Alteration in cardiac output, potential for injury related to cyanide toxicity, alteration in tissue perfusion

1. Obtain baseline hemodynamic parameters, such as pulmonary artery pressures, wedge pressures, arterial pressure, cardiac output, and SVR especially in the normotensive individual. Continue to monitor during infusion.
2. Determine with the physician the critical LVEDP (wedge pressure) and arterial pressure to be achieved.

ACE inhibitors

Captopril (Capoten) and enalapril (Vasotec) are both classified as ACE inhibitors. The most recently introduced agent is lisinopril (Zestril, Prinivil).[4,5,150] The ACE inhibitors dilate both the arterial and venous beds, resulting in a reduction in both preload and afterload. These agents inhibit the renin-angiotensin system and are indicated in the first-line management of hypertension and CHF.[5,7,150,211,214] Renin is secreted in CHF in response to a fall in cardiac output and ultimately results in an increased secretion of aldosterone and intense vasoconstriction. Inhibition of this response results in excretion of sodium and water, retention of K^+, and vasodilation. ACE inhibitors are more effective antihypertensive agents in white and younger patients.[7,8] The hypertensive pa-

3. Prepare prescribed dose of medication. When preparing nitroprusside:
   —Protect from deterioration by light by wrapping the bottle in foil or other opaque material.[4,216]
   —Infuse only with microdrip or infusion pump.
   —Nitroprusside infusion may be prepared by adding 50 mg to 500 cc of D5W for a concentration of 100 mcg/cc.
4. Monitor wedge pressure or PAEDP and arterial pressure frequently during the infusion. Nitroprusside produces a balanced reduction in preload and afterload. Nitroglycerin, however, predominantly affects preload.
5. With nitroprusside therapy, thiocyanate and cyanide levels after 72 hours may be a consideration. Monitor for signs of toxicity, which include acidosis, resistance to therapy, and CNS changes. Nitroprusside may also inhibit platelet function. Monitor patients with bleeding tendencies carefully if they are receiving nitroprusside.

tient can take captopril sublingually by chewing a 25-mg dose.[5]

These agents are often the vasodilators of choice in CHF since they affect both hormonal and vascular responses in CHF. Patients do not develop tolerance to ACE inhibitors, unlike prazosin. This factor makes these agents ideal for both acute and long-term therapy. These agents are also effective with high renin levels. They are ideally combined with non-K^+-sparing diuretics, such as the loop and thiazide diuretics, because of their K^+-retaining effects. Aspirin and other nonsteroidal antiinflammatory drugs may potentiate these K^+-retaining effects.[7]

Two major groups of side effects that occur with ACE inhibitors are renal and immune effects. Drug-induced hyperkalemia may further compromise patients with borderline renal function. Cough is common. Immune effects include loss of taste, rash, and neutropenia.[2,150]

Contraindications for use include renal failure or severe renal disease. Also avoid concomitant use with other agents that can potentially alter immune function, such as procainamide, hydralazine, tocainide, and probenecid.

Hydralazine

Hydralazine hydrochloride (Apresoline) is another peripheral dilator used in the management of both acute and chronic heart failure. The predominant effect of hydralazine is to dilate the arterial bed and thus reduce afterload. As a result, SVR decreases and cardiac output increases. Hydralazine may be combined with a nitrate to achieve a more balanced effect on preload and afterload reduction, particularly in patients with signs of congestion. A major disadvantage is the development of tolerance through long-term therapy.

Side effects associated with the use of hydralazine include intractable headache, nausea, abdominal pain, and potentiation of ischemic events. Potentiation of ischemia without CHF may be caused by a reflex tachycardia. However, in the management of CHF, dilators usually do not induce a reflexive tachycardia. Potential for ischemic events with hydralizine use is a result of a decrease in coronary perfusion gradient induced by marked afterload reduction. Autoimmune disorders, such as lupus, have been reported. An increase in renin may occur secondary to vasodilation, resulting in Na^+ and fluid retention.

Prazosin

Prazosin hydrochloride (Minipress) exerts a vasodilator action by blocking the alpha receptors of the sympathetic nervous system. The alpha-adrenergic receptors are found primarily in blood vessels. Prazosin dilates both the venous and arterial beds and produces a balanced reduction in preload and afterload, as IV nitroprusside does.

Prazosin is currently in use as an oral antihypertensive agent. The drug is under clinical investigation in the management of heart failure associated with acute MI, especially as a potential alternative to IV nitroprusside. Hemodynamic responses to initial doses of prazosin used in the management of heart failure have been favorable. However, rapid development of drug tolerance and complete loss of favorable effects may occur with longer therapy. Further clinical studies will determine if prazosin has a role as a vasodilator in the management of heart failure. Reported side effects include dizziness, headache, nausea, and palpitations.

SUMMARY FIGURES AND TABLES (Figs. 9-12 to 9-14 and Tables 9-5 to 9-7) are presented on pp. 425-435.

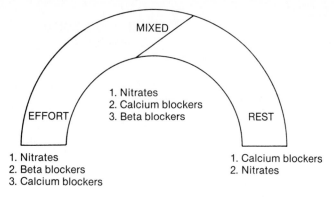

Fig. 9-12   Therapy for anginal syndromes.

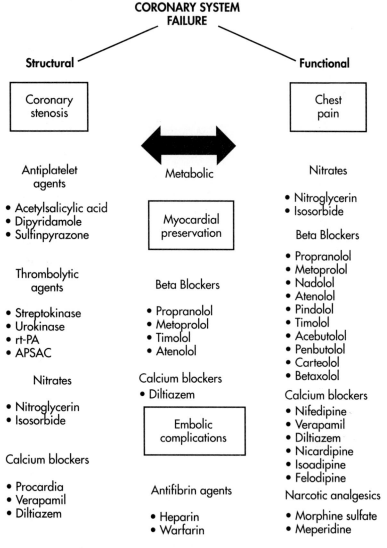

Fig. 9-13   Pharmacologic management of coronary system failure.

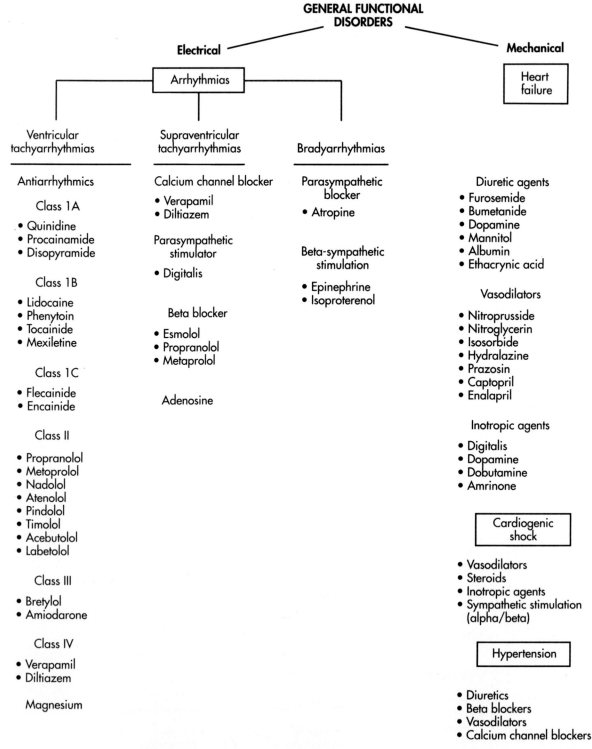

Fig. 9-14 Pharmacologic management of the major cardiovascular complications.

Table 9-5. Common intravenous cardiac agents

Drug	Dosage	Actions	Precautions
INDICATION: Bradyarrhythmias			
Atropine Sulfate	0.5-1 mg repeated up to 3 mg	*Anticholinergic/vagolytic* Increases the sinus rate and heart rate through AV node conduction	Doses lower than 0.5 mg may have paradoxical slowing effect. Do not treat if asymptomatic. Monitor for tachycardia, urinary retention, facial flushing, dryness of mouth, and dilation of pupils. Avoid in patients with glaucoma.
Dopamine (Intropin)	Continuous infusion (e.g., 400 mg in 500 cc D5W) at one of the following rates: • 1-2 μcg/kg/min • 2.5-10 μcg/kg/min* • >10 μcg/kg/min * Set pump at 30 gtts/min (cc/hr)	*Adrenergic stimulator (dopaminergic/beta/alpha)* Dilation of renal arteries, increased urine output (low dosage) Increases contractility (moderate dosage) at upper limits increases heart rate, AV conduction, automaticity Vasoconstriction, increased systemic vascular resistance, systolic and diastolic BP, coronary and peripheral perfusion (high dosage) *Also used in heart failure and shock*	Administer phentolamine (Regitine) 5-10 mg diluted in 10 cc NS SC around the site if infiltration occurs to prevent necrosis and sloughing of tissues. Monitor for tachycardias/ventricular arrhythmias, decreased urine output, and high BP (≥10 μcg/kg/min). Monitor wedge pressure and cardiac output. Administer in central line. Do not administer with alkaline solutions (e.g., Na^+ bicarbonate, aminophylline). Use infusion pump.
Epinephrine (Adrenalin)	*Bradycardia* Continuous infusion at 2-10 μcg/min (e.g., 2 mg in 500 cc D5W at 30 gtts/min)	*Adrenergic stimulator (beta > alpha)* Increases heart rate, AV conduction, contractility, automaticity	Administer phentolamine (Regitine) 5-10 mg diluted in 10 cc NS SC around the site if infiltration occurs to prevent necrosis/sloughing of tissues. Monitor for tachycardia and ventricular arrhythmias.

Continued.

427

Table 9-5. Common intravenous cardiac agents—cont'd

Drug	Dosage	Actions	Precautions
	Asystole 1 mg (diluted 1:10,000) initially, then 1-5 mg q 3-5 min or continuous infusion at 200 μcg/min (e.g., 30 mg in 250 cc D5W at 100 gtts/min or cc/hr)	Mild vasoconstriction, increased systemic vascular resistance, systolic and diastolic BP, coronary and cerebral perfusion *Also used in ventricular fibrillation, EMD/PEA, and shock, especially anaphylactic (dosage in VF/EMD/PEA same as in asystole)*	Administer infusion in central line. Do not administer with alkaline solution (e.g., Na$^+$ bicarbonate, aminophylline) Use infusion pump.
Isoproterenol (Isuprel)	Continuous infusion at 2-10 μcg/min (e.g., 2 mg in 500 cc D5W at 30 gtts/min)	*Adrenergic stimulator (beta)* Increases heart rate, AV conduction, contractility, automaticity	Monitor for tachycardias and ventricular arrhythmias. Do not administer with alkaline solutions (e.g., Na$^+$ bicarbonate, aminophylline) Use infusion pump.

INDICATION: Ventricular Tachyarrhythmias

Drug	Dosage	Actions	Precautions
Lidocaine (Xylocaine)	1-1.5 mg/kg (usually 50-150 mg) repeated q 5-10 min at half the dose up to 3 mg/kg Continuous infusion at 2-4 mg/min (e.g., 2 g in 500 cc D5W at 30 gtts/min)	*Antiarrhythmic (Class 1B)* Decreases ventricular instability by depressing automaticity and/or inhibiting re-entry circuits.	Monitor for hypotension, tremors, changes in sensorium, seizures, or psychosis. If these occur, stop the infusion. For hypotension, have the patient lie flat and raise legs. Use infusion pump. Use with caution in bradycardia—may be preceded or followed with atropine. Initiate infusion with an IV bolus. Drip may be "weaned" by turning off. NEVER GIVE IN VENTRICULAR ESCAPE RHYTHMS.

Drug	Dose	Action	Nursing Considerations
Procainamide (Pronestyl)	100 mg up to 800-1600 mg (17 mg/kg) at a rate not >20 mg per min Continuous infusion at 2-4 mg/min (e.g., 2 g in 500 cc D5W at 30 gtts/min)	*Antiarrhythmic (Class 1A)* Decreases ventricular instability by depressing automaticity and/or inhibiting re-entry circuits. Also effective in the atrial arrhythmias of WPW and indicated in nonspecific wide QRS tachycardia.	Monitor for hypotension and widening of QRS complex. Use with caution in pre-existing wide QRS complexes. Administer Na$^+$/bicarbonate for QRS widening >50% baseline.
Bretylium Tosylate (Bretylol)	5-10 mg/kg (usually 250-500 mg), repeated up to 30 mg/kg, administered rapidly in VF and over at least 8-10 min in VT (e.g., diluted in 50 cc) Continuous infusion at 2-4 mg/min (e.g., 2 g in 500 cc D5W at 30 gtts/min)	*Antiarrhythmic (Class III)* Decreases ventricular instability primarily by inhibiting re-entry circuits.	Monitor for hypotension, nausea, and vomiting. Avoid in single PVCs since these may be aggravated.
Magnesium Sulfate	1-2 g diluted in 100 cc over 1-2 min, followed by 2-4 g after 10-15 min if needed Continuous infusion at 3-20 mg/min until QT <0.50 sec	*Electrolyte* Reversal of torsades de pointes, stimulation of the Na$^+$/K$^+$ pump with restoration of intracellular K$^+$, inhibition of Ca^{++} channels and after depolarizations *Also effective in acute MI — decreases arrhythmias, inhibits coronary spasm, and lowers BP (continuous infusion of 8 g in 500 cc at 8 cc/hr)*	Monitor for bradycardic hypotension and respiratory depression (primarily during infusion). Anticipate flushing sensation during administration. Avoid in patients with renal failure. Monitor deep tendon reflexes during infusion.

INDICATION: Supraventricular Tachyarrhythmias

Drug	Dose	Action	Nursing Considerations
Adenosine (Adenocard)	6 mg administered rapidly, followed after 1-2 min by 12 mg Follow each dose with 10 cc flush	*Endogenous nucleoside* Decreases AV conduction, interrupts AV node re-entry circuits *Also used as a vasodilator in pharmacologic stress testing (Unit 6)*	Anticipate transient flushing, dyspnea, chest pain, and bradycardia — no therapy needed unless sustained.

Continued.

Table 9-5. Common intravenous cardiac agents—cont'd

Drug	Dosage	Actions	Precautions
Verapamil (Isoptin/Calan/Verelan)	2.5-5 mg over 2-3 min, repeated after 15-30 min up to 10 mg (total = 15 mg)	Ca^{++} *channel blocker* Decreases AV conduction, heart rate, and, to a lesser extent, contractility *Also used in angina, hypertension, and some forms of cardiomyopathy (PO)*	Do not give on known sick sinus disease. Never give together with IV inderal. Monitor for bradycardia (antidote—atropine) and hypotension (antidote—dopamine). Avoid in WPW and wide QRS tachycardia.
Diltiazem (Cardizem)	20 mg over 2 min, repeated after 15 min up to 25 mg Continuous infusion of 5-15 mg/hr (e.g., 100 mg in 100 cc or 1 mg/cc at 5-15 cc/hr)	Ca^{++} *channel blocker* Decreases AV conduction, heart rate, and, to a lesser extent, contractility *Also used in angina, hypertension, and non-Q wave infarction (PO)*	Same as with Verapamil.
Esmolol (Brevibloc)	0.5 mg/kg (usually 25-50 mg) over 1 min followed by infusion of 2.5-5 mg/min, repeated q 5 min, increasing the dose by 2.5-5 mg up to a maximum of 10-20 mg/min	*Adrenergic blocker (beta)* Decreases heart rate, AV conduction, contractility, automaticity, cardioselective.	Monitor primarily for bradycardia and hypotension.
Digoxin (Lanoxin)	0.25-0.5 mg (maintenance dose is 0.125-5 mg/day)	*Digitalis glycoside* Decreases heart rate, AV conduction (parasympathetic) Increases contractility and automaticity (inhibition of Na^+/K^+ pump) *Also used in heart failure (same dose)*	Check serum K^+/Mg^{++} Monitor for anorexia, nausea, vomiting, bradycardia, and arrhythmias, such as ventricular bigeminy, junctional tachycardia, and PAT with block. Also note vision changes (halos, yellow-green vision). When side effects appear, check serum digitalis levels. Hold the digitalis for extremely high levels and administer Digibind.
Other: **Pronestyl**	See Ventricular Arrhythmias		

INDICATION: Chest Pain

Drug	Dosage	Action	Nursing Considerations
Morphine Sulfate	1-3 mg at a rate of 1 mg/min, repeated q 5 min as needed	*Narcotic analgesic* Blocks pain perception in CNS, decreases anxiety and O_2 demands, venodilator. *Also used on severe heart failure to decrease pulmonary congestion.*	Monitor for respiratory depression, bradycardia, hypotension, dizziness, nausea/vomiting. Reverse side effects with Narcan.
Nitroglycerin (Tridil)	Continuous infusion at 10-20 mg/min, increasing dose by 5 mg q 3-5 min (e.g., 25 mg in 250 cc D5W = 5 μcg each 3 gtts/min)	*Vasodilator* Decreases O_2 demands primarily by decreasing venous return (preload), relaxes coronary spasm, increases collateral circulation, dilates peripheral arteries decreasing afterload. *Also used in heart failure to decrease pulmonary congestion; decreases afterload.*	Avoid in patients with RV infarction. Monitor BP. Mix in glass containers. Use nonpolyvinyl tubing provided. Use infusion pump.
rt-PA (Alteplase/ Activase)	100 mg over 3 hrs (10 mg over 1-2 min, 50 mg the 1st hr, and 20 mg over each of the next 2 hrs) Consider "accelerated" administration—100 mg over 1½ hrs (15 mg over 1-2 hrs, 50 mg over 30 min, and 35 mg over next hour)[176a]	*Thrombolytic* Activate body's own clot lysis (fibrinolytic) system	Monitor urine, stool, and emesis for bleeding, neurologic states. Note bruising, ecchymosis. Limit IV punctures. Monitor for signs of reperfusion (sudden end to chest pain, arrhythmias, CK peaking) Avoid in patient with history of bleeding, increased BP, surgery within 2 months.
Streptokinase (Kabbinase, Streptase)	1.5 million U over 60 min	*Thrombolytic* Activate body's own clot lysis (fibrinolytic) system	Same as with rt-PA; also monitor for rash/fever (tx with steroids/ antihistamines)
APSAC (Eminase)	30 U over 2-5 min	*Thrombolytic* Activate body's own clot lysis (fibrinolytic) system	Same as with rt-PA and Streptokinase

Continued.

Table 9-5. Common intravenous cardiac agents—cont'd

Drug	Dosage	Actions	Precautions
Metoprolol (Lopressor) Propanolol (Inderal)	5 mg q 5 min up to 15 mg, then oral dosing 0.1 mg/kg (5-10 mg)	*Adrenergic blocker (beta)* Decreases heart rate, AV conduction, contractility. Limits infarction size, extension, and complicates automaticity—BP, O_2 demands. Cardioselective (Lopressor only) Limits infarction size, extension, and complications. *Also used in hypertension and supraventricular arrhythmias*	Monitor for bradycardia and hypotension, CHF and bronchospasm (in higher dosages with Lopressor). Administer Inderal at rate no > 1 mg/min.
Other: Magnesium	See Ventricular Arrhythmias		

INDICATION: Heart Failure/Shock/Hypertension

Drug	Dosage	Actions	Precautions
Furosemide (Lasix)	0.5-1 mg/kg (25-100 mg) initially[3]	*Diuretic* Acts primarily at the loop of Henle to promote Na^+/water excretion, venodilator—decreases pulmonary congestion, preload.	Monitor urine output, lung sounds, wedge pressure, serum K^+/Mg^{++}. ABGs for metabolic alkalosis, BP (long-term).
Dobutamine (Dobutrex)	Continuous infusion (e.g., 500 mg in 250 cc D5W) at 2.5-20 μcg/kg/min. *Note:* Intermittent infusion may also be used in chronic CHF with prolonged effects.	*Adrenergic stimulator (beta)* Increases contractility—at upper limits increases heart rate, AV conduction, automaticity. Mild pulmonary and peripheral vasodilation (↓ afterload/ pulmonary vascular resistance)	Monitor for tachycardia, ventricular arrhythmias. Do not administer with alkaline solutions (e.g., Na^+ bicarbonate, aminophylline) Use infusion pump. Preferred over dopamine in patients with RV infarction.
Amrinone Lactate (Inocor)	0.75 mg/kg (3.75-7.5 mg) over 2-3 min, repeated in 30 min. Continuous infusion of 2-20 μcg/kg/min (e.g., 500 mg in 400 cc NS).	*Phosphodiesterase inhibitor* Increases contractility. Vasodilation—arterial and venous (decreases afterload/preload)	Mix only in saline. Monitor for bleeding, thrombocytopenia, hypotension, tachycardia, ventricular arrhythmias. Monitor liver function tests, BUN, and creatinine.

Drug	Dosage	Action	Nursing Considerations
			Do not administer Furosemide (Lasix) in same line. Use infusion pump.
Norepinephrine (Levophed)	Continuous infusion of 1-30 μcg/min (e.g., 8 mg in 500 cc D5W at 3 gtts/min)	*Adrenergic stimulator (alpha > beta)* Marked vasoconstriction, increased systemic vascular resistance, systolic and diastolic BP, coronary and cerebral perfusion. Increases heart rate, AV conduction, contractility, automaticity.	Administer phentolamine (Regitine) 5-10 mg in 10cc NS. SC around site if infiltration occurs to prevent necrosis. Monitor for high BP, tachycardia, ventricular arrhythmias, decreased urine output. Do not administer with alkaline solutions (e.g., Na$^+$ bicarbonate, aminophylline). Use infusion pump.
Nitroprusside (Nipride)	Continuous infusion of 0.1-5 μcg/kg/ml (e.g., 50 mg in 500 cc D5W).	*Vasodilator* Balanced effect on peripheral arteries and veins (decreases afterload/preload), lowers BP and systemic vascular resistance.	Use lower dose in normotensive patient and monitor more closely. Wrap bottle in foil to protect from light. Monitor BP, wedge pressure, SVR, and cardiac output, especially in normotensive patients. Monitor for hypotension and cyanide toxicity (coma, tinnitus, dilated pupils, shallow breathing, seizures, metabolic acidosis). If this occurs, D/C infusion and administer amyl nitrite by inhalation. Use infusion pump. Do not purge or give boluses through the line.
Other: **Nitroglycerin/ Morphine Sulfate**	See Chest Pain		
Dopamine	See Bradyarrhythmias		
Digitalis	See Supraventricular Tachyarrhythmias		

Table 9-6. Drugs used during cardiopulmonary resuscitation

Arrhythmias	CHF/shock	Chest pain	Metabolic complications	Electromechanical dissociation/PEA
Antiarrhythmics	Diuretic agents	Narcotic	Oxygen*	Epinephrine* (Adrenalin)
Lidocaine* (Xylocaine)	Furosemide (Lasix)	Morphine sulfate	Na$^+$ bicarbonate*	Na$^+$ bicarbonate*
Procainamide* (Pronestyl)	Ethacrynic acid (Edecrin)	Nitrate	Corticosteroids	
Bretylium tosylate* (Bretylol)	Vasodilators	Nitroglycerin	Nitrates (MI)	
Sympathetic (beta) stimulators	Nitroglycerin		Nitroglycerin	
Isoproterenol (Isuprel)	Nitroprusside (Nipride)		Calcium blockers	
Epinephrine (Adrenalin)	Inotropic agents			
Sympathetic (beta) blocker	Digitalis (Digoxin, Lanoxin)			
Propranolol (Inderal)	Amrinone lactate (Incor)			
Parasympathetic stimulator	Sympathetic (beta) stimulators (inotropic agents)			
Digitalis (Digoxin, Lanoxin)	Dopamine (Intropin)			
Parasympathetic blocker	Dobutamine (Dobutrex)			
Atropine sulfate*	Sympathetic (alpha) stimulators			
Magnesium	Norepinephrine (Levophed)			
Adenosine*	Metaraminol (Aramine)			
Calcium blocker				
Verapamil* (Isoptin, Calan)				

*Currently designated as emergency drugs by the American Heart Association.

Table 9-7. Cardiac drug levels

Assay	Therapeutic range	Toxic level
Digoxin	0.9–2.0 ng/ml	>2.5 ng/ml
Lidocaine	1.5–5.0 mcg/ml	>7.0 mcg/ml
Phenytoin (Dilantin)	10.0–20.0 mcg/ml	>25.0 mcg/ml
Procainamide (Pronestyl)	4.0–10.0 mcg/ml	>16.0 mcg/ml
Quinidine	2.0–5.0 mcg/ml	>10.0 mcg/ml

REFERENCES/SUGGESTED READINGS

General

1. ACC/AHA guidelines for the early management of patients with acute myocardial infarction, Circulation 82(2):685, 1990.
2. Braunwald E, editor: Heart disease: a textbook of cardiovascular medicine, ed 3, Philadelphia, 1988, WB Saunders.
3. Guidelines for cardiopulmonary resuscitation and emergency care: part III: Adult advanced cardiac life support, JAMA 268(16):2199, 1992.
4. Olin B, editor: Facts and comparisons, St. Louis, 1993, JB Lippincott.
5. Opie LH et al: Drugs for the heart, ed 3, Philadelphia, 1991, WB Saunders.
6. Textbook of advanced cardiac life support, 1990, American Heart Association.
7. The fifth report of Joint National Committee on detection, evaluation, and treatment of high blood pressure, Arch Intern Med 153:154, 1993.
8. Underhill S et al: Cardiovascular medications for cardiac nursing, Philadelphia, 1990, JB Lippincott.

Adenosine

9. Camm AJ, Garratt CJ: Adenosine and supraventricular tachycardia, N Engl J Med 325(23):1621,1991.
10. Chronister C: Clinical management of supraventricular tachycardia with adenosine, Am J Crit Care 2(1):41, 1993.
11. DiPalma JR: Adenosine for paroxysmal supraventricular tachycardia, Am Fam Physician 44(3):929, 1991.
12. Ely SW, Berne RM: Protective effects of adenosine in myocardial ischemia, Circulation 85(3):893, 1992.
13. Faulds D, Chrisp P, Buckley MM: Adenosine. An evaluation of its use in cardiac diagnostic procedures, and in the treatment of paroxysmal supraventricular tachycardia, Drugs 41(4):596, 1991.
14. Freilich A, Tepper D: Adenosine and its cardiovascular effects, Am Heart J 123(5):1324, 1992.
15. Griffith MJ et al: Adenosine in the diagnosis of broad complex tachycardia, Lancet 672:1988.
16. Hori M, Kitakaze M: Adenosine, the heart, and coronary circulation, Hypertension 18(5):565, 1991.
17. Lerman BB, Belardinelli L: Cardiac electrophysiology of adenosine: basic and clinical concepts, Circulation 83(5):1499, 1991.
18. Merva, J: Adenosine: new treatment of P.S.V.T, Nursing 21(5):32K, 1991.
19. Parker RB, McCollam PL: Adenosine in the episodic treatment of paroxysmal supraventricular tachycardia, Clin Pharm 9(4):261, 1990.
20. Rankin AC et al: Adenosine and the treatment of supraventricular tachycardia, Am J Med 92(6):655, 1992.

Antiarrhythmic agents

21. Anderson JL: Effectiveness of sotalol for therapy of complex ventricular arrhythmias and comparison with placebo and class I antiarrhythmic drugs, Am J Cardiol 65(2):37A, 1990.
22. Birgersdotter-Green U: Propafenone for cardiac arrhythmias, Am J Med Sci 303(2):123, 1992.
23. Colatsky TJ, Follmer CH, Starmer CF: Channel specificity in antiarrhythmic drug action. Mechanism of potassium channel

block and its role in suppressing and aggravating cardiac arrhythmias, Circulation 82(6):2235, 1990.

24. Donnelly AJ: Pharmacist's corner. Part I: Antiarrhythmic agents use in the surgical patient, AORN J 53(5):1261, 1991.

25. Falk RH: Proarrhythmia in patients treated for atrial fibrillation or flutter, Ann Intern Med 117(2):141, 1992.

26. Grant AO Jr: On the mechanism of action of antiarrhythmic agents, Am Heart J 123(4 Pt 2):1130, 1992.

27. Greene HL: The efficacy of amiodarone in the treatment of ventricular tachycardia or ventricular fibrillation, Prog Cardiovasc Dis 31(5):319, 1989.

28. Griffith MJ et al: Relative efficacy and safety of intravenous drugs for termination of sustained ventricular tachycardia, Lancet 336: 670, 1990.

29. Grubb BP: Moricizine: a new agent for the treatment of ventricular arrhythmias, Am J Med Sci 301(6):398, 1991.

30. Horowitz LN: Efficacy of moricizine in malignant ventricular arrhythmias, Am J Cardiol 65(8):41D, 1990.

31. Josephson ME: Antiarrhythmic agents and the danger of proarrhythmic events, Ann Intern Med 111(2):101, 1989.

32. Kopelman HA, Horowitz LN: Efficacy and toxicity of amiodarone for the treatment of supraventricular tachyarrhythmias, Prog Cardiovasc Dis 31(5):355, 1989.

33. Kutalek SP, McCormick DJ: Classification of antiarrhythmic drugs, Am Fam Physician 38(4):261, 1988.

34. Lazzara R: Amiodarone and torsade de pointes, Ann Intern Med 111(7):549, 1989.

35. Levine JH, Morganroth J, Kadish AH: Mechanisms and risk factors for proarrhythmia with type Ia compared with Ic antiarrhythmias drug therapy, Circulation 80(4): 1063, 1989.

36. Levy S: Combination therapy for cardiac arrhythmias, Am J Cardiol 61(2):95A, 1988.

37. Luderitz B, Manz M: Pharmacologic treatment of supraventricular tachycardia: the German experience, Am J Cardiol 70(5): 66A, 1992.

38. Lynch RA, Horowitz LN: Managing geriatric arrhythmias, II: Drug selection and use, Geriatrics, 46(4):41, 1991.

39. Marcus FI: Ventricular arrhythmias. When should they be suppressed? Postgrad Med 90(2):62, 67, 1991.

40. Mattioni TA et al: The proarrhythmic effects of amiodarone, Prog Cardiovasc Dis 31(6):439, 1989.

41. Michelson EL, Dreifus LS: Newer antiarrhythmic drugs, Med Clin North Am 72(2):275, 1988.

42. Morganroth J: Proarrhythmic effects of antiarrhythmic drugs: evolving concepts, Am Heart J 123(4 Pt 2):1137, 1992.

43. Naccarelli GV et al: Advances in the treatment of supraventricular tachycardia. Am J Cardiol 62(19):1L, 1988.

44. Naccarelli GV et al: Pharmacologic therapy of arrhythmias, Hosp Pract [Off] 23(10): 183, 1988.

45. Nattel S et al: What is an antiarrhythmic drug? From clinical trials to fundamental concepts, Am J Cardiol 66(1):96, 1990.

46. Patt MV: Combination antiarrhythmic therapy for management of malignant ventricular arrhythmia, Am J Cardiol 62(14):18I, 1988.

47. Podrid PJ, Beau SL: Antiarrhythmic drug therapy for congestive heart failure with focus on moricizine, Am J Cardiol 65(8):56D, 1990.

48. Podrid PJ, Levine PA, Klein MP: Effect of age on antiarrhythmic drug efficacy and toxicity, Am J Cardiol 63(11):735, 1989.

49. Podrid PJ, Wilson JS: Should asymptomatic ventricular arrhythmia in patients with congestive heart failure be treated? An antagonist's viewpoint, Am J Cardiol 66(4):451, 1990.

50. Pritchett EL: Management of atrial fibrillation, N Engl J Med 326(19):1264, 1992.

51. Ravid S: Antiarrhythmic drug therapy in congestive heart failure. Indications and complications, Postgrad Med 90(8):99, 1991.

52. Ravid S et al: Congestive heart failure induced by six of the newer antiarrhythmic drugs, J Am Coll Cardiol 14(5):1326, 1989.

53. Rehnqvist N: Arrhythmias and their treat-

ment in patients with heart failure, Am J Cardiol 64(20):61J, 1989.

54. Roden DM: Role of electrocardiogram in determining electrophysiologic end points of drug therapy, Am J Cardiol 62(12):34H, 1988.

55. Salerno DM: Quinidine: is it a good drug or a bad drug? Postgrad Med 92(4):131, 1992.

56. Siddoway LA: Initial dosage selection of antiarrhythmic therapy, Am J Cardiol, 62(12): 2H, 1988.

57. Singh BN: Advantages of beta blockers versus antiarrhythmic agents and calcium antagonists in secondary prevention after myocardial infarction, Am J Cardiol 66(9):9C, 1990.

58. Surawicz B: Ventricular arrhythmias: why is it so difficult to find a pharmacologic cure? J Am Coll Cardiol 14(6):1401, 1989.

59. Wellens HJ, Brugada P, Smeets JL: Antiarrhythmic drugs for supraventricular tachycardia, Am J Cardiol 62(19):69L, 1988.

60. Wellens HJ et al: Antiarrhythmic drug treatment: need for continuous vigilance, Br Heart J 67(1):25, 1992.

61. Weller DM, Noone J: Mechanisms of arrhythmias: enhanced automaticity and reentry, Crit Care Nurse 9(5):42, 1989.

62. Wesley RC Jr, Resh W, Zimmerman D: Reconsiderations of the routine and preferential use of lidocaine in the emergent treatment of ventricular arrhythmias, Crit Care Med 19(11):1439, 1991.

63. Wood DL: Potentially lethal ventricular arrhythmias. Minimizing the danger, Postgrad Med 88(6):65, 1990.

64. Zehender M, Kasper W, Just H: Lidocaine in the early phase of acute myocardial infarction: the controversy over prophylactic or selective use, Clin Cardiol 13(8):534, 1990.

Antilipemic agents

65. Betteridge DJ: Lipoproteins and coronary heart disease, J Hum Hypertens 3(suppl 2):13, 1989.

66. Bilheimer DW: The role of lipid regulation in the prevention of coronary heart disease, Eur Heart J 13(suppl B):23, 1992.

67. Denke MA, Grundy SM: Hypercholesterolemia in elderly persons: resolving the treat-

ment dilemma, Ann Intern Med 112(10): 780, 1990.

68. Gotto AM Jr: Rationale for treatment, Am J Med 91(1B):31S, 1991.

69. Gwynne JT: HDL and atherosclerosis: an update, Clin Cardiol 14(2 suppl 1):117, 1991.

70. Jafri SM et al: Medical therapy after acute myocardial infarction, Curr Probl Cardiol 16(9):585, 1991.

71. Kashyap ML: Basic considerations in the reversal of atherosclerosis: significance of high-density lipoprotein in stimulating reverse cholesterol transport, Am J Cardiol 63(16):56H, 1989.

72. Keller KB et al: Management of hyperlipidemia: an update, Heart Lung 19(3):317, 1990.

73. Kuo PT: Management of blood lipid abnormalities in coronary heart disease patients, Clin Cardiol 12(10):553, 1989.

74. Lavie CJ et al: Management of lipids in primary and secondary prevention of cardiovascular diseases, Mayo Clin Proc 63(6):605, 1988.

75. Report of National Cholesterol Education Program Expert Panel on Detection, evaluation, and treatment of high blood cholesterol in adults, Arch Intern Med 148:36, 1988.

76. Secondary prevention of coronary disease with lipid-lowering drugs, Lancet 1(8636): 473, 1989.

77. Stoy DB: Helping patients take cholesterol-lowering drugs, Am J Nurs (12):1631, 1989.

78. Stoy DB: Pharmacotherapy for hypercholesterolemia: guidelines and nursing perspectives, J Cardiovasc Nurs 5(2):34, 1991.

Beta blockers

79. Becker RC, Gore JM: Adjunctive use of beta-adrenergic blockers, calcium antagonists and other therapies in coronary thrombolysis, Am J Cardiol 67(3):25A, 1991.

80. Charlap S, Lichstein E, Frishman WH: Beta-adrenergic blocking drugs in the treatment of congestive heart failure, Med Clin North Am 73(2):373, 1989.

81. Dix-Sheldon DK: Pharmacologic management of myocardial ischemia, J Cardiovasc Nurs 3(4):17, 1989.

82. Egstrup K: Silent ischemia and beta-blockade, Circulation 84(6 suppl):VI84, 1991.

83. Eichhorn EJ: The paradox of beta-adrenergic blockade for the management of congestive heart failure, Am J Med 92(5): 527, 1992.

84. Frishman WH, Lazar EJ: Reduction of mortality, sudden death and non-fatal reinfarction with beta-adrenergic blockers in survivors of acute myocardial infarction: a new hypothesis regarding the cardioprotective action of beta-adrenergic blockade, Am J Cardiol 66(16):66G, 1990.

85. Frishman WH et al: Beta-adrenergic blockade and calcium channel blockade in myocardial infarction, Med Clin North Am 73(2):409, 1989.

86. Gleeson B: Loosening the grip of anginal pain, Nursing 21(1):33, 1991.

87. Gray RJ: Managing critically ill patients with esmolol. An ultra short-acting beta-adrenergic blocker, Chest 93(2):398, 1988.

88. Hampton JR: Secondary prevention of acute myocardial infarction with beta-blocking agents and calcium antagonists, Am J Cardiol 66(9):3C, 1990.

89. Hjalmarson A: International beta-blocker review in acute and postmyocardial infarction, Am J Cardiol 61(3):26B, 1988.

90. Hjalmarson A, Olsson G: Myocardial infarction. Effects of beta-blockade, Circulation 84(6 suppl):VI101, 1991.

91. Lazar EJ, Lazar JM, Frishman W: Angina pectoris and silent ischemia in the elderly: a management update, Geriatrics 47(7):24, 1992.

92. Morganroth J: Management of arrhythmias in ischemic heart disease. The role of beta blockers, Postgrad Med Spec No.:113, 1988.

93. Packer M: Drug therapy. Combined beta-adrenergic and calcium-entry blockade in angina pectoris, N Engl J Med 320(11):709, 1989.

94. Packer M: Pathophysiological mechanisms underlying the effects of beta-adrenergic agonists and antagonists on functional capacity and survival in chronic heart failure, Circulation 82(2 suppl):177, 1990.

95. Pepine CJ et al: Beta-adrenergic blockers in silent myocardial ischemia, Am J Cardiol 61(3):18B, 1988.

96. Pitt B: The role of beta-adrenergic blocking agents in preventing sudden cardiac death, Circulation 85(1 suppl):I107, 1992.

97. Singh BN: Advantages of beta blockers versus antiarrhythmic agents and calcium antagonists in secondary prevention after myocardial infarction, Am J Cardiol 66(9):9C, 1990.

98. Strauss WE, Parisi AF: Combined use of calcium-channel and beta-adrenergic blockers for the treatment of chronic stable angina. Rationale, efficacy, and adverse effects, Ann Intern Med 109(7):570, 1988.

99. Wikstrand J, Berglund G, Tuomilehto J: Beta-blockade in the primary prevention of coronary heart disease in hypertensive patients. Review of present evidence, Circulation 84(6 suppl):VI93, 1991.

100. Wolman RL, Fiedler MA: Esmolol and beta-adrenergic blockade, AANA J 59(6):541, 1991.

101. Yusuf S: Early intravenous beta blockade in acute myocardial infarction, Postgrad Med, Spec No.:90, 1988.

Calcium channel blockers

102. Akhtar M, Tchou P, Jazayeri M: Use of calcium channel entry blockers in the treatment of cardiac arrhythmias, Circulation 80(6 suppl):IV31, 1989.

103. Beller GA: Calcium antagonists in the treatment of Prinzmetal's angina and unstable angina pectoris, Circulation 80(6 suppl): IV78, 1989.

104. Benstein JA et al: Renal vascular effects of calcium channel blockers in hypertension, Am J Hypertens 3(12 Pt 2):305S, 1990.

105. Chan PK et al: The role of nitrates, beta blockers, and calcium antagonists in stable angina pectoris, Am Heart J 116(3):838, 1988.

106. Charlap S, Frishman WH: Calcium antagonists and heart failure, Med Clin North Am 73(2):339, 1989.

107. Cohn PF: Effects of calcium channel blockers on the coronary circulation, Am J Hypertens 3(12 Pt 2):299S, 1990.

108. Crawford MH: Theoretical consideration in the use of calcium entry blockers in silent

myocardial ischemia, Circulation 80(6 suppl):IV74, 1989.

109. Ellenbogen KA: Role of calcium antagonists for heart rate control in atrial fibrillation, Am J Cardiol 69(7):36B, 1992.

110. Fifer MA et al: Techniques for assessing inotropic effects of drugs in patients with heart failure: application to the evaluation of nicardipine, Am Heart J 119(2 Pt 2):451, 1990.

111. Follath F: The role of calcium antagonists in the treatment of myocardial ischemia, Am Heart J 118(5 Pt 2):1093, 1989.

112. Gheorghiade M, Goldstein S: Calcium-channel blockers in postmyocardial infarction patients with special notation to the Danish verapamil infarction trial II, Prog Cardiovasc Dis 34(1):37, 1991.

113. Gibson RS: Current status of calcium channel-blocking drugs after Q wave and non-Q wave myocardial infarction, Circulation 80(6 suppl):IV107, 1989.

114. Heywood JT: Calcium antagonists and left ventricular function, Am J Cardiol 68(12):52C, 1991.

115. Jaffe AS: Use of intravenous diltiazem in patients with acute coronary artery disease, Am J Cardiol 69(7):25B, 1992.

116. Kedas A, Shively M, Burvis J: Nursing delivery of sublingual nifedipine, J Cardiovasc Nurs 3(4):31, 1989.

117. Keogh AM et al: A review of calcium antagonists and atherosclerosis, J Cardiovasc Pharmacol, 16(suppl 6):S28, 1990.

118. Kern MJ: Perspective: the cellular influences of calcium antagonists on systemic and coronary hemodynamics, Am J Cardiol 69(7):3B, 1992.

119. Kowalchuk GJ, Nesto RW: Calcium antagonists and myocardial infarction, Am J Cardiol 64(11):10F, 1989.

120. Lazar EJ, Lazar JM, Frishman W: Angina pectoris and silent ischemia in the elderly: a management update, Geriatrics 47(7):24, 1992.

121. Levy MN: Role of calcium in arrhythmogenesis, Circulation 80(6 suppl):IV23, 1989.

122. O'Malley K, Kelley J, O'Brien E: Clinical benefits of structural and functional changes with calcium antagonists, Am Heart J 122(1 Pt 2):370, 1991.

123. Opie LH, Commerford PJ: The total vascular burden, peripheral and coronary: vasodilator effects of nifedipine, Am Heart J 115(1 Pt 1):228, 1988.

124. Packer M: Pathophysiological mechanisms underlying the adverse effects of calcium channel-blocking drugs in patients with chronic heart failure, Circulation 80(6 suppl):IV59, 1989.

125. Pearle DL: Calcium antagonists in acute myocardial infarction, Am J Cardiol 61(3):22B, 1988.

126. Ram CV: Anti-atherosclerotic and vasculoprotectice actions of calcium antagonists, Am J Cardiol 66(21):29I, 1990.

127. Roberts R: Preventing recurrent myocardial infarction. Use of calcium-channel blockers, Postgrad Med 83(1):249, 1988.

128. Roberts R: Review of calcium antagonist trials in acute myocardial infarction, Clin Card 12:111, 1989.

129. Roberts R: Thrombolysis and its sequelae. Calcium antagonists as potential adjunctive therapy, Circulation 80(6 suppl):IV93, 1989.

130. Salerno DM et al: Efficacy and safety of intravenous diltiazem for treatment of atrial fibrillation and atrial flutter, Am J Cardiol 63:1046, 1989.

131. Scheidt S: Therapy for angina pectoris: comparison of nicardipine with other antianginal agents, Am Heart J 116(1 Pt 1):254, 1988.

132. Schlant RC, King SB III: Usefulness of calcium entry blockers during and after percutaneous transluminal coronary artery angioplasty, Circulation 80(6 suppl):IV88, 1989.

133. Skolnick AE, Frishman WH: Calcium channel blockers in myocardial infarction, Arch Intern Med 149(7):1669, 1989.

134. Sowers JR: Antiatherosclerotic effects of calcium channel blockers, Postgrad Med 92(2):265, 1992.

135. vanZweiten PA: Vascular effects of calcium antagonists: implications for hypertension and other risk factors for coronary heart disease, Am J Cardiol, 64(17):117I, 1989.

136. Walsh RA: The effects of calcium entry

blockade on normal and ischemic ventricular diastolic function, Circulation 80(6 suppl):IV52, 1989.

137. Wei JY: Use of calcium entry blockers in elderly patients. Special considerations, Circulation 80(6 suppl):IV171, 1989.

Inotropic agents

138. Conover MB: Understanding electrocardiography, ed 6, St Louis, 1992, Mosby Year Book.

139. Fabius DB, Rein A: Intravenous amrinone therapy: Nursing implications, Dimens Crit Care Nurs, 9:6:336, 1990.

140. Gheorghiade M, Zarowitz BJ: Review of randomized trials of digoxin therapy in patients with chronic heart failure, Am J Cardiol, 69(18):48G, 1992.

141. Kelley RA: Cardiac glycosides and congestive heart failure, Am J Cardiol, 65(10):10E, 1990.

142. Kelly RA, Smith TW: Recognition and management of digitalis toxicity, Am J Cardiol 69(18):108G, 1992.

143. Lang R: Medical management of chronic heart failure: inotropic, vasodilator, or inodilator drugs? Am Heart J 120(6 Pt 2):1558, 1990.

144. Leier CV: Current status of non-digitalis positive inotropic drugs, Am J Cardiol 69(18):120G, 1992.

145. Man in t, Veld AJ: How to select a drug for the long-term treatment of chronic heart failure, Am Heart J 120(6 Pt 2):1572, 1990.

146. Murphy MB, Elliot WJ: Dopamine and dopamine receptor agonists in cardiovascular therapy, Crit Care Med 18(1 Pt 2):S14, 1990.

147. Nagelhout JJ: Pharmacologic treatment of heart failure, Nurs Clin North Am 26(2):401, 1991.

148. Packer M: Vasodilator and inotropic drugs for the treatment of chronic heart failure: distinguishing hype from hope, J Am Coll Cardiol 12(5):1299, 1988.

149. Paradis NA, Koscove EM: Epinephrine in cardiac arrest: a critical review, Ann Emerg Med 19(11):1288, 1990.

150. Parmley WW: Pathophysiology and current therapy of congestive heart failure, J Am Coll Cardiol 13(4):771, 1989.

151. Sarter BH, Marchlinski FE: Redefining the role of digoxin in the treatment of atrial fibrillation, Am J Cardiol 69(18):71G, 1992.

152. Saunders MR, Kostis JB, Frishman WH: The use of inotropic agents in acute and chronic congestive heart failure, Med Clin North Am 73(2):283, 1989.

153. Tisdale JE, Gheorghiade M: Acute hemodynamic effects of digoxin alone or in combination with other vasoactive agents in patients with congestive heart failure, Am J Cardiol 69(18):34G, 1992.

154. Yusuf S et al: Need for a large randomized trial to evaluate the effects of digitalis on morbidity and mortality in congestive heart failure, Am J Cardiol 69(18):64G, 1992.

Diuretics

155. Khair GZ, Kochar MS: Mild hypertension, diuretics, and cardiac arrhythmias: consensus amid controversy? Am Heart J 116(1 Pt 1):216, 1988.

156. Kruck F: Acute and long term effects of loop diuretics in heart failure, Drugs 41(suppl 3):60, 1991.

157. Mende CW: Current issues in diuretic therapy, Hosp Pract [Off] 25(suppl 1):15, 1990.

158. Parmley WW: Pathophysiology and current therapy of congestive heart failure, J Am Coll Cardiol 13(4):771, 1989.

159. Sica DA, Gehr TG: Diuretics in congestive heart failure, Cardiol Clin 7(1):87, 1989.

160. Stevenson LW: Tailored therapy before transplantation for treatment of advanced heart failure: effective use of vasodilators and diuretics, J Heart Lung Transplant 10(3):468, 1991.

Antithrombotic agents

161. Balsano F et al: Antiplatelet treatment with ticlopidine in unstable angine. A controlled multicenter trial, Circulation 82:17, 1990.

162. Bates ER, Topol EJ: Thrombolytic therapy for acute myocardial infarction, Chest 95(5 suppl):257S, 1989.

163. Belle-Isle C: Patient selection and administration of thrombolytic therapy, JEN 15(2 Pt 2):155, 1989.

164. Benedict CR et al: Thrombolytic therapy: a state of the art review, Host Pract [Off] 27(6):61, 1992.

165. Breed J et al: Commonly asked questions

concerning thrombolytic therapy, JEN 15(2 Pt 2):207, 1989.

166. Briones TL: Tissue-plasminogen activator: nursing implications, Dimens Crit Care Nurs 8(4):200, 1989.

167. Brooks-Brunn JA: Thrombolytic intervention and its effect on mortality in acute myocardial infarction: review of clinical trials, Heart Lung 17(6 Pt 2):756, 1988.

168. Brunelli C et al: Thrombolysis in refractory unstable angina, Am J Cardiol 68(7):110B, 1991.

169. Cairns JA et al: Coronary thrombolysis, Chest 95(2 suppl):73S, 1989.

170. Conti CR: Brief overview of the end points of thrombolytic therapy, Am J Cardiol 68(16):8E, 1991.

171. Davies MJ: Successful and unsuccessful coronary thrombolysis, Br Heart J 61(5):381, 1989.

172. Dunn M et al: Antithrombotic therapy in atrial fibrillation, Chest 96(suppl):85, 1989.

173. Emde KL, Searle LD: Current practices with thrombolytic therapy, J Cardiovasc Nurs 4(1):11, 1989.

174. Faxon DP: The risk of reperfusion strategies in the treatment of patients with acute myocardial infarction, J Am Coll Cardiol 12(6 suppl A):52A, 1988.

174a. Friedman H: Thrombolytic therapy for acute myocardial infarction: GUSTO criticized, N Engl J Med 330(7):504, 1994.

175. Fuster V, Cohen M, Halperin J: Aspirin in the prevention of coronary disease, N Engl J Med 321:183, 1989.

176. Fuster V et al: Antithrombotic therapy after myocardial reperfusion in acute myocardial infarction, J Am Coll Cardiol 12(6 suppl A):78A, 1988.

176a. GUSTO investigators: An international randomized trial comparing four thrombolytic strategies for acute myocardial infarction, N Engl J Med 329(10):673, 1993.

177. Halperin JL, Fuster V: Left ventricular thrombi and cerebral embolism, N Engl J Med 320:392, 1989.

178. Henderson E: Thrombolytic therapy in acute myocardial infarction: an overview, J Emerg Nurs 15(2 Pt 2):145, 1989.

179. Hennekens CH et al: Aspirin and other antiplatelet agents in the secondary and primary prevention of cardiovascular disease, Circulation 80:749, 1989.

180. Heras M et al: Emergency thrombolysis in acute myocardial infarction, Ann Emerg Med 12(11):1168, 1988.

181. Hugenholtz PG, Suryapranata H: Thrombolytic agents in early myocardial infarction, Am J Cardiol 63(10):94E, 1989.

182. Kleven MR: Comparison of thrombolytic agents: mechanism of action, efficacy, and safety, Heart Lung 17(6 Pt 2):750, 1988.

183. Kline EM: Comparison of thrombolytic agents: mechanisms of action, Crit Care Nurs Q 12(2):1, 1989.

184. Martin G, Kennedy JW: Thrombolytic therapy in the management of acute myocardial infarction, part 2—influence on mortality, Mod Concepts Cardiovasc Dis 59(3):13, 1990.

185. Misinski M: Pathophysiology of acute myocardial infarction: a rationale for thrombolytic therapy, Heart Lung 17(6 Pt 2):743, 1988.

186. Mueller HS Et al: Thrombolytic therapy in acute myocardial infarction: Part I, Med Clin North Am 72(1):197, 1988.

187. Mueller HS et al: Thrombolytic therapy in acute myocardial infarction: Part II—rt PA, Med Clin North Am 73(2):387, 1989.

188. ONeill WW, Topol EJ, Pitt B: Reperfusion therapy of acute myocardial infarction, Prog Cardiovasc Dis 30(4):235, 1988.

189. Ouyang P, Shapiro EP, Gottlieb SO: Thrombolysis in post infarction angina, Am J Cardiol 68(7):119B, 1991.

190. Paspa PA, Movahed A: Thrombolytic therapy in acute myocardial infarction, Am Fam Physician 45(2):640, 1992.

191. Rapaport E: Thrombolysis, anticoagulation and reocclusion, Am J Cardiol 68(16):17E, 1991.

192. Resnekov L et al: Antithrombotic agents in coronary artery disease, Chest 95:525, 1989.

193. Selzer A: Does thrombolytic therapy reduce infarct size? J Am Coll Cardiol 13(6):1431, 1989.

194. Sherry S: Thrombolytic therapy for acute myocardial infarction: a critical perspective, part 1, Mod Concepts Cardiovasc Dis

60(4):19, 1991; part 2: Mod Concepts Cardiovasc Dis 60(5):25, 1991.

195. Stein B, Fuster V: Antithrombotic therapy in acute myocardial infarction: prevention of venous, left ventricular and coronary artery thromboembolism, Am J Cardiol 64(4):33B, 1989.

196. Swither CM: Tools for teaching about anticoagulants, RN 51:157, 1988.

197. Tate DA, Dehmer GJ: New challenges for thrombolytic therapy, Ann Intern Med 110(12):953, 1989.

198. Theroux P: Antiplatelet and antithrombotic therapy in unstable angina, Am J Cardiol 68(7):92B, 1991.

199. Tiefenbrunn AJ, Ludbrook PA: Coronary thrombolysis—it's worth the risk, JAMA 261(14):2107, 1989.

200. Topol EJ: Integration on anticoagulation, thrombolysis and coronary angioplasty for unstable angina pectoris, Am J Cardiol 68(7):136B, 1991.

201. Topol EJ: Which thrombolytic agent should one choose? Prog Cardiovasc Dis 34(3):165, 1991.

202. Verstraete M: Thrombolytic treatment in acute myocardial infarction, Circulation 82(3 suppl):II96, 1990.

203. Wasserman AG, Ross AM: Patient selection for thrombolytic therapy, Am J Cardiol 64(4):17B, 1989.

204. White HD: Comparison of tissue plasminogen activator and streptokinase in the management of acute myocardial infarction, Chest 95(5 suppl):265S, 1989.

204a. Zoldhelyi P et al: Recombinant hirudin in patients with chronic, stable coronary artery disease, Circulation 88(5Pt1):2015, 1993.

Narcotic analgesics

205. Buck ML, Blumer J: Opioids and other analgesics—adverse effects in the intensive care unit, Crit Care Clin 7(3):615, 1991.

206. Herlitz J: Analgesia in myocardial infarction, Drugs 37(6):939, 1989.

207. Herlitz J, Hjalmarson A, Waagstein F: Treatment of pain acute myocardial infarction, Br Heart J 61(1):9, 1989.

208. Remetz MS, Cabin HS: Analgesic therapy in acute myocardial infarction, Cardiol Clin 6(1):29, 1988.

Vasodilator agents

209. Abrams J: A reappraisal of nitrate therapy, JAMA 259(3):396, 1988.

210. Abrams J: Mechanism of action of the organic nitrates in the treatment of myocardial ischemia, Am J Cardiol 70(8):30B, 1992.

211. Ambrosioni E et al: Potential use of ACE inhibitors after acute myocaridal infarction, J Cardiovasc Pharmacol 14(suppl 9):592, 1989.

212. Cohn JN: Future directions in vasodilator therapy for heart failure, Am Heart J 121(3 Pt 1):969, 1991.

213. Cohn PF: Total ischemic burden: effect of vasoactive agents, Part I, Am Heart J 115(1):215.

214. Ertk G et al: Influence of angiotensin-converting enzyme inhibition on cardiac function in myocardial infarction, Am J Cardiol 3:65(14)70G, 1990.

215. Flaherty JT: Role of nitrates in acute myocardial infarction, Am J Cardiol 70(8):73B, 1992.

216. Gold ME: Pharmacology of the nitrovasodilators: antianginal, antihypertensive, and antiplatelet actions, Nurs Clin North Am 26(2):437, 1991.

217. Jugdutt BI: Intravenous nitroglycerin unloading in acute myocardial infarction, Am J Cardiol 68(14):52D, 1991.

218. Jugdutt BI: Role of nitrates after myocardial infarction, Am J Cardiol 70(8):82B, 1992.

Electrical Intervention in Cardiac Disease

Laurie Futterman Correa, RN, MSN, CCRN

COUNTERSHOCK

Countershock is the delivery of an electrical current through the heart sufficient to depolarize a critical mass of myocardium.[17,32] This charge may interrupt ectopic tachyarrhythmias, allowing the physiologic pacemaker, the sinoatrial (SA) node, to regain control of the rhythm. There are two types of countershock: cardioversion and defibrillation. You may deliver both types through either manually controlled devices or automatic devices. Power sources for both are internal (automatic implantable cardioverter defibrillator) or external (automatic external defibrillator). Self-induced countershock and cardiopulmonary resuscitation (CPR) by cough have also been documented.[19]

Manual defibrillation and cardioversion

Manual defibrillation and cardioversion utilize similar mechanical equipment. This equipment includes (1) a power generator, which builds up the charge, (2) a set of paddles to deliver the charge, and (3) an oscilloscope with ECG recorder to document the ECG patterns.

One of the most critical factors ensuring the depolarization of a significant mass of ventricular myocardium is proper electrode, or paddle, placement. Standard anterolateral or transverse paddle placement entails placing one paddle to the right of the upper sternum just below the right clavicle and the other paddle just to the left of the nipple in the midaxillary line. With anteroposterior placement, one paddle is positioned anteriorly over the precordium, just to the left of the lower sternal border. The other paddle is positioned behind the heart (Fig. 10-1).[4]

Research does not support the superiority of either method of paddle placement.[17,27a]

Defibrillation and cardioversion differ primarily according to mode of discharge, indications, amount of energy required, and related precautions. Survival from ventricular fibrillation (VF) demands rapid, early electrical countershock. Defibrillation is the random, or unsynchronized, delivery of electricity to the myocardium and is the most effective method of terminating this tachyarrhythmia.

Cardioversion is the delivery of a synchronized charge to the myocardium.[14,17,32] Synchronization implies that the countershock device is programmed to deliver its charge only after sensing the patient's major QRS deflection. A sensing circuit allows the countershock to be delivered during the absolute refractory period, or on the QRS complex of

443

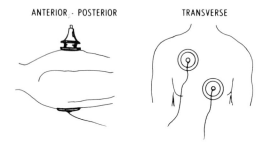

ANTERIOR · POSTERIOR   TRANSVERSE

Fig. 10-1 Paddle placement for manual defibrillation or cardioversion.

the electrocardiogram.[14,17,33] Synchronized cardioversion usually requires less energy and involves fewer complications. The synchronization of the charge to the QRS complex prevents delivery of electricity during the vulnerable period of ventricular repolarization (T wave), thus avoiding further electrical deterioration into VF.

Emergency cardioversion is preferred for hemodynamically unstable or pharmacologically unresponsive ventricular or supraventricular tachyarrhythmias, such as ventricular tachycardia or atrial fibrillation with a rapid ventricular response. Cardioversion is not indicated for arrhythmias such as VF in which there are neither discernible QRS complexes to be sensed nor pulseless rhythm disturbances. In ventricular tachycardia, when the patient is severely unstable (hypotensive, unconscious), unsynchronized countershock is suggested to avoid delays inherent in the synchronization process.[14,17,27a,32] However, other causes of wide QRS tachycardia should be ruled out. The absence of a pulse rules these causes out most effectively.

The amount of energy, or joules (J), required for the delivery of countershock is dependent on the characteristics of the dysrhythmia. Immediate defibrillation with 200 J is recommended in VF and pulseless ventricular tachycardia (VT). If the patient still remains in VF or VT, defibrillation with 200 to 300 J is recommended, immediately followed by a 360 J shock if ineffective.[27a] These initial steps should be followed by CPR, intubation, and pharmacologic support (see Unit 6). Once artificial ventilation and circulation are established, reattempt defibrillation with 360 J alternating with pharmacologic therapy until the arrhythmia is terminated. In a witnessed event, when VF or pulseless VT is confirmed, random or unsynchronized countershock may be delivered initially by a blow to the precordium. This mechanical shock, although of low voltage, may completely depolarize the myocardium and terminate certain arrhythmias. A precordial blow is used in witnessed arrest situations only and is delivered to the center of the sternum with the fleshy part of the fist from a height of no more than 12 inches. If the patient remains pulseless and VF or VT persists, defibrillate immediately with 200 J.

Initial energy level settings for cardioversion of supraventricular tachy arrhythmias or unstable VT should begin with 100 J, followed by 200 J, 300 J, and 360 J, respectively.[27a] If this is unsuccessful, initiate pharmacologic therapy and repeat attempts at cardioversion. Initial energy settings of 50 J may be effective in atrial flutter and paroxysmal supraventricular tachycardia (PSVT).[27a] Unless the clinical situation allows for emergency overdrive pacing, continue pharmacologic and cardioversion interventions per ACLS guidelines until the dysrhythmia is terminated.[14,17,32]

Factors to be considered before cardioversion include preparation of the patient as well as the equipment. After delivery of a countershock charge to the myocardium, there is always a period of electrical instability that may result in arrhythmias. Before elective cardioversion, avoid factors enhancing electrical instability such as hypokalemia, acid-base disturbances, hypoxia, or digitalis toxicity. Short-acting barbiturates, diazepam (Valium), or midazolam (Versed) are often used for transient amnesic effects before and during elective cardioversion. Respiratory depression and hypoventilation can occur after the administration of these drugs. Consequently, adjunctive respiratory or ventilatory equipment should be on hand.

If the SA node is depressed from pharmacologic effects or chronic conduction system disease, or if it has been insulted by an acute ischemic process, it may not resume control of the rhythm. When this occurs, lower pacemaker centers may assume control of the rhythm. If such escape rhythms are ineffective or do not appear, atropine or pacing may be required.

NURSING ORDERS: For the patient undergoing manual defibrillation or cardioversion

RELATED NURSING DIAGNOSES: Alteration in cardiac output, anxiety, potential ineffective ventilation

1. Ensure a stable, patent IV line. However, do not delay initial shocks for VF.
2. If the patient is alert, explain the procedure in friendly, nonthreatening terms.
   — Inform the patient that the procedure will make his or her heart slower and more regular and will relieve his or her symptoms.
   — Some patients may benefit by observing precardioversion and postcardioversion strips of their rhythm.
   — Describe the cardioversion procedure as being analogous to a "message" delivered to the heart.
3. If time allows, ascertain recent K^+ and Mg^{++} levels and digitalis dose or level before countershock intervention.
4. Because of the potential respiratory depressant effects of the various pharmacologic agents employed when cardioverting, oxygen, bag-valve-mask, emergency suction, and intubation equipment should be available in case of hypoventilation or respiratory arrest.

5. Before defibrillation, confirm VF or VT by quick-look paddles or ECG trace and *pulselessness*.
6. Before cardioversion, securely attach electrodes and obtain a clear ECG trace with no artifact. Select a lead other than the paddle lead since some models will not allow synchronization in the paddle lead. Then activate the synchronizer selector. Illuminated QRS complexes will appear on the ECG scope. Have lidocaine (Xylocaine) and atropine at bedside.
7. Apply conductive material to paddles or electrodes, or apply prepackaged conductive pads to chest.
8. Charge the machine to the desired voltage.
9. Confirm proper placement of paddles or electrodes on the chest. If paddle electrodes are used, apply approximately 25 pounds of pressure (do not lean on paddles because they may slip).
10. Call "all clear" and visually confirm that personnel are not in direct contact with the patient or bed.
11. Deliver countershock by depressing both discharge buttons simultaneously. During cardioversion, there may be a slight delay in actual discharge as the sensing mechanism locates the QRS complex.
12. Check for return of pulse and evaluate postcountershock rhythm. When defibrillating, the second pulse check is performed after three rapidly delivered initial shocks.[27a] If the patient remains pulseless and VF or VT persists, continue ACLS protocols for VF. If the rhythm changes to VF following cardioversion, the synchronizer selector must be turned off prior to attempting defibrillation.

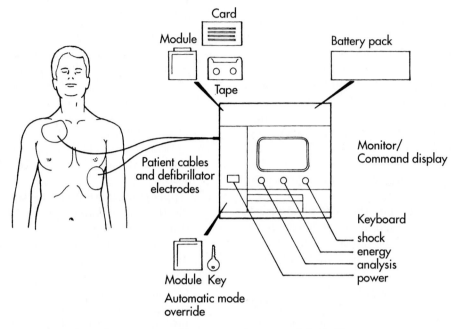

Event documentation

Card

Module

Tape

Battery pack

Patient cables
and defibrillator
electrodes

Monitor/
Command display

Module Key

Automatic mode
override

Keyboard
shock
energy
analysis
power

Fig. 10-2   Components of an automatic external defibrillator (AED).

Automatic external defibrillator[6,17,44]

To expedite effective defibrillation, use an automatic external defibrillator (AED). The AED is an external device composed of a cardiac rhythm system that both senses and analyzes certain cardiac rhythms and an external defibrillator capable of delivering electrical countershock, if necessary. The shock is dispersed through two adhesive pads and may be delivered under the command of a total automatic mode, or a semiautomatic mode (Fig. 10-2). The fully automatic mode requires only the attachment of the defibrillator pads and activation of the device. Once the device is activated, it begins analyzing the rhythm, recommending and/or initiating appropriate therapy automatically. The semiautomatic mode requires the operator to initiate AED analysis of the rhythm and manually activate the delivery of the countershock. CPR must be interrupted to allow for analysis of the rhythm.

The benefits of using an AED include the rapidity of initiation of shock therapy and safety for the operator.[6,17,44] Disadvantages include the inability to apply pressure to the defibrillating pads (which helps to decrease transthoracic resistance) and lack of variability in energy selection. The lowest energy setting is 200 J. This is high for persons of small body weight; therefore, AED use in children is not recommended. ACLS-trained providers should know the protocols and the role of the AED in the cardiac arrest situation.

Implantable cardioverter defibrillator[1,2,12,15,32,39,40,42,50]

The implantable cardioverter defibrillator (ICD) was developed as a life-saving device for patients at risk for sudden cardiac death (SCD). VF, or sustained VT that deteriorates into VF, is believed to be the predominate cause of SCD (see Unit 11). Despite the recent release of new antiarrhythmic agents, and refinement of noninvasive and invasive methods of assessing drug efficacy, many patients remain without effective and identifiable therapy. Arrhythmia surgeries are precluded in many individuals because of an absence of either an inducible tachycardia during electrophysiology studies (EPS) or a discrete left ventricular aneurysm. Some patients who do undergo such arrhythmia surgeries continue to demonstrate postoperative arrhythmias or inducibility rates. Since its approval for clinical use in 1985, the ICD has evolved from an investigational device to an extraordinary technologic tool for the management of malignant ventricular arrhythmias. More than 18,000 units are currently implanted.[1,4,12,32,39,40,42,50]

Recipients of the earliest investigational devices were those at highest risk for SCD, having survived multiple, separate, documented cardiac arrests. These persons had reproducible, hemodynamically unstable VT or VF that could not be suppressed despite many antiarrhythmic trials. Currently, fewer drug trials are performed before considering ICD implantation. Several prerequisites exist for successful application. These include patients with syncope and inducible, drug-refractory sustained arrhythmias during electrophysiologic testing, as well as patients who have survived cardiac arrest but have no inducible arrhythmias. Because of the associated patient discomfort and the limited number of shocks that the battery of the device allows, life-threatening arrhythmias must not occur frequently. Therefore, patients with multiple, daily episodes of VT or VF are not considered candidates.[40,42,50]

Unlike the traditional manual cardioverting-defibrillating systems, the ICD automatically and selectively detects and terminates ventricular arrhythmias by repeated countershocks. It is not, however, indicated for controlling supraventricular arrhythmias.

The ICD detects arrhythmias by sensing electrical activity of these impulses from their intracardiac ECG patterns or electrograms. The electrograms are analyzed for both ECG morphology and/or heart rate by the sensing circuitry in the ICD. The major components of an ICD system, a pulse generator and four electrodes, are similar to those of artificial pacing systems. For this reason, ICD units have been incorporated into the latest proposed revision of the International Pacing Code (see Pacemakers). The pulse generator produces, stores, and releases the charge and contains the sensing circuitry for detection of heart rate and QRS morphology. The pulse generator weighs approximately one-half pound and is surgically implanted within a subcutaneous pocket in the left paraumbilical area. Chest tube placement may be required after certain surgical approaches.[40,43,50]

Two electrodes (one negative and one positive) are used as a bipolar system to detect and transmit the heart rate to the pulse generator. These electrodes may be contained within a single catheter or lead, which is threaded transvenously into the heart and positioned against the inner (endocardial) surface of the right ventricle. These electrodes may also be separately attached to the outer or epicardial surface of the heart (Fig. 10-3). A second set of two electrodes also act as a bipolar system and are used to detect and transmit ECG morphology to the pulse generator and deliver the defibrillation current to the heart. These patch electrodes, known as transcardiac leads, are positioned so that the current will transverse the heart.

The primary mechanism by which the ICD recognizes VF or VT is by *rate criteria,* or when

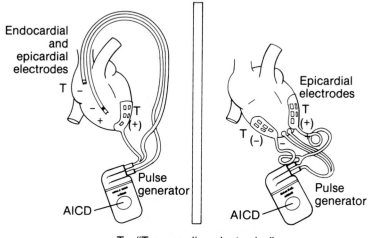

Fig. 10-3 Components of an automatic implantable cardioverter defibrillator (ICD). Alternative electrode systems are illustrated.

the heart rate exceeds a programmable, pre-set value. Any arrhythmia less than the preset cutoff rate is not sensed. A second mechanism for detection of arrhythmia is analysis of other detection enhancement parameters. The most common detection enhancement parameter is ECG complex morphology or *probability density function* (PDF). PDF is based on the time the ECG complex spends on the isoelectric line or baseline. Since the ECG patterns of VT and VF spend little time on the baseline (low PDF), these rhythms are considered abnormal by the pulse generator.[48a] ICDs may be programmed to respond to rate only or to both rate and morphology criteria.[6–11,32,40,42,50] Most physicians prefer to program the device using the simpler single rate criteria. In newer models, rate limits may be programmed from 110 to 200.[48a] Supraventricular tachycardias exceeding the rate limits may trigger an inappropriate "synchronized" shock that may terminate the arrhythmias. These shocks are uncomfortable for the patient and unnecessarily use up the life of the battery. Pharmacologic

suppression of these arrhythmias is indicated to avoid inappropriate ICD activation and discharge. The unit also may be temporarily inactivated.

Recently developed criteria designed to enhance ICD sensitivity include analysis of the prematurity of the first beat of the tachycardia, analysis of the regularity of the arrhythmia, and duration by which the tachycardia exceeds the rate cutoff value. Future devices are likely to assess hemodynamics and the degree of instability caused by the arrhythmia and subsequently customize the discharge energy required to terminate it. Early devices used batteries with life expectancies of 18 to 24 months or about 100 to 200 shocks. Today's batteries last 3 to 4 years or 200 to 400 shocks, before generator replacement is required.[4,12,18,34,37,39,40,42,50,63]

Once a tachycardia that satisfies preprogrammed criteria is detected (5 to 15 seconds), the device's capacitors (energy storage units) begin to charge (5 to 12 seconds). The first shock is then delivered. If the arrhythmia is not terminated by the first shock, the device recharges and delivers up to five more shocks depending on the specific model; this is known as *recycling*.[40,48a] After that time the ICD remains dormant until at least 35 seconds of a rhythm other than VT or VF is sensed. If VT or VF persists after the sixth shock, initiate external cardioversion or defibrillation. Placement of the epicardial patch electrodes may impede transmission of electrical current via standard transverse paddle placement. Anteroposterior positioning is suggested. Because external countershock may affect the device's programming, you should assess the ICD through device interrogation after each external countershock intervention. This is accomplished with a programmer similar to those used with pacemakers (see Pacemakers). New models reconfirm the presence of VT before shocking and "dump" the charge if the arrhythmia terminates before the discharge of the shock. A delay in the delivery of the first shock may be programmed to allow for intermittent arrhythmias.[48a] The energy level of the first shock may also be programmed (0.1–40 J).

The ICD has an *audio function* that signals when it is in the active and inactive modes. When a specialized ring magnet is placed over the upper part of the pulse generator for a minimum of 30 seconds, the device alternately activates or inactivates. When the ICD is in the *active mode*, it beeps with each QRS complex it senses. When the ICD is inactivated, placement of the magnet causes a continuous electronic tone. Nurses caring for patients with an ICD should know how to inactivate the device in case an emergency arises and it fires inappropriately. The change from a beeping sound to a continuous tone confirms inactivation. Leave the generator in the inactive mode the first 24 to 72 hours postoperatively to prevent activation from expected, transient postoperative arrhythmias. Such arrhythmias may occur as a result of decreased pre- and intraoperative antiarrhythmic blood levels or from myocardial irritability secondary to metabolic or electrolyte alterations or mechanical irritation and inflammation. Initial postoperative activation of an ICD should be ordered by the physician.

Before discharge, repeat electrophysiologic testing may be performed to evaluate the ICD's response to induced arrhythmias and subsequent termination capabilities. At this time the patient may experience a shock under supervised conditions. Shocks from the ICD are unpleasant and have been compared to being "thumped on the chest" or an "explosion." Controlled shock experiences have been effective in minimizing both the anxiety related to anticipation of what the shock will feel like, as well as in instilling confidence in the device and its ability to terminate potentially fatal arrhythmias.

Devices now undergoing clinical trials have improvements, including a reduction in pulse generator size and more sophisticated sensing modalities.[12,18,25,43,47,57,58] Lead systems involving various combinations of transvenous and subcutaneous or submuscular electrodes and patches have been successfully developed without the need for a concomitant thoracotomy incision.[43,47] As this text goes to print, these transvenous leads have become available and are in clinical use. The combined decrease in surgical risk from and in cost of a nonthoracotomy procedure is attractive. Devices that function as combined antitachycardia pacemaker, backup ventricular demand pacemaker, and cardioverter defibrillator are discussed later in this chapter.[12,25,32,36,57,58] Other exciting areas of technologic advancement involve enhanced capabilities of data storage, programmability, and telemetric functions, improvements in transvenous lead implantation techniques, and implementation of bidirectional energy waveforms to decrease energy required for successful countershock.[12,25,58]

NURSING ORDERS: For the patient with an ICD[15,34]

RELATED NURSING DIAGNOSES: Alteration in cardiac output, alteration in comfort, knowledge deficit (patient or family) related to ICD function, manual resuscitative measures, activity restrictions, ineffective coping related to unpredictability of discharge, physical and emotional dependency, fear of activity and/or shocks

Preoperatively

1. Explain purpose of the ICD, surgical procedure and basic mode of operation of the ICD. The patient needs to know he or she will have a bulge in the paraumbilical area from the pulse generator. Show model of the ICD pulse generator if possible.

2. Explain reason for chest tube postoperatively, if appropriate, and importance of breathing exercises and coughing postoperatively. Some patients may require ventilator support for short periods depending on prior state of health.

Postoperatively

1. Monitor patient in the immediate postoperative period for incisional pain, recurrence of ventricular arrhythmias, and integrity of the chest drainage system along with amount and consistency of drainage.

2. After the ICD has been activated, monitor, document, and report inappropriate shocks during nonsustained VT and supraventricular tachycardias such as atrial fibrillation. Double or triple sensing of paced beats, pacemaker spikes, and/or T waves may also occur inappropriately and should be reported.[1] Unipolar pacemakers are contraindicated because of the larger spikes.[1]

3. Monitor and document lack of discharge or ineffective discharge during sustained VT or VF. Antiarrhythmias can increase energy requirements or alter the characteristics (rate, QRS morphology) of previously stable or predictable arrhyth-

mias, making successful ICD interventions difficult.[34]

4. If VT or VF persists after a sixth shock, initiate manual cardioversion or defibrillation. Anterior-posterior paddles may be more effective in models with ventricular patches by overcoming some of the impedance associated with these patches.

5. Allow patient to ventilate feelings of dependency, fear, and so on.

6. Provide patient with application for Medic Alert bracelet and explain the importance of wearing it at all times. Also instruct patient to always carry the ICD recipient ID card.

7. Avoid administering subcutaneous injection, such as heparin or insulin, in the area near the device.

8. Instruct patient and family on what to do if the patient receives a shock:
   a. Contact the physician for initial postimplant shock and subsequent shocks as directed by the physician.
   b. Activate the emergency medical service (EMS) system if, after the initial shock, a second shock occurs or if the patient loses consciousness.
   c. If the patient is unresponsive, check for a pulse and initiate CPR if indicated.[17] Encourage family members to become CPR certified. Explain that they may "feel" the shock through the chest wall if they are doing CPR when the device discharges. The feel has been described as a startle-type reaction and is not dangerous to the person performing CPR.

9. If appropriate, instruct patient and family in use of the ring magnet to disarm the ICD in the event of repeated discharges.

10. Tell patients to avoid environmental elements that may generate strong magnetic fields and potentially interfere with functioning of the device. These include arc welders, electrocautery, electric smelting

furnaces, large outboard motors, timer lights, airport metal detectors, and radio frequency transmitters, including radar and power plants.

11. Instruct patient that if the device emits beeping sounds, he or she may be near an electromagnetic field and should walk in the opposite direction. The device could accidentally be inactivated in the presence of an electromagnetic field. Contact the physician or nurse to confirm that the unit is active.

12. Instruct patient to observe for and report any signs of infection (i.e., fever, local redness, excessive tenderness, drainage from the incisions).

13. Tell patients to avoid lifting, isometric-type movements, and driving for the first 6 weeks to allow for healing, depending on the surgical approach used. Instruct patients to avoid wearing constrictive clothing over the generator. A support binder is often suggested to minimize discomfort from the weight of the device and to prevent migration of the device.

14. Instruct patient on the importance of avoiding contact sports after device is implanted because of potential lead wire disruption.

15. Inform patient of the importance of contacting physician for antibiotic prophylaxis before going to the dentist or for any "flulike" or febrile symptoms to prevent subacute bacterial endocarditis (SBE).

16. Inform patient that sexual activity can usually be resumed when he or she is comfortable and that the partner will not be harmed in the event of an inadvertent shock.

17. Inform family of risks of driving. State laws regarding implantable devices vary.

18. Stress compliance with periodic outpatient visits (usually q 2 months).[48a] Since a rise in the need for defibrillating shocks has been demonstrated after the fifth year, defibrillator generators are usually replaced before that time even if the patient has not received a shock.[1,40,42,50,63]

PACEMAKERS

Unlike countershock, pacemakers are used primarily in the management of slow rates. A cardiac pacemaker provides an artificial electrical stimulus when the heart's own electrical system is failing. Pacemakers may be initially categorized as (1) *single-* or *dual*-chamber and (2) *temporary* or *permanent.*

Indications for pacing

Current indications for pacing follow four major categories: (1) symptomatic bradyarrhythmias, (2) prophylaxis, (3) diagnosis, and (4) tachyarrhythmias.[9,16,18,23,26,28,29,31,33,35,38] Symptomatic bradyarrhythmias are the oldest and most important indication for both temporary and permanent pacing. These arrhythmias involve either the SA node or atrioventricular (AV) node conduction system. They can occur in both acute myocardial infarction (MI) and chronic conduction system disease or may be drug induced.

Pacing in acute MI may be employed prophylactically, on a temporary basis, in anticipation of significant bradyarrhythmias or loss of AV synchrony (see Unit 6). Temporary pacing is required in most postoperative cardiac surgical patients either to augment cardiac output, suppress or control supraventricular arrhythmias or to provide rate support in AV blocks. Therefore, prophylactic pacing is routine in this setting. Pacemakers may also be used in postoperative and other settings when a risk of rate suppression exists as a result of adverse effects of drug therapy. During balloon counterpulsation in irregular rhythms such as atrial fibrillation, pacemakers are used to facilitate balloon timing (see Unit 8). Prophylactic pacing may be indicated during cardiac catheterization or invasive procedures to the right side of the heart, especially in the presence of preexisting left bundle branch block (LBBB). Diagnostic uses of pacemakers include (1) assessment of SA and AV conduction in electrophysiologic laboratories, (2) hemodynamic evaluation of varying pacing rates, (3) identification of mechanisms of tachyarrhythmia onset and termination, and (4) assessment of the effectiveness of antiar-rhythmic therapy.[9,16,18,23,26,28,29,31,33,35,38]

Antitachycardia pacing uses temporary or specialized implantable pacing systems, depending on the clinical situation. The mechanism of antitachycardia pacing can be categorized according to those that *prevent* tachycardias (tachycardias caused by prolonged repolarization periods) and those that *terminate* tachycardias.[16] Antitachycardia pacing is discussed thoroughly at the end of this chapter.

Dual-chamber stimulation is most often indicated in AV conduction disease when both the atrial and ventricular contributions to cardiac output are critical or when single-chamber pacing induces pacemaker syndrome (see Hemodynamics of cardiac pacing). Atrial contribution is most easily maintained by the different forms of dual-chamber pacing.[18,26]

Basic components and function

An artificial pacemaker consists of two essential components: a pulse generator, which acts as an energy source for the stimulus, and a minimum of two electrodes, which may be contained within a single catheter (Fig. 10-4) or may remain separate. The electrodes deliver the electrical stimulus to the heart and transmit the signals from the heart to the pulse generator. Some tempo-rary pacing units also use a bridging cable as an extension between the pulse generator and the catheter.

Basic pacemaker function involves (1) release of a stimulus, (2) response to the stimulus (atrial, ventricular, or both), and (3) sensing (of natural impulses). This function is reflected in the specific characteristics of the pulse generator and the ECG assessment of pacemaker patterns.

The pulse generators of permanent pacemakers are implanted internally in a subcutaneous pocket. The pulse generators of temporary pacemakers remain external.[49,51] The electrodes are contained within one or more catheters, also called lead wires. The catheter is positioned in contact with either the endocardium or epicardium. Endocardial positioning is the most common positioning. A variety of catheters are available for single- and dual-chamber use. Stiff Dacron catheters that require fluoroscopy during insertion have been replaced by flexible

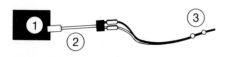

1. Pulse generator
2. Bridging cable
3. Electrodes

Fig. 10-4 Components of an artificial pacemaker. Essential components are the pulse generator *(1)* and two electrodes *(3)*. The electrodes may both be contained within a catheter, as illustrated, or may remain separate. A bridging cable *(2)* is optional.

floating and semifloating catheters that are positioned by ECG guiding equipment. Balloon-tipped pacing catheters are available, as are catheters that combine both pulmonary artery (PA) pressure monitoring and pacing capabilities.[18,30,45,49,51]

Pacemaker catheters may be either unipolar or bipolar.[45,46] Bipolar catheters are more common in temporary pacing. Both unipolar and bipolar catheters are common in permanent pacing. Bipolar catheters contain two electrode sites (distal and proximal) on a single catheter. When the catheter is in the proper position, both electrode sites lie within the heart. The electrical signal stimulating the myocardium exits from the negative terminal of the pulse generator and returns through the positive terminal (Fig. 10-5). With bipolar catheters, the distal electrode (tip) should be initially connected to the negative terminal since the catheter tip is usually in better contact with the myocardium. However, this method of connection is not essential for pacer function. In the event of inadequate stimulation or sensing, the poles may be reversed, allowing the impulse to exit from the proximal electrode. If the proximal electrode is in closer contact with the endocardial wall, better functioning will be achieved. The small interelectrode distance of bipolar

systems restricts the sensitivity range to a small area of myocardium. Advantages of bipolar pacing include reduced probability of skeletal muscle stimulation and low susceptibility to electromagnetic interference or other extraneous intracardiac or extracardiac signals that could inhibit the pacemaker.[45]

Unipolar catheters contain one electrode site on the catheter itself, which functions as the negative electrode when attached to the negative terminal of the pulse generator. The electrical signal exits from this negative electrode. An external site on the pulse generator or outer skin surface serves as the positive electrode. When the catheter is in the proper position, only one electrode lies within the heart. Because of its larger interelectrode distance, the unipolar electrode system is exposed to a greater amount of intracardiac activity. The major advantage of the unipolar system is a greater sensitivity to intracardiac signals. However, a major corresponding disadvantage is a greater sensitivity to outside interference that may inhibit the pacemaker.[45]

Unipolar pacing systems also generate a significantly larger pacing artifact than bipolar systems. Although the more prominent pacing artifact is more easily recognized on the ECG, it distorts the ECG pattern. Emis-

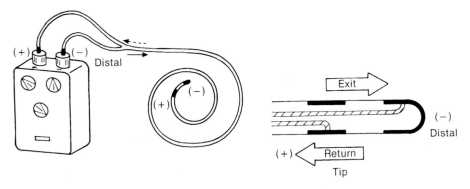

Fig. 10-5 Bipolar catheter systems. The impulse exits from the negative terminal of the pulse generator, which is ideally connected to the distal electrode to allow the impulse to exit from the catheter tip.

sion of larger signals stimulates skeletal muscles, causing patient discomfort. A bipolar system may be converted to a unipolar system, if indicated. However, the converse is not true.

The principles of pacing are similar for both temporary and permanent pacemakers. Both types are currently used in patients with acute MI or chronic conduction system disease and are therefore commonly seen in coronary care and progressive care areas.

Classification of pacemakers: NASPE/BPEG Generic (NBG) code[18]

In 1974, The Intersociety Commission of Heart Disease Resources devised a three-letter code that was used to describe the basic functions of pacing systems available at that time. Since then, pacers have become more sophisticated. Consequently, under the direction of a committee of cardiologists of the North American Society of Pacing and Electrophysiology (NASPE) and the British Pacing and Electrophysiology Group (BPEG), revisions have occurred.

Although the code now consists of five positions, the first three antibradycardia positions are used most frequently (Table 10-1).[9,18,23,28,38] The first position represents the chamber (or chambers) in which stimulation, or pacing, occurs. The options are A—atrium, V—ventricle, D—dual (or both atrium and ventricle), and O—no bradycardia support capabilities (used in antitachycardia pacers that have no bradycardia support). Dual-chamber pacing is also called AV sequential pacing. The second position refers to the chamber(s) in which sensing of natural impulses occurs. Sensing options are similar to the pacing options. The third position refers to the mode in which sensing, or the pacemaker's response to a sensed event, occurs. Option T indicates that an output is *triggered* in response to a sensed event and is also called *synchronous* pacing (see Dual-Chamber Pacing: DDD). Option I indicates that sensed events—i.e., the patient's own natural impulses—*inhibit* the pacer from generating an output, allowing the pacemaker to fire only when needed. For this reason, the inhibited mode of pacing is commonly called *demand* pacing. Option D indicates a combination of inhibition and triggered pacing and is reserved for dual-chamber pacemakers. Option O indicates no sensing. In this mode, the pacemaker fires *continuously* without regard for the patient's own rhythm. This mode of pacing is also called *asynchronous* or *fixed rated* pacing. It is used primarily as an antitachycardia mode.

The fourth position of the code, used most often in permanent pacing, reflects the degree of programmability and the presence or absence of rate modulation capabilities. Commonly programmable, or adjustable, functions include mode of pacing, rate, output, sensitivity, refractory period, hysteresis, and polarity. O indicates that the device is neither programmable nor rate responsive. P indicates simple programmability (only one or two variables can be changed). M indicates multiple programmability (three or more variables). C reflects telemetric ability, or the ability of the pacemaker to noninvasively transmit data from the pulse generator to an external receiver. R denotes rate-responsive capabilities in which the pacemaker rate is automatically adjusted or *modulated* in response to increased physical activity. Physical activity is sensed as muscle vibrations, increased respiratory rate, temperature changes, or other factors (see Hemodynamics of Cardiac Pacing).

Position five indicates the presence of one or more active antitachycardia pacing functions. S indicates that the device is capable of delivering synchronized and unsynchronized countershocks. AD (or D) reflects the capa-

Table 10-1. The NASPE/BPEG Generic (NBG) Pacemaker Code (1987)

Position	I	II	III	IV	V
Category	Chamber(s) paced	Chamber(s) sensed	Response to sensing	Programmability, rate modulation	Antitachyarrhythmia function(s)
	O = None	O = None	O = None (continuous) (asynchronous)	O = None	O = None
	A = Atrium	A = Atrium	T = Triggered (synchronous)	P = Simple programmability	P = Pacing (antitachyarrhythmia)
	V = Ventricle	V = Ventricle	I = Inhibited (demand)	M = Multiprogrammability	S = Shock
	D = Dual (A + V)	D = Dual (A + V)	D = Dual (T + I)	C = Communicating	D = Dual (P + S)
Manufacturer's designation only	S = single (A or V)	S = single (A or V)		R = Rate modulation	

Note: Positions I through III are used exclusively for antibradyarrhythmia function.

bility of performing both antitachycardia pacing and countershock delivery.[18-23]

The most common modes of either temporary or permanent pacing are the following: (1) VVI, (2) AOO/AAI, (3) DVI, and (4) DDD. The pulse generator characteristics and ECG patterns of each of these are discussed further in the remaining sections of this chapter.

Single-chamber pacing systems[18,23,26,28]

Single-chamber pacing refers to systems that stimulate one chamber, either the atrium or ventricle. These systems are either temporary or permanent and deliver their signals to either the inner endocardial wall, or to the outer epicardial wall. These pacing systems use various access routes, such as transvenous insertion or direct surgical implantation of the pacemaker lead electrode.

Temporary versus permanent single-chamber pacing systems differ primarily with regard to the location, accessibility, and complexity of the pulse generator. In contrast with permanent pacemakers, temporary pacemakers use an *external* pulse generator with only essential, more easily accessible control dials.

Transvenous[18,23,26,28,30,51]

The most commonly used form of single-chamber pacing is ventricular endocardial pacing using a transvenous route (Fig. 10-6).[18] The catheter is threaded into the right side of the heart using either antecubital, subclavian, jugular, or femoral veins. The tip is ideally positioned in the right ventricular apex. Temporary transvenous ventricular pacing is the most stable method of emergency pacing. It is preferred when pac-

ing for an extended period of time. Effective transvenous atrial pacing requires specialized catheters adapted to maintain contact with the smoother atrial wall. These adaptations include a J-shaped tip and spikes called *tines*. The catheter tip of an atrial catheter is ideally positioned in the right atrial appendage, which contains some trabeculae or ridges (see Dual-Chamber Pacing Systems, Fig. 10-9).

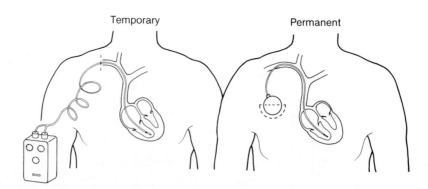

Temporary   Permanent

Fig. 10-6 Single-chamber ventricular pacing: temporary versus permanent. Catheter position is usually the same. The major difference is the location and specific characteristics of the pulse generator.

Transcutaneous[26,64,66]

Because of its high efficacy and virtual absence of complications, transcutaneous transthoracic (TC) pacing is a valuable mode of initial pacing for bradyarrhythmias. Per ACLS protocols, implementation of temporary transcutaneous pacer support is as vital as pharmacologic adjuncts for the treatment of symptomatic or unstable bradyarrhythmias. The technique of TC pacing is quick, safe, easily initiated by minimally trained persons, and offers temporary, emergency support until transvenous pacing can be initiated.

Indications for TC pacing can be categorized into immediate and prophylactic. Immediate TC pacing is indicated during asystole, symptomatic bradyarrhythmias, rhythm support of drug toxicities, or during anesthesia induction.[27a] Standby or prophylactic TC pacing may be indicated during cardiac catheterization, angioplasty, electrophysiologic testing, before and after cardioversion, during replacement of permanent pulse generator, or during insertion of a PA catheter in patients with known LBBB. In the TC pacing system, the electrode configuration (chest electrode pads) remains separate rather than within a catheter. The electrode pads are placed on the skin surface of the outer chest wall in a transverse or anteroposterior fashion (Fig. 10-7). Anteroposterior placement is most commonly used. Although neither electrode is actually in the heart, these electrode pads function as a bipolar pacing system. The electrical signal exits from the negative terminal and respective electrode, delivering the stimulus through the chest wall to both the ventricles and atria simultaneously. Ventricular activation dominates. TC pacing is contraindicated in patients with cervical spine injury and flail chest because skeletal muscle stimulation may exacerbate the injury.

Patient discomfort is the major limitation of TC pacing therapy. The degree of dis-

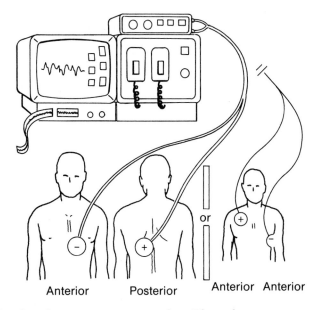

Fig. 10-7 Noninvasive transcutaneous pacing. The pulse generator may attach to cardioverter or defibrillator units as illustrated or may remain separate.

comfort correlates with the amplitude of current needed to obtain effective pacing. Increased chest wall muscle mass, chronic obstructive pulmonary disease (COPD), or pleural effusions may require increased amplitude, leading to further patient discomfort. Recent increases in the size of the electrode pads have helped to minimize output requirements and diminish discomfort.

The pulse generator of transcutaneous pacemakers may attach to cardioverter or defibrillator units as shown in Fig. 10-7 or may remain separate. An attached monitor is optional depending on the specific modes used. Most TC pacing devices feature asyn-

chronous (continuous) and demand pacing modes, as well as widely adjustable rate and current output settings. In the demand mode, the internal circuitry of the pulse generator detects QRS complexes. However, these complexes are usually sensed from the ECG pattern on the attached monitor rather than directly from the patient. Thus, in alert patients, artifact may be misinterpreted as QRS complexes.

You may select various rates and electrical current settings using adjustable dials. Pacing outputs of 75 to 200 milliamperes (mA) may be necessary to overcome the transthoracic resistance associated with TC pacing.

Direct access[17,18]

A direct access approach (thoracotomy or mediasternotomy) is used for temporary epicardial pacing after cardiac surgeries or for long-term pacing associated with the implantation of other devices such as the ICD. Thoracic surgical pacing wires are specially designed, partially insulated suture wires. They may be threaded either through the epicardial (pericardial) lining or through the sutures used to redirect the blood flow dur-

ing cardiopulmonary bypass (Fig. 10-8). Suture these wires only to the outer thoracic wall so that they may be easily removed postoperatively. A minimum of two wires in position are left postoperatively. These wires should be labeled as either atrial or ventricular. An additional skin or ground (G) electrode may be provided to allow for unipolar pacing. Unipolar pacing is most frequently used with atrial pacing (see Fig. 10-8). Nurs-

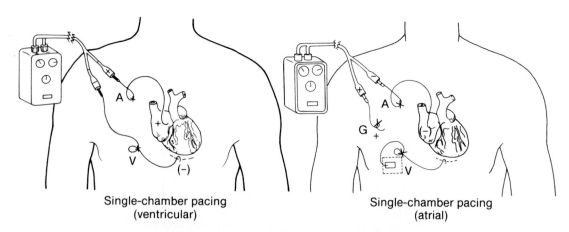

Single-chamber pacing
(ventricular)

Single-chamber pacing
(atrial)

Fig. 10-8 Thoracic surgical pacing: single chamber. An electrode from the chamber to be paced must be connected to the negative terminal of the pulse generator or extension cable. The ground (G) wire may be used to create a unipolar system for either atrial pacing, as illustrated, or ventricular pacing.[39a]

ing of the patient with thoracic epicardial wires includes (1) provision of site care, (2) correct and clear labeling of pacing wires as either atrial or ventricular, and (3) insulation of exposed endings.

Dual-chamber pacing systems[9,18,21,23,26,28,29,31,33,38,49]

Dual-chamber pacing refers to systems that stimulate both the atria and ventricles, thus maintaining normal physiologic AV synchrony. Like single-chamber pacing, these systems may be either temporary or permanent, deliver their signals to either the endocardial or epicardial wall, and use both transvenous and direct access routes.

Transvenous[17,18,23,26,28,30,51]

As in single-chamber pacing, the most commonly used form of dual-chamber pacing is endocardial pacing using a transvenous route. Use two sets of electrodes. Position one set in the atria and the other in the ventricles. These electrodes may be contained within a single catheter, within two separate catheters, within separate catheters but a single sheath, or within a PA catheter for simultaneous hemodynamic monitoring (see Unit 9). As in single-chamber ventricular pacing, the ventricular catheter tip is ideally positioned in the RV apex. The atrial catheter is often J-shaped. One may tie or prong it to facilitate its more stable position in the right atrial appendage (Fig. 10-9).

Direct access[17,18]

Dual-chamber epicardial pacing uses the direct access to the heart available during thoracic surgery. Dual-chamber external (temporary) pacing units are used frequently in conjunction with surgical pacing wires. Four wires may be used—two in the atria and two in the ventricles—mimicking bipolar pacing (Fig. 10-10). A fifth skin electrode may be provided as a ground, particularly if a unipolar atrial system is preferred.

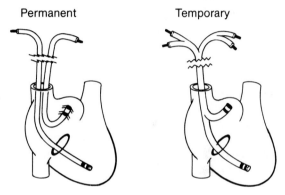

Fig. 10-9 Transvenous catheter placement: dual-chamber pacing.

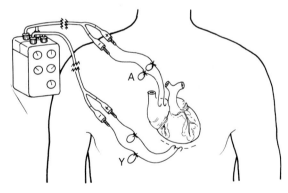

Fig. 10-10 Thoracic surgical pacing: dual-chamber.

Transesophageal[55]

Transesophageal (TE) atrial pacing can be employed to terminate select reentrant supraventricular tachyarrhythmias (SVTs), to evaluate sinus node function, or to accelerate the heart rate for the purpose of studying myocardial ischemia. TE pacing requires oral or nasal introduction of specialized leads. Because of the unreliability and severe discomfort associated with the high energy levels needed for ventricular pacing, TE pacing is not used for elective ventricular pacing.

Specific pacemaker components and function

Both the basic and more complex functions of a pacemaker are controlled by the adjustable parameters of the pulse generator.[30,51] These parameters are reflected in the control dials or buttons of temporary units and the programmable features of permanent, implanted units.

Pulse generators: single-chamber[18,30,51]

The control dials of a typical single-chamber temporary pulse generator correlate with minimal pacemaker function (Fig. 10-11). In newer computerized models, these dials are replaced by similar touchpad selections. The rate dial or selector controls stimulus release and determines the automatic (pulse) interval, or pacemaker rate, on the ECG trace. Therefore, it controls the pulse per minute. You may need to adjust an on/off switch, depending on the manufacturer. Verify that a battery pack is properly positioned within the pulse generator, since it is removable. The battery pack generates the electricity. The physician determines the initial rate at which the pacemaker is set. This rate is usually just above that at which symptoms are anticipated to disappear.

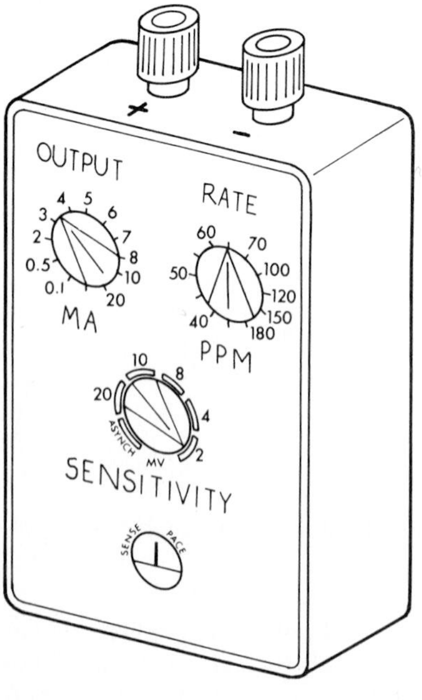

Proper catheter position and adjustment of the *output* dial or selector ensure adequate stimulus response from the myocardium. The output dial controls the strength or intensity of the electrical signal, which is determined by its milliamperage (mA). The physician determines the mA at which the pacemaker is initially set. If the initial setting is 0.2 to 0.4 mA, gradually increase the output until capture is confirmed by the ECG (see ECG Assessment: Normal Function). The output may also be initially set at a higher level of 5 mA and gradually lowered (see Thresholds).

The third key dial or selector controls sensing.[18] The property of sensing may be added, depending on the specific mode of pacing selected. In the inhibited or demand mode, sensing is required. Since ventricular demand pacing is currently the most common mode of temporary pacing, the sensing dial will usually be adjusted. Increase sensing

Fig. 10-11 Pulse generator: single-chamber.

by turning the dial away from the asynchronous position. Sensitivity is the strength of the myocardial signals, usually in millivolts (mV), detectable by the pacemaker. If the pacemaker detects weaker signals (less than 2 mV) as well as strong ones, it is more sensitive. Therefore, if numbers are provided on the sensing dial, the lower numbers indicate greater sensitivity and correspond to positions farther from the asynchronous position. In the newer computerized models only the numbers appear.

Pulse generators: dual-chamber[18,26,29,33]

Temporary dual-chamber pulse generators have four terminals for catheter connection (Fig. 10-12). Two terminals connect to a bipolar atrial catheter or its equivalent. The other two terminals connect to a bipolar ventricular catheter or its equivalent. Both DVI and DDD temporary units are currently

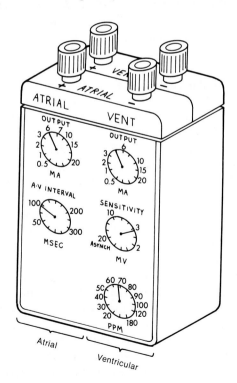

Fig. 10-12 Pulse generator: dual-chamber (DVI).

Pace and sense indicators are provided on external pacing units. The pace indicator moves or lights as each stimulus is released. Released stimuli are visible and best confirmed on the ECG. The sense indicator moves or lights as each stimulus is inhibited as the result of proper sensing. Proper sensing is often assumed with adequate rates but is difficult to confirm on the ECG if paced beats are not seen. One may monitor the sense indicator for reassurance, but accuracy is best obtained from the ECG trace.

available. They are most popular in patients after cardiac surgery.

The DVI unit is the older and simpler model (see Fig. 10-12). The key to the DVI unit is the ventricular component. The dials/selectors of the ventricular component are identical to those of single-chamber units. Stimulus release in the atria, or the atria rate, is determined by both the ventricular rate and *AV interval* dials. The AV interval dial allows for the release of the atrial spike at a prescribed time before each ventricular spike, establishing an artificial P–R interval. The AV internal dial is usually set between 120 and 200 milliseconds (msec). This is the equivalent of 0.12 to 0.20 seconds, the normal P–R interval. Stimulus response in the atria is controlled by an output dial similar to its ventricular parallel. An atrial sensing dial is not provided since only ventricular sensing occurs in the DVI mode.

The temporary DDD unit is the most versatile, but complex, temporary pacing unit.[21,22,49,54] Both the DDD and DVI units can function as single- as well as dual-chamber pacing units by not utilizing the atrial component. However, the DDD pulse generator has many extra features previously available only in permanent implanted or experimental models. The DDD unit initially defaults to the most commonly used VVI or DDD modes (Fig. 10-13). Multiple

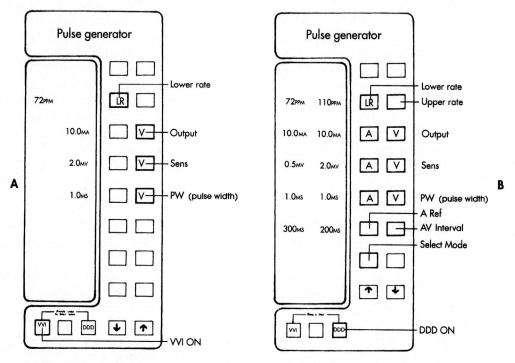

Fig. 10-13 Pulse generator: dual-chamber (DDD). This pulse generator may be used as either a single-chamber (**A**) or dual-chamber (**B**) pacemaker.

modes are available, however, in the model illustrated in Fig. 10-13 by simultaneously pressing the select mode button on the front and the parameter change button on the side. When in the VVI mode, the parameters appearing on the screen are very similar to those available on single-chamber pulse generators (see Fig. 10-11). The ventricular rate selector is called the *lower rate* (LR) rather than pulse per minute. The major difference is the control of stimulus response by pulse width, or stimulus duration as well as output (mA) or strength. Pulse width has been used in permanent pacers for years. In the DDD mode, as in the previously discussed DVI units, the atrial rate and artificial P–R interval are determined from the AV interval option. Stimulus response is controlled by both pulse width and amplitude selectors as on the

ventricular component. A key feature added in the DDD mode is an atrial sensing selector. Since atrial sensing in this mode triggers a ventricular impulse, fast atrial rates could, potentially, result in fast ventricular rates. For this reason, an upper rate limit selector is provided. The atrial refractory period selector also protects against pacemaker tachycardia while in the DDD mode (see Pacemaker-Induced and Pacemaker-Mediated Arrhythmias). As the values decrease for atrial and ventricular sensitivity, the sensitivity increases (i.e., the lower the number, the greater the sensitivity). To provide continuous or asynchronous pacing, turn the sensitivity off by increasing the numbers to their highest setting. The VOO or DOO modes may also be selected more easily by using "select mode" option. Other antitachycardia features are also provided.

Thresholds

The pacing *threshold* is the minimum energy necessary to depolarize or activate myocardial tissue. It is determined and influenced by many factors including the contact, or interface, between the electrode tip and the myocardium, the duration of the pacing stimulus, the design characteristics of the stimulating electrode, and physiologic, metabolic, and pharmacologic effects on myocardial tissue.[45,65] Thresholds are obtained and evaluated clinically by determining the minimum voltage, or MA, producing capture on the ECG pattern (see ECG Assessment: Normal Function). When caring for a patient with a temporary pacemaker, even if on standby, attach the pacing system and check thresholds, along with effective pacing and sensing, at least once per shift. A lower threshold usually indicates a more stable catheter position. Higher thresholds, although sometimes necessary, may result in chest wall twitching and patient discomfort.

Contact between the tip of the pacing catheter and myocardial tissue and resultant threshold levels are more likely to vary with temporary transvenous pacing, where the interface is less stable.[18,45] Variations in pacing thresholds of permanently implanted pacer wires (as well as temporary catheters) are well documented. At implantation, a pacemaker demonstrates its lowest pacing threshold because the electrode is in direct contact with excitable myocardial tissue. During the first 2 to 12 postoperative or postinsertion weeks, the pacing threshold rises to its highest level (three to four times initial energy requirements) because of localized myocardial edema and inflammatory reaction at the electrode interface. As the inflammatory process subsides (after approximately 6 months), a fibrous capsule forms at the catheter tip and the stimulation threshold decreases. This threshold stabilizes at a level two to three times higher than that observed immediately after implantation.[18,45]

To compensate for similar threshold variations after temporary pacer insertion, set the voltage, or mA, of any newly inserted temporary pulse generator at double the energy required for initial capture. To compensate for changes in pacing thresholds of permanent pacemakers, set the pulse amplitude at 5 to 10 times the minimum voltage required to capture the myocardium. Change these settings later to twice the initial settings.

Thresholds may increase as a result of certain metabolic disorders (hypoxia, ischemia, acid-base disorders, hyperglycemia, and hypercapnia), the effects of pharmacologic agents (beta blockers, Ca^{++} channel blockers, class 1A antiarrhythmics), increases in intracellular K^+, and normal physiologic processes (sleeping and eating). Conversely, thresholds, or energy requirements for capture, decrease with exercise. Future pacemakers will be able to automatically detect loss of capture secondary to threshold changes and adjust their output accordingly.[18,29,38]

Reprogramming and interrogating

Permanently implanted pulse generators are more complicated to evaluate and adjust than temporary units. These units are initially set in the operating room by the physician. They are evaluated in the coronary care unit (CCU) or progressive care area. Evaluation includes assessment of the ECG pattern on both rhythm and 12-lead ECG traces using a pacemaker magnet, as indicated (see Magnetic Rates and Evaluation of Catheter Position). Implanted pulse generators are adjusted by external reprogramming. A variety of modes and specific functional parameters may be readjusted or reprogrammed, depending on the manufacturer's specifications.[18] Many of these parameters are unfamiliar to the average coronary care nurse, who works to a greater

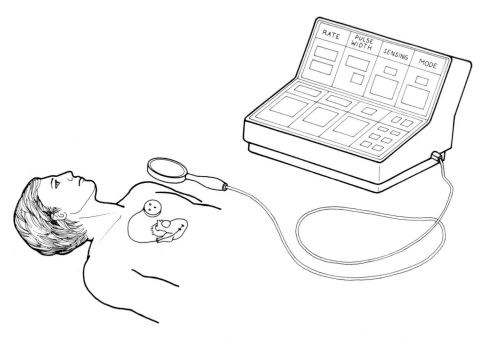

Fig. 10-14   Reprogramming and interrogating permanent pacemakers.

extent with external units that may have only three adjustable dials/selectors. Keep frequently used manufacturer's specifications on file. Common programmable parameters include pulse width and refractory periods, in addition to routine parameters such as rate, output, and sensitivity.[38]

You should be familiar with the general purpose and function of an external programming unit; however, reprogramming is reserved for the physician, manufacturer, or pacemaker nurse specialist trained and experienced in the use of specific units. Unlike pacemaker magnets, programming units are manufacturer-specific and sometimes model-specific. A bedside recorder is preferred during the procedure. The programmer wand is applied over the area of the implanted pulse generator. The desired adjustment is then selected on the computerized programming module (Fig. 10-14) and is verified by the ECG pattern. Pacemakers may also be evaluated initially after reprogramming and at designated intervals by *interrogation*. Interrogation is a commonly available feature whereby a computer printout of the currently set parameters is obtained using the same programming equipment.

Transtelephonic monitoring[62]

Pacemaker follow-up is essential for successful long-term management of patients with pacemakers, especially those with complex dual-chamber pacemakers. Although there are a number of electrocardiographic techniques that enable the pacemaker nurse or physician to assess pacemaker function in the ambulatory patient, the most significant of these is transtelephonic monitoring. Transtelephonic monitoring is used in conjunction with outpatient visits to the pacemaker clinic where physical examination and programming manipulations are performed. Specialized telephone equipment allows the patient to transmit information in between visits to a pacemaker center. Vital information such as the pacing rate, effective capture and sensing, magnetic rate, and pulse width is elicited and evaluated. Unfortunately, no physical examination is possible, and reprogramming activities cannot be carried out.

Magnetic rates

The placement of a magnet over the pulse generator inactivates the sensing mechanism, creating a fixed-rate mode of pacing, known as the magnet rate.[18] In the absence of sensing, the pacemaker fires automatically. This allows you to evaluate the pacing rate and to indirectly assess battery life. Under normal conditions, the magnet rate is usually equal to or slightly faster than the basic automatic rate but is manufacturer dependent. When the rate of the pacemaker generator decreases by 7% to 10% or increases by more than a few beats per minute, replace the generator. Many programmable pacing systems reveal end of battery life by magnet application only, although interrogation also identifies reduced battery voltage.

ECG assessment: normal function[7,18,27,57–59,67]

The ECG is the foundation for pacemaker function assessment. Since normal pacemaker function involved the release of a stimulus, a response to the stimulus, and, frequently, some level of intracardiac sensing, systematic ECG assessment should evaluate at least these parameters.

Stimulus release is indicated by a sharp, narrow deflection (pacing spike) on the ECG. In temporary units, the pace indicator should flash each time a pacemaker spike appears on the ECG. The *automatic,* or pacing, *interval* (interval from spike to spike) corresponds roughly to the rate at which the pacemaker is set to fire on the pulse generator, as well as the prescribed rate (Fig. 10-15). The automatic interval is also called the pulse interval.

In single-chamber pacemakers, the presence of a QRS complex (or P wave) following each pacing spike indicates myocardial response to the pacing stimulus. This response is called ventricular (or atrial) *capture* (Fig. 10-16, *A* and *B*) and indicates the chamber paced. Since a paced impulse does not follow normal conduction pathways, the QRS complex following a ventricular spike is typically wider than and morphologically different from the patient's native QRS complex. P waves following atrial spikes are often not clearly visible (see Fig. 10-16 and Atrial Pacing [AOO/AAI]). The subsequent QRS morphology may provide a clue to atrial capture. Spikes consistently followed by narrow, unchanging QRS complexes after a short delay suggest supraventricular or atrial pacing.

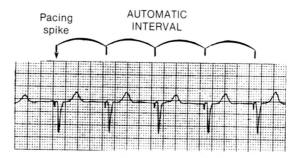

Fig. 10-15 Stimulus release. Normal stimulus release is illustrated by the presence of pacing spikes. The rate of the pacemaker is determined from two pacing spikes, also referred to as the automatic or pulse interval. In this example, the pacemaker is firing at a rate of 72.

A Ventricular

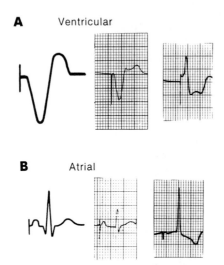

B Atrial

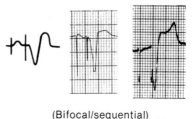

(Bifocal/sequential)

NOTE: The p wave following the atrial spike is usually difficult to see.

Fig. 10-17 Stimulus release/response (capture): dual-chamber pacemakers.

Fig. 10-16 Stimulus response (capture). In single-chamber ventricular pacing, a wide, distorted QRS complex normally follows the spike **(A)**. In single-chamber atrial pacing, a P wave normally follows the spike **(B)** but is often difficult to see. The related QRS complex is narrow and unchanging.

In dual-chamber pacemakers, two pacing spikes appear on the ECG (Fig. 10-17). The second (ventricular) spike should be followed by a QRS complex. The first (atrial) spike should be followed by a P wave. However, as in single-chamber atrial pacing, this P wave is often not clearly visible regardless of the lead. In dual-chamber pacing, the QRS complex configuration is not helpful in confirming atrial capture since it is distorted by the simultaneous ventricular pacing. Actual validation of atrial activity may require esophageal leads, atrial electrograms, or echocardiographic visualization of atrial contraction. Assume atrial capture to be present unless there is clear evidence to the contrary or atrial fibrillation occurs. Since the two spikes fire in sequence,

each activating a different chamber of the heart, dual-chamber pacemakers are also known as *bifocal* or *AV sequential*.

Sensing depends on the mode of pacing selected.[7,18,27,67] The sensing mechanism allows the pacemaker to receive signals from the patient's natural impulses. These signals are then interpreted by the pulse generator and result in altered stimulus release. In demand pacing, the stimulus is inhibited and remains dormant when sensing occurs. If the sensing electrodes are within the ventricle, the pacemaker senses the presence of QRS complexes. If the sensing electrodes are within the atrium, the pacemaker senses the presence of P waves. The automatic, or pacing, interval is reset by any sensed beats; therefore, there will be a pause between a sensed beat and the next paced beat. This interval is called the *escape interval,* and it usually equals the automatic interval (Fig. 10-18). If a second natural impulse occurs before the lapsed time, it may again inhibit and reset the pacemaker. If another impulse does not occur, the pacemaker escapes and automatically fires at an interval corresponding to the minimum, or lower, rate limit.

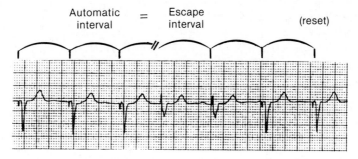

Automatic interval = Escape interval   (reset)

Fig. 10-18 Sensing. In ventricular demand pacing, normal sensing is confirmed when natural QRS complexes inhibit the pacing spike and reset the automatic interval.

Ventricular pacing (VOO/VVI)[18,23,26,28]

In VVI, or QRS-inhibited (demand) ventricular pacing, pacing spikes are immediately followed by QRS complexes, confirming that the ventricle is the chamber paced and that the pacemaker is in capture. Natural QRS complexes inhibit and reset the automatic (pacing) interval, confirming the presence of ventricular sensing and the inhibited mode of response (Fig. 10-19). The reset, or escape, interval is typically equal to the automatic interval. In VOO, or continuous (asynchronous) ventricular pacing, the pattern of stimulus release and ventricular capture is identical. However, since there is no sensing, natural QRS complexes do not inhibit the pacing spikes or reset the automatic interval. As a result, a pacing spike may occur on the vulnerable period (T wave) of a native beat and ventricular tachycardia or fibrillation may be induced (see ECG Assessment: Abnormal and Pseudoabnormal Function).

Atrial pacing (AOO/AAI)[18,23,26,28]

In AOO, or continuous (asynchronous) atrial pacing, pacing spikes followed by P waves or, after a short pause, by QRS complexes suggest a supraventricular origin. This pattern confirms that the atrium is the chamber paced. However, since sensing does not occur, natural P waves do not inhibit or reset the automatic interval (Fig. 10-20).

Spikes may appear after a natural P wave. As a result, atrial fibrillation may be induced. In AAI, or atrial demand pacing, the major ECG difference is the inhibition and resetting of the pacing rate by natural P waves. This pattern is seen in thoracic pacing or permanent pacing systems.

Dual-chamber pacing: DVI[18,23,26,28]

In DVI pacing, two pacing spikes are either intermittently or consistently seen, suggesting that stimuli are released, pacing both the atria and ventricles. The distance between the atrial spike and the ventricular spike is the AV interval. It refers to the time from beginning of atrial activation to beginning of ventricular activation, acting as an artificial P–R interval. Note this interval at the time that stimulus release is evaluated. When stimulus response is adequate, a QRS complex should follow the second (ventricular) spike and a P wave should follow the first (atrial) spike (Fig. 10-21). However, as

Identification code (1981)

Chamber paced	Chamber sensed	Mode of response	Programmable functions	Special tachyarrhythmia functions
V	V	I	Varies with manufacturer	

A

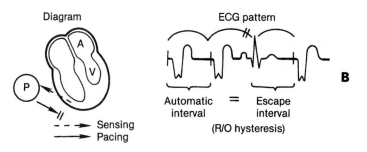

Diagram

ECG pattern

--- → Sensing
——→ Pacing

Automatic interval = Escape interval
(R/O hysteresis)

B

ECG TRACE: NORMAL FUNCTION

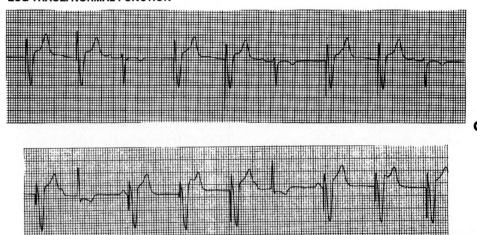

C

Fig. 10-19 Normal ventricular demand (VVI) pacing. The variations in the height of the pacemaker spikes are commonly seen and are probably caused by respiratory artifact.

	Chamber paced	Chamber sensed	Mode of response	Programmable functions	Special tachyarrhythmia functions
A	A	O	O	Varies with manufacturer	

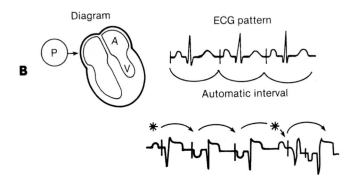

Diagram

ECG pattern

B

Automatic interval

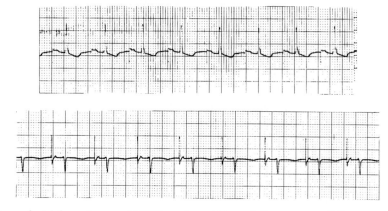

C   **ECG TRACE: NORMAL FUNCTION**

Fig. 10-20   Normal atrial continuous (AOO) pacing. Although P waves are difficult to see following the pacing spikes **(C)**, the presence of related narrow, unchanging QRS complexes suggests a supraventricular (atrial) origin.

with single-chamber atrial pacemakers, the P waves are not apparent following the atrial spike.

All dual-chamber pacers sense ventricular impulses and are QRS inhibited. Naturally occurring QRS complexes can completely in-hibit both pacing spikes (Fig. 10-21). The interval from a paced or natural QRS complex to the atrial spike is the VA interval and is used by many pacemaker manufacturers and clinicians to evaluate effective ventricular sensing (Fig. 10-22). The VA interval is a

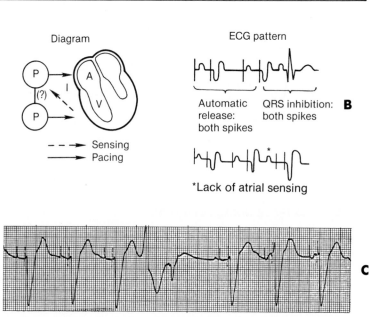

Identification code (1981)

Chamber paced	Chamber sensed	Mode of response	Programmable functions	Special tachyarrhythmia functions
D	V	I	Varies with manufacturer	

A

Diagram

ECG pattern

Automatic release: both spikes   QRS inhibition: both spikes   **B**

--- → Sensing
— → Pacing

*Lack of atrial sensing

C

Fig. 10-21 Normal dual-chamber DVI pacing. Note the presence of ventricular sensing only.

calculated parameter. It is determined in most pacemakers by subtracting the AV interval from the pacer R–R (automatic or pulse) interval. We prefer to focus on the AV interval since it is a directly set parameter. This approach also works effectively in problem solving. Lack of atrial sensing is normal in DVI pacing as indicated by the second letter of the pacing code. Thus, an atrial spike may normally appear after a natural P wave (see Fig. 10-21).

In most currently available temporary and permanent dual-chamber pacemakers, ventricular sensing may occur within the AV in-

terval, or after the atrial spike has already been released. QRS complexes occurring after the release of the atrial spike but before the ventricular spike is due may still inhibit the second, ventricular spike. This phenomenon appears on the ECG as intermittent single-chamber atrial pacing (Fig. 10-23).

When sensing occurs freely within the AV interval, large atrial spikes may be interpreted as ventricular impulses by the pacemaker with subsequent inhibition of the second, most critical, ventricular spike. This phenomenon is called *crosstalk* or *far-field sensing* and occurs more frequently with unipolar

470

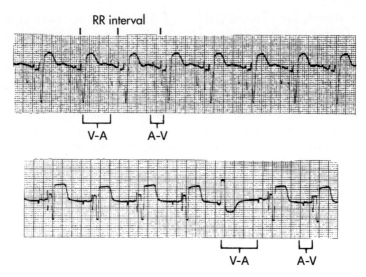

Fig. 10-22 VA interval: evaluating ventricular sensing (VA interval = pacer RR interval − AV interval).

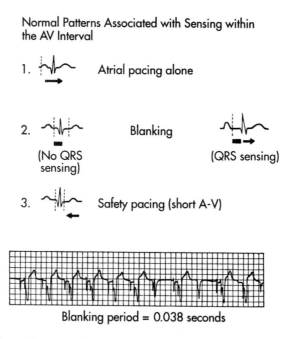

Normal Patterns Associated with Sensing within the AV Interval

1. Atrial pacing alone

2. Blanking
   (No QRS sensing)   (QRS sensing)

3. Safety pacing (short A-V)

Blanking period = 0.038 seconds

Fig. 10-23 Effects of normal sensing within the AV interval and blanking periods. Selective inhibition of ventricular spikes may mimic atrial pacing (1). QRS complexes immediately following the initial (atrial) spike may not be sensed if within the blanking period (2) or may trigger a short AV interval in some models (3). Similar patterns may be seen in DDD pacing when natural P waves do not occur.

pacing since larger stimuli are emitted (see ECG Assessment: Abnormal and Pseudoabnormal Function).[18] Unfortunately, unipolar catheters are commonly used for permanent dual-chamber pacing. To avoid this complication, an extra programmable feature is available on implantable pulse generators. The sensing ability is blocked or "blanked out" for a short period early in the AV interval, referred to as a *blanking period*. QRS complexes occurring within this blanking period are not sensed and thus allow spikes to appear after the QRS complexes (see Fig. 10-23). This infrequent pattern is usually accepted as normal. However, if the AV interval is longer, spikes may fall on the T wave and risk inducing VF. If this occurs, the blanking and/or AV interval may be shortened, the blanking interval may be eliminated, or the system may be reprogrammed to single-chamber pacing.

Unipolar atrial pacing used in temporary pacing after open heart surgery may also induce crosstalk. However, temporary pulse generators do not have blanking intervals or safety pacing. Conversion to a bipolar or single-chamber system will correct the problem in this setting. Ventricular *safety pacing* is provided by at least two popular pacemaker manufacturers in implanted units. It provides an alternative to prevent crosstalk when blanking is ineffective or produces complications of its own.[3,18] The blanking process itself may increase the sensitivity of the pacer to electrical interference in the period immediately after it. With safety pacing, a signal sensed during the crosstalk detection period in the first portion of the AV interval triggers a ventricular output at an abbreviated AV interval. Risk of an "R on T" phenomenon is avoided (see Fig. 10-23). This variation of the AV interval is the diagnostic hallmark on the ECG. Another helpful diagnostic clue is that the shorter AV interval in safety pacing is always 110 msec or 0.11 second.

Dual-chamber pacing: DDD[18]

The ECG patterns of stimulus release, stimulus response, and *ventricular* sensing occurring with DDD pacing are identical to those seen in DVI pacing. Two spikes are released, resulting in a paced AV interval. Ventricular capture is confirmed by a QRS complex immediately after the second (ventricular) spike. Both spikes may be inhibited by QRS complexes occurring before the first (atrial) spike. Patterns mimicking atrial pacing may appear when the ventricular spikes are inhibited by QRS complexes occurring after the atrial spike has been released but within the AV interval (Fig. 10-24). Patterns associated with blanking intervals and safety pacing may also occur with implantable DDD pulse generators.

DDD pacing differs from DVI pacing primarily by the added feature of atrial sensing and tracking. This feature is confirmed by its typical ECG pattern. Atrial sensing prevents the atrial competition and fibrillation seen with DVI pacing. It also provides the necessary ingredient for P wave tracking. When natural P waves are sensed, the atrial spikes are inhibited and the pacemaker converts immediately to atrial triggered (synchronized) pacing or *P wave tracking*. The atrial triggered or tracking mode allows the pacemaker to increase its ventricular rate in response to increased sinus (P wave) rates, further maximizing cardiac output (Fig. 10-25). The resulting ECG pattern intermittently mimics single-chamber ventricular pacing. However, the paced ventricular beats are related to preceding P waves at fixed intervals. The rate of the ventricular spikes normally varies according to the rate of the naturally occurring P waves. The dual response to sensing (inhibited [QRS/P] and triggered)

Dual-sensing, dual function (demand) AV sequential bifocal pacemaker (universal pacing) = DDD

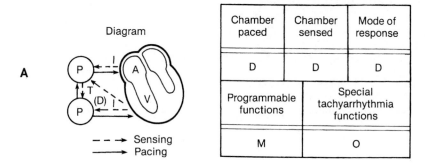

Diagram

--- → Sensing
— → Pacing

Identification code (1981)

Chamber paced	Chamber sensed	Mode of response
D	D	D
Programmable functions	Special tachyarrhythmia functions	
M	O	

ECG PATTERN:

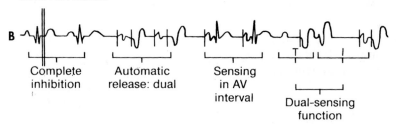

Complete inhibition | Automatic release: dual | Sensing in AV interval | Dual-sensing function

Fig. 10-24 Normal dual chamber DDD pacing. Note the presence of atrial, as well as ventricular, sensing.

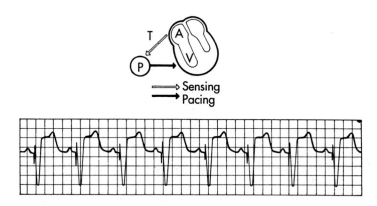

⇒ Sensing
→ Pacing

Fig. 10-25 Atrial sensing and P wave tracking. Note the disappearance of the atrial spike and the constant P to ventricular pacing spike intervals.

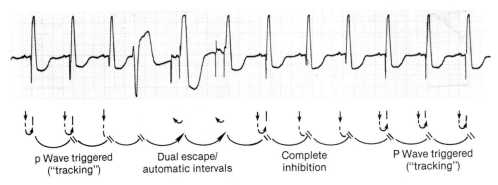

| p Wave triggered ("tracking") | Dual escape/ automatic intervals | Complete inhibition | P Wave triggered ("tracking") |

Fig. 10-26   Summary of common ECG patterns of DDD pacing.

confirms the function described by the third letter of this pacemaker's code. The most

common normal ECG patterns of DDD pacing are summarized in Fig. 10-26.

ECG assessment: abnormal and pseudoabnormal function[7,18,27,67]

The major problems resulting from pacemaker malfunction can be classified as follows: (1) problems related to stimulus release, (2) problems related to stimulus response (capture), (3) problems related to sensing, (4) arrhythmias in pacing, and (5) pseudomalfunctions.

Due to the advanced technology of current pacing systems and multiple programmable functions, not all causes of pacemaker malfunction are easily detected. Failure to sense the intracardiac signal warrants investigation. Cessation of output (stimulus release) and failure to capture are the most potentially dangerous abnormalities encountered in pacemaker-dependent patients.

Stimulus release

Improper stimulus release may be manifested by gross variations in the pacing interval (Fig. 10-27). This phenomenon should be reported as a possible sign of battery and/or pulse generator failure, especially with implanted units. Emergency intervention is not required. When marked acceleration of the stimulus occurs, the pacing unit is referred to as a runaway pacemaker. This problem occurs primarily with permanent pacemakers and requires immediate attention (Fig. 10-28). A magnet may be applied to break the rapid delivery of stimuli until the unit can be interrogated or replaced. In a temporary, external unit, disconnect the pacing unit to terminate arrhythmia.

Improper stimulus release is also mani-

fested by intermittent or sustained absence of pacing stimuli. This pattern can indicate unstable connections between the catheter and pulse generator, catheter fracture, battery depletion, or oversensing (Fig. 10-29). Oversensing is the inappropriate sensing of unwanted signals, which results in inhibition of pacer output. Musculoskeletal myopotentials, external electromagnetic signals, and false signals arising from within the pacing lead system may interfere with sensing function. Electrical activity generated by the contraction of chest wall muscles may reach 3 to 4 mV. This voltage can be detected by the highly sensitive electrodes of a unipolar system, causing inhibition of pacing output. This problem is prevalent in unipolar pacing

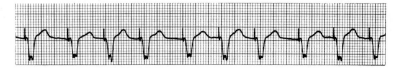

Fig. 10-27 Abnormal stimulus release: variations in spike interval.

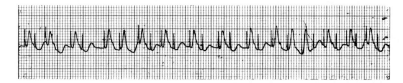

Fig. 10-28 Abnormal stimulus release: runaway pacemaker.

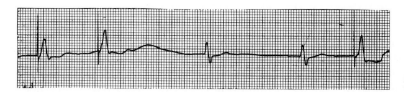

Fig. 10-29 Abnormal stimulus release: intermittent absence of pacing spike.

systems because of the proximity of the anode to the pectoral skeletal muscles and because of the enhanced potential for interference in a unipolar system. To manage myopotential inhibition, reprogram or convert the pacemaker catheters to a bipolar system and/or reduce the sensitivity setting.[7,18,27,67]

Environmental sources of electromagnetic interference can also inhibit pacemaker output; other abnormal responses include conversion from demand pacing to asynchronous pacing. Arc welders, large engines, electrocautery devices, and high-frequency transmitters are some of the devices that interfere with pacemaker function. However, because of combined regulatory standards for microwave oven strength and leakage and the shielding of pacing generator and lead systems, electromagnetic interference from microwave ovens has been virtually eliminated.[3,7] Magnetic resonance imaging should be avoided in patients with permanent pacemakers because it can actually reprogram, dislodge or destroy pulse generator components.

Crosstalk or far-field sensing is a special form of oversensing occurring with dual-chamber pacemakers.[18,23,26,28,38] It usually involves ventricular sensing of atrial pacing signals with subsequent inhibition of ventricular pacing. Only a single pacing spike appears. However, unlike normal P wave tracking where a P wave precedes the single ventricular spikes at a fixed interval, the P wave follows this spike, confirming its atrial origin (Fig. 10-30). When P waves are difficult to see, the atrial origin of the single spike may be confirmed by comparing it to the previous atrial spike interval or atrial escape (V−A) interval. Crosstalk is a more frequent problem in unipolar atrial pacing because of the magnitude of the atrial pacing spike and

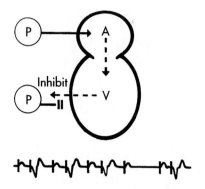

Fig. 10-30 Crosstalk. The large atrial spike is sensed as a QRS complex inhibiting the ventricular spike. The atrial spike can appear out of capture if P waves are not visible.

increased chance of sensing by the ventricular lead. High atrial outputs combined with high ventricular sensitivity settings almost guarantee crosstalk. Bipolar lead configuration is recommended for all dual-chamber pacemakers.[6b] Crosstalk demands immediate attention, since it is potentially life-threatening for the pacemaker-dependent individual.

Crosstalk can be managed in implanted systems by programming a ventricular *blanking* period or extending it. In the presence of a blanking period, the ventricular sensing mechanism is temporarily disabled after release of the atrial pacing stimulus. Crosstalk can also be avoided by ventricular safety pacing windows (see Dual-Chamber Pacing: DVI). A signal sensed during this crosstalk detection period triggers a premature ventricular output at an abbreviated AV interval.

Stimulus response (capture)[7,18,21,49,61,67]

Capture, or myocardial stimulation, depends on the interface between the stimulating electrode(s) and the myocardium. Failure to capture is defined by the presence of a pacing stimulus not followed by a myocardial re-

NURSING ORDERS: For problems with stimulus release[7,18,21,49,61,67]

1. With external (temporary) units, verify that the battery pack is inside the pulse generator, since such packs are currently removable. This is a possible solution when no spikes are released.
2. Check the integrity of the catheter and connections between the catheter and pulse generator, especially the negative terminal.
3. Evaluate the adequacy of the patient's own rhythm: is the patient symptomatic? Have an epinephrine drip on standby and/or have atropine available.
4. To test for oversensing:
   —With external (temporary) units, turn down the sensitivity by adjusting the sensitivity dial or selector, and note the effect on the pauses.
   —With internal (implanted) units, apply the pacemaker magnet over the pulse generator site as a test and note the effect on pauses. Remove the magnet if competition occurs and report to physician. Reapply only if patient is symptomatic from pauses and maintain in place until unit can be reprogrammed.
5. To correct oversensing:
   —With external (temporary) units, turn down the sensitivity dial and replace the battery pack and/or pulse generator. If the system is unipolar and convertible to bipolar, convert it.
   —With internal (implanted) units, reprogram sensitivity down if trained to do so, or contact the physician and/or discuss possible replacement of the pulse generator if the system is not unipolar.

sponse. When a ventricular pacemaker is *out of capture*, the pacing spike fails to produce a QRS complex (Fig. 10-31, *A*). This pattern may also be referred to as *loss of capture*. When an atrial pacemaker is out of capture,

476

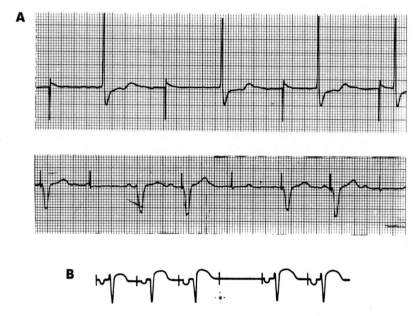

Fig. 10-31 Abnormal stimulus response: out of capture. Ventricular pacemaker out of capture (A), atrial pacemaker out of capture (B).

the pacing spike fails to produce a P wave (Fig. 10-31, *B*). One common cause of loss of capture is an increase in pacing threshold or energy requirements necessary for myocardial depolarization. Contact of the pacing electrode with electrically inactive myocardium may impair impulse transmission, preventing capture. Obtaining ventricular capture may be difficult in the presence of congestive heart failure with intra- and intercellular myocardial edema, metabolic disturbances such as hypoxia, hypercapnia, ischemia, acid-base or electrolyte disturbances, and drugs such as the type I antiarrhythmic agents, verapamil, propanolol, and insulin.

Failure to capture may also occur if stimulating energy is lost before reaching the pacing electrode(s). This may be caused by wire fracture, breaks in lead insulation, or poor generator-electrode connection. Other causes of capture loss are catheter movement or displacement (especially in the first few weeks af-

ter implantation), battery depletion (years after implantation), or myocardial perforation. Ventricular perforation is an uncommon cause of loss of capture and is often accompanied by hiccups (caused by diaphragmatic pacing). Perforation occurs most commonly during insertion or in the first week after insertion.

Since the most common cause of loss of capture is increased pacing thresholds, increasing the pacemaker output or mA usually corrects the problem. If this does not restore consistent capture, reposition the lead either by repositioning the patient or by having the physician reposition it directly. When capture loss is due to battery depletion, replace the pulse generator.

NURSING ORDERS: For problems with stimulus response (capture)
1. With external (temporary) units:
   —Increase the voltage or mA by adjusting the output dial.
   —Reposition the patient.

—Check adherence of transcutaneous electrodes.

—Change the battery pack and/or pulse generator.

—Call the physician to reposition the catheter.

2. With internal (implanted units):

—Reprogram the output if trained to do so or notify the physician and/or discuss possible replacement of the pulse generator.

Sensing[18,27]

The third component of pacemaker malfunction is abnormal sensing. Sensing mechanisms allow the pacemaker to sense the patient's own natural impulses. Generally, sensing malfunctions can be categorized as undersensing and oversensing. Oversensing results in inhibition of the pacing stimuli and is thus more appropriately classified as a problem with stimulus release (see Stimulus Release).

Undersensing is a failure to sense intracardiac signals. It occurs when the pacemaker generator does not adequately sense natural atrial or ventricular signals and consequently does not inhibit its output. Undersensing is most frequently related to pulse generator failure but can also be caused by catheter dislodgement or fracture, loose electrical connections, or poor lead contact with the myocardial tissue. When the sensing mechanism fails, the pacemaker fires without regard for the patient's own beats or rhythm. A pacing spike may fall within the vulnerable period of the cardiac cycle or T wave, precipitating abnormal firing or fibrillation. Complete ventricular activation by the natural beat is usually required to inhibit and reset the pacing spike. Undersensing in a ventricular pacemaker appears as a spike or spikes released after a fully formed QRS complex.

Failure of the sensing mechanism may be manifested by failure to sense occasional im-

3. Evaluate the adequacy of the underlying rhythm: is the patient symptomatic?

—Obtain an order for standby atropine or epinephrine or have transcutaneous pacer at bedside.

—If the patient loses consciousness, start supportive cardiopulmonary resuscitation.

4. With bipolar pacing, try switching polarity.

pulses (Fig. 10-32, *B*) or failure to sense an entire series of beats or rhythm. The pacemaker then competes with the patient for control of the rhythm. This phenomenon is known as *competition* (Fig. 10-32, *A*). With dual-chamber pacemakers, loss of sensing appears as *two* spikes after a fully formed QRS complex (Fig. 10-33). Before assuming malfunction, verify that the pacemaker is not set on continuous mode and that the sensitivity dial has not been accidentally turned off (set on asynchronous).

If undersensing problems are detected in external pulse generators, adjust the sensitivity setting to a more sensitive value. In implanted devices, telemetric communication through a programmer can help to determine the magnitude of the cardiac signal that is being sensed. Sensitivity levels may be increased accordingly.

NURSING ORDERS: For failure to sense/undersensing[10,61,67]

1. Make sure that the pacemaker is not set on the continuous mode.

2. Increase sensitivity by adjusting the sensitivity dial or by reprogramming.

3. Reposition the patient.

4. With failure to sense occasional beats:

—Turn up the pacemaker rate to override.

—Administer lidocaine if the beat is ventricular.

—Change the pulse generator or battery.

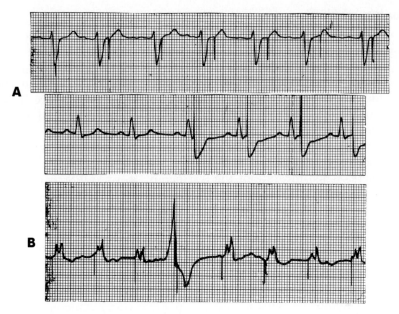

Fig. 10-32 Undersensing: single-chamber ventricular pacing.

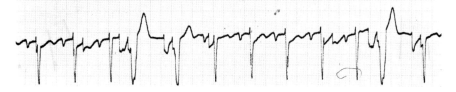

Fig. 10-33 Undersensing: dual-chamber pacing.

5. If the system is bipolar, convert it to unipolar by connecting the positive terminal of the pacemaker to an electrode on the body surface instead of to the proximal catheter electrode (Fig. 10-34).

6. In the presence of sustained loss of sensing or competition:
   —Turn the pacemaker off.
   —Change the pulse generator or battery.

Fig. 10-34 Converting bipolar systems to unipolar. Only one functional electrode remains inside the heart. The catheter end attached to the positive terminal is disconnected and capped, and the negative terminal remains connected to the electrode inside the heart. The positive terminal is connected to a skin or ground electrode.

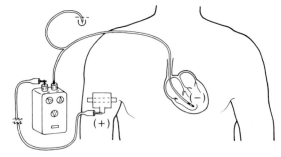

Pseudomalfunctions[3,7,18,53]

Normal pacemaker function that is associated with abnormal-appearing QRS complexes or QRS complex timing is also known as *pseudomalfunction*. The distorted QRS complexes include fusion beats, pseudofusion beats, some transcutaneous pacing patterns, and hysteresis. Fusion beats are the most common form of pseudomalfunction and are typically seen in ventricular or dual-chamber pacemakers. When the rate of the underlying cardiac rhythm (native complexes) is about the same as that of a ventricular pacemaker, or ventricular ectopic complexes, fusion beats can occur. In ventricular endocardial pacing, when the pacing or sensing electrodes are optimally positioned in the right ventricular apex, natural ventricular impulses cannot be sensed until they have completely activated the ventricles and reached the apex. Fusion beats are normal and result from two foci competing for simultaneous depolarization of the same chamber, producing a blending of the two initiating impulses and complexes on the surface ECG (Fig. 10-35). This mutual activation distorts the QRS complex after the pacing artifact or spike and can resemble both the sinus and pacemaker complexes or sinus and ectopic complexes in morphology and in timing (see Unit 6). Assume any change in QRS morphology after a pacemaker spike to be normal and representative of a fusion complex. True loss of sensing (abnormal function) appears as a spike *after* fully formed QRS complexes.

Pseudofusion beats occur when a pacemaker artifact is superimposed on a spontaneous P or QRS complex without any change in the morphology of the native complex.[18,53] Pseudofusion beats occur intermittently. Because the pacing stimulus is delivered after the chamber has already been spontaneously depolarized, the stimulus fails to generate an electrical response. A similar but sustained pattern occurs with at least one popular transcutaneous pacing unit (Fig. 10-36). A sensing marker on the ECG trace confirms sensing. This marker appears with each natural (sensed) QRS complex and mimics pacer malfunction associated with an irregular stimulus release. During ventricular pacing, the marker resembles another pacing spike and may be mistaken for dual-chamber pacing.

Hysteresis ("a lagging behind") is an optional programmable feature available in

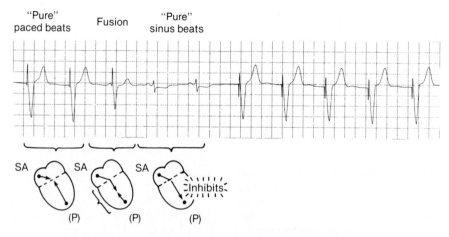

Fig. 10-35 Fusion beats in single-chamber ventricular pacing.

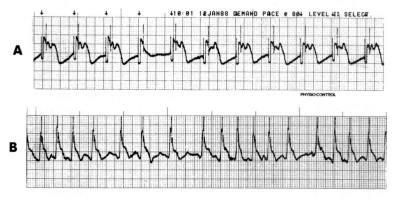

Fig. 10-36 Pseudomalfunction secondary to transcutaneous pacing. During a natural, irregular rhythm, the sensor may mimic pseudofusion or irregular stimulus release **(B)**. During pacing, the sensor mimics dual-chamber pacing **(A)**.

permanent pacemakers. In this feature the escape interval is extended slightly beyond the automatic interval.[18] A longer escape interval gives natural beats a second chance to inhibit the pacemaker; however, undesirable ectopic beats are also given the chance. Therefore, carefully evaluate the appropriate use of hysteresis.

Pacemaker-induced and pacemaker-mediated arrhythmias[18,24,53,56]

Although pacemakers may be used to prevent or correct tachyarrhythmias as well as bradyarrhythmias, they can generate tachyarrhythmias of their own. In *pacemaker-induced* arrhythmias, once the arrhythmia is initiated the pacemaker is inhibited and no longer participates in perpetuating the arrhythmia. Single-chamber *ventricular* pacemakers are most typically associated with ventricular arrhythmias. Pacemaker-induced ventricular arrhythmias are usually right ventricular, producing a negative complex on V_1 similar to that of the paced beat (see Nursing Assessment and Intervention and Unit 7). These beats may be treated with lidocaine and/or by repositioning the catheter. You may also leave PVCs untreated unless sustained VT occurs. Ventricular arrhythmias occurring immediately after pacemaker insertion often subside without therapy.

Atrial arrhythmias are most typically associated with single-chamber *atrial* pacemak-

ers. The most common atrial arrhythmia induced by these pacemakers is atrial fibrillation, due to lack of atrial sensing or competition. The atrial component of a *dual-chambered* pacemaker can also precipitate atrial arrhythmias. Atrial fibrillation is commonly reported in DVI pacing because of the inherent lack of atrial sensing. When this occurs, convert the pacemaker to the VVI mode.

DDD pacing is typically associated with *pacemaker-mediated* arrhythmias. Pacemaker-mediated, or endless-loop, tachycardia (PMT) is a paced tachycardia sustained by continuous pacemaker activity.[18,24,53] In PMT, the pacemaker tracks not only normal P waves, but ectopic or retrogradely conducted P waves as well. There are two major forms of PMT: (1) atrial tachycardia or atrial flutter with antegrade P wave tracking and (2) atrial tachycardia secondary to retrograde P wave tracking (Fig. 10-37). An adjustable upper rate limit

A) Antegrade P-wave Tracking:

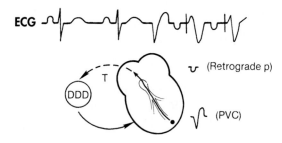

B) Retrograde P-wave Tracking:

Fig.10-37 Pacemaker-mediated tachycardia (PMT) with antegrade tracking **(A)** and retrograde tracking **(B).** These two pacemaker rhythms may be difficult to distinguish without documentation of their onset.

feature provided in both temporary and permanent DDD pulse generators limits the ventricular rate. The first is the result of a normal P wave–triggered response to a spontaneous ectopic tachycardia. The second is caused by unintended tracking of retrogradely conducted P waves, usually associated with premature ventricular contractions (PVCs). When such retrogradely conducted P waves are detected by the pacemaker's sensing lead, the pacemaker appropriately tracks the P wave and paces the ventricle. This induces another retrograde P wave, which is again tracked. The result is an endless-loop tachycardia near or at the pacemaker's present upper rate limit. In patients who have intact ventriculoatrial conduction, the pacemaker becomes an essential component of a reentrant circuit. The pacemaker provides the presenting (or antegrade) pathway for the arrhythmia. The native conduction system provides the retrograde path for its return.

These endless-loop tachycardias may be interrupted or prevented by any measure that prevents the pacemaker from sensing and responding to a retrograde atrial depolarization. One may terminate PMT by magnet application over the generator. This temporarily converts the unit to DOO (fixed rate) mode, whereby both the atria and ventricle are paced sequentially at a determined rate without sensing in either channel. This measure breaks the reentrant cycle as long as the magnet is applied. By externally reprogramming the pacer to a non-sensing atrial pacing mode (VVI/DVI), you avoid all sensing of atrial signals. Unfortunately, this method of *preventing* PMT causes the loss of physiologic rate response, loss of AV synchrony (in VVI), and competitive discharges between spontaneous and paced events leading to atrial arrhythmias (in DVI).

To resolve pacemaker-mediated tachycardia, you may reprogram atrial sensitivity levels, reprogram the upper rate limit to a lower level, or extend the postventricular atrial refractory period (PVARP) to prevent retrograde P waves from being sensed.[3,18,53,56] The PVARP is the time or interval after a ventricular event during which the pacemaker fails to sense an atrial depolarization.[65] Although this is the best solution to prevent PMT, very long atrial refractory periods limit the pacemaker's ability to track physiologic variations of sinus rate. Newer DDD pacemaker models use algorithms that automatically adjust the PVARP or the A–V interval. If a P wave occurs within the PVARP, the next atrial stimulus is omitted. If the next P wave then occurs before the next ventricular output, that P wave will not initiate an A–V interval. Advanced technologic functions of such DDD pacing models demonstrate the ability of these systems to distinguish between and react to physiologic versus pathologic atrial rhythms.[3,18,23,26,29,31,33,38,53]

Hemodynamics of cardiac pacing[5,8,9,11,18,20–23,26,28,29,38,48,49,52,60]

The hemodynamic benefit of dual-chamber AV sequential pacing versus single-chamber ventricular pacing is well documented. Properly timed AV atrial contraction with synchrony facilitates normal AV valve closure, enhances ventricular filling and cardiac output at rest and during exercise, and helps to maintain normal levels of atrial natriuretic peptide (ANP). Lack of AV synchrony can cause inappropriate vasomotor reflexes, resulting in low cardiac output, orthostasis, and syncope. Long-term absence of AV synchrony also increases the incidence of atrial fibrillation, systemic emboli, and overt congestive heart failure. Lack of AV synchrony may reduce patient life expectancy, particularly in patients with impaired ventricular function, idiopathic hypertrophic subaortic stenosis (IHSS), or aortic stenosis. In patients with systolic and/or diastolic dysfunction, proper AV synchrony maintains cardiac output, preserves physiologic cardiac pressures, and prevents backward circulatory flow. Loss of AV synchronization is more pronounced and poorly tolerated in patients with noncompliant ventricles. As heart rates increase, the importance of atrial contraction increases.

Hemodynamic improvement obtained with dual-chamber pacing over single-chamber pacing is readily indicated by a rise in systolic blood pressure and an increase in cardiac output. Both are brought about by the atrial contribution to end-diastolic ventricular volume.

Long-term benefits of rate adaptability and AV synchrony are increased oxygen transport, exercise tolerance, and enhanced quality of life. Despite these positive results, less than one third of permanent pacing systems implanted are dual-chamber devices. Problems and skepticism regarding current atrial lead positioning may be one reason for this trend.

Pacemaker syndrome[11,18,26,52,60]

Pacemaker syndrome describes the pathophysiologic, hemodynamic, and electrophysiologic consequences of permanent single-chamber ventricular pacing. In addition, adverse hemodynamic consequences of single-chamber ventricular pacing, once thought to occur in 10% to 15% of VVI-paced patients, currently exist in more than 80%. These consequences result from three problems that occur during basic ventricular pacing: (1) loss of AV synchrony with atrial contraction against closed AV valves, (2) loss of atrial contribution to ventricular filling and cardiac output, (3) retrograde or VA conduction, and (4) loss of cardiac rate response to activity needs.

Symptoms of pacemaker syndrome range from easy fatigability and lethargy to palpitations, neck vein pulsations, overt congestive heart failure, and syncope. A decrease in systolic blood pressure of 20 mm Hg, or a 20% reduction in cardiac output associated with ventricular pacing compared with AV synchronous pacing confirms the diagnosis of pacemaker syndrome. Therapy includes reducing the frequency of ventricular pacing in patients who are not pacemaker dependent or implantation of a dual-chamber system to maintain AV synchrony.

Rate responsiveness[5,9,18,20,23,29,38,41,48,49,60]

The development of dual-chamber AV sequential pacing has led to more physiologic pacing. However, AV sequential devices are not always capable of adjusting the pacing rate in response to changing metabolic demands. Heart rate response may be a more important factor in generating and sustaining cardiac output during increased metabolic processes than is the preservation of AV synchrony. Sensor-based rate-responsive pacing provides augmented cardiac output and supports metabolic demands during periods of stress, without reliance on SA node function; this type of pacing is also associated with improved functional capacity and thus exercise tolerance. Rate-responsive single-chamber pacemakers may be equivalent to standard dual-chamber pacers in terms of physiologic effectiveness.

The primary indication for a rate-responsive pacemaker is to permit a heart rate increase in the absence of an appropriate spontaneous increase in heart rate. Patients who may benefit most from single-chamber rate-modulated pacing (VVIR) include those with chronic atrial fibrillation. Those with sinus node dysfunction and symptomatic bradycardias would benefit most from dual-chamber rate-modulated pacing (DDDR).[6b] Aggressive rate-responsive pacing may be deleterious to patients with myocardial ischemia and may not be as beneficial for elderly patients with sedentary lifestyles.[6b] VVIR pacing may also worsen

retrograde conduction and, consequently, lead to pacemaker syndrome. The ideal sensor for a rate-responsive pacing system would directly measure a physiologic variable or determinant of sympathetic tone and/or circulating catecholamine levels. However, current sensors only detect and modulate pacing rates by correlating the degree of metabolic demand to the indirect measurement of physiologic parameters. These parameters include activity, temperature, pH, venous oxygen saturation, minute ventilation, and Q–T interval.

Clinical investigations suggest that the most physiologic pacemaker is one that offers a combination of rate modulation (i.e., a pacemaker that can vary its pacing rate according to physiologic demands) and maintenance of synchronized AV electrical activity.[18,19] Currently, the only sensors available for clinical commercial use are based on activity, temperature, oxygen saturation, Q–T interval, and respiratory parameters. The others remain investigational. Because of their simplicity, activity-driven systems are the most frequently used rate-responsive pacemaker systems.

Nursing assessment and intervention[9,10,14,23,28,29,31,38,61,67]

Advances in pacemaker technology present additional challenges in the nursing care of pacemaker patients. As the number of pacing options increases, so does the complexity of properly assessing their functions.

Nursing care of the individual with an external or implanted pacemaker requires a thorough understanding of basic pacing concepts in order to monitor and analyze pacemaker activity and to intervene in any pacemaker complication or malfunction.[31,39] Nurses who care for patients with either temporary or permanent pacemakers must monitor the patient's physiologic response to pacing. Prompt recognition of compromised

hemodynamic function may minimize adverse responses to certain paced rhythms. With knowledge of various pacing modes and an ability to accurately interpret the ECG, the nurse may also detect pacemaker malfunctions. Patient and family teaching is also an integral part of nursing assessment and intervention.

NURSING ORDERS: For the patient with a pacemaker

RELATED NURSING DIAGNOSES: Alteration in comfort, potential for injury related to pacemaker malfunction or electrical hazards, impaired skin integrity, potential for infection, knowledge deficit

1. *Preinsertion:* temporary transvenous pacemakers
   a. Confirm battery is in pulse generator and check battery function by checking battery life indicator by pressing "battery test" button, which indicates how much battery charge remains. A fresh battery may be used each time.
   b. Explain procedure to patient.
   c. Position patient.
   d. Assist physician with obtaining venous access.
2. *During and after insertion:* temporary transvenous pacemakers
   a. Monitor for right ventricular PVCs (negatively deflected QRS complexes in lead V1) caused by mechanical stimulation. Have lidocaine and countershock equipment available for emergencies.
   b. Once the catheter is in position, connect the pacing catheter(s) to the pulse generator, proximal lead or electrode to positive terminal, distal lead or electrode to negative terminal.
   c. Turn on the pacemaker and select the pacing rate and mode.
   d. Determine the pacing threshold by adjusting the output strength (mA) dial until capture is obtained.
   e. Determine the sensitivity threshold with the sensitivity dial at the most sensitive position (clockwise—farthest away from asynchronous). Slowly, or at the lowest number, move the sensitivity dial in a counterclockwise fashion (or increase the MV setting) to a position where the pacemaker starts to fire pacing stimuli. At this point, turn the dial clockwise again until the sense indicator starts to flash and pacing stops.
   f. Assess patient's tolerance to the pacing mode:
      —Determine and document tolerance level of loss of AV synchrony if single-chamber ventricular demand (VVI) pacing.
      —Document intrinsic heart rate and rhythm, as well as paced rate and rhythm.
      —Assess chronotropic response to activity, cardiac output, and tissue perfusion parameters (mental status, pulses, urine output, blood pressure, heart sounds) at rest as well as with activity.
3. *Postinsertion:* both temporary and permanent pacemakers
   a. Obtain and analyze 12-lead ECG to confirm lead placement, pacing, capture, and sensing function.
   b. Obtain chest radiograph to confirm anteroposterior and lateral lead placement.
   c. Monitor for potential complications:
      —Bleeding or hematoma formation
      —Pneumothorax
      —Sepsis at insertion site
      —Perforation of the right ventricle (loss of capture, stimulation of diaphragmatic muscle with hiccups)
4. After surgical implantation, confirm that data regarding the pacemaker's parameter is available and documented in the chart. This information includes (a) date of implant or insertion, (b) manufacturer, model or serial number, end-of-life indicators, and (c) timing cycles and settings (e.g., lower and upper rates, A–V interval, pulse width, sensitivity, mA, refractory periods).
5. Since pacing thresholds may change gradually or abruptly, it is recommended to perform routine threshold assessment every 8 hours with temporary pacemakers.
6. Cap or cover exposed uninsulated catheter endings to prevent inadvertent electrical stimulation and fibrillation.
7. If DC cardioversion or defibrillation is necessary, place paddles at least 3 to 5 inches away from the pulse generator.

Thoroughly evaluate pacemaker function after cardioversion or defibrillation.

8. *Patient and family education:* temporary pacing
   a. Inform patient and family of the purpose of, insertion process, and possible complications associated with temporary pacemaker insertion.
   b. Instruct patient in activity limits for the first 24 hours or as determined by site (femoral insertion site may require more restriction).

9. *Patient and family education:* permanent pacing
   a. *Preoperatively,* instruct patient and family about the heart and its conduction system, method of implantation, operative site, components of the pacer system, preoperative orders, duration of surgery, type of anesthesia, postanesthesia recovery, postoperative routine and expectations (pain and analgesia, activity restrictions, pressure dressing, incentive spirometry, postoperative ECG monitoring, and chest radiograph).
   b. *Postoperatively,* instruct patient and family about:
      —Routine wound care, symptoms of potential postoperative complications (s/s of infection at the pacemaker site, shortness of breath, dizziness, fainting ankle swelling, chest pain, prolonged hiccuping), and importance of prompt recognition and treatment
      —Purpose and description of external reprogramming procedures, when indicated
      —Pulse taking with meanings of increased or decreased pulse tailored to the individual patient
      —Concerns (avoidance of trauma to pacemaker pocket, awareness of sources of electromagnetic interference, effects of medication changes on pacemaker function, importance of routine follow-up care, dental prophylaxis, importance of carrying ID and pacemaker information at all times)
      —Importance of follow-up clinic. Follow-up visits are usually scheduled for the first 1, 3, and 6 months, and then every 6 months for the life of the pacemaker. Transtelephonic monitoring may be added to follow-up protocols to ensure close surveillance of older pacing system function.[62]
      —Local and national patient and family support groups

Systematic approach to ECG assessment

I. Evaluate stimulus release ("automatic interval").
   A. Is there ever too long a pause without a stimulus being released?
   B. Identify pacing spikes and automatic pacing interval, including discharge rate and regularity and A–V interval with dual-chamber pacemakers.
   C. Problems identified
      1. Absence of stimulus (intermittent/sustained)
      2. Changes in stimulus rate and/or regularity

II. Evaluate stimulus response ("capture").
   A. Does each pacemaker stimulus away from a potential refractory period produce a myocardial response ("capture")?
   B. Is the response atrial, ventricular, or both (dual)?: Classification criterion 1 (chamber paced)
   C. With variations in QRS response R/O fusion
   D. Problem identified: loss of capture

III. Evaluate adequate sensing.
   A. Is the pacemaker given the oppor-

tunity to sense (presence of natural beats from same chamber or chambers)?: Classification criterion 2 (chamber sensed)

B. Evaluate ventricular sensing.
  1. Is/are the spike(s) ever completely inhibited by natural QRS complexes?: Classification criterion 3 (mode of sensing)
  2. Is the automatic interval reset by these natural QRS complexes?
  3. Identify escape interval and correlate it with automatic interval. (With dual-chamber pacing correlate with A–V or V–A interval.)
  4. Is there ever a spike or spikes after a fully formed natural QRS complex?
  5. With dual-chamber pacing, evaluate sensing within the A–V interval to explain loss of ventricular spike.

C. Evaluate atrial sensing.
  1. Can natural P waves be clearly seen? On any other lead?
  2. Do atrial spikes appear after these natural P waves?
  3. Do the P waves appear to be "tracking" single-chamber ventricular spikes?: Classification criterion 3 (mode of sensing)
D. Problem identified: Loss of sensing or competition

IV. Evaluate any arrhythmias present (independent or pacemaker-induced).
V. Determine if the pacemaker is implanted.
  A. Are programmable options available?
  B. Does it have antitachycardia capabilities?
    1. Primary: major pacemaker function
    2. Secondary: programmable functions (Fig. 10-38)

Evaluation of catheter position

After initiation of permanent or temporary TV pacing, optimal positioning of the pacing catheter is confirmed in the antero-posterior and lateral views of the chest radiograph and 12-lead ECG patterns. When the catheter is properly positioned in the right ventricular apex, pacing should generate a positive complex in lead I and a negative complex in leads II and aVF (see Unit 7). The QRS complex in lead V_1 should also be negative (Fig. 10-39).

Antitachycardia pacing[4,11,13,18,33,59]

Major forms of antitachycardia pacing include (1) external antitachycardia pacing, (2) normal rate competition, (3) overdrive, (4) scanning, and (5) bursting. These antitachycardia pacing functions are referred to by the letter *P* in the fifth position of the NASPE/BPEG Generic (NBG) pacing code (see Classification of Pacemakers).

Antiarrhythmic agents may affect conduction characteristics of the myocardium, influencing the function of antitachycardia pacing. By increasing tissue refractoriness, antiarrhythmic drug therapy can make termination of tachyarrhythmias by pacing difficult. Antitachycardia pacing remains contraindicated in those persons who demonstrate the following: acceleration of VT during antitachycardia pacing, incessant VT, hemodynamic instability or ischemia due to rapid pacing, unreproducible tachycardia termination, and unreproducible tachycardia.

External antitachycardia pacing refers to

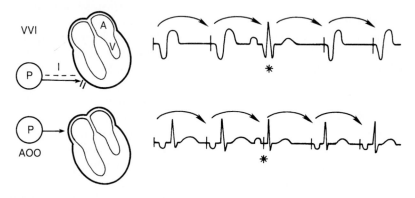

Stimulating ⟶   ■ Blanking

Sensing ┈▸

SINGLE-CHAMBER PACING:

VVI

AOO

DUAL-CHAMBER PACING:

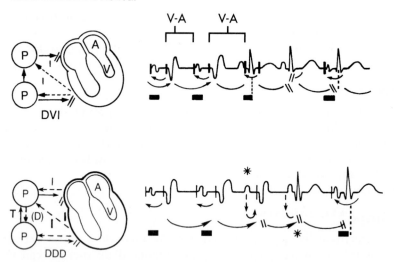

V-A   V-A

DVI

DDD

Fig. 10-38 Summary of normal ECG patterns: common single- and dual-chamber pacing modes.

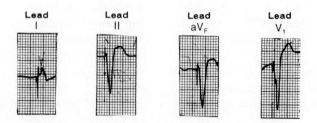

Lead I   Lead II   Lead aV$_F$ Lead V$_1$

Fig. 10-39 Right ventricular apical pacing.

external activation of antitachycardia function. To activate the fixed-rate (nonsensing) or continuous-stimulus release mode, apply a magnet or telemetry unit over the pulse generator during a tachyarrhythmia. The patient or physician can also initiate this maneuver. The pacemaker signal falls at different times in the tachycardia sequence, eventually interrupting its circuit. Since all demand pacemakers are magnetically responsive, this is an easy and effective method for interrupting a tachycardia. It is not recommended for sustained use. However, fixed-rate, nonsensing pacing is effective in emergency situations.

Normal-rate competition antitachycardia pacing is similar to external antitachycardia pacing and is available as a programmable function in certain DDD units.[18] Tachycardia of a certain rate automatically activates the pacemaker's magnetic fixed-rate pacing mode without external influence or control. Similar to externally activated methods, this pacing mechanism delivers fixed-rate stimuli (at a normal rate range). These stimuli fall at different times within the tachycardia cycle, eventually interrupting the tachycardia circuit.

Temporary *overdrive* pacing, using an external pulse generator, prevents tachycardias that emerge from sinus bradycardias, AV block, or prolonged Q–T interval or repolarization syndrome.[13,18,28] Insert the pacemaker wire as you do for conventional temporary pacing.[17,30,66] Once you have secured contact, pace the chamber synchronously or asynchronously at a rate faster than the tachycardia (usually around 10 to 15 beats per minute faster) until the tachycardia is terminated. Unfortunately, this approach has become clinically unappealing because it can result in hemodynamic compromise.

Scanning and burst pacing are forms of programmed stimulation.[18] Programmed extrastimuli are the introduction of one or more extrastimuli at a set rate and time during the tachycardia cycle. *Scanning* is the delivery of carefully timed pacemaker stimuli during the tachycardia. The pacemaker automatically recognizes the rapid rate and emits timed stimuli at progressively longer coupling intervals until the tachycardia is interrupted. Burst pacing refers to short, rapid bursts of 7 to 10 stimuli released at a rate at least 10 beats per minute faster than the tachycardia (Fig. 10-40). Use fixed-rate pacing with progressive hysteresis, or progressively longer automatic intervals. If the tachycardia persists and the patient remains stable, extend the burst pacing length until the dysrhythmia is terminated or countershock is indicated. You may access tachycardia control in at least one popular VVI

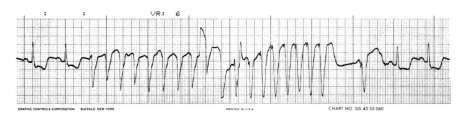

Fig. 10-40 Antitachycardia pacing. Implanted antitachycardia pacemaker, which recognized the ventricular tachycardia and then delivers a "burst" of stimuli at a fixed interval that interrupts the tachycardia. This pacemaker is also a VVI antibradycardia pacer, which escapes at a rate of approximately 60 after termination of VT.

temporary (external) unit by pressing an "X5" button on the pulse generator. The rate of stimulus release is briefly increased to five times the rate indicated on the rate dial.

A major problem in most forms of antitachycardia pacing is the potential acceleration of the tachycardia or deterioration of either a supraventricular or ventricular tachycardia to ventricular fibrillation (VF).[13,18] Because of the faster pacing rate, the risk of tachycardia acceleration is greatest with burst pacing. Generally, this pacing is closely monitored in an electrophysiology laboratory. Because of the associated risks, most patients who require implanted antitachycardia pacmakers also require concomitant AICD implantation. This is necessary for rescue countershock to terminate tachycardias that are not responsive to antitachycardia pacing, or those that accelerate and become hemodynamically unstable.[12,25,57,58]

GLOSSARY

AV interval—in a dual-chamber pacemaker, the period of time between an atrial event (sensed or paced) and the succeeding ventricular paced or sensed event (electronic PR interval).

AV synchrony—the sequence of cardiac activation, where the atria contract first, followed by, after an appropriate delay, the ventricles.

automatic, or pacing, interval—the rate at which an implanted pulse generator emits pacing stimuli in the absence of intrinsic cardiac activity; interval between the spikes of two consecutively paced beats; also referred to as the *pulse interval* or *lower rate limit.*

bipolar—having two electrodes or poles that are located within the heart.

blanking intervals—in a dual-chamber pacemaker, short insensitive portions of the pacing cycle, immediately following the atrial stimulus, designed to avoid oversensing of the atrial stimulus as if it were a ventricular event.

capture—depolarization of the atria and/or ventricles by an electrical stimulus delivered by an artificial pacemaker.

crosstalk (far-field sensing)—inappropriate ventricular sensing of atrial pacing signals in dual-chamber pacemakers with subsequent inhibition of ventricular pacing.

dual-chamber pacing—pacing in both the atria and ventricles in order to preserve or restore synchronized cardiac activities.

end-of-life (EOL)—the point at which a pacemaker generator signals that it should be replaced as a result of near battery depletion.

escape interval—the time, in milliseconds, between a spontaneous event and the first paced complex that follows it.

hysteresis—an optional programmable parameter where the escape interval exceeds the automatic interval in order to facilitate the opportunity for spontaneous cardiac activity.

lower rate limit—the minimum pacemaker rate, synonymous with the automatic or pulse interval.

pacemaker syndrome—a collection of signs/symptoms related to the adverse hemodynamic effects of ventricular pacing.

pulse amplitude—the intensity or strength of an electrical stimulus.

pulse width—time or duration of stimulus delivery.

rate modulation or responsiveness—artificial pacing in which pacemakers change pacing rate in response to detected changes in physiologic parameters which reflect increased metabolic demands.

refractory period—the period after a sensed or paced event (atrial or ventricular) during which the pacemaker's sensing mechanism is insensitive to incoming signals.

safety pacing—an abbreviated AV interval (0.11 sec) triggered by ventricular sensing within the early portion of the AV intervals.

thresholds—usually used to refer to the minimum amount of energy or milliamperes (mA) necessary to generate myocardial depolarization or capture (i.e., the stimulation threshold); the amount of millivolts needed to inhibit a demand pacemaker from firing may be referred to as the sensitivity threshold. The higher the number, the less sensitive the pacer becomes (asynchronous); the lower the number, the greater the sensitivity (demand).

upper rate limit—the maximum pacemaker rate, available in DDD pacemakers, that limits the ventricular response to fast atrial rates.

VA interval—the interval from a paced or natural QRS complex to the atrial spike; also referred to as the *atrial escape interval*.

SELF-ASSESSMENT

1 Defibrillation is indicated primarily to convert _____. Cardioversion refers to the delivery of a _____ charge to the myocardium. The mechanical equipment used for both of these is (similar/different).

VF
synchronized

similar

2 The primary mechanism by which an ICD recognizes VT or VF is by (rate/ECG morphology). Wide QRS complexes with fast ventricular rates trigger (synchronized/unsynchronized) shocks. These shocks (are/are not) felt by the patient.

rate
synchronized; are

If VT or VF persists after six sequential shocks from an ICD, _____ cardioversion, defibrillation, or CPR should be initiated.

external

If an ICD fires inappropriately, it may be inactivated by placing a specialized _____ over the upper part of the pulse generator for a minimum of _____ seconds. When inactivated, the AICD emits a (beeping/continuous) tone.

magnet
30
continuous

3 In the pacing code VVI, the first letter refers to the chamber _____, the (atria/ventricles); the second letter refers to the chamber _____, the (atria/ventricles); the third letter refers to the _____ sensing mode.

paced; ventricles
sensed; ventricles
inhibited

4 When connecting a temporary pacing system, the distal electrode or at least one electrode in the chamber to be paced should be connected to the (negative/positive) terminal.

negative

5 The effect of a magnet placed externally on an implanted demand pacemaker is to turn off the _____, allowing the pacing spikes to (fire/be inhibited) in the presence of normal heart rates.

sensitivity
fire

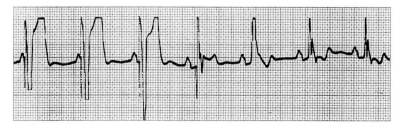

Fig. 10-41   Self-assessment trace #1.

6 *Interpretation:* Normal ventricular demand (VVI) pacing
   Action: None
   Comments: Ventricular pacemaker in capture firing at a rate of
_____. Sensing well as indicated by the natural QRS complexes,   63
which inhibit the pacing spike and resent the automatic intervals (beats #
_____ from the left). Beat # _____ is a fusion   5, 6, 7; 4
beat.

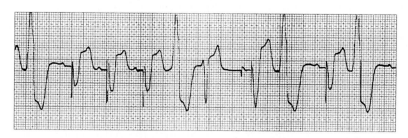

Fig. 10-42   Self-assessment trace #2.

7 *Interpretation:* Normal DDD pacing with frequent PVCs
   Action: None
   Comments: Dual-chamber pacing (as indicated by the two pacing spikes
in beat # _____ from the left) firing at a rate of _____   7; 80
and A–V interval of _____. Note: Since two consecutive   140 msec (0.14
dual-paced beats are not available, the rate may be estimated from the   seconds)
ventricular escape interval (V–A + A–V intervals). The ventricular component (second spike) is in capture. Atrial capture cannot be confirmed
on this trace but can be assumed to be present unless complications arise.
Ventricular sensing is confirmed by the natural QRS complexes, which inhibit the pacing spike and reset the automatic interval (beats #
_____ from the left). Beats # _____   1, 5, 6, 8, 10;
indicate normal atrial sensing and tracking. The PVCs are not caused by   2, 3, 4, 9
the pacer, since they do not have the same configuration as the captured
beats.

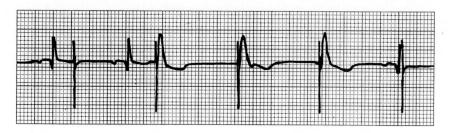

Fig. 10-43   Self-assessment trace #3.

8 *Interpretation:* Ventricular pacemaker undersensing or loss of sensing (competition)

Action: Since there appears to be a natural underlying rhythm, the pacemaker (if external) may be turned off. Increase the sensitivity. Change the battery and/or pulse generator. Notify the physician. If undersensing or loss of sensing recurs, can convert to a unipolar system. If pacemaker is implanted, notify physician immediately to reprogram.

Comments: Spikes follow the fully formed QRS complexes (beats # _____ from the left). Spikes within the refractory period (beat # _____) are not followed by a response. However, those falling outside the refractory period (beats # _____) are followed by a response, confirming effective capture.

1, 2
1
2, 3, 4, 5

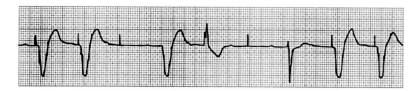

Fig. 10-44   Self-assessment trace #4.

9 *Interpretation:* Ventricular pacemaker out of capture

Action: Increase the mA. Reposition the patient. If patient is symptomatic, support the ventricular rate with an external pacemaker, atropine, or isoproterenol (Isuprel). Notify the physician to reposition the catheter. Change battery and/or pulse generator. If unresolved, try switching the polarity of the electrodes.

Comments: Spikes well away from refractory periods are not followed by a myocardial response (spikes #3, #4 from the left).

REFERENCES

1. Ahern TA, et al: Device interaction—antitachycardia pacemakers and defibrillators for sustained ventricular tachycardia, PACE 14: 302, 1991.
2. Ajiki K et al: A case of pseudomalfunction of a DDD pacemaker, PACE 14:1456, 1991.
3. Anonymous: Microwaves and pacemakers, J Occup Med 34:250, 1992.
4. Arteaga WJ, Drew BJ: Device therapy for ventricular tachycardia or fibrillation: the implantable cardioverter defibrillator and anti-tachycardia pacing, Crit Care Nurs Q 14(2):60, 1991.
5. Baig MW et al: One-year follow-up of automatic adaptation of the rate response algorithm of the QT sensing, rate adaptive pacemaker, PACE 14:1598, 1991.
6. Barbiere CC, Liberatore K: Automated external defibrillators: an update of additions to the ACLS algorithms. Crit Care Nurse 11:17, 1992.
6a. Barbiere CC: From emergent transvenous pacemaker to permanent implant follow-up, Crit Care Nurs 13(2):39, 1993.
6b. Barold SS: The evolution of cardiac pacing: where have we been—where are we going? Medtronic News 21(2):15, 1993.
7. Barredo J: What really interferes with pacemakers? Am J Nurs 90:24, 1990.
8. Benedek ZM, Gross J: Rate modulated pacemakers, Newspaper of Cardiology 2:10, 1992.
9. Blumberg SM, Gross J: Permanent pacemaker implantation: indications, technique and follow-up, Hosp Med 27:24, 1991.
10. Brunner LS, Suddarth DS: Cardiac pacing. In Lippincott Manual of nursing practice, Philadelphia, 1986, JB Lippincott.
11. Buckingham TA, Janosik DL, Pearson, AC: Pacemaker hemodynamics: clinical implications. Prog Cardiovasc Dis 34:347, 1992.
12. Cannom DS: Implantable cardioverter defibrillator: the promise and perils of an evolving technology, PACE 15:1, 1992.
13. Cavanaugh JA: Overdrive pacing: an approach to terminating ventricular tachycardia, J Cardiovasc Nurs 5:58, 1991.
14. Clark A, Cotter L: DC cardioversion, PACE 46:114, 1991.
15. Cooper D, Futterman L, Valladares B: Care of the patient with the implantable cardioverter-defibrillator: a guide for nurses. J Heart Lung, 16:640, 1987.
16. Dreifus LS, Fisch C, Griffin JC, et al: Guidelines for implantation of cardiac pacemakers and antiarrhythmia devices, J Am Coll Cardiol 18:1, 1991.
17. Electrical therapy in the malignant arrhythmias. In Textbook of advanced cardiac life support, 1987, 1990, American Heart Association.
18. Ellenbogen KA: Cardiac pacing, Boston, 1992, Blackwell Scientific Publications.
19. Eorgan PA, Greer JL: Cough CPR: a consideration for high-risk cardiac patient discharge teaching, Crit Care Nurse 12:21, 1992.
20. Fabiszewski R, Volosin KJ: Rate-modulated pacemakers, J Cardiovasc Nurs 5:21, 1991.
21. Ferguson TB, Cox JL: Temporary external DDD pacing after cardiac operations, Ann Thorac Surg 51:723, 1991.
22. Ferguson TB: Temporary DDD pacing after open heart surgery: indications, techniques and performance, Medtronic News 20:15, 1991.
23. Finkelmeier NE: Pacemaker technology: an overview, AACN Clin Issues 2:99, 1991.
24. Folland ED: Cardiac pacemakers, Choices in Cardiology 6(3):108, 1992.
25. Fromer M et al: Experience with a new implantable pacer-cardioverter-defibrillator for the therapy of recurrent sustained ventricular tachyarrythmias: a step toward a universal ventricular tachyarrhythmia control device, PACE 14:1288, 1991.
26. Furman S, Gross J: Dual-chamber pacing and pacemakers, Curr Probl Cardiol 15:162, 1990.
27. Goldschlatger N: Evaluation of pacemaker function: general principles, J Arrhythmia Management 12:15, 1992.
27a. Guidelines for cardiopulmonary resuscitation and emergency care: part III—Adult advanced cardiac life support, JAMA 268(16):2199, 1992.
28. Harthorne JW: Cardiac pacemakers, Curr Probl Cardiol 12:654, 1987.

29. Hayes DL: The next five years in cardiac pacemakers: a preview, Mayo Clin Proc 67:379, 1992.
30. Hickey CS, Baas LS: Temporary cardiac pacing, AACN Clin Issues 2:107, 1991.
31. Hummel J et al: The natural history of dual chamber pacing, PACE 14:1745, 1991.
32. Klein LS, Miles WM, Zipes DP: Antitachycardia devices: realities and promises, J Am Coll Cardiol 18:1349, 1991.
33. Kleinschmidt KM, Stafford MJ: Dual-chamber cardiac pacemakers, J Cardiovasc Nurs 5:9, 1991.
34. Kuiper R: The automatic implantable cardioverter defibrillator as a therapeutic modality for recurrent ventricular tachycardia: a case study, Progr Cardiovasc Nurs 5(1):6, 1990.
35. Kuiper R, Nyamathi AM: Stressors and coping strategies of patients with automatic implantable cardioverter defibrillators, J Cardiovasc Nurs 5(3):65, 1991.
36. Kutalek SP, Michelson EL: Cardiac pacing and antiarrhythmic devices: newer modes of antibradyarrhythmia pacing, Mod Concepts Cardiovasc Dis 60:31, 1991.
37. Kutalek SP, Michelson EL: New technologies for implantation and follow-up of antibradyarrhytmias pacemakers, The Heart House Learning Center Highlights 7:2, 1991.
38. Levine PA: Benefits of dual-chamber pacemakers, West J Med 156:70, 1992.
39. Luderitz B: The impact of antitachycardia pacing with defibrillation, PACE 14:312, 1991.
39a. Manion PA: Temporary epicardial pacing in the postoperative cardiac surgical patient, Crit Care Nurs 13(2):30, 1993.
40. Manolis AS, Rastegar H, Estes III NA: Automatic implantable cardioverter defibrillator, JAMA 262:1362, 1989.
41. Markewitz A, Hemmer W: What's the price to be paid for rate response: AV sequential versus ventricular pacing? PACE 14:1782, 1991.
42. Mason P, McPherson C: Implantable cardioverter defibrillator: a review, Heart Lung 21:141, 1992.
43. McCowan R et al: Automatic implantable cardioverter-defibrillator implantation without thoracotomy using an endocardial and submuscular patch system, J Am Coll Caridol 17:415, 1991.
44. McDanial CM et al: Automated external defibrillation of patients after myocardial infarction by family members: practical aspects and psychological impact of training, PACE 11:2029, 1988.
45. Mond HG, Stokes KB: The electrode-tissue interface: the revolutionary role of steroid elution, PACE 15:95, 1992.
46. Mond HG: Unipolar versus bipolar pacing—poles apart, PACE 14:1411, 1991.
47. Moore SL et al: Implantable cardioverter defibrillator implanted by nonthoracotomy approach: initial clinical experience with the redesigned transvenous lead system, PACE 14:1865, 1991.
48. Morton PG: Rate responsive cardiac pacing, AACN Clin Issues 2:140, 1991.
48a. Hoser SA, Crawford D, Thomas A: Updated care guidelines for patients with automatic implantable cardioverter defibrillators, Crit Care Nurs 13(2):62, 1993.
49. Moungey S: Temporary AV sequential pacing, Progr Cardiovasc Nurs 4:49, 1989.
50. O'Donoghue S: Core curriculum: the automatic internal defibrillator: 1991, Intelligence Reports in Cardiac Pacing and Electrophysiology 10:1, 1992.
51. Owen A: Keeping pace with temporary pacemakers, Nursing 91 21:58, 1991.
52. Pavlovic SU, Kocovic D, Djordjevic M: The etiology of syncope in pacemaker patients, PACE 14:2086, 1991.
53. Perrins EJ, Sutton R: Arrhythmias in pacing, Med Clin North Am 68:1111, 1984.
54. Quick Operation Checklist: Medtronic Dual Chamber Temporary Pulse Generator Model 5345, 1991.
55. Res JC et al: Transesophageal atrial pacing, PACE 14:1359, 1991.
56. Rognoni G et al: A new approach in the prevention of endless loop tachycardia in DDD and VVD pacing, PACE 14:1828, 1991.
56a. Rogove H, Hughes C: Defibrillation and cardioversion, Critical Care Clinics 8(4):839, 1992.
57. Saksena S et al: Experience with a third-generation implantable cardioverter-defibrillator, Am J Cardiol 67:1375, 1991.

58. Singer I et al: The initial clinical experience with an implantable cardioverter defibrillator/antitachycardia pacemaker, PACE 14:1119, 1991.

59. Spittell PC, Hayes DL: Venous complications after insertion of a transvenous pacemaker, Mayo Clin Proc 67:258, 1992.

60. Stafford MJ, Kleinschmidt KM: Physiologic cardiac pacing: the DDD pacemaker system and rate-responsive modes, Cardiovasc Nurs 27:13, 1991.

61. Stewart JV, Sheehan AM: Permanent pacemakers: the nurse's role in patient education and follow-up care, J Cardiovasc Nurs 5:32, 1991.

62. Strathmore NF, Mond HG: Noninvasive monitoring and testing of pacemaker function, PACE 10:1359, 1987.

63. Tchou P et al: When is it safe not to replace an implantable cardioverter defibrillator generator? PACE 14:1875, 1991.

64. Teplitz L: Transcutaneous pacemakers, J Cardiovasc Nurs 5:44, 1991.

65. Tworek DA et al: Interference by antiarrhythmic agents with function of electrical cardiac devices, Clin Pharm 11:48, 1992.

66. Weiner I, Conover MB: Pacemakers. In Tilkian AG, Daily EK, editors: Cardiovascular procedures: diagnostic techniques and therapeutic procedures, St. Louis, 1986, CV Mosby.

67. Witherell CL: Questions nurses ask about pacemakers. How they work—and what to do when they don't, Am J Nurs 90:20, 1990.

The Patient without Coronary Artery Disease in the Coronary Care Unit

Chronic electrical or mechanical cardiac disorders often occur in the absence of acute coronary artery disease. Patients with these disorders can present with potentially life-threatening complications. They may thus require the acute monitoring and intervention or diagnostic expertise provided in the coronary care unit (CCU). Two frequently seen electrical disorders are torsades de pointes and Wolff-Parkinson-White (preexcitation) syndrome. Two frequently seen mechanical disorders with both electrical and mechanical complications are mitral valve prolapse and cardiomyopathy. Although the complications of mitral prolapse are usually benign, they can be disturbing enough to warrant evaluation in a coronary care unit.

Sudden cardiac death (SCD) is usually a manifestation of chronic cardiac disorders and may not necessarily be associated with coronary artery disease. Survivors may be admitted to a coronary care unit for further monitoring and evaluation. Each of the previously addressed disorders is associated with some risk of SCD.

SUDDEN CARDIAC DEATH

SCD is most commonly defined as unexpected death from cardiac causes occurring within 1 hour of the onset of symptoms.[1,3,4,11,12] In most cases, the terminal event is ventricular fibrillation, presenting as abrupt loss of consciousness and sudden collapse. Bradyarrhythmias and asystole and electrical-mechanical dissociation (EMD) are reported in a small percentage of cases. The incidence of sudden death is highest in the early waking hours, suggesting a circadian rhythm.[11,26] A little less than half of the victims consult a physician within the prior month with nonspecific complaints such as fatigue or dyspnea.[1,4]

Although SCD occurs most frequently in the setting of coronary artery disease (75-90%),[1,3,6,12,22] it has also been reported in other cardiac disorders. SCD is usually a manifestation of both structural and functional cardiac abnormalities.[1,12] The structural changes may be either electrical or mechanical. Structural abnormalities, other than coronary artery disease and myocardial infarction, associated with SCD include left ventricular hypertrophy, dilated or hypertrophic cardiomyopathy, dissecting aortic aneurysm, aortic stenosis, mitral valve prolapse, congenital coronary artery malformations including bridging, and Wolff-Parkinson-White syndrome.[1,4,12,16,24] The risk in mitral valve prolapse is the least relative to the total number of cases with this disorder.[1] In athletes less than 35 to 40 years of age, hypertrophic cardiomyopathy is associated with the highest risk, whether obstructive or nonobstructive.[1,16,24] Episodes of nonsustained ventricular tachycardia (VT) have the highest predictive value in this setting (see Cardiomyopathies).[6,16]

The risk is significantly increased in the presence of left ventricular dysfunction with or without coronary artery disease.[20,22,26] Other functional disorders contributing to SCD include ischemia, electrolyte imbalance, catecholamine release due to stress, autonomic dysfunction or imbalance, and drug toxicity (especially from digitalis, antiarrhythmics). Prolonged QT syndrome may be a manifestation of many of these functional changes or may reflect extracardiac influences (e.g., hypothermia, CNS injury) on cardiac electrical activity. This syndrome is associated with an increased risk of sudden death related to torsades de pointes (see Torsades de pointes).

Noncardiac causes of sudden death in adults include subarachnoid hemorrhage, pulmonary embolism, choking, and pulmonary hypertension in pregnancy.[3] Ventricular fibrillation is the most frequently reported terminal event in these settings as well.

As might be expected, certain risk factors associated with coronary artery disease are also reported as risk factors for sudden cardiac death. These include hypertension, smoking, hypercholesterolemia, obesity, and stress.[1,3,26] At least two vessels with more than 75% stenosis are found in most patients.[1,3,4,7a,11,12] Plaque fissures or tears, thrombosis, platelet aggregation, and spasm have also been implicated (see Unit 5).[1,3,7a,12] In patients with coronary artery disease, complex premature ventricular contractions (PVCs) are associated with an increased risk of

sudden death.[3] Markers of SCD after myocardial infarction include left ventricular dysfunction, frequent or complex ventricular arrhythmias, ventricular aneurysm, and bundle branch block.[1,3,6,16,21,22] The risk associated with left ventricular dysfunction is greatest in the first six months, and the risk associated with bundle branch block is greatest in the first 6 weeks. A higher incidence of complex ventricular arrhythmias is reported in patients with ejection fractions less than 40%.[3,4,15,21] Multiple small foci of myocardial necrosis are typically present. These necrotic foci are similar to those occurring in reperfusion injury, within the ischemic zone surrounding acute infarction, or secondary to catecholamine release in stress.[3,4]

The specific electrophysiologic mechanism triggering ventricular fibrillation (VF) is currently disputed. However, the association with positive findings on signal-averaged electrocardiography and inducible ventricular tachycardia in electrophysiologic studies (EPS) suggests a reentrant mechanism in most patients (see Unit 6).[6,12] Signal-averaged electrocardiography is helpful in identifying high-risk patients with acute myocardial infarction, syncope, and possibly hypertrophic cardiomyopathy but is not predictive in dilated cardiomyopathy.[6,16,21] A negative study may be more helpful than a positive study.[11]

Ambulatory Holter monitoring or exercise testing may also help identify and evaluate high-risk patients. Exertional hypotension, ventricular ectopy, and inability to complete level II of the Bruce protocol are associated with increased risk in patients with coronary artery disease. Holter monitoring may be used effectively to guide drug therapy if frequent spontaneous arrhythmias are present, allowing for a meaningful end point to be established.[3,11,20,22] Echocardiography is performed to determine the ejection fraction, which in turn reflects the extent of left ventricular dysfunction or heart failure.[34]

Echocardiography may also rule out myopathy in young athletes.[16,24]

The risk of *recurrent* SCD is highest in the same populations in which initial SCD occurs. These populations include patients with left ventricular dysfunction (congestive heart failure or previous MI), coronary artery disease, atrioventricular (AV) or intraventricular conduction abnormalities, inducible VT on EPS, exercise-induced hypotension, or angina.[4,6,15] Smoking and male sex are also associated with high risk. The highest incidence of recurrent arrest is within the first 1 to 2 years following the initial episode, even in patients without previous MI.[4] Factors affecting survival after in-hospital resuscitation include homebound life-style, arrest duration greater than 15 minutes, hypotension, pneumonia, and coma following resuscitation.[1]

Effective management of SCD focuses on basic cardiopulmonary resuscitation (CPR) and rapid defibrillation.[2,3] Automatic external defibrillators are an integral component (see Unit 10). Control of risk factors may be effective in preventing SCD.[3] Recurrent SCD may be prevented by the administration of antiarrhythmic agents, use of implantable cardioverter defibrillators (ICDs), antitachycardia pacemakers, correction of functional disorders, and surgical intervention.

Antiarrhythmic drug therapy was formerly the initial treatment of choice for malignant ventricular arrhythmias. However, the traditional class 1 antiarrhythmic agents have not been consistently effective.[6,13,26] As reported by the Cardiac Arrhythmic Suppression Trial (CAST), proarrhythmic effects limit the use of class IC agents. The incidence of proarrhythmic effects is higher in patients with left ventricular dysfunction and sustained ventricular arrhythmias.[15] The class IC agent propafenone (Rhythmol) is currently under further investigation.[13] The class II antiarrhythmics (beta blockers) have proved effective primarily after acute myocardial infarction and in some patients with long QT syndrome (torsades de pointes).[3,6,22] Beta blockade is the only mode of therapy effective in preventing the initial episode of sudden death.[26] The incidence of VF decreases, although the incidence of PVCs may not. The major significant contributing factors are thought to be a decrease in rate and catecholamine release.

Preliminary studies with the class III antiarrhythmic agent amiodarone (Cardarone) shows some promise after acute myocardial infarction and in the patient with congestive heart failure (CHF) and hypertrophic myopathy. Amiodarone decreases heart rate and sympathetic responses similar to beta blockers.[26] The incidence of proarrhythmia, primarily torsades de pointes, is low even in the presence of QT prolongation. This characteristic is thought to be due to calcium antagonism, which partially inhibits the early afterdepolarizations of torsades (see Torsades de pointes). However, amiodarone is associated with serious side effects (see Unit 10).[6,22] Further studies are in progress with this agent and another class III agent, sotalol.

Antiarrhythmic therapy may be prescribed alone or in combination with an implantable device.[23] Antiarrhythmic therapy alone is considered primarily in patients with ejection fractions greater than 30%, inducible VT or VF, and frequent spontaneous ventricular arrhythmias. Its effectiveness is monitored by either EPS or Holter monitoring.[13,15] Antiarrhythmic agents are helpful in preventing recurrences of sustained, asymptomatic VT. However, in SCD survivors, there is a 10% to 15% recurrence of VT or VF over the next 2 years in the presence of drug therapy alone.[13] In patients with normal hearts, chronic drug therapy is not necessary.[13] Episodes of VT can be managed with intermittent, acute drug therapy or electrical intervention.

The current trend is toward nonpharmacologic alternatives, particularly the implantable devices. In patients with decreased ejection fractions, the use of an implantable cardioverter defibrillator is preferred.[15] An ICD is also indicated in patients with noninducible ventricular arrhythmias, or VT or VF refractory to drug therapy, especially in patients who are not surgical candidates. SCD survivors with normal hearts may also benefit.[13] Antiarrhythmic therapy may be prescribed in combination with an ICD to decrease the number of shocks required. Shocks not only deplete the battery but also cause patient discomfort. Drug therapy may also be added to slow the ventricular response of supraventricular tachycardia (SVT) to prevent its being mistaken for VT.

The preferred mode of therapy varies to some extent with the specific setting. Surgical intervention for malignant ventricular arrhythmias in the setting of coronary artery disease includes coronary bypass and aneurysectomy.[6,15,19] Indications include significant multivessel obstruction on coronary arteriography with ischemia documented on a thallium scan.[13] Coronary reperfusion is less likely to be effective in the presence of previous infarction or positive signal-averaged ECGs.[13] Coronary bypass surgery may provide a cure, although sometimes temporary, if the arrhythmias are ischemic in nature. In high-risk patients with hypertrophic cardiomyopathy, an ICD or amiodarone is preferred.[6,13] Specific therapies for patients with long QT syndrome (torsades de pointes), Wolff-Parkinson-White syndrome, and mitral valve prolapse are discussed in their respective sections of this chapter.

Surgical ablation is reserved for those patients in whom drug therapy is ineffective in preventing recurrence or inducibility on EPS as an alternative to ICD insertion (see Unit 6). Both surgical ablation and aneurysectomy offer the advantage of a permanent cure not found with ICD insertion or bypass surgery.[9,13] Major adjustments in life-style are also not required. EPS "mapping" of the arrhythmia is a prerequisite to guide the accuracy and effectiveness of the surgical intervention. If the ventricular tachycardia cannot be mapped, the patient is not considered a surgical candidate. Catheter ablation is not well tolerated in the SCD survivor.[13] This procedure is effective primarily in Wolff-Parkinson-White syndrome.

Once the patient is physiologically stabilized, the nursing care of the SCD survivor centers on the preparation and follow-up for diagnostic tests, pharmacologic management, and therapeutic procedures. These tests and procedures include signal-averaged electrocardiography, exercise stress testing, Holter monitoring, echocardiography, EPS, surgery, and ICD insertion. Psychological support to the patient and family is also crucial.[5] Feelings such as anger, frustration, fear, and depression are frequently reported. After returning home, the patient may experience fatigue, memory loss, sleep disturbances, and sexual dysfunction. These feelings and symptoms may be related to drug side effects, underlying left ventricular failure, the effects of ICD shocks, or the psychological impact of recurring ventricular arrhythmias and sudden death.[5] Patients should be encouraged to talk about their feelings with the family, friends, and health care professionals. Support groups of other patients with recurrent ventricular arrhythmias and/or an ICD are helpful. Two other helpful strategies are balanced activity with rest periods and participation in diversional activities such as hobbies.[5]

In the event the patient does not survive the SCD episode, the focus of nursing care shifts toward the family. The family are escorted to the patient's room, are encouraged by example to touch their loved one, and are given time to say goodbye. The chaplain's assistance is offered. A follow-up call within 2 weeks by the nurse or chaplain is also helpful.[7]

Role of electrophysiologic studies

Electrophysiologic studies evaluate the electrical characteristics of the conduction system, tachyarrhythmias, and bradyarrhythmias from multiple recording sites on specialized catheters threaded transvenously into the heart.[11,14,17] The intracardiac patterns obtained include atrial and His bundle electrograms. These patterns are correlated with the surface ECG. Sites and pathways of abnormal electrical activity may be identified more clearly than from the surface ECG. Although initially used extensively for the evaluation of bradyarrhythmias, these studies are currently used to a greater extent to evaluate and assist in the management of tachyarrhythmias.[14]

Arrhythmias may be induced in this controlled situation with specialized artificial pacing systems that deliver single and/or multiple electrical stimuli to different sites within the heart. This technique is referred to as *programmed electrical stimulation* (PES). Rapid atrial or ventricular pacing may also be used to evaluate normal and accessory conduction pathways or trigger tachyarrhythmias.[16] Triggered or induced arrhythmias are safely terminated by these same pacing techniques, cardioversion, or defibrillation.[11,14] Hemodynamic responses may be evaluated by monitoring level of consciousness, blood pressure, skin temperature and moisture, and by obtaining simultaneous arterial blood gases.[16] Arterial O_2 saturation is monitored by pulse oximetry.

Electrophysiologic testing is currently used for both diagnostic and therapeutic purposes. Indications include diagnosis of wide QRS tachycardia, diagnosis and/or catheter ablation in supraventricular tachycardias in cluding those associated with Wolff-Parkinson-White syndrome, and monitoring the effectiveness of drug therapy in patients with episodes of sustained VT too infrequent to evaluate with Holter monitoring.[4,14,20,25] Suppression of inducible arrhythmias or slowing of their ventricular rate is the usual end point when evaluating drug therapy.[11,14,15,22] A negative study suggests electrophysiologic mechanisms other than reentry and indicates EPS is not a reliable method to guide therapy in that patient. EPS is also indicated before and after nonpharmacologic therapy for ventricular arrhythmias and in the evaluation of patients with structural heart disease and unexplained syncope.[17,20,25] According to the recently published American Heart Association Guidelines, electrophysiologic testing is recommended in all SCD survivors without acute Q wave infarction or with an episode of SCD occurring more than 48 hours after acute myocardial infarction.[25] However, the results of studies on the value of routine prophylactic EPS after acute myocardial infarction are contradictory.[11,16,20] EPS is not beneficial in idiopathic cardiomyopathy or prolonged QT syndrome.[17,20,25] Reentry probably does not play a role in these settings. The benefits of EPS in patients with hypertrophic myopathy have not been clearly established. Findings are primarily meaningful in SCD survivors.[16]

Atrial or ventricular mapping is included as part of the electrophysiologic studies performed before electrical or surgical intervention. The atrial or ventricular chamber is divided into 10 to 20 areas, each designated by a number. Recordings are obtained from each site during sinus rhythm and the tachycardia using the multiple electrode endocardial catheters.[10] A diagram, or "map," of the tachycardia origin and activation sequence is thus obtained. Epicardial mapping requires a thoracotomy and is performed primarily before surgical procedures.[10] Epicardial mapping uses both a stationary and mobile electrode, which is attached to the surgeon's finger.[4,11]

When EPS is used to evaluate either pharmacologic or nonpharmacologic management, an initial baseline study is usually performed. Effects of various drugs may be evaluated in this same study.[14] Antiarrhythmic drugs or drugs used to control the ventricular rate are discontinued for a few half-lives before the study. The patient should be carefully monitored during this period for spontaneous recurrence of significant arrhythmias. Acute ischemia, electrolyte imbalance, and severe CHF are contraindications since they enhance electrical instability.[14] Aortic stenosis is also associated with increased risk.[10,14]

The insertion procedure is similar to that for a cardiac catheterization (see Unit 5).[4,10] Two to six intracardiac dual-purpose pacing or recording catheters may be inserted. Multiple electrode sites may be present on each catheter. Typical catheter tip locations include the high right atrium, the great cardiac vein between the left atrium and left ventricle accessed via the coronary sinus, the area of the His bundle near the tricuspid valve, and the right ventricular apex.[4,10,14] Left ventricular recordings are also performed prior to surgery or catheter ablation of left ventricular sites or if PES from the right ventricular apex or outflow tract is ineffective.[14] As in cardiac catheterization, anticoagulation with heparin is used to decrease thromboembolic complications.[4] The duration of the study usually varies from 1 to 4 hours depending on specific purpose.[4]

Before the procedure, the reasons for the study are explained to the patient and family. Explanations of the room, personnel, equipment, and procedure are included. The experience can be related to prior catheterizations. The importance of lying still during the procedure is stressed. Sedation with diazepam (Valium) may be provided.[4] The patient and family are made aware of the duration of the procedure. The patient should be prepared to expect the recurrence of his or her arrhythmias and symptoms during the procedure. Patch electrodes for defibrillation are usually placed on the patient's chest prophylactically.[14] The nurse should frequently reassure the patient and encourage questions. The patient is instructed to report complaints of chest pain, palpitations, dizziness, or any discomfort immediately to the physician during the procedure. Related nursing diagnoses include alteration in cardiac output, anxiety, fear, knowledge deficit, and alteration in family processes.[4,23]

Postprocedural nursing care is similar to the care of a patient following cardiac catheterization.[4,10] The patient is kept on bedrest with the head elevated 30 degrees for 6 to 24 hours depending on whether an arterial or venous access site has been used.[14] The affected extremity is immobilized, and the the patient is instructed not to bend the knee. Peripheral pulses are assessed frequently, and the site is monitored for hematoma and signs of infection. The patient is instructed to report increased shortness of breath, chest pain, syncope, and new or increased palpitations. Medic-Alert bracelets are encouraged. Families may be trained in CPR.[17,23] Both the patient and family are encouraged to verbalize fears related to recurrence of the arrhythmia. Support groups are available and may be contacted. Control of risk factors such as smoking, weight, cholesterol, and stress should also be emphasized.[23]

Torsades de pointes

Torsades de pointes is a malignant ventricular tachyarrhythmia associated with a prolonged QT(U) interval. Torsades de pointes is commonly classified as a form of ventricular tachycardia.[1,30,35,36,42–45] However, its ECG pattern may mimic that of either VT or VF. Torsades de pointes rhythm is named for its characteristic ECG appearance of

QRS complexes cyclically *twisting* from upright to negative or negative to upright and back. This ECG feature is easiest to see in the pattern mimicking VT, which is distinctly different from the usual pattern of VT (Fig. 11-1). The typical pattern of torsades de pointes may appear only on selected leads, so obtaining a 12-lead ECG or multilead trace may be helpful.

Torsades may also present with a spindle-like pattern identical to the pattern seen in true VF (Fig. 11-2).[32,37] The spindle pattern

is thought to be produced by a more gradual shift in the polarity of the deflections. Caution is indicated to avoid misinterpreting and mistreating true VF as torsades de pointes. A prolonged Q–T interval is necessary for a definitive diagnosis of torsades. Progressive deterioration in amplitude favors true VF.[28]

Since the ECG pattern in torsades de pointes can mimic both VT and VF, it has been labeled multiform (polymorphous) VT, atypical VT, ventricular fibrilloflutter, and paroxysmal or transient VF.[36,37] Torsades

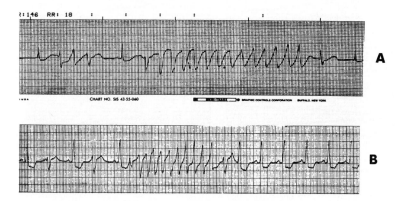

Fig. 11-1 Torsades de pointes mimicking VT. In **A,** the Q–T interval is greater than 0.5 second without correcting for heart rate. Torsades de pointes is triggered by a PVC late in diastole. In **B,** the Q–T interval does not appear prolonged until corrected for heart rate (QTc). The typical long-short cycle sequence is evident in both examples.

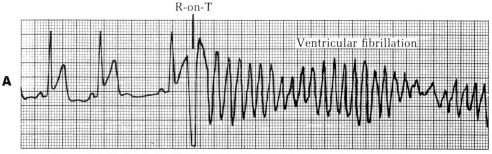

(From Conover MB: Understanding Electrocardiography, ed. 5, St. Louis, 1988, The CV Mosby Co.)

Fig. 11-2 Torsades de pointes mimicking VF versus true VF. Note the spindle pattern in both. The Q–T interval is normal in **A,** ruling out Torsades de pointes, whereas the Q–T interval is prolonged in **B,** confirming Torsades de pointes.

Continued.

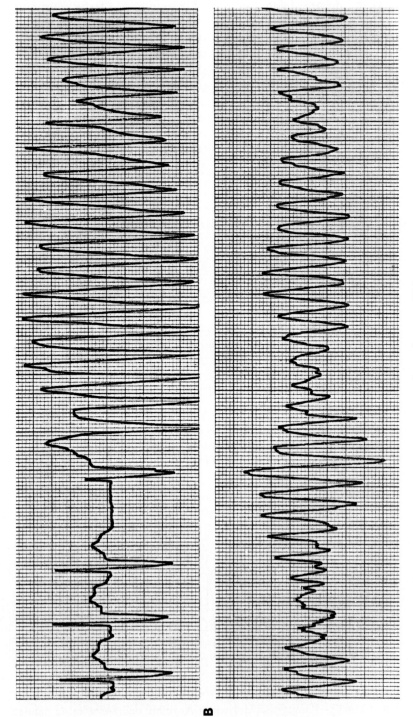

B

Fig. 11-2 For legend, see p. 503.

de pointes has also been referred to as cardiac ballet and delayed repolarization syndrome.[37] The pattern mimicking VT has been reported with a normal Q–T interval in the setting of coronary artery disease and cardiomyopathy.[27,33,37] The treatment and clinical significance in these settings are very different from those in settings in which the Q–T intervals are prolonged. For this reason, most authorities suggest that the term *polymorphous VT* be used only to describe the pattern with a normal Q–T interval. The term *torsades* is reserved instead for characteristic patterns occurring in the presence of a prolonged Q–T interval.[36,37,42,43]

The normal Q–T interval is less than 0.40 second for men and less than 0.44 second for women at a heart rate of 60 beats per minute. It is measured from the beginning of the QRS complex to the end of the T wave (see Unit 2). The Q–T interval prolongs with slower heart rates and shortens with faster heart rates. Q–T(U) intervals greater than 0.50 second are diagnostic for torsades.[1,27,36,37,42] However, intervals greater than 0.60 second carry the highest risk.[33,35,41,44] Borderline Q–T intervals should be corrected for heart rate by calculating the "QTc," or Q–T interval *corrected* for heart rate, or using available conversion charts. QTc intervals greater than 0.44 second are considered diagnostic for torsades (see Fig. 11-1B).[1,27,41,44] Patients who have a prolonged QTc only with exercise are equally at risk.[27] A screening exercise stress test has been suggested before prescribing medications that might prolong the Q–T interval. The most popular method of calculating the QTc is the Bazett formula, in which the measured Q–T interval is divided by the square root of the R–R interval in seconds.[30,33,41,45] However, this method usually requires a calculator to be done quickly at the bedside. However, if the Q–T interval is less than half the R–R interval, it may be quickly determined to be normal.[27,30,36,38]

This method of estimating the Q–T interval is accurate at normal heart rates of 60 to 100. The appearance of broad T waves is another clue to the presence of a prolonged Q–T interval. The longest Q–T intervals in patients with acute myocardial infarction are measured on leads V2 or V3.[36] Accurate measurements may also be obtained on the lead where the end of the T wave is most clearly seen.[41]

An R on T phenomenon is usually the triggering factor. In the presence of a prolonged Q–T interval, PVCs do not have to be significantly early to create this phenomenom. A typical characteristic of torsades de pointes is the initiation of the arrhythmia by a PVC late in diastole.[36,37] The last supraventricular beat before the onset of a torsades de pointes episode is usually preceded by a long R–R cycle, often following an ectopic beat (see Fig. 11-1).[27,33,35,36,42,44,45] The torsades occurs after a shorter cycle, producing a "long-short" cycle sequence. The lack of a pause at the onset and/or a close coupling interval at the onset favors true VF or polymorphous VT.[28]

Torsades de pointes occurs secondary to delayed repolarization. Recent evidence indicates that the most likely mechanism is triggered activity related to afterdepolarizations (see Unit 6).[1,27,33,39,42] Sympathetic stimulation and intracellular calcium movements may play a role in the production of these afterdepolarizations.[40,42] Reentry due to disparity of refractory periods is another still popular theory.[30,35,37,42,44,45] However, unlike typical reentrant arrhythmias, torsades de pointes is not induced during EPS.[1,33,42] It is possible that triggered activity generates the arrhythmia, which is then sustained using reentry circuits.[33] A third, less popular proposed mechanism is bifocal and/or multifocal ventricular activity in competition with biventricular tachycardia. The concept of bifocal or biventricular ectopy may explain the directional changes in the ECG pattern.[37,44]

The mechanism is still not clearly established at this time.[28,43]

Torsades often terminates spontaneously. According to Dessertenne, who is credited with labeling torsades, this characteristic helps differentiate torsades from true VF.[28] Torsades has been associated with episodes of syncopy, seizures, and sudden death if prolonged or not terminated spontaneously. It is usually unresponsive to conventional antiarrhythmic therapy and may actually be caused or aggravated by it.[35,44] Countershock remains an effective mode of therapy. However, the arrhythmia tends to recur.[33]

QT prolongation may be either acquired or congenital. Although the pattern of torsades is the same in both, the specific causes and treatment vary.[1,28,43,45] Congenital QT prolongation is thought to be due to autonomic imbalance with dominant sympathetic activity from the left stellate ganglion.[1,33] Precipitation of torsades in acquired QT prolongation is more likely to be "pause dependent." In contrast, precipitation of torsades in congenital QT prolongation is more likely to be significantly "adrenergic dependent," or dependent on sympathetic stimulation. Torsades is typically triggered by loud noises, sudden exertion, fear, pain, or emotional stress.[33] The theory of afterdepolarizations links both syndromes.

Acquired QT prolongation occurs from a variety of clinical factors that temporarily prolong the Q–T interval. These factors include class IA or class III antiarrhythmics, electrolyte imbalance, selected psychotropic agents, bradycardia, central nervous system (CNS) disorders, high protein diets, hypothermia, insecticide poisoning, coronary spasm, and occasionally mitral valve prolapse.[1,27,30,33,35,36,37,44,45] Electrolyte imbalances associated with prolonged Q–T or Q–U intervals include hypokalemia, hypocalcemia, and hypomagnesemia (see Unit 4). Psychotropic agents producing torsades de pointes include the phenothiazines such as Thorazine, Compazine, Trilafon, and Mellaril and tricyclic antidepressants such as Elavil, Tofranil, and Nardil.[1,30,36] Congenital QT prolongation has also been recognized and associated with torsades. Changes in sympathetic tone, bradycardia secondary to elevated systolic blood pressure, or both are implicated in CNS disorders. Prolonged Q–T intervals in patients with coronary artery disease and myocardial infarction have also been associated with an increased risk of sudden death.[36,41,44,45] Results of the Beta Blocker Heart Attack Trial (BHAT) suggest that the risk is highest if the prolonged Q–T interval persists months after acute myocardial infarction.[41]

Antiarrhythmic agents are particularly notorious for producing malignant ventricular arrhythmias—the very type of arrhythmia they are supposed to effectively treat. This ability of a drug to produce arrhythmias is logically referred to as a *proarrhythmic* effect. One of the most common proarrhythmic effects is the production of torsades des pointes. Proarrhythmic effects are more likely to occur in the presence of severe left ventricular dysfunction.

The antiarrhyhmic drugs most commonly producing torsades are the class IA agents. Examples of these agents include quinidine, procainamide (Pronestyl), and disopyramide (Norpace). These drugs act to prolong ventricular repolarization/refractory periods as evidenced by their effect on the Q–T interval. The effect on repolarization has been referred to as quinidine effect and is not thought to be associated with toxic levels of these drugs. It represents a sensitivity to the drug instead, which may occur with even the first dose.[33,37] If the Q–T interval is exceedingly prolonged (i.e., >0.50 second or >0.44 second if QTc), an episode of torsades de pointes may be triggered. Serum drug concentrations are usually normal or low.[27,33,35,36,37]

When any of these drugs is initiated, individuals should be carefully monitored in a CCU or telemetry unit. About half of the episodes of torsades occur in the first 4 days.[32] Baseline normal Q–T intervals and serum electrolyte levels should be validated.[35] Q–T intervals should be checked every 4 to 8 hours for the first 2 days, than daily thereafter.[30,36] If an episode of torsades occurs or the Q–T interval exceeds 0.50 second, the drug is best discontinued. Episodes of torsades after prolonged therapy are unusual unless another complicating factor such as electrolyte imbalance or bradycardia occurs.[36] Patients taking class IA antiarrhythmics should also be regularly monitored for bradycardia and electrolyte imbalance.

Class III antiarrhythmic agents also act to prolong ventricular refractory periods. QT prolongation with torsades de pointes has been associated with amiodarone therapy. However, the incidence of torsades de pointes is low, even in the presence of significant QT prolongation.[27,33,35,38a] If torsades de pointes does occur, the long half-life of this drug necessitates that therapy for torsades be continued up to 5 to 10 days. The newer, experimental class III agent sotalol is associated with a significant incidence of torsades de pointes.[1,27,44] Ironically, the other major class III agent bretylium does not cause torsades de pointes and may actually be effective in its therapy.[33,45] This may be explained by its differential effect on normal versus ischemic or abnormal cardiac tissue, which, unlike amiodarone, may promote uniformity of refractoriness. One calcium channel blocking agent (class IV antiarrhythmic), bepridil (Vasocor), is reported to produce significant QT prolongation with torsades de pointes.[30,33,44]

Magnesium sulfate is currently recommended by the American Heart Association as the treatment of choice for torsades de pointes.[2] However, the pulseless patient is treated initially as if the rhythm were true VF. The therapeutic effect of magnesium occurs without any alteration in the Q–T intervals or magnesium blood levels.[33,34,42,43] One possible mechanism of action is stimulation of the Na^+/K^+ pump with restoration of intracellular K^+. Magnesium is important in the breakdown of ATP for energy, and thus is necessary for the normal functioning of the $Na^+–K^+$ pump. A second possible mechanism of action is inhibition of calcium channels and afterdepolarizations.[42–44] Magnesium acts as nature's calcium channel blocker (see Unit 4).[32,39,42] Calcium channel blocking agents may theoretically be beneficial as well, but further studies are needed. An IV bolus of 1 to 2 g of magnesium is administered over 1 to 2 minutes.[2,32] Although undiluted by Iseri,[32] according to current ACLS guidelines, this bolus should be diluted in 100 ml of D5W.[2,30,34] A second bolus of 2 to 4 g may be administered after 10 to 15 minutes if necessary.[33,36,42] The only reported side effect is a flushing sensation during administration.[35,36,42] Magnesium is contraindicated in patients with renal failure.[35] An infusion of 3 to 20 mg may be administered until the Q–T interval is less than 0.50 second.[35,36] Low serum K^+ levels should be corrected by K^+ administration.[35,36] Magnesium is effective in both congenital and acquired QT prolongation.

If magnesium is ineffective, therapy for torsades de pointes is directed at shortening the Q–T interval by increasing the heart rate. The heart rate may be increased with overdrive pacing, isoproterenol (Isuprel), or atropine.[43] Although overdrive atrial pacing is preferred, cautious ventricular overdrive pacing at the lowest effective VR (approximately 90 to 150) may be more practical in this emergency setting. The use of the newer external transcutaneous pacing systems can further facilitate this mode of treatment (see Unit 10). After the normal rhythm is restored, transvenous pacing may be used to prevent further bradycardia that may trigger torsades de pointes or until the Q–T

(QTc) interval has returned to normal.

Class IB agents may also be effective in therapy for torsades de pointes since they act to shorten repolarization and the Q–T interval.[1,33] Examples of class IB agents include xylocaine (Lidocaine), phenytoin (Dilantin), and mexiletine (Mexitil). Reports are currently available primarily on the use of Xylocaine, although the use of Dilantin and Mexitil has also been successful. Xylocaine is usually unsuccessful[34,37,38a,42] because of a different effect on normal versus ischemic or abnormal cardiac tissue.[44] Xylocaine shortens refractory periods primarily in normal tissues. Because of this differential effect also, Xylocaine occasionally has been reported to actually cause or enhance torsades de pointes.[36,44,45] Further studies are needed in this area, particularly with regard to the effects of the other class IB agents.

Patients with congenitally prolonged Q–T interval, mitral valve prolapse, and CNS disorders exhibit an increased sensitivity to autonomic stimulation. Therefore, in these patients the sympathetic stimulating agent isoproterenol (Isuprel) is not indicated. These patients respond best to sympathetic blocking agents such as the beta blockers.[33,35,36,40] Alpha receptor blockade may also be helpful. Combined alpha and beta blockade with agents such as labetalol (Trandate) can be offered as an alternative to surgery.[29,33,40] Surgical removal of the left stellate ganglion or lidocaine block can be performed as a last resort if there is no response to beta blockade.[33,36] There is little effect on the resting Q–T(U) interval with either sympathetic blocking drugs or surgery.

In contrast to torsades de pointes, polymorphous VT with a normal Q–T interval is responsive to conventional class Ia antiarrhythmic therapy.[36,43] Magnesium is likely to be ineffective.[35,42] Therapy with sympathetic agents such as Isuprel is often harmful, triggering VF.[35,36,42] This rhythm behaves clinically as true VT or VF and is best treated as such. If the QT is unknown, normal, or doubtful, the rhythm is best diagnosed as polymorphous VT or VF *resembling* torsades de pointes and should be initially treated as classic VT or VF.

In our opinion, the use of Isuprel is best avoided since negative effects may occur in the presence of a normal Q–T interval, congenitally prolonged Q–T interval, or CNS disease. Alternate approaches such as overdrive pacing or the administration of magnesium sulfate, class IB agents, or bretylium tosylate (Bretylol) are associated with far less risk.

PREEXCITATION SYNDROME

Preexcitation syndrome refers to the presence of a congenital bypass of part or all of the normal AV conduction system. Since the normal AV delay is avoided, atrial impulses can reach the ventricles through this extra pathway earlier than through the normal conduction pathways. The ventricles may thus be preexcited by atrial impulses using this pathway, predisposing the patient to supraventricular tachyarrhythmias.

Because these congenital pathways bypass part or all of the normal conduction system, they are referred to as extra or *accessory* pathways or bypass tracts. A second major characteristic of an accessory pathway is its insertion into either the free ventricular wall or the normal conduction system. The term *tract* is more strictly reserved for pathways with one end attached to normal conductive tissue.[4,61] There are three major forms of preexcitation syndrome: Wolff-Parkinson-White, Lown-Ganong-Levine, and Mahaim. They are differentiated by the characteristics of their accessory pathways or bypass tracts (Fig. 11-3).

The congenital pathway in Wolff-

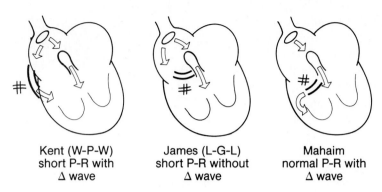

Kent (W-P-W)	James (L-G-L)	Mahaim
short P-R with	short P-R without	normal P-R with
Δ wave	Δ wave	Δ wave

Fig. 11-3   The three major forms of preexcitation. Location of the accessory pathways and corresponding ECG characteristics.

Parkinson-White syndrome is referred to as the *Kent bundle*.[4,48,57,58,63] It completely bypasses the normal AV conduction system, inserting into the ventricular wall, thus connecting the atria directly into the ventricles.

The congenital pathway in Lown-Ganong-Levine syndrome is referred to as the *James bundle*. It partially bypasses the AV node, inserting into the normal AV conduction system below the node and thus connecting the atria directly to the lower portion of the AV node.[4,48,63] This pathway may also be referred to as a bypass tract in the strictest sense since one end remains attached to the normal conductive tissue.

Mahaim fibers originate below the AV node, bypass part or all of the ventricular conduction system, and insert into the ventricular wall. They thus connect the lower AV node or bundle of His directly to ventricular muscle.[4,48,63]

Accessory pathways that bypass the AV node eliminate the major part of the AV delay, resulting in a short P–R interval. Accessory pathways that insert directly into ventricular muscle produce a *delta* (Δ) wave pattern in sinus rhythm or sinus tachycardia. The Kent bundle of the Wolff-Parkinson-White syndrome bypasses the AV node. Therefore, the P–R interval is short. The

Kent bundle also inserts directly into ventricular muscle. Therefore, a delta wave pattern should be expected in sinus rhythm or sinus tachycardia.

The James bundle of the Lown-Ganong-Levine syndrome also bypasses the AV node. Therefore, the P–R interval is short. However, because the James bundle inserts into the lower portion of the normal conduction system (the AV node), a delta wave pattern should not be expected in sinus rhythm or sinus tachycardia.[61]

Because Mahaim fibers do not bypass the AV node, the P–R interval is normal. However, Mahaim fibers insert directly into the ventricular wall, so a delta wave pattern should be expected in sinus rhythm.

Delta waves are seen with both Kent and Mahaim pathways. The delta wave is the result of a *fusion complex*.[1,4,49,50,52,57] Fusion beats occur when two or more impulses attempt to control the ventricles at the same time (see Unit 6). During sinus rhythm in Wolff-Parkinson-White syndrome the atrial impulse travels down both the normal conduction and Kent pathways simultaneously (Fig. 11-4). However, the ventricles are activated by the accessory pathway first since there is no AV delay.

The Kent pathway inserts into the ventri-

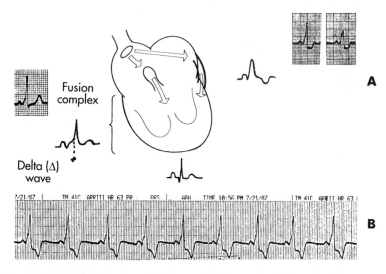

Fusion complex

Delta (Δ) wave

A

B

Fig. 11-4 Mechanism of fusion complex and delta waves in Wolff-Parkinson-White syndrome.

cles which conduct slowly. Thus, the initial part of the QRS complex is wide. The remainder of the QRS complex is produced by activation through the normal conduction pathways and is therefore narrow. The completed QRS complex reflects a blending or fusion of the two potential complexes. The initial slurring of this fusion complex mimics the Greek triangular symbol—delta (Δ)—and it is thus referred to as a *delta wave*. This initial part of the QRS complex reflects activation through the Kent pathway.[1,61]

The delta wave becomes more pronounced during either very slow or rapid atrial rates due to increased refractoriness and delay within the normal AV conduction system. When conduction through the normal AV pathway is delayed, conduction through the accessory pathway is unopposed for a longer period, causing the delta wave to become more pronounced. The delta wave may be totally dormant during normal sinus rates, when the AV node conduction time is normal. The delta wave may decrease or disappear with the normal increases in si-

nus rates occurring during exercise.[46,62,66] Improved AV conduction secondary to sympathetic stimulation is implicated. In contrast, rapid atrial pacing or vagal stimulation prolongs AV conduction time and can be used to elicit the delta wave in a patient with a suspect history.[1,52,62] Complete activation by the accessory pathway can occur at rapid atrial rates, producing a totally wide QRS complex (see Fig. 11-4). The delta wave is completely absent, regardless of the heart rate, in accessory pathways capable of only retrograde conduction. This form of Wolff-Parkinson-White syndrome is referred to as *concealed*.[1,48,50,52,55,57,58,66] The presence of these accessory pathways is detected during electrophysiologic studies. The location of an accessory pathway may also influence its ability to be detected on the surface ECG.[62]

Either single or multiple pathways may exist in a given individual. Although a variety of potential locations exist, the most common locations for accessory pathways are right free wall, left lateral (free wall), posteroseptal, and anteroseptal.[1,2,52,53,57,62,63] Left free wall pathways are more common in in-

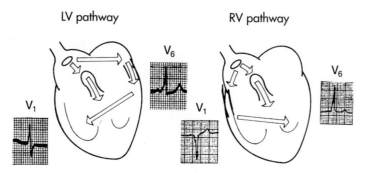

LV pathway RV pathway

V₆

V₁

V₁

V₆

Fig. 11-5 Detection of left ventricular versus right ventricular pathways. Analysis of the polarity of the delta waves in the chest leads.

dividuals with single pathways, and posteroseptal pathways are more common in individuals wtih multiple pathways.[47] Right-sided pathways are the least common.[62] The characteristics of the tachycardia and effectiveness of certain modes of therapy vary with the location of the pathway(s). The former, more simplistic designation of type A and type B Wolff-Parkinson-White syndrome according to right- or left-sided pathways has been abandoned.[1,48,52,61,62]

The 12-lead ECG is helpful in identifying the presence and approximate location of the accessory pathway(s). The direction of the delta wave on the chest and limb leads suggests the location. The direction or axis of the delta wave and QRS complex on V1 may be analyzed initially in V1 to determine a right ventricular versus left ventricular location (Fig. 11-5).[1,4,50] With a right ventricular pathway, the impulse travels away from the positive electrode of V1, producing a negative deflection. Conversely, with a left ventricular pathway, the impulse travels toward the positive electrode of V1, producing a positive deflection. Evaluation of the complex at maximal preexcitation provides more accurate information.[1] The direction of the delta wave in the limb leads can assist in determining a septal versus free wall location.[1,53,61] A negative delta wave in leads II,

III, and aVF (left axis deviation) suggests a posteroseptal location, although a right free wall pathway must be ruled out. Normal axis is more typical of an anteroseptal pathway. A left lateral (free wall) pathway typically produces a negative delta wave in lead I (right axis deviation), aVL, V5, and V6.[1,61] The delta wave may not be seen and identified in leads where it is isoelectric.[48] Multilead assessment is also recommended for this reason.

Wolff-Parkinson-White syndrome is the most common form of preexcitation. The most common tachyarrhythmias occurring in patients with Wolff-Parkinson-White syndrome are AV reentrant paroxysmal supraventricular tachycardia (PSVT), which presents most typically with a narrow QRS and atrial fibrillation, which presents most typically with a wide QRS (Fig. 11-6).[1,4,50] These arrhythmias are less common in right free wall pathways and more common with anteroseptal pathways.[2] Symptoms include palpitations, dizziness, diaphoresis, syncope, or occasional SCD.[2,63] Wolff-Parkinson-White syndrome may be tolerated asymptomatically or with minimal symptoms in up to 50% of individuals with this ECG pattern.[1,51,62] Related nursing diagnoses in symptomatic patients include alteration in cardiac output, impaired cerebral tissue per-

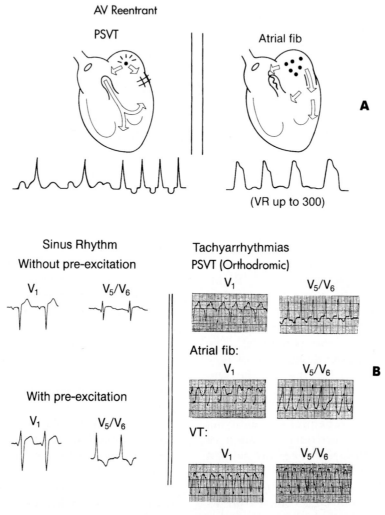

AV Reentrant

PSVT

Atrial fib

A

(VR up to 300)

Sinus Rhythm

Without pre-excitation

V_1 V_5/V_6

Tachyarrhythmias

PSVT (Orthodromic)

V_1 V_5/V_6

Atrial fib:

V_1 V_5/V_6 **B**

VT:

V_1 V_5/V_6

With pre-excitation

V_1 V_5/V_6

Fig. 11-6 Common supraventricular tachyarrhythmias in Wolff-Parkinson-White syndrome. Note the narrow, regular QRS complexes in orthodromic AV reentrant tachycardia and the wide, irregular QRS complexes in atrial fibrillation. The wide complexes mimic the complexes in sinus rhythm with pre-excitation. Ventricular tachycardia is differentiated from atrial fibrillation in the same patient by the regular, wide complexes. Antidromic PSVT is unlikely because of the presence of negative concordance.

fusion, anxiety related to palpitations, risk of sudden death, unknown prognosis, and diagnostic tests.

AV reentrant supraventricular tachycardia (PSVT) is reported more frequently than atrial fibrillation in Wolff-Parkinson-White syndrome and is also referred to as *circus movement tachycardia* (CMT).[48,55,61,68] Patients with a James pathway (Lown-Ganong-Levine syndrome) may also present with this form of supraventricular tachycardia.[58] Reentry is one of the major mechanisms of arrhythmia formation. Reentry is defined as the ability of an impulse to reexcite a region of the heart through which it has already passed (see Unit 6). AV reentry uses macrocircuits connecting the atria and ventricles to reexcite either the atria or ventricles after already leaving the chamber. Thus, the exciting impulse may originate in either the atria or the ventricles.

In Wolff-Parkinson-White syndrome, the macrocircuit is formed by the AV node, bundle branches, and accessory (Kent) pathway. During sinus rhythm, the impulse travels simultaneously through both the normal conduction system and the Kent pathway, colliding with itself in the ventricles. However, ectopic impulses do not always travel simultaneously down both pathways.

Premature atrial contractions (PACs) are often selectively unable to conduct through the accessory pathway because of its longer refractory period. Kent pathways typically conduct faster but recover more slowly than the AV node.[50] Thus, *block* occurs selectively within the accessory pathway. The PAC is transmitted exclusively through the AV node and bundle branch system to the ventricles. At the same time, the impulse is conducted in a retrograde fashion to the atria via the accessory pathway (see Fig. 11-6).[48,58] Since the AV node has a natural *delay*, the atria are given the time to recover and be able to again accept this impulse. The atria are thus reexcited by the original impulse, limited only by the refractory period of the accessory pathway and atria. This impulse can easily recycle again and again, resulting in a tachycardia.

The ECG characteristics of this form of AV reentrant tachycardia are (1) a premature P at the onset, (2) a P wave that changes direction during the tachycardia, (3) a long P–R interval at the onset, and (4) a short R–P interval during the tachycardia.[52,55] The P wave changes direction since the atria are activated initially in an antegrade direction and subsequently in a retrograde direction. This change may be seen on any lead with clear P waves depending on the exact location of the accessory pathway (see Unit 6).[48] Alternating heights of the R waves or depths of the S waves (QRS alternans) are also typical of PSVT in Wolff-Parkinson-White syndrome and may indicate the presence of concealed pathways.[48,55,61,62] The polarity of the retrograde P wave on the limb leads or chest leads can help locate the accessory pathway.[61,62]

The *R–P interval* is the distance from the beginning of the QRS of one impulse to the P wave of the next impulse. It reflects retrograde conduction from the ventricles through the Kent pathway in contrast with the P–R interval, which reflects antegrade conduction to the ventricles through the AV node and bundle branches. The natural delay at the AV node is reflected in the normal P–R interval of up to 0.20 second. Since there is usually no natural delay within the Kent pathway, the R–P interval is shorter than the P–R interval. The R–P interval may be longer in patients with concealed pathways.[62] The delta wave is not present during the tachycardia since the ectopic impulses are usually conducted to the ventricles using only the normal AV conduction pathway. Therefore, the QRS complex during the tachycardia is usually narrower than in sinus rhythm.

AV reentrant tachycardia with antegrade conduction through the normal conduction pathways in the patient with Wolff-Parkinson-White syndrome is also referred to as *orthodromic*.[1,46,50,52,57,58,63] Orthodromic reentrant tachycardia may be triggered, less commonly, by a PVC as well as a PAC.[1,46,50,58] The PVC conducts selectively through the accessory pathway in a retrograde fashion, then antegrade back into the ventricle through the normal AV conduction system. Narrow QRS (orthodromic) tachycardia also typically occurs in concealed Wolff-Parkinson-White syndrome. Concealed Wolff-Parkinson-White syndrome is uncommon in right free wall or anteroseptal pathways.[49]

Antegrade conduction through the accessory pathway with retrograde conduction through the normal conduction pathway occurs less commonly in Wolff-Parkinson-White syndrome. This form of AV reentrant tachycardia is referred to as *antidromic* and characteristically occurs in the presence of multiple accessory pathways.[1,46,47,50,57,58,63] With multiple accessory pathways, antegrade conduction may occur in one pathway with retrograde conduction through another.[1,46,49] Since the ectopic impulses are conducted to the ventricles using the accessory pathway, the QRS complexes during this tachycardia are usually wider than in sinus rhythm. This regular wide QRS tachycardia associated with antidromic conduction is particularly difficult to differentiate from ventricular tachycardia (see Unit 7). EPS is usually required.[48] QRS complexes changing abruptly from narrow to wide during the tachycardia suggest both orthodromic and antidromic tachycardias and the presence of multiple pathways.[47,62,68]

AV reentrant orthodromic PSVT may result in a wide QRS, mimicking antidromic conduction, when rate-dependent bundle branch block occurs.[1,62] The further delay in the AV macrocircuit associated with the bundle branch block may trigger a reentrant tachycardia that could not be triggered in the presence of AV node delay alone.[55,66]

Since the original impulse *returns* to the initial chamber via either the accessory pathway or the normal AV conduction system, AV reentrant PSVT, whether orthodromic or antidromic, is also referred to as a *reciprocating tachycardia*.[1,46,47,57,58,62] A single reciprocal beat or the first beat of a potential reciprocating tachycardia is called an *echo beat*, since as in a true echo, the same message that is sent out is returned to its source. This beat has also been referred to as a *sandwiched*

beat because the QRS complex appears to be sandwiched between the two related P waves when triggered by a PAC. If triggered by a PVC, the P wave appears sandwiched between the two related QRS complexes.

Atrial fibrillation is the second most commonly occurring arrhythmia in Wolff-Parkinson-White syndrome. The multiple, rapid impulses of atrial fibrillation bombard the AV node, prolonging its refractory period to a greater extent than that of the accessory pathway. These impulses are therefore preferentially conducted exclusively through the accessory pathway. The ventricular rate is rapid, limited only by the refractory period of the accessory pathway. In atrial fibrillation, the accessory pathway does not act as part of a circuit. It is merely a point of entry to the ventricles, controlling the ventricular response. Therefore, this rhythym does not represent an AV reentrant tachycardia. The QRS complex remains irregular. Since ventricular conduction occurs totally by means of the accessory pathway, the resulting QRS complex is wide. The irregular, rapid QRS complexes are the only ECG changes clearly differentiating this rhythm from ventricular tachycardia. The differential diagnosis is particularly difficult in very rapid rates in which this irregularity is not so easily seen. The major helpful 12-lead finding is the absence of negative concordance in the chest leads (see Unit 7). With multiple pathways, different QRS complexes and fusion beats may be present, depending on which pathway or pathways activate the ventricles.[48,68] The preexcitation pattern may also change after procainamide (Pronestyl) administration in multiple pathways.[68]

The rapid ventricular response in atrial fibrillation may eventually deteriorate into ventricular fibrillation and therefore is a particularly significant, though only potentially life-threatening, rhythm.[4,48,52,58,63] Atrial flutter occurs less commonly with characteristics similar to those of atrial fibrillation.[4,49,52] When a VR of 300 or more is sustained in a wide QRS tachycardia without immediate deterioration into VF, Wolff-Parkinson-White syndrome should be highly suspected. The risk of ventricular fibrillation and sudden death in Wolff-Parkinson-White syndrome is highest in the presence of an accessory pathway with a short antegrade refractory period or in multiple accessory pathways.[47,52,65] The presence of syncope does not correlate with the risk of sudden death.[65] Atrial fibrillation with wide, rapid QRS complexes is not possible in concealed Wolff-Parkinson-White syndrome since antegrade conduction does not occur over the accessory pathways.[50,61]

The length of the refractory period of the accessory pathway can be estimated noninvasively by observing the length of the shortest R−R cycle in spontaneous or induced atrial fibrillation. R−R intervals less than 250 msec during atrial fibrillation indicate short refractory periods.[50,52,57−59,62,63,65] Blocking of accessory pathway conduction during exercise testing or with procainamide (Pronestyl) administration indicates a long refractory period and low risk of sudden death.[52,59] Disappearance of the delta wave in sinus rhythm or sinus tachycardia (intermittent preexcitation) also suggests an adequately long refractory period of the accessory pathway.[48,52,59,62]

The supraventricular tachycardias of Wolff-Parkinson-White (preexcitation) syndrome may be treated pharmacologically, electrically, or surgically. Asymptomatic patients require no intervention, since the risk of sudden death is very small.[51,60,66] However, some physicians believe that the patient should be informed of this small risk and be allowed to decide whether to pursue diagnostic screening.[59] If a short antegrade refractory period is documented on EPS, both medical and surgical intervention are acceptable, although research does not support the effectiveness of either at this time.[66] Asymptomatic patients should be instructed in signs and symptoms of tachycardia to report, so that intervention can be provided if needed.[59]

According to ACLS guidelines in symptomatic patients, cardioversion is the initial treatment of choice for supraventricular arrhythmias with a ventricular response greater than 150[2] (see Unit 6). Subsequent management differs according to whether the tachycardia is associated with a narrow or wide QRS complex.

Orthodromic (narrow QRS), AV reentrant tachycardia is prevented and/or interrupted by drugs that prolong the refractory period of the AV node (Fig. 11-7). Vagal maneuvers such as carotid sinus pressure, Valsalva maneuvers, gagging, squatting, or elevation of the legs are also effective in the narrow complex PSVT of Wolff-Parkinson-White syndrome as in other forms of PSVT.[1,4,48,52] Examples of drugs that prolong the refractory period of the AV node include adenosine (Adenocard), verapamil (Isoptin, Calan, Verelan), diltiazem (Cardizem), and esmolol (Brevibloc). These drugs are effective in the acute management of the narrow complex PSVT of Wolff-Parkinson-White syndrome.

Administration of these same agents may be contraindicated in the presence of atrial fibrillation with a wide QRS in Wolff-Parkinson-White syndrome.[62] Agents prolonging the refractory period of the AV node can facilitate conduction via the accessory pathway, thus further increasing the ventricular response. These rapid ventricular responses can deteriorate into ventricular fibrillation. The drug-induced acceleration of the ventricular response in atrial fibrillation occurs primarily in patients with short antegrade refractory periods of the accessory pathway (i.e., less than 250 msec). The risk is greatest with digitalis, which also has a direct effect on the accessory pathway, shortening its refractory period. Increased risk of inducing a rapid ventricular response has

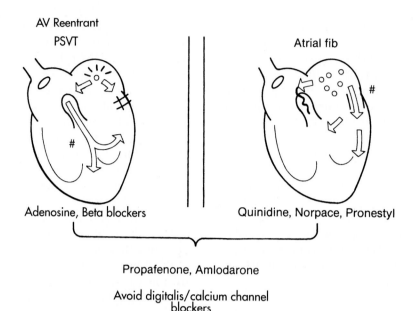

AV Reentrant
PSVT

Atrial fib

Adenosine, Beta blockers

Quinidine, Norpace, Pronestyl

Propafenone, Amiodarone

Avoid digitalis/calcium channel
blockers

Fig. 11-7 Pharmacologic therapy in Wolff-Parkinson-White syndrome.

been reported with verapamil and is assumed to occur with diltiazem because it is also a calcium channel blocker. Since AV tachycardia can progress to atrial fibrillation, digitalis and the calcium channel blockers are best avoided in all patients with Wolff-Parkinson-White syndrome.[1] Calcium channel blockers or beta blockers can be used in the presence of a documented long refractory period of the accessory pathway.[52,66] However, beta blockers are the preferred drugs for long-term management.[52,62]

The ventricular response of atrial fibrillation in Wolff-Parkinson-White syndrome is decreased by agents that prolong the antegrade refractory period of the accessory pathway or totally block antegrade conduction via this pathway. These drugs are also effective in the antidromic (wide QRS) tachycardia of Wolff-Parkinson-White syndrome. Examples of drugs that prolong the antegrade refractory period of the accessory

pathway include quinidine, procainamide (Pronestyl), and disopyramide phosphate (Norpace). These drugs are all class IA antiarrhythmic agents. Class I agents are less effective in the presence of a short accessory pathway refractory period.[1,58] Of these drugs, only Pronestyl can be administered intravenously to quickly control the ventricular rate. The wide QRS tachycardias of WPW can mimic ventricular tachycardia and flutter, which are also controlled by this drug. Thus the initial drug of choice in the management of wide QRS tachycardia due to Wolff-Parkinson-White syndrome is the class IA agent Pronestyl.[46,62]

Class IB antiarrhythmics such as lidocaine have variable effects on the accessory pathway. Lidocaine prolongs the refractory period and blocks conduction in the accessory pathway primarily in the presence of long initial refractory periods (greater than 380 msec). However, lidocaine has also been reported to shorten the refractory period of the accessory pathway in individuals with short initial refractory periods, resulting in an increased ventricular response and deterioration into ventricular fibrillation. It is best avoided in patients with Wolff-Parkinson-White syndrome.

Examples of drugs that prolong the refractory period of both the AV node and the accessory pathway include the class III agents amiodarone (Cordarone) and sotalol and the class IC agents flecainide (Tambocor), encainide (Enkaid), and propafenone (Rhythmol).[52,62] These agents are effective in *both* the paroxysmal atrial tachycardia and atrial fibrillation of Wolff-Parkinson-White syndrome. They may be preferred when the properties of the accessory pathway are unknown. However, these agents are associated with significant side effects of their own and require further study. The diffuse effect of amiodarone on the conduction system as well as its delayed onset of action, long half-life, and side effects limits its use in this setting because less toxic agents are now available. Propafenone (Rhythmol) is associated with the fewest side effects.[52]

Both surgical and catheter (electrical) ablation are used successfully in the management of Wolff-Parkinson-White syndrome. Ablation refers to the partial or complete destruction of conduction structures (see Unit 6). Electrical intervention with antitachycardia pacemakers is no longer recommended because of the risk of triggering atrial fibrillation.[63,66]

Surgical ablation in Wolff-Parkinson-White syndrome consists of division of the accessory pathway or pathways after precise electrophysiologic mapping to determine the location.[53,57] Epicardial cryoablation has also been used recently during surgery, minimizing the need for cardiopulmonary bypass.[53,63] Surgical ablation is indicated in patients with atrial fibrillation R–R cycles of less than 250 msec, survivors of SCD, indi-

viduals refractory to drug therapy or limited by side effects, and young, otherwise healthy individuals with recurrent symptomatic tachyarrhythmias who might require lifetime antiarrhythmic therapy.[50,53,57,58,63] Transient ST–T wave changes present preoperatively take time to disappear postoperatively and do not represent ischemia.[57] Temporary pacing wires can be left in place.[57] Repeat electrophysiologic studies with mapping are performed 5 to 7 days after the surgery. The pacing wires are then removed. Nursing care, including patient teaching, is similar to that for the patient following open heart surgery.

The more recently introduced catheter ablation provides an alternative to surgical intervention or long-term antiarrhythmic therapy but is not currently approved by the Food and Drug Administration (FDA) for this purpose.[46] General anesthesia is not required. Ablation using radiofrequency energy is most promising. Ablation is effective in multiple as well as single pathways.[18] The effectiveness is higher for left-sided (greater than 95%) than right-sided or septal (greater than 90%) pathways.[58] Catheter ablation can be performed in conjunction with standard EPS, combining diagnosis and therapeutic intervention into one study.[58,67] This procedure can take up to 8 to 10 hrs.[46]

The patient is sedated with Versed or fentanyl. Earphones playing relaxing music may be worn during the procedure. Mild discomfort is felt when the current is applied. Atrial fibrillation occurs immediately after catheter ablation but terminates spontaneously and is associated with a slower ventricular rate.[17] A follow-up study of only about 1 hour duration is usually performed in 4 to 6 weeks.[1] The patient should be instructed that sinus tachycardia is normal with exercise, but abrupt-onset tachycardia should be reported.[46] The patient should also be encouraged to wear a Medic Alert bracelet.[50]

Electrophysiologic studies are used in

Wolff-Parkinson-White syndrome to confirm the presence of an accessory pathway, precisely locate the pathway(s) in order to guide surgical or catheter ablation, and confirm the effectiveness of surgical or catheter ablation[62] (see Role of Electrophysiologic Studies). Atrial fibrillation is induced or triggered during EPS to determine the shortest R–R cycle, which in turn allows for the selection of the most appropriate form of therapy.[58] Multiple pathways are best located in the electrophysiologic laboratory. Indications for EPS in Wolff-Parkinson-White syndrome include atrial fibrillation or antidromic tachycardia, VF (sudden death), syncope, and tachycardias unresponsive to pharmacologic intervention.[63] Routine screening of asymptomatic patients using EPS is not recommended because the risk of sudden death is so low.[51,52,59,60] However, routine screen-

ing of all symptomatic patients has been suggested.[52]

Noninvasive diagnostic tests helpful in the initial evaluation and follow-up of the patient with Wolff-Parkinson-White syndrome include 12-lead ECG, body surface mapping, exercise stress testing, two-dimensional echocardiography, radionuclide ventriculography, and Holter monitoring.[63] Body surface mapping using 32 to 196 unipolar leads has been used with sufficient accuracy to locate an accessory pathway.[63] Intermittent preexcitation can be documented with Holter monitoring or exercise stress testing or after procainamide (Pronestyl) administration. These findings are particularly helpful in confirming probable low risk of sudden death in asymptomatic patients in whom EPS is not indicated.[52,59,60,62,66]

CARDIOMYOPATHIES

Laurie Futterman Correa, RN, MSN, CCRN

The cardiomyopathies are diseases of the heart muscle, occurring independently of any other cardiovascular pathology.[3,69,71,79] Myocardial changes secondary to coronary artery disease, hypertension, or congenital or valvular disease are excluded from this classification.[1,4,69,71,79] Therefore, myocardial infarction is not typically considered a form of cardiomyopathy.

The cardiomyopathies are separated into three distinct groups according to their structural and functional or hemodynamic changes: dilated, hypertrophic, and restrictive (Fig. 11-8). Common factors include abnormal calcium handling, myofibril changes, and stiff, noncompliant left ventricular walls.[1,3,4,72] The decreased compliance results in difficulty in filling and a rise in left ventricular diastolic pressure. Myofibril changes may be detected by endomyocardial

biopsy, but specific patterns vary, so it is usually not indicated.[1]

Structural and hemodynamic differences between the cardiomyopathies focus on left ventricular cavity and systolic changes (see Fig. 11-8). In *dilated* cardiomyopathy, the left ventricular cavity is enlarged. Dilated cardiomyopathy is associated with decreased contractility and ineffective emptying in systole. Cardiac output and ejection fractions are decreased.[1,3,4,80]

In *hypertrophic* cardiomyopathy, the muscle wall is thickened at the expense of the left ventricular cavity.[73,75,79,84,95] These changes result in a hyperdynamic state with increased ejection fractions, although some authorities question a true increase in contractility.[4,72,88] The thickening or hypertrophy of the muscle wall may be asymmetrical or symmetrical (usually only 5% to 10%). The asymmetrical

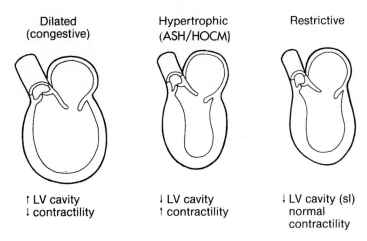

Fig. 11-8   Major forms of cardiomyopathy.

hypertrophy may be apical or midventricular involving the papillary muscle. However, in 55% to 90% of the cases, it is located in the septal area and is referred to as *asymmetric septal hypertrophy* (ASH).[1,88,97] Since septal hypertrophy results in a narrowing or stenosis of the left ventricular outlet below the aortic valve, ASH was formerly referred to as *idiopathic hypertrophic subaortic stenosis* (IHSS).

Hypertrophic cardiomyopathy may be obstructive (HOCM) or nonobstructive. The nonobstructive form is characterized by a thin, pointed left ventricular free wall, whereas the obstructive form is characterized by thickening of the posterior basal left ventricular free wall under the posterior mitral leaflet.[3,4] In the obstructive form, a pressure gradient develops late in systole after most of the volume has been ejected. This obstructive pressure gradient is thought to be related to abnormal anterior motion of the posterior mitral valve leaflet during systole and plays a somewhat controversial role in the severity of the related symptoms.[1,4,72,88,97]

Restrictive cardiomyopathy is associated with an increased wall thickness and small cavity size similar to but not as small as the

left ventricular cavity size associated with hypertrophic cardiomyopathy. The left ventricular compliance changes are more pronounced. Contractility and ejection fraction during systole are normal. However, the cardiac output is decreased secondary to impaired filling or diastolic changes.

Although causes may not always be clearly identified in any of the myopathies, mechanisms implicated at least as precipitating or predisposing factors include infective myocarditis, genetic factors, metabolic disturbances or toxins, and immunopathies.[1,79,92,97] Specific risk factors for dilated cardiomyopathy include viral diseases, alcoholism, selected chemotherapy agents such as doxorubicin hydrochloride (Adriamycin) and 5-fluorouracil, diabetes, and peripartal immunopathy.[3,92] Hypertrophic cardiomyopathy is familial in nearly 60% of cases and is thought to be related to a disturbance in the sympathetic nervous system with loss of fetal regression of hypertrophy.[1,71,84,96] The strong genetic link associated with hypertrophic cardiomyopathy can make the evaluation of family history a crucial component of the diagnosis. Restrictive cardiomyopathy is the rarest form. Specific risk factors include endocardial fibrosis, amyloidosis, and neoplastic processes.

Both dilated and restrictive cardiomyopathy are associated with a poor long-term prognosis.[92] One- and two-year mortality rates of 23% and 48%, respectively, have been reported in dilated cardiomyopathy after the diagnosis has been established. Unfortunately, dilated cardiomyopathy is the most frequently occurring type of cardiomyopathy. End-stage CHF may be reached within 2 years of the initial diagnosis. At that time, the only effective mode of therapy is cardiac transplantation. Statistically, most patients with restrictive hemodynamic patterns have a systemic disease process and thus are not candidates for cardiac transplantation. Consequently, these patients tend to deteriorate rapidly in their clinical course, requiring a significant amount of emotional support.[4] Since restrictive cardiomyopathy is rare, the remainder of this discussion will focus on a comparison between dilated and obstructive hypertrophic myopathy.

Many symptoms of dilated and obstructive hypertrophic myopathy are similar, although the mechanisms, significance, and management may differ (Tables 11-1 and 11-2).[74,80,83,89,95,97] Related nursing diagnoses include alteration in cardiac output, activity intolerance, impaired gas exchange, alteration in comfort, chest pain, impaired tissue perfusion, anxiety or depression related to treatment, prognosis, and knowledge deficit.[73,75]

Cardiac dysrhythmias and sudden death may occur in both dilated and hypertrophic myopathy before hemodynamically significant left ventricular dysfunction develops.[3,69,72,81,86,89,95] Both ventricular and supraventricular arrhythmias are common. There is also an increased incidence of conduction system disease and AV block.

The frequency of malignant ventricular arrhythmias and SCD in dilated cardiomyopathy is very high and may not correlate with, or predict, the clinical or hemodynamic course. The presentation and clinical course of hypertrophic cardiomyopathy are highly variable.[95] The individual may be mildly symptomatic for years, may become more symptomatic as the disease progresses, or may experience sudden death as the first manifestation of the disease.[1,4] There is an increased risk of sudden death in obstructive hypertrophic myopathy with younger patients, documented syncope, ventricular tachycardia, or family history of sudden death.[1,3,72] Sudden death typically occurring during strenuous exercise such as athletic activity.[24] An ICD may be indicated in either hypertrophic or dilated myopathy if ventricular arrhythmias cannot be effectively managed with antiarrhythmic therapy (see Sudden Cardiac Death and Unit 10).

Supraventricular arrhythmias occur secondary to increases in left atrial pressure and atrial enlargement.[36] Because of impaired relaxation and filling, patients with hypertrophic cardiomyopathy are highly sensitive to atrial flutter and fibrillation and the corresponding loss of atrial contribution to cardiac output.[72,97] A rapid ventricular rate may contribute to further hemodynamic deterioration by shortening diastolic filling time. Pharmacologic or electrical restoration of sinus rhythm should be attempted.[1,3,72] Antiarrhythmic therapy may be effective in the management of both ventricular and supraventricular arrhythmias. The class IA agents (quinidine, Pronestyl, Norpace) and the class III agent amiodarone (Cardarone) may be used in both dilated and hypertrophic myopathy.[1,72,74,78,82,97] However, these agents should be used with caution due to their negative effect on contractility. Antiarrhythmic therapy in hypertrophic myopathy is reserved for high-risk patients. Amiodarone may be contraindicated if AV block is present.[3] Norpace may provide hemodynamic benefit as well because of its effect in decreasing contractility.

Table 11-1. Dilated versus obstructive hypertrophic cardiomyopathy: signs and symptoms

Signs and Symptoms	Dilated	Hypertrophic (Obstructive)
Arrhythmias (ventricular/supraventricular)	+	+
Congestive heart failure (CHF)	+	Sensitivity to atrial fibrillation
• S$_3$ • JVD • crackles		
• weight gain • edema • dependent		
• dyspnea • orthopnea • hepatomegaly		
Hemodynamic changes		
• LVEDP, PCWP, PAEDP	↑	↑
• cardiac output, cardiac index	↓	↓ (exercise)
• Ejection fraction	↓	↑
Mitral regurgitation	+	+
S$_4$	+	+
Chest pain, angina	+	+
Mural thrombi, emboli	+	Rare in patients without atrial fibrillation
Nonspecific signs (fatigue, syncope)	2° CHF, arrhythmias	2° arrhythmias, ↓ LV filling/cardiac output
Sudden death	+	+
ECG changes	LVH LBBB nonspecific Q waves/St-T changes	Apical LVH giant negative T waves Q waves II, III, aVF + tall R waves − right precordium

↑ = elevated; ↓ = decreased; LVEDP = left ventricular end-diastolic pressure; PCWP = pulmonary capillary wedge pressure; PAEDP = pulmonary artery end-diastolic pressure.

Table 11-2. Dilated versus obstructive hypertrophic cardiomyopathy: therapy

Therapy	Dilated	Hypertrophic (obstructive)
Antiarrhythmics (class IA—quinidine, Pronestyl, Norpace) (class III—amiodarone)	+ (Use with caution)	+ In high-risk patients
Beta blockers	Early stages only	+
Calcium channel blockers	− (Usually)	+
Vasodilators/inotropic agents	+	−
Diuretics	+	Combined with beta blockers/Ca^{++} channel blockers
Anticoagulation	+	In patients with atrial fibrillation
Surgery	Cardiac transplantation	Septal myotomy/myectomy
Other	Steroids, IABP, Vitamin E Rest/energy conservation/O_2	Exercise restriction Rest/energy conservation

+ = indicated; − = not indicated.

Chest pain (angina) is common in both major forms of cardiomyopathy and may be at least partially caused by decreased small vessel coronary flow. Other possible mechanisms include narrowing of intramural vessels, increased left ventricular diastolic pressures, limited coronary vasodilation, decreased capillary density, increased myocardial O_2 consumption, and left ventricular outflow obstruction.[1,72,92]

Signs of both pulmonary congestion and right ventricular failure are present secondary to the increased left ventricular diastolic pressures. However, left ventricular failure is present in dilated myopathy and is usually absent in hypertrophic myopathy.[1] Specific signs and symptoms include crackles (rales), dyspnea, orthopnea, jugular venous distention, hepatomegaly, dependent edema, and decreased exercise tolerance. Hormonal responses may cause Na^+ and water retention, weight gain, and further increases in the work load of the heart (see Unit 8). The treatment of the heart failure varies significantly for dilated and hypertrophic myopathy. Inotropic agents such as digitalis or dopamine, diuretics, and vasodilators, though indicated in the management of heart failure secondary to dilated myopathy, may be contraindicated in the management of hypertrophic myopathy. Both inotropic agents and afterload reducing agents (arterial dilators) such as the ACE inhibitors and direct vasodilators such as hydralazine (Apresoline) and nitroprusside (Nipride) are helpful in the presence of the decreased systolic function associated with dilated myopathy.[1,78,82,92] However, in obstructive hypertrophic myopathy, these same agents further stimulate the already hyperactive systolic function, increasing the pressure gradient.[1,72] Patients with hypertrophic myopathy are highly sensitive to decreases in left ventricular diastolic volume (preload) occurring with diuretics or venodilators. However, diuretics may be helpful when combined with a beta blocker or calcium channel blocker.[1,72]

Beta blockers are the drugs of choice for the arrhythmias, chest pain, and pulmonary congestion (dyspnea) of hypertrophic obstructive myopathy. Potential mechanisms of action include decreased heart rate with improved diastolic function, decreased contractility, decreased myocardial O_2 demands, and inhibition of sympathetic responses.[3,72,80] Exercise tolerance improves as a result of the prevention of outflow obstruction or pressure gradients typically occurring with exercise.[1,80] The use of beta blockers in dilated myopathy is more controversial but may be helpful in preserving compensatory beta receptor responses (see Unit 8).[1]

Calcium channel blockers are indicated as an alternative to beta blockers in hypertrophic myopathy.[1,72,88] Therapeutic effects include increased muscle relaxation and decreased heart rate with improvement in diastolic function. Systolic gradients may also be decreased secondary to the decreased contractility, and coronary blood flow is increased. Verapamil (Isoptin, Calan) is the calcium channel blocker most often used.[1,72] In a small percentage of patients with wedge (left ventricular diastolic) pressures greater than 20 mm Hg and rest obstruction, calcium channel blockers should be administered with caution if at all since their use may be associated with pulmonary edema, hypotension, and sinoatrial (SA) and AV block.[3,97] Surgical intervention is preferred in these settings when beta blockers are ineffective.[72] Either calcium channel blockers or beta blockers can be used prophylactically in high-risk asymptomatic patients with significant obstruction (pressure gradients).[72] The use of calcium channel blockers in dilated myopathy is more controversial, although diltiazem (Cardizem) has been effective in some cases as a result of

the prevention of abnormal Ca++ loading.[1]

Fatigue, syncope, and thromboembolic complications occur in both dilated and hypertrophic myopathy. Fatigue and syncope are nonspecific since they may represent decreased cardiac output due to heart failure or decreased left ventricular filling, arrhythmias, or a combination of these.[15] Formation of mural thrombi with thromboembolic complications is common in dilated myopathy but rare in hypertrophic myopathy in the absence of atrial fibrillation. Anticoagulation is recommended in patients with hypertrophic myopathy who present with intermittent or sustained atrial fibrillation.[1] In dilated myopathy, anticoagulation is recommended in patients with CHF if no other contraindications are present, even if mural thrombi are not identified.[1,4,80]

Mitral regurgitation has been reported in 40% to 60% of patients with dilated myopathy due to enlargement of the mitral ring.[1] In hypertrophic cardiomyopathy, mitral regurgitation is associated with abnormal bending of the papillary muscle due to anterior leaflet compression.[3]

Auscultatory findings include the presence of S_3 and S_4 gallops, and a systolic murmur. The S_4 gallop occurs in all forms of myopathy secondary to compliance changes (see Unit 8).[1,4] An S_3 gallop occurs secondary to the significant increases in diastolic pressure typical of heart failure. Unlike the blowing, holosystolic murmur typical of mitral insufficiency, the systolic murmur of hypertrophic obstructive myopathy is midsystolic, correlating with the late onset of the pressure gradient. It is loudest at the apex and lower left sternal border.[1,3,4] Again, unlike with the typical murmur of mitral insufficiency, the intensity of the murmur increases with decreases in venous return associated with standing, Valsalva maneuvers, tachycardia, exercise, or the administration of amyl nitrite. In contrast, the intensity of the murmur decreases with increases in venous return (preload) or afterload associated with lying, squatting, and hand grip maneuvers.[1,4]

Typical ECG changes include signs of left ventricular hypertrophy (LVH) in both major forms of myopathy.[9] In addition, left bundle branch block (LBBB), nonspecific Q waves, and ST–T wave abnormalities may be seen in dilated cardiomyopathy. Giant negative T waves along with Q waves in leads II, III, aVF, and V4–V6 and tall R waves in the right precordial leads are typical of apical hypertrophic myopathy.[1,3,4,73] Other useful diagnostic tests include chest radiograph, ecchocardiography, and radionuclide angiography. Thallium imaging may also be used to detect potentially infarcted areas.

Surgical intervention for hypertrophic obstructive myopathy consists of septal myotomy and myectomy.[72,91] Benefits are primarily a reduction in the pressure gradient since the coronary arteries compliance and left ventricular diastolic pressure changes are not affected.[72] Indications are primarily patients with symptoms at rest or with ordinary physical activity and outflow gradients at rest or with provocation of more than 50 mm Hg in spite of treatment with beta blockers or verapamil.[3,72] Coronary bypass may also be performed.[1] Mitral valve replacement is rarely indicated.[4] Surgical intervention for dilated myopathy consists primarily of cardiac transplantation.

Other modes of intervention include the use of steroids such as prednisone and immunosuppressants such as azathioprine (Imuran) in dilated myopathy when lymphyocyte infiltration is present on biopsy.[1] An intraaortic balloon pump (IABP) may be used in the patient with severe heart failure as a temporary measure. Vitamin E has also shown some benefit. Cessation of alcohol consumption is beneficial in alcoholic cardiomyopathy.[1,80] Patients with hypertrophic cardiomyopathy should be instructed to avoid strenuous exercise, other situations causing tachycardia, and dehydration.[1,80] Competitive sports should be avoided in patients with significant resting outflow obstruction, ventricular or atrial arrhythmias on Holter monitoring, history of syncope, or family history of sudden death and in those who have had medical or surgical treatment.[24] Rest and other energy conservation measures should be stressed in dilated cardiomyopathy, and supplementary O_2 may be necessary.[3,4]

Cardiac transplantation

Cardiac transplantation, once a scientific curiosity, is now the treatment of choice for end-stage heart disease no longer responsive to conventional therapeutic modalities. Most transplantations are performed in patients with either dilated cardiomyopathy or heart failure secondary to extensive coronary artery disease.[77] The idea of cardiac transplantation should be explored while the individual is free from secondary organ failure and before changes in the systemic and pulmonary vasculature become irreversible.

The timing of cardiac transplantation as a therapeutic option and the struggle to support hemodynamically fragile individuals until an appropriate donor organ becomes available remain constant challenges.[70,76,81] Appropriate timing requires knowledge of transplant science and the natural history of the illness for which transplantation is indicated.

Although no formulas can precisely predict the prognosis of any individual, certain physiologic and hemodynamic risk factors allow stratification of patients into high-, intermediate-, or low-risk subsets for sudden death or hemodynamic demise.[76] The presence of malignant ventricular dysrhythmias, diminished functional capacity (NYHA class

III or IV), ejection fractions less than 20%, and abnormal neurohormonal activity seem to be associated with the highest risk.[70,85]

Maximizing the use of scarce donor organs makes selection of potential transplant candidates a critical process. Pretransplant assessment and selection criteria remain essentially the same for all potential candidates, despite etiologic differences. Candidacy must be a consensus decision of the primary physician, transplant surgeon, transplant nurse coordinators, cardiologists, social worker, and others who may be involved in the patient's care. The current approach to selection of cardiac transplant candidates is based on the determination of those patients most likely to demonstrate a significant improvement in symptoms, functional capacity, and life expectancy after transplantation.[70,76,81,87]

A comprehensive evaluation is performed, although specific protocols may vary between institutions. Generally, this evaluation includes measurement of right-sided heart pressures to rule out pulmonary hypertension, an echocardiogram or radionuclide angiography to assess wall motion and ejection fraction, and general renal, hepatic, hematologic, and metabolic studies.[93] A psychological assessment is also performed. A willingness to adhere to strict medication use, diet, and long-term follow-up care should be understood and accepted. It is crucial to ascertain that the candidate is not actively abusing drugs, alcohol, or tobacco. Psychiatric instability must also be ruled out.[85,93]

Absolute contraindications to cardiac transplantation include fixed or irreversible pulmonary hypertension, recent or unresolved pulmonary infarction, evidence of uncontrolled infection, and neoplastic processes.[85,93] When all test results are complete and absolute contraindications are ruled out, the patient's name, weight, ABO type, and priority status are entered into the United

Network for Organ Sharing (UNOS) donor computer.[77,93]

Relative physiologic contraindications include insulin-dependent diabetes, age, moderate to severe renal or liver failure, chronic obstructive pulmonary disease, and impaired cerebral or peripheral circulation.[85,93] Chronic corticosteroid therapy usually exacerbates the diabetic process, increasing the chance for infection, delayed wound healing, and vascular complications. Age restrictions (above 55 to 65 years of age) remain controversial, although many individuals over 60 have undergone transplantation. Adequate peripheral circulation is critical to ensure access for bypass, biopsy, and frequent blood samples. The patient with impaired cerebral circulation is at risk for a CVA, which would ultimately affect the quality of life after transplantation.

Ideally donors should be less than 40 to 45 years of age and screened for human immunodeficiency (HIV) and hepatitis, systemic infection, malignancies other than those of the CNS, and significant hemodynamic instability.[93] Both cortical and brainstem function must be absent. Because of these CNS changes, cardiovascular and oxygenation parameters, temperature, and fluid and electrolyte balance must be carefully monitored in the donor patient.[77]

Nursing care of the pretransplant patient with end-stage heart disease is multifaceted. The complex and chronic hemodynamic and psychological demands of these individuals are a constant challenge for the critical care nurse.[77] Related nursing diagnoses include alteration in cardiac output, alteration in tissue perfusion, impaired gas exchange, potential for infection, alteration in fluid and electrolyte balance, alteration in nutrition, anxiety or knowledge deficit, alteration in body image, powerlessness, and sleep pattern disturbances.[77]

Nursing intervention in pretransplant patients includes managing vasoactive drugs and mechanical assist devices, preventing infection, maintaining optimum oxygenation and fluid homeostasis, and preventing complications associated with heart failure and chronic hypoperfusion (see Units 8 and 9). Emotional support to the patient and family is a priority during the unpredictably long and tumultuous wait for a suitable donor heart. Increasing dependency, role changes, and the threat of impending death are common, realistic concerns. Identification and support of the patient's coping mechanisms may help him or her to adapt to the many uncontrollable events and may optimize his or her chances for survival.

The average duration of the surgical procedure is about 4 hours.[93] After successful transplantation, most recipients will have no functional limitations (NYHA I) or only mild limitations (NYHA II). The current expectation for 1- and 5-year survival after cardiac transplantation is 80% to 90% and 60% to 70%, respectively.[77,85,93] Posttransplant patient problems and related nursing diagnoses include alteration in comfort, alteration in cardiac output, impaired renal tissue perfusion, potential for injury related to rejection, potential for infection, potential nutritional deficit, fear and anxiety, and knowledge deficit.[77] The patient's nutritional status significantly affects the postoperative recovery and should be supported. Fresh, unpeeled fruits and vegetables should be avoided for up to 6 to 8 weeks to prevent infection.[77] Stress ulcers may form secondary to steroid administration, postoperative stress, and infectious or ischemic processes.

Several variables require attention postoperatively to achieve optimal results. These include monitoring of the response of the denervated transplanted heart, prevention and management of rejection and infection, and the provision of patient and family education.[77,86] Since autonomic innervation is severed during transplantation, the hemodynamic responses of the transplanted heart differ greatly from those of the normal, innervated myocardium. Cardiac output is subsequently compromised. Vagal influence, which normally controls basal heart rate, is absent, resulting in a higher resting heart rate. Neurally mediated cardiac responses, such as those elicited by carotid massage, Valsalva maneuvers, or abrupt changes in posture, will not be accompanied by the usual physiologic, reflexive changes in heart rate. In addition, drugs that work via the vagal pathways (atropine, digitalis) will no longer be effective. Necessary changes in heart rate in response to stress or exercise become dependent on an increase in circulating catecholamines. Administration of intravenous catecholamines is often necessary in the early postoperative period. During the rehabilitation process, circulating catecholamines are increased by having the patient do warm-up exercises before physically demanding activities.

Because the donor heart is not immunologically identical to that of the recipient, the recipient's body mounts an immunologic response against the foreign tissue. This immunologic response is known as *rejection* and is classified as either hyperacute, acute, or chronic. Although much investigative effort is under way to find a reliable, noninvasive method to detect and confirm rejection, the only reliable method to date is achieved by a transvenous endomyocardial biopsy. Samples of right ventricular tissue are taken for histologic examination. Biopsies are performed weekly for the first 6 weeks, then are tapered down to monthly and eventually every third or fouth month.[77,93] A biopsy can also be performed if symptoms suggestive of rejection emerge. These symptoms are usually nonspecific and include fatigue, lethargy, pump failure with PACs, and complaints of "just not feeling right."

Chronic rejection produces atherosclerotic changes in the coronary arteries, referred to as *accelerated graft atherosclerosis*.[77,93] Cytomegalovirus infection has also been implicated. Denervation often renders the patient incapable of perceiving anginal pain. Therefore, yearly coronary angiograms and close clinical follow-up are necessary to monitor the progression of coronary disease. These atherosclerotic changes begin to occur around the second to third posttransplant year. Characteristically, this concentric and diffuse process produces narrowing of the small, distal coronary arteries, rendering bypass and/or percutaneous transluminal coronary angioplasty (PTCA) ineffective.

Current immunosuppressive therapy pauses on a triple drug regimen which now includes corticosteroids (prednisone), azathioprine (Imuran), and cyclosporine (Sandimmune).[93] Other agents are under clinical trials. Use of a triple drug regimen enables the patient to benefit from the effect of these medications without the major side effects seen with the higher doses of single agents. Side effects include bone marrow depression, hepatic toxicity or nephrotoxicity, and seizures.[93] T cell antibodies in the form of antithymocyte globulin (ATG) have also been used but are more toxic.[77,93] Immunosuppression is generally guided by the white blood cell (WBC) count, blood levels of cyclosporine, and previous biopsy results. These agents may be used either to treat or to prevent rejection. Immunosuppressive techniques currently under investigation include monoclonal antibodies and extracorporeal radiation of the WBCs.[93]

Although morbidity and mortality due to infection have decreased since the introduction of cyclosporine, it is well known that immunosuppression makes the patient vulnerable to a multitude of potential pathogens and opportunistic infections.[77,94] Therefore, prevention of infection is a top priority for all persons interacting with the transplant recipient. Isolation and infection control protocols continue to vary among institutions. If personnel traffic is controlled, strict handwashing techniques and donning of masks have been shown to provide adequate hygienic protection for the recipient.[77,87]

The transplant procedure also results in unusual but characteristic changes in the baseline ECG. The presence of two independently discharging sinus nodes (one from the native remnant posterior right atrium and the other from the donor right atrium) results in two P waves. The native, innervated P wave remains independent from the donor P–QRS–T complex.

A comprehensive educational program for patients and their families, beginning preoperatively, is most likely to facilitate a successful postoperative recovery. Essential topics include descriptions of the waiting period, preoperative preparation, early postoperative period, medications, diet, activity, routine follow-up visits, psychological responses, financial concerns, and other aspects of the rehabilitation process. Physiologic characteristics of the transplanted heart and immunologic complications (rejection, infection) should also be discussed.[77]

MITRAL VALVE PROLAPSE

Mitral valve prolapse (MVP) is the most common valvular disorder and may be defined functionally, clinically, and anatomically. It is defined *functionally* as a disorder in which there is a pronounced displacement of one or both of the mitral leaflets back up into the left atrium during systole.[105,109,110,113]

The posterior leaflet is most often affected. Unlike the cardiomyopathies, MVP is considered a primary systolic disorder. The heart muscle may not be directly affected. MVP is defined *clinically* by its auscultatory findings. Both the functional and clinical definitions of MVP can be confirmed diagnostically. Neither is considered more accurate. The presence of both has the highest accuracy and may be considered major criteria in the diagnosis of significant MVP.[1,111]

MVP is defined *anatomically* as degenerative changes in the mitral valve and chordae tendineae. These changes produce weakened leaflets with a larger than necessary ("redundant") surface area. The redundant leaflets act similar to a furled sail, unfurling during systole (Fig 11-9). In classic MVP, the leaflets are thickened as well as redundant, whereas in the nonclassic form, there is minimal or no thickening or redundancy.[106,109] The chordae are thin and long and are further weakened by the strain of the prolapsing valve. The diameter of the AV opening into the left ventricle is larger than the diameter of the left ventricular cavity itself in prolapse with significant mitral regurgitation.[3,4,103,106,115]

The most commonly proposed mechanism for the degenerative changes is a genetic biochemical abnormality in valve colla-

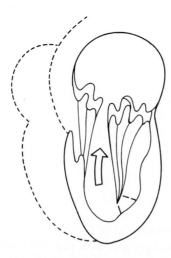

Fig. 11-9 Anatomic and functional changes in MVP. Note the extra, billowing surface area of the mitral valve and elongated chordae, which facilitate systolic displacement of the mitral valve back into the left atrium.

gen.[4,98–100,105,109,110,115] The onset is in late childhood or adolescence. Skeletal deformities are common in these individuals, confirming the presence of systemic connective tissue disease. MVP also occurs secondary to congenital or acquired disorders such as Marfan's syndrome, Duchenne's muscular dystrophy, atrial septal defect, rheumatic heart disease, coronary artery disease, hypertophic cardiomyopathy, and anorexia nervosa.[1,98,99,103,105,110] Because of its functional, clinical, and anatomic characteristic, this syndrome has also been referred to as *Reid-Barlow's syndrome, floppy mitral valve syndrome, billowing mitral leaflet syndrome, flailed mitral valve,* or *mitral click-murmur syndrome.*[1,99,100,115]

The *functional* diagnosis of MVP is confirmed by visualization of valve movements on M-mode or two-dimensional echocardiogram. The incidence of false-negative diagnoses is greater in M-mode (10-20%).[99,115] Because of the availability of both forms of echocardiography, MVP is now diagnosed more frequently and is recognized as highly prevalent in many otherwise normal individuals. If echocardiograhic findings alone are required, the incidence is as high as 20% or even greater in young patients (ages 10 to 18).[99,105,110,113] It is currently recognized that some degree of prolapse is normal, especially in women.[100,110] Color-flow Doppler studies may also be ordered to detect the presence and evaluate the extent of mitral regurgitation[1,100,113,115] (see Unit 5).

The *clinical* diagnosis is confirmed by the presence of positive auscultatory findings. These findings focus on a systolic murmur preceded by a characteristic mid- to late systolic "click."[98,103,110,113,115] This click-murmur combination can be the first diagnostic clue in asymptomatic patients. The systolic murmur occurs secondary to mitral regurgitation and is heard best over the apex.[3,4,99,105,115] Although some arching back into the left atrium is normal during systole, pronounced displacement can prevent the valve leaflets from approximating and closing tightly, thus predisposing to mitral regurgitation. The click is produced by a sudden tightening of the chordae tendineae with ventricular contraction.[99,113] It has been said to sound similar to a parachute snapping open. When accentuated, the murmur may also sound like a "whoop" or "honk."[3,98,99,103,115] This sound is thought to be produced by thin jets of regurgitant blood striking the nonprolapsed leaflet.[99]

The click-murmur characteristically varies in intensity and timing in the same individual at different times.[98,105,109,110,113] Changes in venous return (preload), systolic effort, and afterload affect the timing, duration, and intensity of the click and murmur (Fig. 11-10). These changes can also make the click-murmur easier or more difficult to identify.

The degree and extent of prolapse are accentuated by maneuvers that decrease venous return, left ventricular volume, and left ventricular size, allowing for a greater discrepancy between the diameter of the AV opening and that of the left ventricular cavity.[3,99,103,110,115] Examples of such maneuvers are standing or sitting, performing a Valsalva maneuver, administration of amyl nitrate, and tachycardia.[1,98,99,105,115] Both the click and murmur occur earlier, are longer in duration, and may be louder in intensity depending on the specific maneuver.[1,105] These characteristics allow them to be more clearly heard, facilitating their identification. The degree and extent of prolapse are also accentuated by an increase in the force of contraction or systolic effort. Examples are sympathetic stimulation related to stress or exercise and tachycardia related to sympathetic stimulation or other factors.[1,99,115]

The degree and extent of prolapse are decreased by maneuvers that increase venous return, left ventricular volume, and left ventricular size, reducing the discrepancy between the diameter of the AV opening and that of the left ventricular cavity. Examples of such maneuvers are lying flat, elevating the legs, and bradycardia.[1,99,115] Both the click and murmur occur later, are shorter in duration, and are often silent or absent.[1,99] The auscultatory changes may disappear in

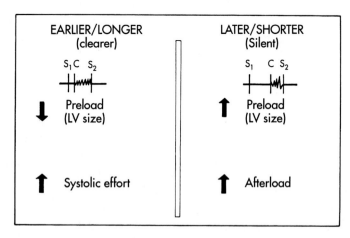

Fig. 11-10 Systolic click-murmur of MVP. Changes in timing and duration with maneuvers affecting left ventricular size (preload/afterload) and systolic effort.

the last trimesters of pregnancy because of an increased circulating volume, returning after delivery.[99,103] An increase in afterload also decreases the degree and extent of the prolapse as a result of reduced left ventricular emptying. Examples are squatting and isometric hand grip.[1,99,115] In the presence of these maneuvers, the click-murmur frequently disappears.

A variety of additional signs and symptoms are associated with the MVP syndrome. However, MVP is generally considered a benign disorder. Patients should be reassured that these symptoms, although frequently disturbing, are more of a nuisance than life-threatening.[100,103] A significant number of patients with this disorder are asymptomatic. Perloff refers to all findings other than those documented by auscultation or echocardiography as nonspecific.[1,99,115] Signs and symptoms of MVP that correlate most consistently with echocardiographic findings include arrhythmias, dizziness or syncope, autonomic dysfunction, skeletal abnormalities, low body weight, and hypomastia (small breast size) in women.[99,100,105,107]

The arrhythmias of MVP may be either ventricular or supraventricular and are typically referred to by the patient as palpitations. These arrhythmias are often triggered by emotions or exercise.[100] The most common arrhythmias are PVCs. Malignant ventricular arrhythmias, although rare, have been associated with sudden death. Multiple mechanisms are implicated. These include stretching of the papillary muscle or valve leaflets, stimulation of the left atrium or left ventricle by valve movements, impact of regurgitant jets on the atria, autonomic dysfunction, and the presence of beta receptors or pacemaker tissue in the mitral leaflets.[1,99,105,108,115] Prolonged Q–T intervals have also been reported in MVP, especially in symptomatic patients.[1,4,98,99] This finding was not supported by two recent studies.[101,104] Prolonged Q–T intervals may con-

tribute to the presence of ventricular arrhythmias and/or sudden death, but more studies need to be done since current findings are contradictory. Since there is a strong association with Wolff-Parkinson-White syndrome, the existence of this disorder should be ruled out in the presence of supraventricular arrhythmias.[1,4,99,108] Evidence of delta wave indicating a left-sided bypass tract may be present on the ECG (see Preexcitation Syndrome).

Dizziness or syncope in MVP is usually related either to arrhythmias or to autonomic dysfunction. Psychological factors have also been implicated. The autonomic dysfunction may be manifested as either parasympathetic (vagal) or sympathetic (adrenergic) hypersensitivity.[4,99,114] Bradycardia, irregular pupil size, and orthostatic hypotension may be present because of vagal sensitivity. Adrenergic sensitivity may be manifested as hypersensitivity to noise or cold, paresthesias of the extremities, and tachyarrhythmias. Urinary and plasma catecholamines are often elevated.[113]

Characteristic skeletal abnormalities include scoliosis, pectus excavation, and narrow anteroposterior chest diameter. Individuals with MVP are most typically tall and slender with long arms, consistent with the association with Marfan's syndrome.[99] These changes, together with the hypomastia, or small breast size, may be explained by the embryonic development of the vertebral column, thoracic cage, breasts, and mitral valve at about the same time.[99]

Nonspecific signs and symptoms of MVP syndrome include chest pain, dyspnea, anxiety or panic disorders, and ECG changes.[99,113] Although they are commonly reported in MVP, multiple studies have shown the incidence of these signs and symptoms to be no greater than in the general population[99,105,107,115] more commonly reported in women.[105] A high incidence of migraine has also been reported.[1,107]

The chest pain can be precordial, either sharp or dull, often localized, can occur during rest and exertion, and may be relieved by lying down.[1,98–100,113] It most typically occurs during times of combined physical and emotional stress, lending support to an autonomic component. The pain can last for seconds, hours, or days.[98,113] The specific cause of the chest pain is not known at this time.[98] Multiple mechanisms may be involved. The most popular theory is tension on the papillary muscles resulting in ischemia.[4,98,99] Ischemia secondary to compression of the circumflex branch of the left coronary artery has also been proposed. Metabolic changes including epinephrine and norepinephrine have been implicated, as well. Coronary spasm has also been implicated, although this is inconsistent with the benefit derived from beta blockade.[98,103] Ischemia by any of these mechanisms may be further aggravated in the presence of increased blood pressure, rate, and force of contraction due to an imbalance between O_2 supply and demand. These changes occur in the presence of a stress response. Research studies to date have been unable to document the presence of ischemia on thallium imaging.[98] Other proposed nonischemic mechanisms for the chest pain include dysfunctional esophageal motility or chest wall muscle changes.[98,102,103]

Psychological neuroses have long been attributed to the mitral prolapse syndrome. Anxiety and panic disorders including sensations of choking, smothering, dyspnea, diaphoresis, and dizziness have been commonly reported.[98,102] These have been also explained by the presence of autonomic dysfunction. These patients may be merely more "psychologically vulnerable" to the natural fear that accompanies palpitations and chest pain. Blood lactate levels have also been implicated. Findings from actual studies correlating mitral prolapse with anxiety disorders are contradictory.[98,102,114] A sense of sustained fatigue seemingly unrelieved by rest may be accompanied by unexplained depression. Antidepressants such as amitriptyline hydrochloride (Elavil) or imipramine hydrochloride (Tofranil) may be helpful.

Nonspecific ECG changes include T wave inversion in leads II, III, and aVF with or without ST changes, and left precordial changes.[1,98,99,101,105] These changes may be accentuated with exercise.[1] The T wave inversion in leads II, III, and aVF is thought to correlate with stretching and ischemia to the inferoposterior papillary muscle. The valve leaflet most typically involved in mitral prolapse is the posterior leaflet. This leaflet is supported by the posterior papillary muscle, which is attached to the inferior wall of the left ventricle. Leads II, III, and aVF reflect the inferior wall of the left ventricle. These changes may occur after hyperventilating in patients with MVP.[101] Autonomic dysfunction has also been implicated as a mechanism for the ECG changes of MVP. This theory is supported by improvement in the ECG changes following propranolol (Inderal) administration.[99]

In addition to the symptoms of chest pain, palpitations, and syncope, potential complications of MVP include CHF secondary to mitral regurgitation, infective endocarditis, transient ischemic attacks (TIAs) secondary to thrombotic emboli, and sudden death.[1,103,106,115] Infective endocarditis has been the most extensively studied complication. A dental origin is common. The risk of TIAs is six times higher than normal in women under 40 years of age with MVP.[105] Sudden death has been reported primarily in patients with severe mitral regurgitation and significant ventricular ectopy. In these individuals the risk is 50 to 100 times greater than the usual risk for sudden death.[104,105,108] In the absence of mitral regurgitation, the risk of sudden death is similar to that of the normal population. Related nursing diagnoses include alteration in comfort, alteration in cardiac output, potential for infection, knowledge deficit, anxiety, and potential altered cerebral perfusion.

Asymptomatic prolapse without auscultatory findings does not require therapy. Complications are unusual especially in individuals presenting with low body weight and hypotension.[105] Limited therapy is usually indicated in asymptomatic individuals with auscultatory findings.[1,99,105] Antibiotic prophylaxis is recommended before dental work and any invasive procedure including cystoscopy, colonoscopy, or drainage of infected wounds.[99,105,113] The usual antibiotics prescribed are penicillin and erythromycin. Classic prolapse is associated with a higher prevalence of moderate to severe mitral regurgitation and endocarditis.[103,109,115] Males over 45 years of age without low body weight and hypotension also have a greater risk of endocarditis and significant mitral regurgitation.[1,105,106,109,110] In these high-risk individuals antibiotic prophylaxis is even more important. Repeat echocardiograms are recommended at least every 3 years to evaluate the progression of mitral regurgitation.[99] Hypertension should be kept under control since it may predispose to ruptured chordae and progression of mitral regurgitation.

Beta blockers are the treatment of choice in the symptomatic patient with chest pain or arrhythmias.[1,99,100,105,110,113] Both of these symptoms are thought to be associated at least in part with increased sympathetic activity. Beta blockers act to block sympathetic effects on the heart, resulting in decreased autonomic tone, heart rate, and contractility. The decreased heart rate and contractility decrease left ventricle volume and systolic effort, causing less prolapse and stretch of the chordae and papillary muscles.[4] The currently available beta blockers are discussed in Unit 9. Additional antiarrhythmic therapy is frequently required with malignant ventricular arrhythmias. The class III agent amio-

darone (Cardorone) is particularly effective in refractory ventricular arrhythmias.[100,108] The new class III agent sotalol with beta blocking properties has also proved effective but has significant proarrhythmic effects.[100] Levy suggests that electrophysiologic studies be performed in all patients with complex ventricular arrhythmias. Additional antiarrhythmic therapy is prescribed in patients with inducible arrhythmias only.[108] Calcium channel blockers may also be used in the management of arrhythmias and migraine.[113] Phenytoin (Dilantin) has been used in patients with ventricular arrhythmias and prolonged Q–T intervals.[1,99] In patients unresponsive to antiarrhythmic therapy, mitral valve repair (valvuloplasty) or replacement may be considered.[100,108]

Maneuvers that increase venous return, left ventricle volume, and/or afterload may also be helpful in relieving the chest pain of mitral prolapse, because of an increase in left ventricle size and decrease in left ventricle emptying. Examples of these maneuvers are raising the legs, lying flat, squatting, and isometric exercises. Stress management should be a goal of therapy in the management of all patients with symptomatic mitral prolapse. Relaxation techniques such as pursed lip breathing are also helpful in relieving symptoms such as dyspnea.[113] MVP support groups are available. A regular exercise program can help regulate the sympathetic response to activity and stress. A high fluid intake should be encouraged unless hypertension is present.[113] The patient should be instructed to avoid diuretics and stimulants such as caffeine, alcohol, and over-the-counter drugs. Nitrates should also be avoided since they decrease venous return and left ventricle size, accentuating the prolapse.[1] Calcium channel blockade is an alternative to nitrates in patients in whom beta blockade is not effective.[103]

Additional pharmacologic agents used in the management of symptomatic MVP include phenobarbital, antibiotics, and anti-platelet agents. Vagal sensitivity may respond to small doses of phenobarbital, which has a central effect on the vagal system. Antibiotic prophylaxis is indicated in symptomatic patients to prevent bacterial endocarditis. Alprazolam (Xanax) or lorazepam (Ativan) may be prescribed to reduce anxiety. Patients with symptoms of TIAs should receive antiplatelet therapy to prevent stroke.

Examples of antiplatelet agents are dipyridamole (Persantin) and ASA.[1,103]

Significant mitral regurgitation and CHF are unusual unless the chordae tendineae have ruptured. Symptoms of fatigue and shortness of breath are common but do not necessarily correlate with the presence of CHF. Treatment for severe mitral regurgitation is mitral valve repair or replacement.[99,103]

SELF-ASSESSMENT

1 Death from cardiac causes occurring within 1 hour of the onset of symptoms is referred to as _____ sudden cardiac death. Regardless of the presence or absence of coronary artery disease, left ventricular dysfunction (increases/decreases) the risk of sudden death. The most common cause of sudden cardiac death in young athletes is _____ cardiomyopathy.

    The only mode of therapy proven effective in preventing the initial episode of sudden death is _____ blockade following _____ _____.

sudden

increases

hypertrophic

beta
acute myocardial infarction

2 Positive findings on signal-averaged electrocardiography and _____ studies (EPS) suggest a _____ mechanism. In the presence of these findings, initial management with antiarrhythmic therapy (is/is not) indicated.

    In the presence of severe left ventricular dysfunction, infrequent or noninducible ventricular arrhythmias, and the absence of significant coronary artery disease, surgical _____ or _____ implantation is indicated. Functional causes (should/should not) be initially ruled out.

    EPS correlates _____ electrograms with the surface ECG during spontaneous or _____ arrhythmias. These studies are routinely performed before surgical or catheter _____.

electrophysiologic; reentrant

is

ablation; ICD
should

intracardiac
induced

ablation

3 The ECG pattern of torsades de pointes mimics that of (VT/VF/both) and is associated with a (prolonged/short) Q–T interval. QT(U) intervals > _____ second or QTc intervals > _____ second are considered diagnostic for torsades. Q–T intervals are also considered prolonged when greater than _____ the R–R interval. Torsades de pointes is also typically initiated by a(n) (early/late) PVC, preceded by a (long/short) R–R cycle.

    The antiarrhythmic agents most commonly producing torsades de pointes are the class (IA/IB/IC) agents.

both

0.50; 0.44

half
late
long

IA

4 The current treatment of choice for torsades de pointes is _____. Overdrive pacing may also be used to (shorten/prolong) the Q–T interval. Patients with congenitally prolonged Q–T intervals respond best to (calcium channel/beta) blockade.

magnesium; shorten

beta

5 The accessory pathway in Wolff-Parkinson-White syndrome is known as the bundle of (Kent/James/Mahaim). Major ECG characteristics include a (short/long/normal) P–R interval and _____ wave, which result from a _____ complex in sinus rhythm.

Kent
short; delta
fusion

The location of the accessory pathway is suggested by the direction (polarity) of the _____ wave on the chest and _____ leads.

delta; limb

6 The two most common arrhythmias associated with the Wolff-Parkinson-White syndrome are AV _____ supraventricular tachycardia, which presents most typically with (narrow/wide) QRS complexes, and atrial (flutter/fibrillation), which presents most typically with (narrow/wide) QRS complex. PSVT with narrow complexes in Wolff-Parkinson-White syndrome is commonly referred to as (orthodromic/antidromic) tachycardia.

reentrant
narrow
fibrillation
wide
orthodromic

R–R intervals < _____ msec during atrial fibrillation indicate a short antegrade _____ period and an increased risk of (SVT/VT/VF).

250
refractory
VF

7 In the presence of atrial fibrillation in Wolff-Parkinson-White syndrome, the administration of _____ and _____ _____ blockers should be avoided. The drug of choice for wide QRS tachycardia in Wolff-Parkinson-White syndrome, whether regular or irregular, is (Xylocaine/Pronestyl). The initial drug of choice for narrow QRS tachycardia is _____. The preferred agents for long-term management are (calcium channel/beta) blockers.

digitalis,
Ca^{++} channel

Pronestyl
Adenocard
beta

Alternatives to long-term drug therapy are _____ and _____ ablation.

surgical
catheter

8 The cardiomyopathies are diseases of the heart _____, occurring independently of any other _____ pathology. The three major forms of cardiomyopathy are restrictive, _____, and _____. A common physiologic finding is a rise in left ventricular (systolic/diastolic) pressure.

muscle,
cardiovascular

dilated; hypertrophic
diastolic

9 Two common complications of both hypertrophic and dilated myopathy are _____ _____ and _____. Patients with hypertrophic cardiomyopathy are highly sensitive to atrial _____ or _____. The ventricular and supraventricular arrhythmias of both hypertrophic and dilated myopathy

chest pain; arrhythmias

flutter; fibrillation

may be treated with class (IA/IC) antiarrhythmic agents and the class III agent _____. However, the treatment of choice for the complications of hypertrophic myopathy is _____ blockade. Surgical intervention is indicated in symptomatic patients with rest _____.

    The long-term prognosis in both dilated and restrictive cardiomyopathy is (favorable/poor). The only effective mode of therapy for end-stage heart failure in these disorders is cardiac _____.

10 The two major indications for cardiac transplantation are myopathy and end-stage _____ _____ disease. Cardiac transplantation is contraindicated in patients with irreversible _____ _____ or uncontrolled _____. Relative contraindications include impaired _____ or cerebral circulation and _____ or _____ failure.

    After cardiac transplantation, a major goal is the prevention and management of infection and _____. The hemodynamic responses are the (same as/different from) those of a normal heart. Impaired (sympathetic/parasympathetic) responses are present. In the baseline ECG, two _____ waves are typically present.

11 Mitral valve prolapse (MVP) is a (benign/malignant) disorder. A common, although nonspecific, presenting symptom is _____ _____. Other typical signs and symptoms include arrhythmias, _____ dysfunction, _____ abnormalities, (increased/decreased) body weight, and anxiety or _____ disorders.

    Nonspecific ECG findings associated with MVP are _____ wave inversion on leads _____.

12 The diagnosis of MVP is made by the presence of a characteristic _____ on auscultation and _____ findings. The auscultatory findings are most easily heard in the presence of maneuvers that (increase/decrease) venous return or increase _____ effort.

    Potential complications in MVP include mitral (stenosis/insufficiency), infective _____, and _____ secondary to thrombotic emboli. These complications are (frequent/infrequent).

Answer column:

IA
amiodarone
beta

obstruction

poor
transplantation

coronary artery
pulmonary hypertension
infection
peripheral
renal; liver

rejection
different from
parasympathetic
P

benign
chest pain

autonomic; skeletal
decreased; panic

T
II, III, aVF

click-murmur; echocardiographic

decrease,
systolic
insufficiency
; TIAs
infrequent

REFERENCES/SUGGESTED READINGS
General
1. Braunwald E, editor: Heart disease: a textbook of cardiovascular medicine, ed 4, Philadelphia, 1992, WB Saunders.

2. Guidelines for cardiopulmonary resuscitation and emergency care: Part III. Adult cardiac life support, JAMA 268(16):2199, 1992.

3. Hurst WJ, Schlant RB, editors: The heart, arteries, and veins, ed 6, New York, 1990, McGraw-Hill.
4. Underhill S et al: Cardiac nursing, ed 2, Philadelphia, 1989, JB Lippincott.

Sudden death/electrophysiologic studies

5. Burke L et al: Living with recurrent ventricular dysrhythmias, Focus on Crit Care 19(1):60, 1992.
6. Chang-Sing P, Peter T: Sudden death— evaluation and prevention, Cardiol Clin 9(4):653, 1991.
7. Collins S: Sudden death counseling: a compassionate protocol, Nursing 21(7):32C, 1991.
7a. Davies MJ: Anatomic features in victims of sudden coronary death: coronary artery pathology, Circulation 85(1):I19, 1992.
8. Fletcher RD: Sudden cardiac death after myocardial infarction, Drugs 41(suppl 2):1, 1991.
9. Geha A et al: Strategies in the surgical therapy of malignant ventricular arrhythmias, Ann Surg 216(3):309, 1992.
10. Huang SH et al: Coronary care nursing, ed 2, Philadelphia, 1989, WB Saunders.
11. Hurwitz JL, Josephson ME: Sudden cardiac death in patients with chronic coronary heart disease, Circulation 85(1):I43, 1992.
12. Jimenez RA et al: Sudden cardiac death. Magnitude of the problem/substrate/trigger interaction and populations at high risk, Cardiol Clin 11(1):1, 1993.
13. Josephson ME: The role of the electrophysiologist in the treatment of malignant ventricular tachyarrhythmias, Medtronic News 21(2):4, 1993.
14. Kay GN, Bubien RS: Clinical management of cardiac arrhythmias, Gaithersburg, MD, 1992, Aspen Publishers.
15. Knilans TK, Prystowsky EN: Antiarrhythmic drug therapy in the management of cardiac arrest survivors, Circulation 85(1):I118, 1992.
16. Meinertz T et al: Can we predict sudden cardiac death? Drugs 41(suppl 2):9, 1991.
17. Mercer ME: The electrophysiology study: a nursing concern, Crit Care Nurs 7(2):58, 1988.
18. Moss AJ: Prevention of sudden cardiac death, Hosp Pract [Off] 27(1):165, 1992.
19. O'Rourke RA: Role of myocardial revascularization in sudden cardiac death, Circulation 85(1):I112, 1992.
20. Ruskin JN: Role of invasive electrophysiological testing in the evaluation and treatment of patients at high risk for sudden cardiac death, Circulation 85(1):I152, 1992.
21. Simson MB: Noninvasive identification of patients at high risk for sudden cardiac death: signal-averaged electrocardiography, Circulation 85(1):I1465, 1992.
22. Singh BN: When is drug therapy warranted to prevent sudden cardiac death? Drugs 41(suppl 2):24, 1991.
23. Starks-Bledsoe D, Vespe M: Heading off sudden cardiac death, Nursing 22(11):53, 1992.
24. Vaska PL: Sudden cardiac death in young athletes: a review for nurses, AACN Clin Issues in Crit Care Nurs 3(1):243, 1992.
25. Zipes DP et al: Guidelines for clinial intracardiac electrophysiologic studies, J Am Coll Cardiol 14(7):1827, 1989.
26. Zipes DP: Sudden cardiac death: future approaches, Circulation 85(1):I160, 1992.

Torsades de pointes

27. Conover MB: Understanding electrocardiography, ed 6, St. Louis, 1992, Mosby–Year Book.
28. Dessertenne F: Ventricular fibrillation and torsades de pointes, Cardiovasc Drug Ther 4(4):1177, 1990.
29. Grubb BP: The use of oral labetalol in the therapy of arrhythmias associated with the long QT syndrome, Chest 100(6):1724, 1991.
30. Handerhan B: Taking a closer look at torsades de pointes, Crit Care Choices 13:30, 1993.
31. Hii J et al: Precordial QT interval dispersion as a marker of torsades de pointes: disparate effects of class Ia antiarrhythmic drugs and amiodarone, Circulation 86(5):1376, 1992.
32. Iseri LT: Role of magnesium in cardiac tachyarrhythmias, Am J Cardiol 65(23):47K, 1990.

33. Jackman WM et al: The long QT syndromes: a critical review, new clinical observations and a unifying hypothesis, Prog Cardiovasc Dis 31:115, 1988.
34. Keller KB, Lemberg L: The importance of magnesium in cardiovascular disease, Am J Crit Care 2(4):348, 1993.
35. Keren A, Tzivoni D: Torsades de pointes: prevention and therapy, Cardiovasc Drug Ther 5(2):509, 1991.
36. Lefor N et al: Recognizing and treating torsades de pointes, Crit Care Nurse 12(5):23, 1992.
37. Lessig ML et al: Torsades de pointes—a cardiac ballet, Crit Care Nurse 11(10):63, 1991.
38. Marriott HJL: Practical electrocardiography, ed 7, Baltimore, Williams & Wilkins, 1988.
38a.Rankin AC et al: Acute therapy of torsades des pointes with amiodarone: proarrhythmic and antiarrhythmic association of QT prolongation, Am Heart J 119:185, 1990.
39. Roden DM: Magnesium treatment of ventricular arrhythmias, Am J Cardiol 63(14):436, 1989.
40. Schwartz PJ et al: Stress and sudden death: the case of the long QT syndrome, Circulation 83(suppl 4):I71, 1991.
41. Sweitzer P: The values and limitations of the QT interval in clinical practice, Am Heart J 124(4):1121, 1992.
42. Tzivoni D et al: Treatment of torsades de pointes with magnesium sulfate, Circulation 77:392, 1988.
43. Tzivoni D et al: Terminology of torsades de pointes, Cardiovasc Drug Ther 5(2):505, 1991.
44. Vukmir RB: Torsades de pointes: a review, Am J Emerg Med 9:250, 1991.
45. Wines LM et al: Torsades de pointes: a critical care nurse's dilemma, Heart Lung 19(5P1):500, 1990.

Preexcitation syndrome
46. Berry VA: Wolff-Parkinson-White syndrome and the use of radiofrequency catheter ablation, Heart Lung 22(1):15, 1993.
47. Chen SA et al: Reappraisal of radiofrequency ablation of multiple accessory pathways, Am Heart J 125(3):760, 1993.
48. Conover MB: Understanding electrocardiography, ed 6, St. Louis, 1992, Mosby Year Book.
49. de Chillou C et al: Clinical characteristics and electrophysiologic properties of atrioventricular accessory pathways: importance of the accessory pathway location, J Am Coll Cardiol 20(3):666, 1992.
50. Erickson SL: Wolff-Parkinson-White syndrome: a review and an update, Crit Care Nurse 9(5):28, 1989.
51. Fisch C: Clinical electrophysiological studies and the Wolff-Parkinson-White pattern 82:1872, 1990.
52. Gaita F et al: Wolff-Parkinson-White syndrome. Identification and management, Drugs 43(2):185, 1992.
53. Gallagher JJ et al: Surgical treatment of arrhythmias, Am J Cardiol 61:27A, 1988.
54. Hood MA et al: Operations for Wolff-Parkinson-White syndrome, J Thorac Cardiovasc Surg 101(6):998, 1991.
55. Josephson ME, Wellens HJJ: Differential diagnosis of supraventricular tachycardia, Cardiol Clin 8:411, 1990.
56. Kalbfleish JJ et al: Safety, feasibility and cost of outpatient radiofrequency catheter ablation of accessory atrioventricular connection, J Am Coll Cariol 21(3):567, 1993.
57. Kater KM: Wolff-Parkinson-White syndrome: discharge planning, Dimension Crit Care Nurs 9(4):243, 1990.
58. Kay GN, Bubien RS: Clinical management of cardiac arrhythmias, Gaithersburg, MD, 1992, Aspen Publishers.
59. Klein GJ et al: Asymptomatic Wolff-Parkinson-White. Should we intervene? Circulation 80(6):1902, 1989.
60. Leitch JW et al: Prognostic value of electrophysiology testing in asymptomatic patients with Wolff-Parkinson-White pattern, Circulation 82(5):1718, 1990.
61. Marriott HJL, Conover MB: Advanced concepts in arrhythmias, ed 2, St. Louis, 1989, CV Mosby Co.
62. Michelson EL: Clinical perspectives in management of Wolff-Parkinson-White syndrome, part 1: recognition, diagnosis, and arrhythmias, Mod Concepts Cardiovasc Dis

58(8):43, 1989; part 2: diagnostic evaluation and treatment strategies, Mod Concepts Cardiovasc Dis 58(9):49, 1989.

63. Morscher JH: Wolff-Parkinson-White syndrome, AACN Clin Issues in Crit Care Nurs 3(1):180, 1992.

64. Pacetti PE et al: Advances in ablation surgeries for dysrhythmias associated with WPW syndrome, Crit Care Nurs Clin North Am 3(4):733, 1991.

65. Pietersen AH et al: Atrial fibrillation in the Wolff-Parkinson-White syndrome, Am J Cardiol 70(5):38A, 1992.

66. Walso AL et al: Appropriate electrophysiologic study and treatment of patients with Wolff-Parkinson-White syndrome, J Am Coll Cardiol 11:1124, 1988.

67. Wathen M et al: Initiation of atrial fibrillation in the Wolff-Parkinson-White syndrome: the importance of the accessory pathway, Am Heart J 125(3):753, 1993.

68. Wellens HJL et al: The electrocardiogram in patients with multiple accessory atrioventricular pathways, J Am Coll Cardiol 16(3):745, 1990.

Cardiomyopathies

69. Abelman WH, Lorell BH: The challenge of cardiomyopathy, J Am Coll Cardiol 13(6):1219, 1989.

70. American Heart Association, Council on Cardiac Transplantation of the Council on Clinical Cardiology: Cardiac transplantation: recipient selection, donor procurement, and medical follow-up. Draft, 1992.

71. Becker AE: Pathology of cardiomyopathies, Cardiovasc Clin 19(1):9, 1988.

72. Bonow RO et al: Medical and surgical therapy of hypertrophic cardiomyopathy, Cardiovasc Clin 19(1):221, 1988.

73. Casey PE: Pathophysiology of dilated cardiomyopathy: nursing implications, J Cardiovasc Nurs 2:1, 1987.

74. Cohn JN: Current therapy of the failing heart, Circulation 78(5):1099, 1988.

75. Courtney-Jenkins A: The patient with hypertrophic cardiomyopathy, J Cardiovasc Nurs 2(1):33, 1987.

76. Edwards BS, Rodeheffer RJ: Prognostic features in patients with congestive heart failure and selection criteria for cardiac transplantation, Mayo Clin Proc 67:485, 1992.

77. Futterman L: Cardiac transplantation: a comprehensive nursing perspective (Part 1/Part 2), Heart Lung 17(5):499; 17(6):631, 1988.

78. Gilbert EM et al: Therapy of idiopathic cardiomyopathy with chronic beta-adrenergic blockade, Heart Vessels Suppl 6:29, 1991.

79. Goodwin JF: Overview and classification of the cardiomyopathies, Cardiovasc Clin 19(1):3, 1988.

80. Jessup M, Brozena SC: Identification and management of potential heart transplant recipients, Cardiol Clin 8(1):11, 1990.

81. Johnson J, Knowlton WP: Managing cardiomyopathies in the elderly, CV Nurse 4(1):4, 1991.

82. Kawai C: Pharmacotherapy of dilated cardiomyopathy: current status and future directions, Cardiovascular Drugs and Therapy 6(1):7, 1992.

83. Kleber FX: Therapeutic alternatives in dilated myopathy-a review of current options, Eur Heart J 12(suppl D):197, 1991.

84. Kothari SS: Pathogenesis of hypertrophic cardiomyopathy: another viewpoint, Int J Cardiol 30(1):9, 1991.

85. Levine AB, Levine B: Patient evaluation for cardiac transplantation, Prog Cardiovasc Dis 33(4):219, 1991.

86. Maron BJ, Fananapazir L: Sudden cardiac death in hypertrophic cardiomyopathy, Circulation 85(suppl 1):I57, 1992.

87. McGregor CGA: Cardiac transplantation: surgical considerations and early postoperative management, Mayo Clin Proc 67:577, 1992.

88. Murgo JP: The hemodynamic evaluation in hypertrophic cardiomyopathy: systolic and diastolic function, Cardiovasc Clin 19(1):193, 1988.

89. Purcell JA: Advances in the treatment of dilated cardiomyopathy, AACN Clin Issues in Crit Care Nurs 1(1):31, 1990.

90. Sanzobrino B, Lemberg L: The cardiomyopathies, Heart Lung 15:416, 1986.

91. Seiler C et al: Long-term follow-up of medical versus surgical therapy for hypertrophic

cardiomyopathy: a retrospective study, J Am Coll Cardiol 17(3):634, 1991.

92. Stevenson LW, Perloff JK: The dilated cardiomyopathies: clinical aspects, Cardiol Clin 6(2):187, 1988.

93. Tanio JW, Eisen HJ: Medical aspects of cardiac transplantation, Hosp Pract [off] 28(3A):61, 1993.

94. Vaska PL: Common infections in heart transplant patients, Am J Crit Care 2(2):145, 1992.

95. von Doohlen TW, Frank MJ: Current perspectives in hypertrophic cardiomyopathy: diagnosis, clinical management, and prevention of disability and sudden cardiac death, Clin Cardiol 13(4):247, 1990.

96. Watkins LO, Williams RA: Cardiomyopathy in blacks, Cardiovasc Clin 21(3):279, 1991.

97. Wigle ED: Hypertrophic cardiomyopathy 1988, Mod Concepts Cardiovasc Dis 57(1):1, 1988.

Mitral valve prolapse

98. Alpert MA et al: Mitral valve prolapse, panic disorder, and chest pain, Med Clin North Am 75(5):1119, 1991.

99. Ansari A: Syndrome of mitral valve prolapse: current perspectives, Prog Cardiovasc Dis 32(1):31, 1989.

100. Barlow JB et al: Mitral leaflet billowing and prolapse. Implications for management, Cardiovasc Drug Ther 1(5):543, 1988.

101. Bhutto ZR et al: Electrocardiographic abnormalities in mitral valve prolapse, Am J Cardiol 70(2):265, 1992.

102. Carney RM et al: Major depression, panic disorder, and mitral valve prolapse in patients who complain of chest pain, Am J Med 89:757, 1990.

103. Cheng TO: Mitral valve prolapse: when is it serious? Postgrad Med 88(7):93, 1990.

104. Cowan MD: Prevalence of QTc prolongation in women with mitral valve prolapse, Am J Cardiol 63(1):133, 1989.

105. Devereux RB: Mitral valve prolapse: causes, clinical manifestations, and management, Ann Intern Med 111(4):305, 1989.

106. Devereux RB: Diagnosis and prognosis of mitral valve prolapse, N Engl J Med 320(16):1077, 1989.

107. Levy D, Savage D: Prevalence and clinical features of mitral valve prolapse, Am Heart J 113:1281, 1987.

108. Levy S: Arrhythmias in the mitral valve prolapse syndrome: clinical significance and management, PACE 15(7):1080, 1992.

109. Marks AR: Identification of high-risk and low-risk subgroups of patients with mitral valve prolapse, N Engl J Med 320(16):1031, 1989.

110. Perloff JK, Child JS: Clinical and epidemiologic issues in mitral valve prolapse, Am Heart J 113:1324, 1987.

111. Perloff JK et al: New guidelines for the clinical diagnosis of mitral valve prolapse, Am J Cardiol 57:1124, 1986.

112. Schaal SF: Ventricular arrhythmias in patients with mitral valve prolapse, Cardiovasc Clin 22(1):307, 1992.

113. Scordo KA: Helping your patient cope with mitral valve prolapse syndrome, Nursing 22(10):34, 1992.

114. Weissman NJ et al: Contrasting patterns of autonomic dysfunction in patients with mitral valve prolapse and panic attacks, Am J Med 82:880, 1987.

115. Wooley CF et al: The floppy, myxomatous mitral valve, mitral valve prolapse, and mitral regurgitation, Prog Cardiovasc Dis 33(6):387,1991.

Index

Defibrillator(s)
 automatic external, 446
 implantable cardioverter, 446
Deflation, 354
Dehydration, 91-92, 92
Delayed afterpolarizations (DAD), 212
Delayed pericarditis, 130
Delta wave pattern, 509, 510
Demand pacing, 454
Demerol (meperidine), 417
Depolarization, 17, 95-96, 99
Depression, post-myocardial infarction and, 188
Desferal (deferoxamine), 128
Dextran, 92
Diabetes mellitus
 coronary artery disease and, 135
 familial hyperlipidemia and, 135
 hypertonicity or hyperosmolality of plasma and,
  87-88
Diabetic ketoacidosis, 101
Diamox (acetazolamide), 77, 78
Diarrhea, 77
Diastole, 309, 340
 changes in coronary ischemia/reperfusion, 126
 electrical, 98
 in myocardial infarction, 319-320
Dicrotic notch, 326-327
Diffusion, 52, 86, 87
Digibind (Digoxin immune Fab), 179, 408
Digitalis (Digoxin; Lanoxin), 407-410
 for atrial fibrillation, 240-241
 indications, 407
 myocardial contractility and, 407-408
 nursing orders for, 409-410
 for supraventricular tachyarrhythmias, 430
 toxicity, 408-409
  paroxysmal atrial tachycardia and, 234
  treatment of, 408-409
  Wenckebach blocks and, 247
Digoxin immune Fab (digibind), 179
Dihydropyridine vasoactive agent, mechanism of
  action, 404-405
Dilated cardiomyopathy, 518, 519
Diltiazem (Cardizem), 235, 402
 for acute myocardial infarction, 405
 for atrial flutter, 237
 contraindications, 404
 indications, 403
 mechanism of action, 403
 for supraventricular tachyarrhythmias, 430
 toxic effects, 404
 in wide QRS tachycardia, 293
Dilutional hyponatremia, 91, 100
2,3-Diphosphoglycerate (2,3-DPG), 61
Dipyridamole, 391
Dipyridamole (Persantine), 175, 176
Direct access pacing
 dual-chamber, 459
 single-chamber, 458-459
Disopyramide, for arrhythmias, nursing orders for,
  379

Disseminated intravascular coagulation (DIC), 348
Distress, 185
Distributive shock, 345, 346
Diuretic therapy
 excessive, 91-92
 hypomagnesemia and, 113
Diuretics, 92, 412-416
 classification, 412-413
 loop, 413
Dobutamine (Dobutrex), 411, 420, 432
Dopamine (Intropin), 410-411, 415-416
 for bradyarrhythmias, 427
 for cardiogenic shock, 349
Dopaminergic stimulation, 371
Double product, 158
Downregulation, of sympathetic beta$_1$ receptors, 310
Dressler's syndrome, 130
Dromotropic effects
 negative, 369, 403
 positive, 369
Dual-chamber pacemaker
 DDD pacing, 472-474
 DVI pacing, 467-472
 electrocardiogram assessment of pacing, 467-472
 pacing, 490
 pulse generators, 461-462
Dyspnea, 313
Dysrhythmias, 208

E

Early afterpolarizations (EAD), 212
Ecainide (Enkaid), 381-382
ECF (extracellular fluid), 85
Echo beat, 514
Echocardiography, 162-165
Echoes, 162
ECMO (extracorporeal membrane oxygenation), 356
Ectopic arrhythmias, 208
Ectopic beats
 nursing orders for, 296-297
 reentry and, 214-215
Ectopic supraventricular arrhythmias, 229-230
 atrial fibrillation, 238-241
 atrial flutter, 236-238
 atrial tachycardia, 233-236
 junctional or nodal arrhythmias, 241-243
 nursing orders for, 243-245
 premature atrial complexes and, 230-233
Edema, 85
 formation, 93-94
 peripheral, in heart failure, 314
 pulmonary, with left ventricular failure, 316
Egophony, 59
Ejection fraction, 180-181, 310
Elderly, hypovolemia and, 92
Electrical diastole, 98
Electrical systole, 98
Electrocardiogram (ECG), 1, 17
 alarms, 38

Fibrin split products (FSP), 390
Fibrin thrombus formation, 122
Fibrinolytic agents, 393
Fibrinolytic system, 393
Fick principle, 64
First-degree AV block, 247, 269
Fixed acids, 72, 74
Flailed mitral valve, 528
Flecainide acetate (Tambocor), 381-382
Flipped LDH pattern, 143
Floppy mitral valve syndrome, 528
Fluid
  compartments, 86, 87
  depletion, 91-92
  imbalances, 90-92
  intravenous therapy, for hypovolemia, 92
  overload, 90
Fluoro-2-deoxyglucose (FDG), 182
Foot electrode (F), 28
Fowler's position, high, 316
Fraction of inspired air, 49
Fraction of inspired oxygen (FIO$_2$), 49
Fractional inspired oxygen, alveolar-arterial oxygen
      difference and, 56
Free fatty acids, 125-126
Frontal plane, 28
FSP (fibrin split products), 390
Full compensatory pause, 220, 221
Functional capacity, 159
Furosemide (Lasix), 316, 413, 432
Fusion beats, 289
Fusion complex, 509

G

Gallops, 341-343
Gastrointestinal disease, chest pain, 139
Gemfibrozil (Lopid), 134, 386
General adaptation syndrome, 185-187
Glucose, potassium and, 102
  for hyperkalemia, 107
Glycolysis, 186
Graded exercise testing (GXT), 157-162

H

Haber-Weiss reaction, 127
HDL (high-density lipoprotein), 132-134
Headaches, from nitrates, 421
Heart
  auscultation, 339-344
  electrical activity, 1-2
  functions of, 1
  left side, 3
    function of, 2
    musculature of, 2-3
  mechanical activity, 1-2
    electrical activity and, 1-2
    normal, 4-6

mechanical structures of, 2-4
  pumping function, determinants of, 308-309
  right side, 3
    function of, 2
    musculature of, 2
  transplantation, 524-527
  valves, 3
  wall, layers of, 2
Heart block(s)
  AV. *See* AV block
  defined, 245
  SA, 245, 246
Heart failure, 148, 308-317
  diuretics for, nursing orders for, 416
  left ventricular, 311-313
  nitroprusside for, nursing orders for, 423
  nursing orders for, 317
  pharmacologic agents for, 432-433
  therapy, 314-317
Heart rate(s)
  calculating, from ECG graph, 20-23
  defined, 1
  maximal predicted, 158
  stroke volume and, 1
Heart rhythm
  accelerated idioventricular, 226-227, 270
  idioventricular, 226, 270
  junctional, 242, 243, 270
  quadruple, 342
Heart sounds
  correlation with mechanical/electrical events, 340
  first (SI), varying intensity of, in AV dissociation, 255
  normal variations, 339-341
Hemiblock, 275, 285-286
Hemodynamic monitoring, 317-318
  of cardiac output, 336-337
  of cardiac pressures, 320-324
  of distorted pressure waveforms, 328-332
  flow-pressure-resistance relationship and, 318-319
  in myocardial infarction, 319-320
  normal pressure waveforms and, 325-328
  nursing orders for, 337-339
  pulmonary artery catheter for, 332-335
Hemodynamics, of cardiac pacing, 483-484
Hemoglobin
  abnormal, 65
  binding with oxygen, 61-62
  cyanosis and, 60
  deoxygenated, 65
  oxygen carrying capacity of, 60
  oxygen pressure and, 61
Hemostasis, 387-388
Heparin, 391-392
Hepatic failure, hypotonic plasma and, 88
Hetastarch (Hespan), 92
Hexaxial reference system, 30
Hibernating myocardium, 182
Hibernation, 127
High-density lipoprotein (HDL), 132-134
High-density lipoproteins (HDL), cigarette smoking
      and, 131

LVEP. *See* Left ventricular end-diastolic pressure (LVEDP)
Lymphatic system, 53

M

Macrophages, 52
Mafenide (Sulfamylon), 78
Magnesium
    calcium and, 111-112
    imbalances, 111-115, 115
    in intracellular fluid compartment, 85
Magnesium sulfate, for ventricular tachyarrhythmia, 429
Magnetic resonance imaging (MRI), 182-183
Mahaim syndrome, 508, 509
Mannitol, 415
MAP (mean arterial pressure), 327-328
Marfan's syndrome, 530
Maximal predicted heart rate, 158
MCL leads, 37, 38
Mean arterial pressure (MAP), 327-328
Mediators, chemical, 185
Menopause, coronary artery disease and, 136
Meperidine (Demerol), 417
Metabolic acidosis, 73
    anion gap in, 78-79
    causes, 78
    clinical signs, 77
    therapy for, 77-78
    treatment interventions, 78-79
Metabolic alkalosis, 73-74
    clinical signs, 79
    therapy for, 79
Metabolic imaging, 172, 181-182
Metabolism, 125, 347
Methemoglobin, 65
Metoprolol (Lopressor), 400, 432
METs, 158
Mexiletine, 380-381
Microatelectasis, 59
Minipress (prazosin), 419, 424
Minute ventilation, 53
Mitral click-murmur syndrome, 528
Mitral valve, 3
    insufficiency, 129, 309, 343
    prolapse, 527-533
        clinical diagnosis, 528
        diagnostic maneuvers for, 529-530
        electrocardiogram changes, 531
        functional diagnosis, 528
        premature atrial complexes and, 230
        signs/symptoms, 530-532
        treatment, 532-533
    regurgitation
        cardiomyopathy and, 523
        pressure waveforms, 330
Mobitz I block, 247, 269
Mobitz II block, 247, 248-250, 269
Modified bipolar chest leads, 36

Monitoring cable, 36
Monoclonal antibodies, for cardiac myosin, 179
Monofascicular block, 275
Moricizine, 376
Morphine, 416-417
    for chest pain, 431
    for heart failure, 316
MRI (magnetic resonance imaging), 182-183
MUGA (multigated acquisition), 179
Multigated acquisition (MUGA), 179
Mural thrombi, 130, 388
Murmurs, 343
MVP. *See* Mitral valve, prolapse
Myocardial contractility, digitalis and, 407-408
Myocardial infarction, acute, 122, 124
    anxiety and, 188
    cardiac enzymes and, 140-141
    chest pain, 137
        differential diagnosis, 137-139
    depression and, 188
    diltiazem for, 405
    edema formation and, 93-94
    electrocardiogram changes in, 143-146
    factors altering automaticityin, 208, 209
    hemodynamic patterns in, 324
    left ventricle and, 44
    nontransmural, 143
    nursing management, 189-194
    post-infarction period, 188-189
    Q wave vs. non-Q wave, 146-147
    transmural, 124, 143-144
        anterior wall, 147-149
        inferior wall, 149-154
    ventricular aneurysm and, 129
Myocardial oxygen consumption
    beta blockers and, 400
    in myocardial infarction, 320
Myocardial steal syndrome, 176
Myocardial stunning, 126-127
    calcium overload and, 127
    oxygen radicals and, 127-129
Myocardium, 2, 309
Myoglobin levels, 143

N

Na^+-K^+ pump, 96, 126, 212
NAIDS (nonsteroidal antiinflammatory agents), hyperkalemia and, 104
Narcotic analgesics, 416-417
NASPE code (North American Society of Pacing and Electrophysiology code), 454
Necrosis, 144
Negative image, 174
Neurogenic shock, 346
Neurologic control, of respiration, 54, 55
New York Heart Association Classification system, for congestive heart failure, 311
Niacin (nicotinic acid), 134, 386
Nifedipine, sublingual, 406

PVCs. *See* Premature ventricular complexes (PVCs)
PVR (pulmonary vascular resistance), calculation, 337

Q

Q-T interval, 19, 212
  in torsades de pointes, 505-506
Q wave myocardial infarction, 146-147
Q waves, abnormal, in necrosis, 144-145
QRS complex, 17-18, 24, 97
  in aberrant conduction, 287-288
  analysis, 215-216
  chest leads and, 33
  delta wave of, 509-510
  dropped, 247
  duration or width, 19, 24
    calculating from ECG graph, 19, 20-21
    class IA drugs and, 378
    differential diagnosis, 295-296
  in ectopic supraventricular arrhythmias, 229
  in hyerkalemia, 104
  in junctional arrhythmias, 241, 242
  late potentials in, 215
  morphology, deduction from ECG limb leads, 30-31
  negative, 293-294
  premature, 231
  sinus rhythms and, 23
  of third-degree AV block, 252
  triphasic, 277
  upright, 293
  in ventricular arrhythmias, 216-217
  in ventricular escape beats, 226
  in ventricular fusion beats, 228-229
  wide tachycardias. *See* Wide QRS complex
    tachycardias
QS complex, 18
Quadrant method, for ventricular axis estimation, 279-281
Questran (cholestyramine), 385-386
Quinidine, 378-379

R

R on T phenomenon, 219
R-P interval, in Kent pathway, 513
R-R interval, calculating, 20-21
R wave, 18, 353
Rabbit ears, 295
Race, hypertension and, 132
RAD (right axis deviaion), 279, 284
Rade modulation or responsiveness, 490
Radionuclide angiography, 172, 179-181
  nursing orders for, 183-184
Radiopharmaceuticals, 172
Rales, 58, 312
Range of motion exercises (ROM), 197
Rate pressure product (RPP), 158
RBB (right bundle branch), 275
RBBB. *See* Right bundle branch block (RBBB)

Receptors, homeostasis and, 88
Reciprocating tachycardia, 514
Recorder, 36
Recycling, 449
Reentry, 212-215
  alternate models, 214
  conditions for, 212-213
  macrocircuits, 213
  microcircuits, 213
  process, 208
  unidirectional block, 214
Reflection spectrophotometry, 67
Refractory periods, 19-20, 490
  absolute, 20
  relative, 20
Regular sinus rhythm (RSR), 24
Reid-Barlow's syndrome, 528
Rejection, of cardiac transplantation, 526-527
Relative refractory period, 20
Relaxation techniques, 187-188
Renal failure, hypotonic plasma and, 88
Renal medulla, hypercalcemia and, 110
Renin, 89
Renin-angiotensin-aldosterone system, in heart failure, 310-311
Renovascular dilator, 414
Repetitive firing, 20
Repolarization, 17, 96, 97
  refractory periods and, 19-20
  syndrome, 489
  ventricular, 17
Resistance
  blood flow and, 318-319
  blood pressure and, 318-319
  pulmonary vascular, 337
  systemic vascular. See Systemic vascular resistance (SVR)
Respiration
  external vs. internal, 52
  neurologic control, 54, 55
Respiratory acidosis, 72
  clinical signs, 75-76
  intervention, 76
Respiratory airways, 52, 53
Respiratory alkalosis, 72
  clinical signs, 76
  intervention for, 76-77
Respiratory center suppression, in respiratory acidosis, 75
Respiratory failure, 57
Respiratory rate, 53
Resting state, 95
Restrictive cardiomyopathy, 519-520
Retrograde atrial depolarization, 241
Return to work, cardiac rehabilitation and, 195-196
Rhonchus, 58
Right axis deviation (RAD), 279, 284
Right bundle branch block, 276-277, 286
  atypical ECG patterns, 277, 278
Right bundle branch block (RBBB), 275
  aberrant conduction, 287-288

Thrombosis, 387-388
  lipidemia, vasospasm and, 394
Thrombus formation, atherosclerosis and, 122
Thyrocalcitonin, 108
Ticlopidine (Ticlid), 391
Tidal volume, 53
TIMI II trial, 248
Tines, 56
Tissue oxygen extraction, impairment, 69
Tissue oxygenation, 47
  determinants, 47, 48
  evaluation of, 62-65
  inadequate, symptoms of, 47-48
Tissue plasminogen activator (t-PA), 393-394
Tocainamide, 380
Tomography
  angiographic, nursing orders for, 183-184
  computed, 172, 182-183
  for thallium and technetium perfusion imaging, 177
Torsades de pointes, 502-508
  antiarrhythmic drugs for, 506-508
  electrocardiogram of, 502-506
Torsades de points, hypomagnesemia and, 113
Trandate (labetalol), 399
Tranquilizers, post-myocardial infarction, 188
Transcutaneous pacing, 457-458
Transducer, 162
Transesophageal echocardiography (TEE), 163, 164-165
Transesophageal pacing, 460
Transtelephonic monitoring, of pacemaker, 464-465
Transvenous pacing
  dual-chamber, 459
  single-chamber, 456
Treadmill exercise protocols, 158
Tricuspid valve, 3
Tricyclic antidepressants, after acute myocardial infarction, 188
Tridil. See Nitroglycerin (Tridil)
Trifascicular block
  bifascicular block and, 284-285
  defined, 275
Trigeminy, ventricular, 219
Triggered activity, tachyarrhythmia formation and, 212
Triglycerides, coronary artery disease and, 132-135
Trousseau's sign, 108
12-lead electrocardiogram system, 27-35
Two-dimensional echocardiography, 163
Type A personality, 136, 187

U

Unidirectional block, of reentry, 214
Unipolar catheters, for pacemaker, 453
Unipolar leads, 30, 31
Unstable angina, 125
Upper rate limit, 491
Urokinase (Abbokinase; Breokinase; WinKinase), 394
Usurpation, AV dissociation and, 253

V

V leads, 32
V or chest lead position, 37
V wave, 326
VA interval, 491
Vagal sensory pathways, 27
Vagolytic drugs, 371. See Anticholinergic drugs
Vagomimetic effects, 371
Vagus nerve, 89
Valve disease, premature atrial complexes and, 230
Valves, heart, 3
Vasodilators, 417-424. *See also specific vasodilators*
  categories of, 418
  in pharmacologic stress testing, 175-176
Vasogenic shock, 345
Vasopressin (antidiuretic hormone), 88-89, 91, 186
Vasospasm, lipidemia, thrombosis and, 394
Vasotec (Enalapril), 419, 423-424
Venous saturation, 65
Ventilation
  external respiration and, 52
  in respiratory acidosis, 75
  structures of, 52
Ventilation/perfusion mismatch (V/Q mismatch), 54, 55, 56
Ventricle, 3
Ventricular aneurysm, 129
Ventricular arrhythmias, 216, 222-229. *See also specific ventricular arrhythmias*
  clinically significant, 209
  defined, 216
  differential diagnosis, 298
  premature ventricular complexes and, 218-222
  QRS complex in, 216-217
  recognition matrix, 271
  reentrant, 214
  ventricular aneurysm and, 129
Ventricular assist devices (VADs), 356-358
Ventricular automaticity, class I B drugs and, 380
Ventricular axis
  defined, 279
  deviations, 279-284. *See also* Left anterior hemiblock; Left posterior hemiblock
  normal, 279, 280
  quadrant estimation method, 279-281
Ventricular bigeminy, 219
Ventricular bradyarrhythmias, 218
Ventricular capture, 465, 466, 472
Ventricular depolarization, 34
Ventricular ectopy, 282
  patterns, 289-291
  right vs. left, 290-291
  suppression, 375
  width of beats, 216-217
Ventricular escape beat, 226
Ventricular fibrillation, 209, 226, 498
  clinical significance, 267
  coarse fibrillatory waves, 224
  ECG criteria, 267